SECOND EDITION

NURSING ADMINISTRATION

Managing Patient Care

Edited by:

Jacqueline A. Dienemann, PhD, RN, CNAA, FAAN
Associate Professor
Coordinator, Nursing Systems and Management
School of Nursing
The Johns Hopkins University
Baltimore, Maryland

APPLETON & LANGE
Stamford, Connecticut

Copyright © 1998 by Appleton & Lange
A Simon & Schuster Company
Copyright © 1990 by Appleton & Lange

98 99 00 01 02 / 10 9 8 7 6 5 4 3 2 1

Prentice Hall International (UK) Limited, *London*
Prentice Hall of Australia Pty. Limited, *Sydney*
Prentice Hall Canada, Inc., *Toronto*
Prentice Hall Hispanoamericana, S.A., *Mexico*
Prentice Hall of India Private Limited, *New Delhi*
Prentice Hall of Japan, Inc., *Tokyo*
Simon & Schuster Asia Pte. Ltd., *Singapore*
Editora Prentice Hall do Brasil Ltda., *Rio de Janeiro*
Prentice Hall, *Upper Saddle River, New Jersey*

Library of Congress Cataloging-in-Publication Data
Nursing administration: managing patient care /
    edited by Jacqueline A. Dienemann.—2nd ed.
        p.   cm.
    Includes bibliographical references.
    ISBN 0-8385-6986-2 (case : alk. paper)
    1. Nursing services—Administration. 2. Nurse administrators.
    I. Dienemann, Jacqueline A.
    [DNLM: 1. Nurse Administrators. 2. Nursing Services—organization
& administration. 3. Administrative Personnel. WY 105 N9742 1998] RT89.N768 1998
362. 1'73'068—dc21
DNLM/DLC
for Library of Congress   97-14107
                                                            CIP

Acquisitions Editor: Patricia Casey
Editorial Assistant: Elisabeth Church
Production Editor: Lisa M. Guidone
Designer: Mary Skudlarek

ISBN 0-8385-6986-2

PRINTED IN THE UNITED STATES OF AMERICA

9 780838 569863   90000

*To my students, who develop and
test new case applications daily in their
nursing administration practice.*

Contents

Contributors . . . . *ix*

Reviewers . . . . *xiii*

Preface . . . . *xv*

Introduction . . . . *xvii*

**PART I   EXTERNAL FORCES SHAPING HEALTH CARE
DELIVERY ORGANIZATIONS** 1

Chapter 1.   Ethical Frameworks into the 21st Century 3
Mary Cipriano Silva and Joy Kroeger-Mappes

**Application 1–1.
Moral Reasoning in Personnel Decisions** 23
Patricia Snyder

Chapter 2.   The Health Policy Process and Nursing 31
Barbara K. Redman

**Application 2–1.
A Voice in the Wilderness: What Can I Do?** 49
Nancy J. Sharp

**Case 2–1.
It's Politics, Not Policy . . . People!** 54
Nancy J. Sharp

Chapter 3.   Legal Aspects of Patient Care Administration 59
Marjorie Barter and Marva L. Furmidge

**Application 3–1.
Managing Unionized Nurses** 85
Mary Suzanne Hudec

**Application 3–2.
Designing a Patient Care Risk Management
System** 91
George D. Velianoff and Diana K. Hobbs

Chapter 4.   Cultural Diversity in the Workplace 101
Arlene J. Lowenstein

Case 4–1.
A Workplace of Difference 125
Anne Dickinson Cohen

Case 4–2.
Feminist Management at a Community
Health Center 131
Katrina H. Clark and Elizabeth Magenheimer

PART II   ORGANIZATIONAL STRATEGIES 139

Chapter 5.   Managing Change in Health Care Organizations 141
Joyce E. Johnson and Molly Billingsley

Case 5–1.
The Human Side of Change:
Transition to Teams 163
Barbara Balik and Ethel Muchlinski

Case 5–2.
Strategic Implementation: A 10-Year
Retrospective on Opening a Continuing
Care Retirement Center 176
Alice Story Biache

Chapter 6.   Marketing in the New Health Care Environment 185
James W. Harvey

Case 6–1.
Initiating Marketing in a County
Health Department 207
Joanne M. Jorgenson

Case 6–2.
Integrating Marketing into the Psychiatric
Clinical Specialist's Job Responsibilities 213
Carol A. Patney

Chapter 7.   What's Your Niche? Starting a New Venture 225
Belinda E. Puetz and Karen J. Kelly Thomas

Case 7–1.
Establishing a Care Management Business 247
Ann E. O'Neil

Case 7–2.
Consulting. 256
Barbara A. Happ

PART III   STRUCTURING HEALTH CARE ORGANIZATIONS 265

Chapter 8.   Assessing Organizations. 267
Jacqueline A. Dienemann

Case 8–1.
Choosing Partners 284
Emilie M. Deady

Chapter 9.   Financial Skills for Department Managers 293
Michelle Robnett and Alissa Schaub-Rimel

Case 9–1.
**Financial Issues in Opening a New Patient
Care Program** 313
Alejandra M. Dreisbach

Chapter 10.   Information Systems for Managing Patient Care. 323
Susan K. Newbold

Case 10–1.
**Cutting the Gordian Knot: Implementing
OrderNet in an Academic Health Center** 339
Cynthia A. Dolan and Linda Kisamore

Chapter 11.   Job Design and Work Processes in Patient Care 359
Theodore L. Gessner

Case 11–1.
Challenges in Evaluating Redesign 379
*Marcelline Harris, Alice P. Weydt, Holly Frohling,
and Annette McBeth*

Case 11–2.
**Integrating the Work of Nurse Practitioners
in an Acute Care Setting** 394
Marie Collins Donahue

PART IV   NURSING ADMINISTRATION **403**

**Chapter 12. Leadership and Management in
Patient Care Delivery Systems** **405**
Karen B. Haller

**Case 12–1.
Shared Governance in an Academic
Health Center** **417**
Linda M. Herrick

Chapter 13. Professional Development **427**
Brenda S. Cherry

**Case 13–1.
Sustaining a Family Research Team
in an Academic Health Center** **445**
Charmaine Kleiber

**Case 13–2.
From Staff Nurse to Charge Nurse—Introducing
a Management Viewpoint** **452**
Michelle Sly Smith and Sally A. Zuel

Chapter 14. Performance Management **461**
Betsy Frank

**Case 14–1.
Changing Rewards to Match Expectations** **485**
Carolyn A. Taylor

Chapter 15. Evaluation, Quality, and Outcomes **493**
Barbara Barth Frink

**Application 15–1.
Preparing for a JCAHO Accreditation Visit** **510**
Donna Richards Sheridan and Carol Ruth Yocum

**Case 15–2.
Measuring Outcomes of a Spine Evaluation
Service in a Managed Care Setting** **522**
Margaret Fisk Mastal and Carshal A. Burris

Index *529*

Contributors

Barbara Balik, MSN, RN
Vice President, Patient Care
Chief Nurse Executive
United Hospital
St. Paul, Minnesota

Marjorie Barter, EdD, RN
Associate Professor
School of Nursing
University of San Francisco
San Francisco, California

Alice Story Biache, MSN, LNHA, RN, C
Senior Vice President of
Professional Services
Goodwin House Inc.
Alexandria, Virginia

Molly Billingsley, EdD, RN, ANP
Administrative Director
Nursing and Patient Care Services
Washington Hospital Center
Washington, D.C.

Carshal A. Burris, MHA, CHE
Medical Facilities Administrator
Kaiser Permanente
Springfield, Virginia

Brenda S. Cherry, PhD, RN
Dean
College of Nursing
University of Massachusetts, Boston
Boston, Massachusetts

Katrina H. Clark, MPH
Director
Fairhaven Community Health
Center
New Haven, Connecticut

Emilie M. Deady, MSN, MGA, RN
President and CEO
VNA of Northern Virginia
Arlington, Virginia

Anne Dickinson Cohen, MA, RN, C
Staff Development Coordinator
Beth Israel Medical Center
New York, New York

Jacqueline A. Dienemann, PhD, RN, CNAA, FAAN
Associate Professor
Coordinator, Nursing Systems and
Management
School of Nursing
The Johns Hopkins University
Baltimore, Maryland

Cynthia A. Dolan, MS, RN
Project Leader, Information Services
The Johns Hopkins Hospital
Baltimore, Maryland

Marie Collins Donahue, MPH, MS, RN, CPNP
Columbia Presbyterian Medical
Center
Women and Children's Care Center
New York, New York

Alejandra M. Dreisbach, MBA
Director
Value Management, Budget and
Reimbursement
Robert Wood Johnson University
Hospital
New Brunswick, New Jersey

Betsy Frank, PhD, RN
Chair, Department of Health
Restoration
Associate Professor
School of Nursing
Indiana State University
Terre Haute, Indiana

**Barbara Barth Frink, PhD, RN,
FAAN**
Director of Nursing
Systems and Research
The Johns Hopkins Hospital
Baltimore, Maryland

Holly Frohling, MBA, RN
Director, Patient Care Services
Immanuel St. Joseph's Hospital
Mayo Health System
Mankato, Minnesota

Marva L. Furmidge, JD, MS, RN
Director, Administrative Services
and Managed Care
Palm Drive Hospital and Columbia
Healdsburg General Hospital
Healdsburg, California

Theodore L. Gessner, PhD
Associate Professor
Department of Psychology
School of Arts and Sciences
George Mason University
Fairfax, Virginia

Karen B. Haller, PhD, RN, FAAN
Director of Nursing
Department of Medicine
The Johns Hopkins University
Baltimore, Maryland

Barbara A. Happ, PhD, RN
Birch Davis & Associates, Inc.
Falls Church, Virginia

Marcelline Harris, MS, RN
Doctoral Candidate
College of Nursing
University of Nebraska
Omaha, Nebraska

James W. Harvey, MBA, PhD
Associate Professor
Department of Marketing
School of Business Administration
George Mason University
Fairfax, Virginia

Linda M. Herrick, MS, RN
Director, Section of Nursing
Research
Mayo Clinic
Rochester, Minnesota

Diana K. Hobbs, BA, RN, C
Corporate Director, Risk
Management and Legal Services
Upper Chesapeake Health Systems
Fallston, Maryland

Mary Suzanne Hudec, MSN, RN
Associate Director for Patient Services
Veterans Administration Medical
Center
Washington, D.C.

Joyce E. Johnson, DNSc, RN, FAAN
Senior Vice President
Nursing and Patient Care Services
Washington Hospital Center
Washington, D.C.

Joanne M. Jorgenson, BSN, MPH, RN
Director of Patient Care Services
Fairfax County Health Department
Fairfax, Virginia

Linda Kisamore, BSN, RN
Nurse Manager, Osler 8
The Johns Hopkins Hospital
Baltimore, Maryland

Charmaine Kleiber, MS, RN, CPNP
Advanced Practice Nurse
Pediatric/OB Nursing
University of Iowa Hospitals
Iowa City, Iowa

Joy Kroeger-Mappes, PhD, RN
Associate Professor
Philosophy and Women's Studies
Frostburg State University
Frostburg, Maryland

Arlene J. Lowenstein, PhD, RN
Director and Professor
Graduate Program, Nursing
MGH Institute of Health
Professionals
Boston, Massachusetts

Elizabeth Magenheimer, MA, RN, FNP, CNM
Director of Nursing
Fairhaven Community Health Center
New Haven, Connecticut

Margaret Fisk Mastal, PhD, RN
Clinical Coordinator Specialties
Kaiser Permanente
Springfield, Virginia

Annette McBeth, MS, RN, FAAN
Vice President
Immanuel St. Joseph's Hospital
Mayo Health System
Mankato, Minnesota

Ethel Muchlinski, MSN, RN
Project Manager for Shared
Decision Making
United Hospital
St. Paul, Minnesota

Susan K. Newbold, MS, RN, C
Manager, Database Administration
University Physicians
Baltimore, Maryland

Ann E. O'Neil, MSN, RN, CS
President
Care Options for the Elderly and
Disabled
Falls Church, Virginia

Carol A. Patney, MSN, RN, CS-P
Director, Quality Management
and Education
Mental Health Advisor Services
Health Management Strategies
Alexandria, Virginia

Belinda E. Puetz, PhD, RN
President and CEO
Puetz and Associates
Pensacola, Florida

Barbara K. Redman, PhD, RN, FAAN
Dean and Professor
School of Nursing
University of Connecticut
Storrs, Connecticut

Michelle Robnett, PhD, RN
President
Medical Group Management
Company
Baltimore, Maryland

Alissa Schaub-Rimel, LWSA, MHA
Management Analyst
Johns Hopkins Bayview Medical
Center
Baltimore, Maryland

Nancy J. Sharp, MSN, RN
President
Sharp Legislative Resources
Bethesda, Maryland

Donna Richards Sheridan, MBA, PhD, RN
Vice President, Patient Care Services
Chief Nurse Executive
Division of Nursing
San Francisco Memorial Hospital
San Francisco, California

Mary Cipriano Silva, PhD, RN, FAAN
Professor
Director, Center for Health Care
Ethics
College of Nursing and Health
Science
George Mason University
Fairfax, Virginia

Michelle Sly Smith, MSN, RN
Hospice Services Director
Hospice of the Wabash Valley
Terre Haute, Indiana

Patricia Snyder, PhD, RN
Director, Professional Practice
Development
Glens Falls Hospital
Glens Falls, New York

Carolyn A. Taylor, MSN, MBA, RN, C
Director, Maternal Child Health
Services
Holy Cross Hospital
Silver Spring, Maryland

Karen J. Kelly Thomas, PhD, RN, CNAA
Director, Practice and Research
Association of Women's Health,
Obstetric, and Neonatal Nurses
Washington, D.C.

George D. Velianoff, DNS, RN, CHE
Vice President, Patient Services
Upper Chesapeake Health Systems
Fallston, Maryland

Alice P. Weydt, MN, RN, CNAA
Director, Patient Care Services
Immanuel St. Joseph's Hospital
Mayo Health System
Mankato, Minnesota

Carol Ruth Yocum, MA, RN, CNAA
Quality and Utilization
Management
Daughters of Charity, National
Health System
La Honda, California

Sally A. Zuel, MSN, RN
CPR Coordinator
Educational Services
Union Hospital
Terre Haute, Indiana

Reviewers

Jan V. R. Belcher, PhD, RN
Assistant Professor
School of Nursing
Old Dominion University
Norfolk, Virginia

Peggy McCall, MSN, RN
Assistant Professor
Houston Baptist University
Houston, Texas

Sylvia Price, PhD, RN
Professor
College of Nursing
University of Tennessee Memphis
Memphis, Tennessee

Kay Sackett, EdD, RN
Assistant Professor
College of Nursing and Health
Sciences
Winona State University
Winona, Minnesota

Preface

This book is intended for graduate students in schools of nursing studying the organization and delivery of health care and for nurses in management and administrative positions. Nurses at all levels of management and in advanced practice can use this book as a guide to integrating knowledge about organizations from related disciplines into their practice. The chapters are not intended to be specific to any setting, and the cases illustrate application in a wide variety of settings across the United States. This book provides information on business practices and application of management theory for delivery of patient care services. Nursing leaders can use this book in strategic planning, designing systems to implement new ventures or change, and the evaluation of health care delivery.

Health care organizations are evolving into health care delivery systems at a rapid rate. The center of care services is moving from hospitals to primary care and payors are demanding to know the value received for their expenditures. Through mergers, acquisitions, networks, and alliances, health care delivery is becoming more integrated and community-based services are expanding. With these changes, the roles and functions of more and more nurses in management and administration are expanding beyond hospital nursing care.

Increasingly, nurses are patient care administrators of services to target populations. The challenges for these roles go beyond acquiring business skills and building on the human relations skills and clinical knowledge gained from nursing practice. Guided by the values that originally attracted them to nursing, nurses are seeking innovative ways to structure care, configure a mix of skills, identify the best clinical practices, and design care across the life span to maintain and restore health. In this second edition, several changes have been made to assist nurses in patient care administration in these tasks. New chapters on change, cultural diversity, entrepreneurship, and leadership have been added. The focus within the chapters on ethics, evaluation, performance appraisal, work flow, and open systems was shifted to reflect current trends toward interdisciplinary teamwork and data-based decision making. All the other chapters have been completely revised.

This book continues to use an open systems perspective and prescribes no specific actions. The authors assume there is no one right way to act. Rather, nurses in administration must be guided by their values and their analysis of facts, stakeholders, situational factors, and strategic goals in choosing their actions. The authors also believe that a whole organization perspective supports wise decision making that is in congruence with organizational goals and strategic initiatives. The focus remains primarily at the system level and not the individual transaction level. Chapters are organized in a framework of external factors interacting with and shaping possibilities for organizations, the organizational strategies chosen to carry out a mission, and infrastructures supporting an effective organization.

Aspects of this book that make it unique have been retained. The contributors are experts within and outside of nursing. The information provided integrates research, theory, and practices from related disciplines and industries, thus giving the manager fluency in the language and perspectives of colleagues throughout the organization. One or more actual cases or applications written by nurses from across the country and the spectrum of patient care services accompanies each chapter. The 19 cases illustrate the problems encountered, the solutions found, and the human factors involved in implementing programs. The five applications offer guidance, based on experience, on how to apply the information from the chapter in administrative practice. Many contain actual forms used in practice.

The major lesson to be learned from this book is that nurses need theory and research from many disciplines to develop a broad perspective to guide them in resolving system problems. It is only by moving to this broader perspective that nurses in patient care administration and advanced practice will gain the competencies necessary to achieve power and advance their careers.

As with any endeavor of this magnitude, I am indebted to many people. Thanks to Rita Carty, Dean of the School of Nursing at George Mason University, who originally urged me to write the first edition. For this edition, I owe thanks to my Dean at The Johns Hopkins University School of Nursing, Sue K. Donaldson, for creating a scholarly atmosphere that values the blending of research and experience to guide scholarly practice. My other internal adviser was Dorothy Gordon who inquired, listened, and generally kept me focused. My greatest debt is to my husband, Paul, who as an experienced writer offered guidance and an overall view of the purpose of this effort.

Finally, I must recognize the major contribution of nursing leaders practicing in health care administration and education who were my authors and advisers. First and foremost of these is Maryann F. Fralic, Vice President for Nursing at The Johns Hopkins Hospital and Associate Dean, School of Nursing, The Johns Hopkins University. Her networks and ideas were a fantastic resource and inspiration. I thank my colleagues from the Council on Graduate Education for Administration in Nursing (CGEAN) for acting as a support group for this book. Lastly, I value my conversations with nurse administrators in the Baltimore–Washington area, who regularly help me comprehend the current maelstrom of change in patient care delivery. The openness, ideas, patience with my edits, and commitment to this book by all the authors is greatly appreciated.

Jacqueline A. Dienemann

Introduction

Health care organizations are in the midst of a significant transformation. Health care administration texts reflect these changes by moving from a focus on how to control and direct others to how to lead and collaborate with others. Nursing is no longer delivered within a nursing context, but within an interdisciplinary system. Thus, nurses in advanced practice and patient care administration need more knowledge about organizations and how to manage care within them. This book recognizes the complexity of today's practice and the lack of stability in health care delivery systems. It directs you to look ahead—to focus on the future you want to create. It offers no solutions, but provides the information and tools to make wise decisions.

The book is organized in four parts: (1) external forces shaping health care delivery systems, (2) organizational strategies, (3) structuring health care organizations, and (4) administration.

Part I examines selected forces including ethics, health policy, law, and cultural diversity, and how they interact with the U.S. health care delivery system. They are chosen as being representative of the many forces contributing to the American definition of health care and how it is delivered. The authors do not offer a simplified, single point of view that is an amalgam of their comprehension of primary sources. Rather, they present a synthesis of several theories, suggest further reading, and provide illustrative case applications for analysis and personal application. They assume the reader has a basic knowledge of the subject and recommend basic texts for review. In this way, many paths to the same goal are suggested. This approach assists nurses to hone their critical thinking skills to better analyze uncertain situations where there is no one right answer.

Part II provides information and guidance on organizational strategies. These strategies include managing change, strategic marketing, and starting new ventures. The authors include information originally developed in other disciplines, with well-developed applications in health care and nursing. Together, they assist the nurse in developing and implementing a vision for the organization. Parts I and II provide the theoretical underpinnings for a macro perspective in analyzing managerial dilemmas. They also reinforce the importance of boundary-spanning activities such as political action, competitor analysis, professional association leadership, and community service.

Part III examines the infrastructure that supports or acts as a barrier to effective and efficient achievement of desired outcomes. Organizational assessment as a precursor to major commitments, financial skills, use of management information systems, and job design are all key competencies. These competencies are essential for administrators and clinicians to work together productively to deliver quality health care in ways that are more cost-effective.

Nursing is the primary service offered by inpatient facilities and home health agencies. More and more, it is also being recognized as essential to quality primary and community health care services. Part IV focuses on the human factors in the delivery and evaluation of quality patient care. Leadership, professional development, performance management, and evaluation of quality and outcomes are necessary precursors to the professional practice of nursing within the context of a health care delivery organization. Because of the interdisciplinary nature of health care, these activities cannot be carried out in isolation, but must include all those within the organization.

Nurses who master the ideas presented in this book will become more aware of the ramifications of their actions for the whole organization. This understanding will change the thrust of their energies from within nursing to the entire organization and its environment. They will act for their profession and their clients by political action, community involvement, and networking to influence decisions that impact the processes of care and patient outcomes. They will possess the business and leadership skills and speak the language used throughout health care administration. They will be better able to articulate clinical issues to board members and executives who have no clinical background. They will also be better prepared to collaborate with non-nurses to clarify the clinical implications of financial and marketing decisions.

Acting with this world view, nurses in patient care administration and advanced practice will gain power and their careers will encompass wider responsibilities. Many cases in this book are provided by nurses in nontraditional administrative positions in organizational development, managed care, risk management, informatics, patient care administration, and quality management. Some authors are also consultants and entrepreneurs. As our new health care delivery system evolves, opportunities will only increase for nurses prepared to do systems thinking and to develop systems management competencies.

ONE

External Forces Shaping Health Care Delivery Organizations

Ethical Frameworks into the 21st Century

Mary Cipriano Silva and Joy Kroeger-Mappes

Nursing, like other professions, is responsible for ensuring that its members act in the public interest in the course of providing the unique service society has entrusted to them.

—American Nurses Association (ANA), 1995a, p. 17

The preceding quote from *Nursing's Social Policy Statement* sets the stage for this chapter. This call is an *ethical* mandate. The quote makes clear that a reciprocal social relationship exists between nursing and society. The nursing profession is "owned by society" (ANA, 1995a, p. 2) and thus has an ethical responsibility to appropriately provide those unique nursing services that a changing society needs.

That society is changing is a truism; that health care is changing is an understatement. Consequently, all nurses are caught in the current political and economic currents in health care; however, our focus will be on those nurses who are patient care administrators. What specific political and economic turmoil do these nurses face as they enter the 21st century? As a result, what ethical frameworks and nursing standards will best help them to act in the best interests of the public?

■ POLITICAL AND ECONOMIC TURMOIL

Health care and politics cannot be separated. As Elizabeth Harrison Hadley (1996) noted, the two collided in the 103rd Congress. Congress was too embroiled in questions of who should pay for employee health insurance and how generous employer benefit packages should be to address critical nursing issues. Three of these issues noted by Hadley involved restrictions on the scope of nursing practice, restrictions on direct reimbursement for all clinical nurse specialists and nurse practitioners, and obtaining money to retrain nurses who have lost their jobs as a result of institutional downsizing and restructuring. The first and second issues focus on the ethical principles of autonomy and respect for autonomy, while the third issue focuses on justice, in particular, the allocation of scarce resources.

A major stumbling block affecting these three issues was the divisive roadblocks placed by some nurses in the way of efforts to attain nursing's legislative goals. Restated in ethical language, some nurses demonstrated a lack of respect and a lack of caring for one another, thus sabotaging a united political voice on Capitol Hill. Such behavior is not limited to nurses or nurse administrators. H. George Frederickson (1993, pp. 244–247) writes about the integrity (or lack thereof) of administrative persons in public administration. His perspective leads us to character traits or virtue ethics (Hart, 1994, pp. 107–123) and the relevance of this ethical stance for nurses as patient care administrators.

The economic health care marketplace is in turmoil. Managed care is growing dramatically. Hospitals are downsizing, merging, or closing. Numbers of underinsured and uninsured persons are substantially increasing. Health care facilities now turn away those who cannot pay for treatment judged not to be a medical emergency (Hadley, 1996; Hicks, Stallmeyer, & Coleman, 1993; Snook, 1995). According to Suzanne Smith Blancett and Dominick Flarey (1995), "The image of the health care institution was changing from concerned, community caretaker to inept, fragmented, inefficient, and perhaps, unethical provider" (p. 4). These trends denote, at the minimum, unspoken changes in the standards of care and a need for an ethical assessment of health care delivery by nurses in both administration and practice.

■ EMERGING AND EVOLVING ETHICS

This chapter will offer an alternative ethical framework from classical ethical theories. We will focus on feminist ethics because this framework offers a genuinely new approach to ethics and because of its relevance to nursing, a field in which the vast majority of practitioners are women. We will close with a discussion of the relationship between law and ethics and of the standards of care and professional performance for nurses who are patient care administrators. Readers desiring information on the classical ethical theories of utilitarianism, deontology, virtue, and casuistry and on the ethical principles of respect for autonomy, beneficence (doing good), nonmaleficence (preventing harm), and justice are referred to nursing ethics texts such as

Ethical Decision Making in Nursing, by Gladys Husted and James Husted (1995), and the many bioethics texts such as *Principles of Biomedical Ethics,* by Tom Beauchamp and James Childress (1994).

Feminist Theory and Feminist Ethics

Alison Jaggar (1991) points out two common assumptions from feminist theory that underlie feminist ethics. First, women's moral experiences are worthy of respect and count fully in any theorizing about morality, and, second, the subordination or oppression of women is morally wrong (p. 95). Much of the work of feminists is an attempt to show the overt and insidious ways in which the oppression of women is perpetuated and the ways of eliminating the oppression. Susan Sherwin (1992) addresses the question directly in the first chapter of *No Longer Patient: Feminist Ethics and Health Care.* According to Sherwin, in the economic sphere, women's earnings, job benefits, and job security are less than those of men; positions held by women are ones of less authority and political power than those held by men; women in traditionally male fields or professions (e.g., medicine, law, engineering, business, and politics) tend to be concentrated at the lower end of the pay scale; and women and their children make up a majority of the poor in the developed world (1992, pp. 14–15). Martha Nussbaum and Jonathan Glover (1995), using data drawn from a United Nations study (United Nations, 1993), go beyond economic oppression to reveal the ways in which a significant gap exists between the general well-being of large numbers of women and men in both industrial and developing countries. Because of this gap, Nussbaum supports Catherine McKinnon's claims that "[b]eing a woman is not yet a way of being a human being" (1995, p. 61), and "[w]omen in much of the world lack support for the most central human functions, and this denial of support is frequently caused by their being women" (p. 104).

Many observers are quick to point out that there are several varieties of feminism. Liberal, radical, or socialist feminism are perhaps the most commonly referred to; however, psychoanalytical, traditional Marxist, phenomenological, ecological, anarcha, and postmodernist feminist perspectives have contributed significantly to our current understandings of feminism (Jaggar, 1983; Tuana & Tong, 1995). As Margaret Little (1996) points out, the diversity within feminist thought has led those persons who take a policy-oriented view of feminism to question how feminist theory can contribute to, say, bioethics, until it resolves which variety of feminism is correct. This objection, she claims, "sets the stage for far too flat a conception of how feminist theory can enrich bioethics" (p. 2).

Feminist theory—moral, social, and political theory—is an attempt to show how conceptions of gender distort our views of the world and are particularly hurtful not only to females of all ages, but also to males. Fundamental concepts such as rationality, emotion, and autonomy are shaped by basic assumptions of gender. As Little (1996) notes, feminist theory looks at how "distorted and harmful conceptions of gender have come to affect the very ways in which we frame our vision of the world, affecting what we notice, what we value, and how we conceptualize what does come to attention" (p. 2). In particular, androcentrism, or a male-centered perspective, has resulted in false generics in everyday life. For example, in medicine, women are underrepresented in clinical trials (Little, 1996). A critique of the practices constituting women's oppression, stressing the anti-woman and masculine bias in the basic constructs of moral theory, as well as in theories of knowledge and social–political theory, forms a part of feminist analysis and spurs the development of alternative theories and practices.

Margaret Walker (1992) raises pivotal questions regarding the juridical models of ethics such as utilitarianism and deontology that have been dominant in the last four or five centuries. She asks, "Which interests do they serve, and what do they enable doing" (p. 31)? Historical and contemporary examples cited in her work suggest the importance of exploring links between the rise of these models of ethics and certain features of the last few centuries known as the modern period, including "the extended political enfranchisement of white European males, emergence of a production-oriented market economy, colonialism, industrialization, and increasing bureaucratic centralization of political, educational, medical, and other social authorities. Feminist critique of ethics targets something disturbing about theories of a *certain historically specific kind,* modern theories that seem (intentionally or not) to model hierarchical and bureaucratic structures of administrative control" (p. 31). According to Walker (1992), this kind of theory is not the only form ethics can take; she outlines an expressive–collaborative conception of ethics as an alternative form. The moral logic here is a "logic of interpersonal acknowledgment" (p. 33); the moral understanding is a constructive and flexible process drawing on interpersonal skills (e.g., perceptive, discursive, and communicative) and emotional responses, and these "linked capacities to attend, describe, inquire relevantly, feel appropriately, and respond reliably to situations of a certain kind are the sorts of complex dispositions usually called 'virtues'" (p. 33). However, Walker's thinking does not reflect the usual understanding of virtue theory in ethics.

Integral to feminist ethics is a social–political dimension. Feminist ethicists reveal the ways in which ethical theory has been and remains embedded in certain social structures and understandings, and in political institutions. According to feminist ethicists, an understanding of social and political forces is necessary to understand and alter any moral theory's impact on and import for women. According to Jaggar (1992), those who adopt a feminist approach to ethics are committed to three practical goals: (1) to articulate moral critiques of actions and practices that perpetuate women's subordination, (2) to prescribe morally justifiable ways of resisting such actions and practices, and (3) to envision morally desirable alternatives that will promote women's emancipation (p. 361).

Feminist Ethics and the Ethic of Care

The dominant utilitarian and deontological theories of ethics, which Monique Deveaux (1995) and others have referred to as "grand moral theory," are most commonly called the *ethic of rights* or the *justice* perspective. With the work of moral psychologist Carol Gilligan in the early 1980s, the *ethic of care* was widely discussed as an alternative ethic that had been invisible to and devalued by moral theorists.

The ethic of justice or rights, as Gilligan and others frame it, embodies an obligation theory and posits individuals as opponents in contests of rights. In this logic, morality consists of a hierarchy of rights and rules used to resolve moral conflicts or problems by weighing claims and acting on whichever is the strongest claim. Images of winning and losing are common. There is potential for violence—resulting, in part, from seeing others as opponents and seeing oneself in contests to obtain, or win, one's rights and to maintain them. Individual rights are primary and universal. Actual moral dilemmas are conceived of as "math problems with humans," and the solution is rationally arrived at so that anyone following reason will arrive at more or less the same conclusion. Abstracting from the interpersonal situation and solving hypothetical dilemmas are means of arriving at objective criteria and objectively deciding who will win in the contest of rights. An underlying premise of the ethic of rights is that individuals are separate from one another. Relationships are viewed, then, as developing among individuals who see themselves as separate from any other person, and connections with others are experienced as freely contracted.

The ethic of care and relationship, articulated by Gilligan (1982) and as commonly understood, rejects the preceding rule-based morality and instead emphasizes responsibility within a context of relationship or connection. The image is that of a web that ultimately connects everyone. Responsibility is equated with the need to respond. Individuals need to respond when they recognize that others are counting on them and when they are in a position to help. The ideal of care is an activity of relationship, of seeing and responding to need. The moral imperative is to care, namely, to discern and alleviate trouble in the world. Communication is the principal means of resolving conflict. Because the activity of care is seen as enhancing both others and self, and violence is viewed as destructive to all, conflict resolution is nonviolent. No single specific principle or set of principles, as moral principles are generally thought of, apply to situations or settle disputes. Rather, a guiding principle relates responsibility to caring about others and oneself.

According to Joan Tronto (1993), three distinguishing characteristics separate this ethic of care from the ethic of justice: (1) the ethic of care revolves around responsibility and relationships instead of rights and rules; (2) the care ethic is not formal and abstract but, rather, tied to concrete circumstances; and (3) care morality does not consist of a set of principles but is an activity of caring grounded in the everyday moral problems of actual people

(p. 79). However, Tronto also points to studies that indicate that what is at stake here is not merely a gendered morality, because the differences between the two ethics may describe differences not only between men and women, but also between people in the middle class and working class and between white and ethnic minorities (p. 82).

How are we to understand the ethic of care relative to feminist ethics? Many moral theorists argue that the ethic of care is a *feminine* ethic rather than a *feminist* one. Sherwin (1992), for example, describes feminine ethics as consisting "of observations of how the traditional approaches to ethics fail to fit the moral experiences and intuitions of women" (p. 42), and feminist ethics, because of the explicitly political perspective of feminism, "involves more than recognition of women's actual experiences and moral practices; it incorporates a critique of the specific practices that constitute their oppression" (p. 49). Rosemarie Tong (1993) prefers to speak of feminine and feminist approaches to ethics, highlighting the multiplicity of both. Feminine approaches to ethics, for example, Gilligan's (1982) and Noddings's (1984) ethics of care, employ a feminine consciousness that "regards the *gender* traits that have been traditionally associated with women—in particular, nurturance, compassion, caring—as positive *human* traits" (p. 5).

As we have seen, feminist ethics employs a consciousness that is political, seeing women as subordinated, and seeking to eliminate the subordination (Tong, 1993, p. 6). Included in this effort is asking whether, or to what extent, "feminine traits" and virtues contribute to women's oppression (p. 159). As Tong (1993) points out, however, both feminine and feminist approaches to ethics are ways of doing ethics that depart significantly from traditional approaches to ethics. Those adopting feminine approaches, in particular, have an interest "in exploring the ethical implications of allegedly feminine concepts such as care and connectedness and contrasting them with the ethical implications of allegedly masculine concepts such as justice and autonomy" (p. 10). In addition, feminist approaches are committed to the normative goals of critiquing, resisting, and working on alternatives to "actions and practices that perpetuate women's subordination" (pp. 10–11). Further, regardless of the position taken by these two approaches on the ethic of care, certain ontological and epistemological presuppositions tend to be shared, namely, a belief "that the self is an interdependent being rather than an atomistic entity" (p. 80), "that knowledge is 'emotional' as well as 'rational' and that thoughtful persons reflect on concrete particularities as well as abstract universals" (p. 8).

Difficulties that Arise in Adopting an Ethic of Care

The ethic of care has been widely discussed and adopted by many nurses. The central question is the extent to which fully embracing the ethic of care will result in full respect for the caring work that is so much a part of nursing and in transformation of and improvement in how patients experience that care. Not everyone views the ethic of care as devoid of a political dimension.

According to Monique Deveaux (1995), the care perspective "states that human relatedness and the practices that support it shape us in profound ways. It also states that taking this fact seriously in political terms would precipitate fundamental changes in our social arrangements" (p. 115) and, further, that it "relies centrally on a conception of human good and entails a deep commitment to a transformative politics" (p. 117). Two issues naturally arise for those advocating an ethic of care: (1) how this ethic might gain moral legitimacy and become visible after being rendered invisible for so long, and (2) how the experiences of women might be given respect and be granted full moral worth. Alisa Carse and Hilde Lindemann Nelson (1996) argue that we need the ethic of care if we honestly acknowledge what is required for human flourishing. According to them,

> Women's traditional labor—a vastly disproportionate share of the work of caring—has been important moral labor. It is labor that underscores the moral significance of human *interdependence,* raising ethical concerns about aloneness, abandonment, neglect, and isolation—concerns that arise especially when we are in special states of vulnerability, as are those who are young, ill, frail, disabled, or otherwise in need of others' care. Human thriving requires a world in which there are loving parents and caring citizens: trustworthy and responsible nurses, physicians, political representatives, teachers, neighbors, and cabbies. (pp. 31–32)

As Carse and Nelson also point out, benevolence, compassion, kindness, imagination, and trustworthiness are requirements of a stable social order.

Attempts to garner recognition, let alone respect, for the ethic of care are fraught with difficulties. The problem has been characterized as having to choose between an *assimilation* and a *valorization* approach to obtain recognition for the ethic of care (Kroeger-Mappes, 1994). Neither one of these approaches is effective. The assimilation approach brings the ethic of care into the ethic of justice, claiming that the ethic of care qualifies as a moral theory and can stand on equal footing with, say, utilitarianism and deontology. It assumes that in so doing, an appropriate balance can now be struck, bringing in women's perspectives. However, the assimilation approach clearly underestimates the depth and significance of the problems embedded in traditional moral theory. To subsume care under, say, benevolence misses the point; nothing really would change. Women would remain largely invisible and devalued in all that they do, and moral agents in this theory would have, as they do now, largely "masculine" (taken to be "human") qualities. Another approach is to elevate the ethic of care above the ethic of justice, thereby valorizing it and showing how different it is from standard moral theory. Joan Ringelheim's (1985) questions about this approach echo those taking feminist approaches to ethics: "Is women's culture liberating? How can it be if it was nourished in oppression? Can we ever forget the price we pay as oppressed women? Should we? If we glorify the feminine from a presumably feminist perspective, how do we avoid valorizing oppression in order to criticize and organize against it" (p. 759)? The ethic of care when not viewed in a social and political context serves to maintain the status quo, fails to recognize the oppression of women, and fails to contribute to the process of eliminating oppressive forces.

Joan Tronto (1993) puts the dilemma in a similar way and extends the analysis. The effort among feminist theorists is to end women's marginal status. If some people are marginal, then others are in the powerful center of society. Those who are marginal wish to participate and share power. However, they cannot simply demand to be admitted, having less power, so the only remaining alternative is to persuade those in the center of the circle that they also should be admitted. Only two persuasion strategies are available, namely, "to claim that they should be admitted to the center of power because they are the same as those already there, or because they are different from those already there, but have something valuable to offer to those already there" (p. 15). According to Tronto there is no escape from the *sameness–difference* debate, from this "difference dilemma," because the terms of the debate have been both "historically and theoretically constructed" by those in the center (p. 15). Furthermore, both options are catastrophic. Regardless of which strategy is chosen, the truth of the many different heritages and backgrounds of women—racial, ethnic, religious, class, sexual orientation, and ability—must be denied. It is then easy for those in the center with power to use a number of "divide and conquer" strategies against women. Many women of color, among them Angela Davis (1983) and Gloria Anzaldúa (1990), have written about the effects of these strategies. They also reveal the many ways race and gender often melt together, along with class and other differences.

Tronto (1993), too, points out that "care is gendered, raced, and classed [and] has mainly been the work of slaves, servants, and women in Western history" (pp. 112–113). She nevertheless argues that the dichotomy between care and justice is a false one, one that has been socially constructed along with other moral boundaries. Until we see the boundaries themselves, there is no solution. And seeing the boundaries and removing them requires not only political awareness but also political effort.

■ MULTICULTURAL/GLOBAL PERSPECTIVES AND WESTERN ETHICAL THEORY

To many women of African, Asian, Latino, and Native American heritage, Western "grand moral theory," Western feminist theory, and the ethic of care are far less than the whole story. Indeed, they believe, stories and women's literary works may give the richest understanding of ethical values. According to Katie Cannon (1988), Black women's literature is the best way to understand the ethical values Black women have created and cultivated in this society. She writes, "[l]ocked out of the real dynamics of human freedom in America, they implicitly pass on and receive from one generation to the next moral formulas for survival that allow them to stand over against the perversions of ethics and morality imposed on them by whites and males who support racial imperialism in a patriarchal social order" (p. 7). Katie Cannon's work can be seen as revealing a deep commitment to caring within the African American religious tradition (Tronto, 1993, p. 83). Patricia Hill Collins (1991) also views the ethic of caring as inherently a part of African American culture. She identifies three interrelated components of the ethic of care in the African tradition: an emphasis on individual uniqueness, appropriateness (even requirement) of emotions in dialogues, and developing the capacity for empathy (pp. 215–216). However, many Black women readily point out the ways in which caring has been wanting in their relationships with White women and men, currently and in the past. Bell Hooks (1981), for example, speaks in all of her numerous works of White women's exclusion of Black women from their caring, particularly in *Ain't I a Woman: Black Women and Feminism.*

Because gender pervades every minute of our lives, as Marilyn Frye (1983) reveals, it is sometimes easy to forget that women's experiences do not always center around being female. Gender does deeply affect who we are, how we are treated by others, and how we think of ourselves, but so do the socioeconomic circumstances in which we grew up; the religious upbringing we experienced; the cultures and countries our parents, grandparents, or more distant ancestors came from; and much more. In a widely reprinted article discussing the effects and permutations of colonizations, María Lugones (1987) eloquently and forcefully speaks of the need of women to understand and affirm plurality. They may do so by lovingly "traveling" to one another's "worlds," a term she uses to refer to others' lives of thoughts and interests. This kind of traveling involves "playfulness," which gives meaning to an activity and includes openness to surprise and to self-construction and creativity; here rules are not sacred (pp. 16–17). Without this kind of traveling, we cannot cross ethnic, racial, or any other boundaries.

Uma Narayan (1995) speaks of colonization directly in the context of the debate about justice and care in ethics. She poses the following question: "How did the vast majority of people in the colonizing countries motivate themselves to participate in the large-scale phenomena of slavery and colonialism, not only embracing the idea that distant lands and peoples should be subjugated, but managing to conceive of imperialism as an *obligation . . .*" (p. 133)? In answering this question, we are forced to see the collaboration of elements of the discourse about colonial rights/justice with the discourse on care. It is a self-serving discourse and Narayan points out that the "colonizing project was seen as being *in the interests of, for the good of,* and as *promoting the welfare of* the colonized" (p. 133). Thinking about care in the colonizing context reveals the roles it played in supporting and "justifying relationships of power and domination between *groups of people*" (p. 134). Care has import here, as well as for personal relationships to particular others. Sandra Bartky (1990) points to the disturbing example of Teresa Stangl, wife of Fritz Stangl, Kommandant of Treblinka: "Teresa, anti-Nazi and a devout Catholic, was appalled by what she knew of her husband's work; nevertheless, she maintained home and hearth as a safe harbor to which he returned when he could" (p. 113). Claudia Koonz's (1987) in-depth study of the relationships among particular Jewish and non-Jewish women and groups of women in Nazi Germany is another example of how care often follows power relationships among groups of people. Narayan's point is that any ethical theory can be used for ideological purposes; she is uncertain about the possibility of preventing any ethical theory from being used ideologically, including the ethic of care.

■ WHAT KIND OF ETHICS DO WE NEED?

If any ethical theory can be used for ideological purposes and has been so used, should we get rid of ethics? Some lesbian feminist theorists believe we should (Card, 1991; Tong, 1993). Other feminist theorists argue for a transformation of ethical theory and respond to the challenges directly. The difference dilemma remains. One response to this formidable problem is a postmodernist one. However, according to many, including Joan Tronto (1993), while deconstructing categories well and carefully may help us understand why certain categories of analysis do not work well, postmodernism has not been particularly helpful in understanding why some people are more powerful and privileged than others, and it provides no assistance at all in revealing why "essential activities of caring [are] not well regarded, theorized, supported, and respected in our society" (p. 19). We will now discuss the arguments of three feminist theorists, Joan Tronto, Martha Nussbaum, and Judith Kay, in favor of the transformation of ethics.

Joan Tronto's (1993) response to the challenge of articulating a transformative ethic and the difference dilemma is a specific understanding of the ethic of care for which she gives a *political argument*. The ethic of care she outlines is to be understood as complex and as involving both particular acts of caring and a general "habit of mind" to care. Although it involves dangers and is not intended as a total account of morality, a care ethic "might more quickly expose how the powerful might try to twist an understanding of needs to maintain their positions of power and privilege" (p. 140). Tronto details four elements of care: "caring about, noticing the need to care in the first place; taking care, assuming responsibility for care; care-giving, the actual work of care that needs to be done; and care-receiving, the response of that which is cared for to the care" (p. 127). These elements give rise to four ethical elements of care, namely, attentiveness, responsibility, competence, and responsiveness (considering others' positions as they express them and not as we might in that situation), which fit together as a whole (pp. 127–137). In making the views of those cared for a central requirement of the ethic of care, Tronto is attempting to prevent the infliction of harm while claiming to care. Finally, she sees the *practice* of care as a political idea as well as a moral concept that "describes the qualities necessary for democratic citizens to live together well in a pluralistic society, and that only in a just, pluralistic, democratic society can care flourish" (p. 162).

Martha Nussbaum (1995) also responds to the challenge of a transformative ethic and the difference dilemma. Both Tronto and Nussbaum accept and extend Aristotle's view that morality and politics are intertwined. "Aristotle described political association as the way in which societies created the capacities for ethical practices and modes of existence" (Tronto, 1993, p. 7). Nussbaum (1995) takes a directly feminist approach as well as an Aristotelian stance (although Aristotle did not accord women full membership in human functioning). She views the idea of human functioning or capacities as a powerful moral and political tool for women (p. 96). "Being a woman is indeed not yet a way of being a human being. Women in much of the world lack support for the most central human functioning and this denial of support is frequently caused by their being women" (p. 104).

The conception of a common humanity has great power as a source of moral claims, Nussbaum (1995) argues, and is most helpful in solving the problem of women's "unequal failure in capability" (p. 104). Women, like all other human beings "have the potential to become capable of these human functions, given sufficient nutrition, education, and other support" (p. 104). Viewing the problem in this way, she believes, gives us the leverage to see what is wrong with the many deprivations and abuses women experience and how to proceed in eliminating them. Her account directly addresses the difference dilemma. It is a universalist and "essentialist" proposal that "focuses on what is common to all, rather than on differences (although . . . it does not neglect these)," and . . . "see[s] some capabilities and functions as more central, more to the core of human life, than others" (p. 63). It does so in order to give everyone a moral starting point, one she believes that can be particularly valuable to women everywhere in the world.

According to Nussbaum (1995), "universal ideas of the human do arise within history and from human experience, and they can ground themselves in experience" (p. 69). In other words, it is commonly held in both Western and non-Western philosophical traditions "that there is some determinate way the world is, apart from the interpretive workings of the cognitive faculties of living beings" (p. 68). In providing a "sketch for an account of the most important functions and capabilities of the human being, in terms of which human life is defined" (p. 72), Nussbaum is clear that this is a working list which is to generate debate, as it already has, and to be revised. This sketch "is a story about what seems to be part of any life we will count as a human life" (p. 75).

- *Mortality.* All human beings face death . . . , know [at some point] that they face it . . . , and have an aversion to it.
- *The Human Body.* We live all our lives in bodies of a certain sort. These bodies, similar far more than dissimilar . . . are our homes . . . giving us certain needs and also possibilities for excellence. The experience of the body is culturally shaped. . . . But the body itself sets limits on what can be experienced and valued.
- *Capacity for Pleasure and Pain.* Experiences of pain and pleasure are common to all human life (though, once again, both their expression and, to some extent, the experience itself may be culturally shaped).
- *Cognitive Capability.* All human beings have sense perception, the ability to imagine, and the ability to think.
- *Early Infant Development.* All human beings [experience a] common structure to early life—which is clearly shaped in many different ways by different social arrangements and that gives rise to a great deal of overlapping experience central in the formation of desires, and of complex emotions such as grief, love, and anger.
- *Practical Reason.* All human beings participate (or try to) in the planning and managing of their own lives, asking and answering questions about what is good and how one should live.
- *Affiliation with Other Human Beings.* All human beings recognize and feel some sense of affiliation and concern for other human beings.
- *Relatedness to Other Species and to Nature.* Human beings recognize that they are not the only living things in their world.
- *Humour and Play.* Laughter and play are frequently among the deepest and also the first modes of our mutual recognition.
- *Separateness.* However much we live with and for others, we are, each of us, 'one in number'.
- *Strong Separateness.* Because of separateness, each human life has, so to speak, its own peculiar context and surroundings. . . . (pp. 76–80)

Although Nussbaum's work draws on Aristotle's virtue ethics, it is transformative. Tronto (1993), in contrast, sees an ethic of care as necessary as a context for the moral capabilities and functionings Nussbaum describes. "Care puts moral ideals into action"; the care focus is one that is on the process of sustaining life, on human actors acting (Tronto, p. 154).

Judith Kay (1994), another feminist ethicist, sees the ethical and political as intertwined and also attempts a reconstruction of a common humanity. She highlights difficulties in arriving at a liberatory ethic for women and for everyone. "Too often, universal claims represent only the perspective of the group (usually ruling class males) doing the theorizing. Such claims can also support violent suppression of difference, reify the status quo as natural, and make the natural appear static, beyond the reach of human agency and change" (p. 22). Included among these universal claims are those made about women by feminists themselves, as we pointed out earlier. As a result, Kay argues, many feminists have adopted postmodernism's "rejection of all claims about human nature as essentialist and inevitably oppressive to women" (p. 22). However, the difficulty arising here is a recurring detachment from political engagement of postmodernist thinkers (p. 22).

Kay (1994) puts forward twenty working hypotheses about common humanity. Included are the following: Humans are social and necessarily interdependent; are dynamic and changing; are able to learn from mistakes and change their course of action; are motivated to seek the good appropriate to their being and find certain things harmful; and have the capacity for practical intelligence, that is, the ability to perceive and respond flexibly to new situations (p. 39). So far this list of working hypotheses is quite similar to the capabilities Nussbaum describes. But Kay includes hypotheses about how humans are hurt, in particular by being oppressed, and how humans also have the capacity to heal from the pain of oppression. For example, this list notes that humans "can have their capacity for flexible intelligence disrupted. People are susceptible to the imposition of patterns that replace a portion of their ability to perceive reality and to respond appropriately" (pp. 39–40). People then respond with a rigid pattern, although they originally attempted to resist disempowerment and disrespect. Their attempts at resisting oppression generally go unacknowledged. "[Once] saddled with patterns, they often 'choose' to act on the basis of their patterns due to reinforcing discourses [claims and concepts of dominating groups] and lack of opportunities to heal" (p. 40). They also "find that patterns interfere with the ability to feel, remember, think, be aware, set goals, and act effectively" (p. 40). However, humans "have the capacity to heal the painful emotions that keep patterns in place" (p. 40). In addition, humans "have to be mistreated [first themselves] before they will oppress others" (p. 40).

This understanding of humanity is historical and situated. At the same time it is universal. Kay (1994) is attempting to show that humans are capable of dismantling oppression that has been internalized, that is, beliefs about ourselves that were or are held by people in dominant positions or roles in our lives. She is also showing that everyone is in a dominant position relative to some other humans, for example, adults to children, and that humans are also capable of dismantling the domination they also internalized as a result of mistreatment, say, as a child. Practice or engagement in concrete struggles can lead to flexible thinking outside rigid patterns if people are allowed "to retell their stories with the goal of releasing the painful emotions that 'freeze' their memories in place" (p. 38). Success in healing involves seeing possibilities outside the patterns, not simply recounting stories of pain. This is an ongoing process; "[p]raxis leads to reflection which leads to altered action and renewed reflection" (p. 39).

In showing the capabilities humans have for healing from the wounds inflicted by oppression, resulting in a release from rigid patterns, Kay (1994) can be seen as responding to Narayan's (1995) point that any ethical theory can be used for ideological purposes, namely, to gain and/or maintain domination over other human beings. Women have been dominated and oppressed and have also not only survived but have created, led, inspired, and cared in countless brilliant ways. This is true of women of different groups in different ways, each woman with her own separate or unique intelligence and experiences. Some actions are reactions coming out of rigid patterns; others are fresh appropriate responses to the current situation, which are called virtues (p. 49). Kay is arguing that unless feminist theorists develop a way of thinking about subjectivity and our common humanity that is emancipatory, the installed patterns will be easily employed for ideological purposes. A transformative feminist ethics for Kay and Nussbaum is open to revision. For Kay, it must be a continuing process as we act, heal, reflect, and learn.

■ INTERRELATIONSHIPS OF ETHICS AND LAW

Although there is ongoing turmoil with regard to ethical theory, there are compelling practical reasons to seek some understanding of the relationship between ethics and law. Neither ethics nor law is an exact science; thus, neither ethicists nor lawyers always are able to predict with precision what the outcome of an ethical or a legal conflict may be. Both, however, are sensitive to established, sanctioned, and sometimes changing rules that are culturally transmitted through values.

How, then, do ethics and law interface in nursing practice and administration? According to Smith and Davis (1980), there are four situations in which ethics and law interface:

1. That which is ethical is legal (e.g., informed consent).
2. That which is ethical is illegal (e.g., some would say euthanasia).
3. That which is unethical is legal (e.g., some would say abortion).
4. That which is unethical is illegal (e.g., involuntary medical treatment in nonemergency situations). (p. 1465)

Two of the preceding situations are congruent and two are in conflict. These middle two situations often produce conflict for the nurses as patient care administrators.

Although there is no easy answer on how to resolve the preceding conflicts, the following statements serve to put the two in perspective:

- The conflict between ethical and illegal and unethical and legal will probably always be with us. Ethics cannot be bound by the law when ethical considerations override legal ones. Law cannot be held hostage to ethics in the sense that a law cannot be enacted to control every immoral act. Therefore, the nurse as patient care administrator must expect this tension between ethics and law.

- The role of the institutional lawyer and that of the nurse as patient care administrator may conflict. A primary purpose of institutional lawyers is to protect the institution and the people who work there from legal entanglements. The primary purpose of the nurse as patient care administrator is to ensure that patients receive the best possible care. Therefore, a nurse administrator might reduce this conflict by recommending that a health care institution hire additional lawyers as advocates for patients. This other legal opinion would be helpful in achieving a balanced perspective.
- Lawyers use basic tenets of ethics in formulating laws, and ethicists use laws or court decisions as part of their database in arriving at morally justified decisions. Ethics, however, is not the final determinant of law, and law is not the final determinant of ethics.
- If a conflict about resolution of an ethical dilemma exists among lawyers and nurses, then both should consider how the decision will affect those persons most affected by it. Sometimes one must take a solitary stance but, at other times, reasonable compromise or acquiescence to a majority decision may be in the overall best interest of all.

As advances in science and technology precipitate more ethical and legal dilemmas, nurses as patient care administrators need greater understanding of the interrelationships between law and ethics. Jacquelyn Kay Hall (1996), a nurse lawyer, shows us these interrelationships in a snapshot fashion:

1. Good nursing practice is ethical and legal.
2. The shared values (ethics) of a people are the basis of their law.
3. Law is a *minimum* standard of morality.
4. The ethics incorporated into good nursing practice are more important than knowledge of the law; practicing ethically saves the effort of trying to know all the laws.
5. Nurses who follow specific legal mandates that violate good nursing practice and ethical principles could be legal but not right (and eventually, not even legal).
6. Good practice reflects ethical behavior that results in action that is legal—this is a theory of law.
7. A legal duty does not exist without a higher ethical duty, but there may exist an ethical duty without a lower legal duty.
8. The minimum behavior required by law is not the same as the maximum of ethical behavior. (p. 2)

■ STANDARD OF CARE AND OF PROFESSIONAL PERFORMANCE

Standards of care and of professional performance help nurses as patient care administrators ensure that they are creating and maintaining a professional nursing system within their health care settings. Standards of professional performance are not static; they reflect changes in society, technology, and the professions. Nursing's reflection of these changes, however, must always be a responsible one that ultimately is accountable to ethics, law, and the social contract between nursing and society (ANA, 1995a).

Recently, the ANA (1995b) published its *Scope and Standards for Nurse Administrators*. This document focuses both on standards of care and on standards of professional performance. Regarding standards of care, the following categories are addressed: assessment, diagnosis, identification of outcomes, planning, implementation, and evaluation. Regarding standards of professional performance, the following categories are addressed: quality of care and administrative practice, performance appraisal, education, collegiality, ethics, collaboration, research, and research utilization. Although ethics has been designated in a separate category, the other standards of care and of professional performance all have ethical undertones and implications.

This standard is stated as follows:

The nurse administrator's decisions and actions are based on ethical principles.

Measurement Criteria
The nurse administrator:

1. Advocates on behalf of recipients of services and personnel.
2. Maintains privacy, confidentiality, and security of patient, client, staff, and organization data.
3. Advocates organizational adherence to the *ANA Code for Nurses.*
4. Fosters a non-discriminatory climate in which care is delivered in a manner sensitive to sociocultural diversity.
5. Supports the system to address ethical issues within nursing and the organization. (ANA, 1995b, p. 19)

The preceding measurement criteria of professional performance provide beginning ethical guidelines for nurses as patient care administrators. Nurse administrators, however, must recognize the limitations of the standards. They are based in large part on more traditional ethical principles and do not explicitly incorporate the emerging and evolving ethics discussed in this chapter. We encourage nurses as patient care administrators also to incorporate the insights of multicultural and global feminist ethics and the ethic of care into their administrative practices.

■ SUMMARY

Both nursing and ethics are in a state of profound transition. Regarding nursing, the scope of nursing practice and the ways in which nurses are reimbursed for their care are changing. In addition, managed care has affected how and where nurses, including nurses as patient care administrators, practice. Hospitals are closing or downsizing, and nurses are being retrained for new jobs with a community-based focus. Nurses also are becoming increasingly active in the political arena where they are helping to shape policy that affects how health care is rendered, allocated, and paid for in the United States. To facilitate the practice of nurses as patient care administrators, they must understand the interrelation between ethics and law; in effect, that good administrative practice is both ethical and legal. Finally, nurse administrators can turn to the 1995 ANA *Scope and Standards for Nurse Administrators* as a starting point for ethical professional practice.

Regarding ethics, new ethical frameworks are evolving. During the past several decades, classical ethical theories and associated principles dominated. Today, emerging and evolving ethical frameworks (i.e., feminist ethics and the ethic of care) are coming into their own. Whereas feminist ethics focuses largely on the moral wrongs of the oppression of women because of their gender and on developing liberatory theories and practices, the ethic of care focuses largely on the interpersonal processes of connectedness and on the value of the caring experiences of women. Both feminist ethics and the ethic of care may be seen as transformative ethics and, at least arguably, either of these frameworks might be best articulated and developed from the outset with a keen awareness of multicultural and global perspectives in a search for and an understanding of a common humanity.

▪ BIOGRAPHICAL SKETCHES

Mary Cipriano Silva received her BSN and MS from the Ohio State University and her PhD from the University of Maryland. In addition, as a Kennedy Fellow in Medical Ethics for Nursing Faculty, she undertook postdoctoral study in ethics at Georgetown University. She also has been a Visiting Scholar at the Hastings Center, Briarcliff Manor, New York. From 1984 to 1989, Dr. Silva served as Project Director on a Special Project Grant funded by the Division of Nursing on ethical decision making for nurse executives. She has authored an award-winning book on ethical decision making for nurse administrators and has written extensively in the field of ethics. In 1995, she authored the ANA's new guidelines on ethics in nursing research. In 1996, she was selected to be a member of the ANA Code of Ethics Project Task Force to revise the current *Code for Nurses with Interpretive Statements*.

Joy Kroeger-Mappes received her diploma in nursing from Michael Reese Hospital and Medical Center, her BSN from DePaul University, and her MA and PhD in philosophy from Georgetown University. She has written in feminist ethics; served as coordinator in establishing a women's studies minor; taught women's studies courses including feminist philosophy; founded and been first chair of the University of Maryland System Women's Forum; led coalition work on campus and in the community; founded, chaired, and served on an advisory council to the president of Frostburg State University on diversity; served as a member of a hospital ethics committee for 12 years; been a member of the board for the area safe house for women and children serving as chair for 3 years; and been awarded the university's community service award.

■ SUGGESTED READINGS

Code and Ethical Guidelines

American Nurses' Association. (1985). *Code for nurses with interpretive statements.* Kansas City, MO: Author.

Bibliographies and Encyclopedias

Silva, M.C., & Goldstein, D.M. (1995–1996). Training and information sources. In S. Fry-Revere, J. Sorrell, & M. Silva (Eds.), *Issues and answers in home health care: Practical guidelines for dealing with bioethical issues in your organization.* Fairfax, VA: George Mason University Center for Health Care Ethics in cooperation with the Regis Group, Inc. and the National Association for Medical Equipment Services.

Walters, L., & Kahn, T.J. (Eds.). (1984–1996). *Bibliography of bioethics.* (Vols. 10–22). Washington, DC: Kennedy Institute of Ethics, Georgetown University. (Published yearly.)

Reich, W.T. (Ed.). (1995). *Encyclopedia of bioethics* (rev. ed., Vol. 1–5). New York: Simon & Schuster, Macmillan.

Books

Bowie, G.L., Michaels, M.W., & Solomon, R.C. (1996). *Twenty questions: An introduction to philosophy.* New York: Harcourt Brace College.

Cole, E.B. (1992). *Explorations in feminist ethics: Theory and practice.* Bloomington, IN: Indiana University Press.

Held, V. (1995). *Justice and care: Essential readings in feminist ethics.* Boulder, CO: Westview Press.

Holmes, H.B., & Purdy, L.M. (1992). *Feminist perspectives in medical ethics.* Bloomington, IN: Indiana University Press.

Larrabee, M.J. (1993). *An ethic of care: Feminist and interdisciplinary perspectives.* New York: Routledge.

Okin, S.M. (1989). *Justice, gender, and the family.* New York: Basic Books.

Wolf, S.M. (1996). *Feminism and bioethics: Beyond reproduction.* New York: Oxford University Press.

■ REFERENCES

American Nurses Association. (1995a). *Nursing's social policy statement*. Washington, DC: American Nurses Publishing.

American Nurses Association. (1995b). *Scope and standards for nurse administrators*. Washington, DC: American Nurses Publishing.

Anzaldúa, G. (1990). *Making face, making soul: Creative and critical perspectives by women of color*. San Francisco: Aunt Lute Foundation Books.

Bartky, S.L. (1990). *Femininity and domination: Studies in the phenomenology of oppression*. New York: Routledge, Chapman, and Hall.

Beauchamp, T.L., & Childress, J.F. (1994). *Principles of biomedical ethics* (4th ed.). New York: Oxford University Press.

Blancett, S.S., & Flarey, D.L. (1995). *Reengineering nursing and health care: The handbook for organizational transformation*. Gaithersburg, MD: Aspen.

Cannon, K.G. (1988). *Black womanist ethics*. Atlanta: Scholars Press.

Card, C. (1991). *Feminist ethics*. Lawrence, KS: University Press of Kansas.

Carse, A.L., & Nelson, H.L. (1996). Rehabilitating care. *Kennedy Institute of Ethics Journal, 6,* 19–35.

Collins, P.H. (1991). *Black feminist thought: Knowledge, consciousness, and the politics of empowerment*. New York: Routledge.

Davis, A.V. (1983). *Women, race & class*. New York: Random House.

Deveaux, M. (1995). Shifting paradigms: Theorizing care and justice in political theory. *Hypatia, 10* (2), 115–119.

Frederickson, H.G. (1993). Ethics and public administration: Some assertions. In H.G. Frederickson (Ed.), *Ethics and public administration*. Armonk, NY: M.E. Sharpe.

Frye, M. (1983). *The politics of reality: Essays in feminist theory*. Trumansburg, NY: The Crossing Press.

Gilligan, C. (1982). *In a different voice: Psychological theory and women's development*. Cambridge, MA: Harvard University Press.

Hadley, E.H. (1996). Nursing in the political and economic marketplace: Challenges for the 21st century. *Nursing Outlook, 44,* 6–10.

Hall, J.K. (1996). *Nursing ethics and law*. Philadelphia: Saunders.

Hart, D.K. (1994). Administration and the ethics of virtue. In T.L. Cooper (Ed.), *Handbook of administrative ethics*. New York: Marcel Dekker.

Hicks, L.L., Stallmeyer, J.M., & Coleman, J.R. (1993). *Role of the nurse in managed care*. Washington, DC: American Nurses Publishing.

Hooks, B. (1981). *Ain't I a woman: Black women and feminism*. Boston: South End Press.

Husted, G.L., & Husted, J.J. (1995). *Ethical decision making in nursing* (2nd ed.). St. Louis: Mosby.

Jaggar, A.M. (1983). *Feminist politics and human nature*. Totowa, NJ: Rowman & Allanheld.

Jaggar, A.M. (1991). Feminist ethics: Projects, problems, prospects. In C. Card (Ed.), *Feminist ethics*. Lawrence, KS: University Press of Kansas.

Jaggar, A.M. (1992). Feminist ethics. In L. Becker & C. Becker (Eds.), *Encyclopedia of ethics*. New York: Garland Press.

Kay, J.W. (1994). Politics without human nature? Reconstructing a common humanity. *Hypatia, 9* (1), 21–52.

Koonz, C. (1987). *Mothers in the fatherland: Women, the family, and Nazi politics.* New York: St. Martin's Press.

Kroeger-Mappes, J. (1994). The ethic of care vis-à-vis the ethic of rights: A problem for contemporary moral theory. *Hypatia, 9* (3), 108–131.

Little, M.O. (1996). Why a feminist approach to bioethics? *Kennedy Institute of Ethics Journal, 6,* 1–18.

Lugones, M. (1987). Playfulness, "world"-traveling, and loving perception. *Hypatia, 2* (2), 3–19.

Narayan, U. (1995). Colonialism and its others: Considerations on rights and care discourses. *Hypatia, 10* (2), 133–140.

Noddings, N. (1984). *Caring: A feminine approach to ethics & moral education.* Berkeley, CA: University of California Press.

Nussbaum, M. (1995). Human capabilities, female human beings. In M. Nussbaum & J. Glover (Eds.), *Women, culture, and development: A study of human capabilities.* New York: Oxford University Press.

Nussbaum, M., & Glover, J. (1995). *Women, culture, and development: A study of human capabilities.* New York: Oxford University Press.

Ringelheim, J. (1985). *Women and the holocaust: A reconsideration of research. Signs, 10* (4), 741–761.

Sherwin, S. (1992). *No longer patient: Feminist ethics and health care.* Philadelphia: Temple University Press.

Smith, S.J., & Davis, A.J. (1980). Ethical dilemmas: Conflicts among rights, duties, and obligations. *American Journal of Nursing, 80,* 1462–1466.

Snook, I.D., Jr. (1995). Hospital organization and management. In L.F. Wolper (Ed.), *Health care administration: Principles, practices, structure, and delivery* (2nd ed.). Gaithersburg, MD: Aspen.

Tong, R. (1993). *Feminine and feminist ethics.* Belmont, CA: Wadsworth.

Tronto, J.C. (1993). *Moral boundaries: A political argument for an ethic of care.* New York: Routledge.

Tuana, N., & Tong, R. (1995). *Feminism and philosophy: Essential readings in theory, reinterpretation, and application.* Boulder, CO: Westview Press.

United Nations. (1993). *Human development report.* New York: United Nations Development Program.

Walker, M.U. (1992). Feminism, ethics, and the question of theory. *Hypatia, 7* (3), 23–38.

APPLICATION 1–1   Moral Reasoning in Personnel Decisions

Patricia Snyder

The highly challenging nature of the health care industry today presents nurses at all levels of administration with numerous ethical dilemmas. Decisions about the use of resources in organizing and managing systems to deliver patient care are obviously at issue, but the moral implications of human resource management also demand sensitivity, thoughtful analysis, and careful decision making to ensure that choices are made that consider the well-being, rights, and dignity of the staff.

An effective nurse administrator must give careful consideration to the use of an ethical framework that leads to decisions soundly based on moral principles, which thus will serve the needs of the organization and its members well. Whether an ethic of care or of justice predominates, it is important that the nature of each be understood and that the implications for the culture of the organization which follow from that approach be considered. It is possible that under different circumstances one may more fully inform the moral reasoning process.

An ethic of care, based on nurturance, connection, and relationship may be more attractive to many in nursing, as it is often seen as an administrative expression of the caring in nursing practice (Brandt, 1994; Nyberg, 1993). The ethic of justice, on the other hand, speaks clearly of fairness, equity, and autonomy, which are firmly established values in management theory and for our society in general. In considering a justice framework, we become aware of some of the ethical principles that must be applied to relationships with employees, as well as with patients: confidentiality, autonomy (defined as independent decision making); nonmaleficence (avoidance of harmful actions); and beneficence. Truthfulness and respect for the employee's dignity as an individual must also apply. These same elements, however, are involved in using an ethic of care, intertwined as they are in building relationships and considering right actions in the context of the situation as it presents.

Ethical dilemmas arise in all areas of personnel management. Patient care delivery issues notwithstanding, the staff has a legitimate claim on administration for decisions that recognize and provide for individual needs and rights as employees and as persons, and for the professional responsibilities of the staff to patients, and to the profession of which they are members.

Decision making in personnel management is commonly discussed in relation to the organization's need to secure adequate numbers of motivated staff who are qualified and competent to carry out their duties, and to organize and assign staff in a manner that maintains costs within budgeted levels. The reward system is considered, often with an emphasis on motivation and achievement of the organization's goals and strategic direction. Legal and risk management

APPLICATION 1–1   *Continued*

considerations involved in employer–employee relationships receive considerable attention, as well.

Another dimension of the issue that merits attention is the rights of the staff in the ethical consideration of their welfare as individuals and their need for growth as professionals through their association with the health care organization. Whether the issue is selection, orientation, staff development, promotion, performance appraisal, discipline, or the components of the reward system, a clear understanding of the ethical principles involved is critical to appropriate concern for each nurse's rights as an individual with inherent dignity. Will the working environment be created to enhance the opportunities of each individual to grow and develop as a person and as a professional? Will there be opportunity to use skills and abilities fully? Will individual interest in adding to a repertoire of skills be nurtured? By the way questions such as these are answered, the organization and its administrative staff express a philosophical stance in relation to employees.

Structuring the organization to promote professional practice emphasizing collaboration, self-direction, and accountability is a manifestation of efforts to achieve such a goal. Perhaps another, even more profound expression, because it exists at the individual level, is the nature of the supervisory relationship of each manager with the members of the staff. When that relationship is caring and just, it will both allow and nurture growth in the nurse as a professional and as an individual. The relationship will become moral in its thrust toward development and ever-expanding ability and skill.

The strategies adopted by health care organizations to adjust to the new circumstances in which they find themselves today have profound effects on the staff, the professions to which the staff belong, and ultimately the patients who are provided care. Mergers of units, services, or institutions; formation of integrated networks; or major restructuring efforts in individual facilities, all give rise to difficult, serious considerations that may well present ethical dilemmas to a sensitive observer. When the primary duty of the health care facility to patients and community is given due consideration during the search for solutions, these issues become even more demanding.

Consider the case of two small hospitals that are being consolidated by a parent corporation. The new facility is planned to be considerably smaller than the aggregate of the two existing facilities. Thus, many current positions will be redundant. It is anticipated that a significant number of current employees will not be required to staff the consolidated organization. In addition, the consolidated facility will be a third distinct entity, not a re-creation of either, and will thus cause a major change in the work life of all involved.

A serious consideration for management will be what amount and level of attention will be paid to the social and psychological effects of such profound organizational change. How will success be determined in making human re-

APPLICATION 1–1 *Continued*

source decisions? Will the organization see itself as highly pragmatic and dispassionate, focused on strictly objective criteria related to strategic and financial issues? Or will it adopt a philosophy of care or justice for the employees that permits it to appropriately consider their welfare as planning and implementation are completed? What will be the implications of the choice that is made for the ability of the organization to carry out its primary mission of caring for patients?

Although a number of personnel decisions must be made jointly by senior management for the whole organization in order to provide equity for all, the nurse administrator will want to ensure that input developed within an ethical framework informs the decision making process. Furthermore, nursing administration will need to consider the manner in which it will carry out organization-wide policies, and how managers will relate to the staff in terms of their dignity and humanity.

In what way will staff be informed of plans as they develop? How will trust be preserved? Will information be made available as quickly as it is produced, allowing staff maximum opportunity to use it to make decisions in their own interests, or will it be provided in such a way as to increase the likelihood that staff will act in a manner that maximizes benefit to the organization? Is it ethically sound to do the latter, given the possible consequences for quality of care if large numbers of particularly expert, highly employable staff decide to seek other employment? Can they be retained while still protecting their interests? Are there

benefits to staff in staying through the transition period? How can these be identified and communicated?

What of the anxiety that staff experience as they contemplate the prospect of changes in their employment? What is the responsibility of the facility in allaying that distress? And at what point does an approach that endeavors to be caring and humane undermine the right and responsibility of the employee to be, and act as, a mature individual rather than a recipient of caretaking by the employer? How is care versus caretaking expressed in such circumstances?

In addition to deciding about the distribution of information, management must plan for selection of staff for the consolidated facility. An overall staffing plan based on the anticipated organizational structure will be constructed as part of the financial plan. After job descriptions have been written, decisions must be made about the nature of the selection process to be used. Will staff, including senior management be given the opportunity to apply for positions? Or will these selections be made in another way? What will be the long-term ethical implications for the organization if any selections are determined through an essentially political process? How will the staff at each level of the organization be selected to ensure that employees from each organization have a fair opportunity to continue employment?

When selection decisions are made, will they be completed fairly based on known qualifications and the expressed interest of the staff, or will some decisions be used to channel individuals in

APPLICATION 1–1 *Continued*

particular directions without their knowledge of the process? Will staff who are occupied with special duties related to the change be fully informed of their ultimate employment status?

When will these selections be made? Will the designated staff have sufficient time to plan thoroughly for new clinical and administrative systems? If so, what of those who know they have not been selected? Their services will still be needed until the physical consolidation occurs to continue appropriate operations of both facilities. What compensation will be provided to reward staff who will ultimately leave the organization for their length of service and for their continuing, but temporary, employment? Will it be set at levels that are just? How will just compensation be determined? What other assistance will be provided to assist in transition and finding other employment?

A consolidation, such as we are considering, involves intricate planning and development of clinical and administrative systems for the new entity. The most important consideration in developing the delivery system will be the needs of the patients and how quality care can best be provided. The organization will also rightly consider the resources that are available to it, and how it can operate efficiently as well as effectively. Cost structure is necessarily a part of the determination of that quality, both in terms of the success of the organization and stewardship of the resources of patients who are served. Ensuring that the choices made in designing the system will facilitate sound relationships among the staff, and create work that

provides satisfaction, inherent gratification, and stimulus to growth becomes an expression of the ethical posture of the organization toward its employees.

Some of the new approaches to organizing care delivery, such as multiskilling, present significant challenges to staff. The implementation of a case management model, for example, often affects the roles of employees in social work, discharge planning, and utilization review. If an agency adopts this process to manage care, not only will there be excess staff in these departments, but redesigned positions will require new skills, and a new approach to organizing care and relating to patients. Considerable training is usually involved—a costly undertaking. To what extent is there an ethical obligation to provide that training? Can it be focused on procedures, simply leaving it to the employee to seek out other resources as needed to enhance skill development? And what is the obligation of the employee? Can that employee expect to look to his employer for expansion of skills? Or does each professional—indeed, each staff member—have a responsibility to actively seek out new knowledge? Is an organization that requires such individual effort acting in a caring manner? Knowing that specific employment is more often a transitory event in today's workplace, what is the responsibility of the organization and of the individual to improve and expand skills and knowledge? Is the future employability of staff with other organizations an ethical obligation of the current employer?

APPLICATION 1–1   *Continued*

The issue of an administrator's ethical duty to employees can be studied further through exploration of another example whose themes are commonly encountered in supervision. An important function of a manager is working with staff to ensure that performance meets accepted standards. At times, individual staff members may find themselves challenged to meet those standards, not only by limitations in the skill set and knowledge base that they possess, but by factors inherent in their interactions with others. In our increasingly diverse society, people may come to the workplace with understandings of proper relationships and behavior that vary from those of the dominant culture.

Suppose that a very talented and accomplished bedside nurse decides to take a new direction in her practice by assuming the role of the regular charge nurse. Although she undertakes her new position with enthusiasm and works hard to perform well, it becomes apparent very quickly that she experiences considerable difficulty in giving direction in a clear and convincing manner. Particularly troublesome is the new charge nurse's problem in dealing with an assertive male member of the staff. The manager endeavors to teach more effective methods, but improvement is slow. The manager recognizes that the nurse is a member of a cultural group that expects women to subordinate themselves to male authority, and the patient care assistant with whom she is having difficulty is a member of another group that does not expect men to take direction from women.

Both these individuals are attempting to relate to co-workers using personal, culturally determined sets of interpersonal rules. What are the ethical issues in relation to assisting both to perform satisfactorily in their work? What kind of assistance should they be given? Should the performance standards to which they are held be altered to accommodate their backgrounds? Should they simply be considered unsuited for the demands of these positions? What of the effects on the other staff and on operations of the unit? What effect might modifying their work behavior have on interactions with family and friends? Are these legitimate concerns for the nurse manager?

The conflict between the needs of the individual and of the work group and organization can be seen, as well, in the following situation. A nurse administrator selects a successful charge nurse for a position as manager of two large units. She is provided with an orientation to her new position and receives ongoing training and supervision. But, as often happens, she is faced early on with difficult problems. She works energetically to master her new role, but finds it very hard to remove herself sufficiently from the day-to-day work to adequately see the overall situation on these two complex units. As time goes by, the administrator sees deterioration in the functioning of the units, and is forced to conclude that the promotion may have been an inappropriate one.

For how long, and how intensively, does justice demand that additional training and support be provided to

APPLICATION 1–1 *Continued*

maintain the new manager in her role? On the other hand, to what extent can the staff be expected to function in a troubled situation? Removing the manager from her position must be considered. But when—to minimize harm to all concerned? Is this a situation rightly defined as a performance problem? Is discipline in order? How else can the problem be addressed? What of the nurse manager herself? She has accepted the role in good faith and tried hard to fill it but is apparently not well suited to it. What impact does leaving it feeling unsuccessful have on her, personally and professionally? How can she be assisted to feel competent to pursue another course better suited to her talents?

In this example, the nurse administrator is concerned not only with justice to all, but also with the good of a professional whose efforts have been energetic and well-motivated, if ineffective. She must also consider the need of society and the profession to preserve this individual as a valuable asset in another area of practice. All of these considerations may make intervention more complex and demanding of time and energy than a less thoughtful resolution of the problem might. The nurse administrator must decide how much of the organization's resources can rightly be invested in this effort, balancing the claims of all.

Nurse administrators will find that the beneficial outcomes of using an ethical approach to decision making in dilemmas such as those identified above extends beyond the individual situations to which it is applied. An important responsibility of nurse administrators in leading staff to achieve high standards is to assist them to thoroughly incorporate moral reasoning into all aspects of practice, including relationships with other professionals and not just in regard to ethical issues that receive wide attention.

Achieving this goal requires development of a certain sensitivity to the presence of ethical concerns, as well as the ability to think in such terms. Nurses in administration will find that including ethical principles in a clear and explicit manner in their rationale for the decisions they make will have a positive influence on the ability of the staff to do likewise. By role modeling moral reasoning in problem solving, especially in personnel matters, nurse administrators will demonstrate for the staff, with the special clarity gained through personal experience, the salutary effects of acting in accordance with an ethical framework. Having experienced it themselves, and seeing it taught as an inherent part of the philosophy of the nursing department, staff members will be prepared and supported to grow in their ability to respond to ethical dilemmas in their own areas of practice.

■ BIOGRAPHICAL SKETCH

Patricia Snyder is Director, Professional Practice Development, at Glens Falls Hospital in Glens Falls, New York. She has served as nurse executive at two hospitals and has a clinical background in psychiatric nursing and a research interest in organizational development. Her doctoral work in nursing was com-

APPLICATION 1–1   *Continued*

pleted at George Mason University. She is active in the American Organization of Nurse Executives and is a member of several other professional associations.

Kahn, W. (1993). Caring for the caregivers: Patterns of organizational caregiving. *Administrative Science Quarterly, 38,* 539–563.

■ SUGGESTED READINGS

Christensen, P. (1988). An ethical framework for nursing service administration. *Advances in Nursing Science, 10* (3), 46–55.

Curtin, L. (1996). Ethics, discipline and discharge. *Nursing Management, 27* (3), 51–52.

■ REFERENCES

Brandt, M. (1994). Caring leadership: Secret path to success. *Nursing Management, 25* (8), 68–72.

Nyberg, J. (1993). Teaching caring to the nurse administrator. *Journal of Nursing Administration, 23* (1), 11–17.

2

The Health Policy Process and Nursing

Barbara K. Redman

America's nurses have long supported our nation's efforts to create a health care system that assures access, quality, and services at affordable costs.

—*Nursing's Agenda for Health Care Reform,* 1992, p.1

Health policy creates the context within which nursing must practice. Thus, the profession is both dependent on health policy and affects health policy by means of the services it delivers as well as by direct lobbying. Health policy in place at a particular time reflects the social contract for the nation's health between professionals and the public, including its governments.

Broadly speaking, policy decisions regulate behavior and determine the distribution of costs and benefits. At their base, policy questions are moral questions, frequently reflecting different views about equity—for instance, does it consist of equal treatment, equal access, or equal outcomes for various populations and individuals? In a democracy, public debate leading to a consensus is a necessary condition for policy development. Policy questions are often cast as economic issues, avoiding the moral questions because it is so difficult to get agreement on them.

This has clearly been true in health care, where the dominant pressure point for policy has been the financing of health services. Casting of the issues as economic is underscored by the commonly understood fact that the United States has by far the most expensive health care system in the world, but far from the best indicators of health status or outcomes from health services. Yet at the base of the health policy debate is the moral question of what we owe each other, especially the most disadvantaged among us, since a certain level of health is necessary to a reasonable chance to reach one's life goals.

This chapter is organized in four sections: professions and health policy; theory about how policy is made; the nature of cracks in the old health policy paradigm; and how the new health policy paradigm is forming. Case examples of the concepts and issues being discussed will be found in italics throughout the chapter. At the conclusion of the chapter, readers should be able to articulate a conception of policy and how it is formed and suggest ways in which the profession of nursing and individual nurses in patient care administration can develop policy that will support the mutual goals of the public and the profession. Many treatises already exist describing federal and state policy programs in health and especially analyzing the 1993–94 federal action toward health care reform (see suggested reading). This chapter will not repeat this material but will instead focus on development of conceptual skills for influencing policy. Examples are illustrative and not comprehensive.

▪ HEALTH POLICY AND THE PROFESSIONS

In addition to the obvious locus in legislative bodies, policy is also made by other authorities. These include courts, private organizations, and government agencies that create regulations to implement laws. The courts, in particular, make health policy about questions of constitutionality or administrative procedure. While relatively more immune to partisan politics, court decisions set precedents for future policy decisions and cannot so easily be changed. Private organizations influencing health policy in the United States, include the Joint Commission for Accreditation of Health Care Organizations (JCAHO), whose decisions about quality are accepted by the federal government as a basis for payment of Medicare and Medicaid funds.

Professions not only exist within the policy context for their field but play a greater or lesser role in creating the policy. Many observers would argue that health policy has largely been defined by the medical profession and that society has allowed it to do so by providing it with a legal monopoly. Many would also argue that the health care system now represents medical values and self interest taken to an extreme degree and that part of what the evolving paradigm of health care is all about is the public reclaiming its ability to define its health care system with its own values.

The evolution of the new paradigm is very important for nursing for two reasons. First, nursing's values represent those toward which the public wants to move—a focus on health, within a social context of family and community, with self-care as a part of everyday life being the dominant mode of caregiving and the role of health professionals being negotiated to fit within the patient's values. Second, nursing's ability to get its services to the public has been seriously thwarted by medicine's legal monopoly to define health and treat deviations from it.

Professions exist in a system in which jurisdictional boundaries between them are constantly changing and under dispute. Interprofessional competition is simply a fundamental fact of life that has shaped the history of each profession. Control of knowledge and its application means dominating outsiders who attack that control. Medicine continues to be the dominant health profession, and it has recently expanded its control into new areas such as substance abuse, mental illness, hyperactivity in children, obesity, and other conditions by using a claim of research-based expertise.

A profession's success in expanding its social mandate reflects as much the situation of its competitors and the system structure as it does the profession's own efforts. Jurisdictional claims are made in the legal system, in public opinion, and in the workplace. In America, it is ultimately through public opinion that professions establish the social power that enables them to achieve legal protection. Professional claims to jurisdiction develop over a period of a decade or more and, once granted, typically last for decades (Abbott, 1988).

Particularly at this time of dramatic change in the health care system, Abbott's (1988) notion of how professions fare rings very true. Nursing needs to accept competition and assertiveness within the political arena as useful tools in order to maintain and expand its mandate. Abbott emphasizes a dynamic of constant competition with other health professions, which should be viewed as healthy and not as noncollegial. In addition, a social mandate demands definition of distinct bodies of knowledge and specific services, along with documented improvement in health outcomes, to use in establishing a significant place in the new paradigm of health care that is evolving.

■ THEORY ABOUT HOW POLICY IS MADE

Although the policy sciences are relatively young, they provide important insights into the processes by which policy is made. Especially in our system of government, policy changes are usually incremental. This is the case for a number of reasons. Often, available information does not provide clarity about the effects and side effects of policy that would be radically different from the present. Since it is necessary to bargain and compromise in order to achieve political support for new initiatives, those who wish to retain the present policy mute those who want significant change. In addition, fundamental changes frequently undermine capitalist interests and benefits to current businesses, which in turn threaten political support for changes that would remove these benefits. There are usually significant sunk costs in the present policy apparatus that may not be retrievable under new policy. For all of these reasons, policy change is usually an amalgam of several approaches and occurs in small increments.

The assumption that a series of adjustments can be made in subsequent policy cycles to complete the move toward the original policy design is dependent on long-term continuance of the political will to do so. Policy windows of support for making certain changes present themselves and stay open only for short periods because leaders and their ideologies change, because other issues are either resolved or new issues capture the stage, and because more and more people recognize how costly a particular solution would be to them. As a result, initial incremental changes often are left in place without other originally intended changes. Thus, governmental policies frequently lack internal coherence and contain multiple partial changes from several policy designs.

Policy Process

One of the most basic ideas in policy theory is the policy process—the series of stages by which an issue is defined and placed on the agenda; options for its resolution are considered; and a policy is adopted, later implemented, and still later evaluated. Most issues are recycled when a past policy becomes unworkable and a new solution must be crafted and agreed upon. Although each stage is perilous—in that failures can put the issue on the back burner, where it languishes indefinitely—each also offers opportunity for influence.

Many issues are problematic but do not achieve sufficient public attention to be placed on a crowded agenda. A triggering event that grabs public attention may precipitate this step. How the issue is defined always has major import for its political standing and for the design of public solutions. The way a problem is defined invariably entails some statement about its origins, causality, culpability, and severity, including its incidence among certain population groups who are generally thought to be worthy of assistance (e.g., children or the frail elderly). Certain problems are defined very simply, specifying single causal agents; others include a variety of influences. Generally, narrowing the focus to just one or two causal factors is a signal that the agent defining the problem is ready for action; more complex formulations may represent a strategy to head off a prompt response. How strongly the severity label gets applied is pivotal to capturing the attention of public officials and the media (Rochefort & Cobb, 1994).

A decision about problem causality can construct the framework for understanding an issue. For example, the recent drug policy debate included three groups, those who defined this issue as a problem of criminality, as ill-conceived prohibitive legislation, or as a disease. Each position carried its own assumptions about why people use drugs, what the core of drug policy should be, and the consequences of policy failure (Rochefort & Cobb, 1994).

The struggle for ownership of a problem is a high stakes game because the group whose definition is accepted has an increased probability of seeing its solution accepted. One policy issue today that features an obvious unresolved struggle for problem ownership is homelessness. At least three major viewpoints have been expressed: that homelessness is a response to a housing shortage, that it represents an economic dislocation, and that it is a product of the deinstitutionalization of mental hospital patients. Each perspective has its well-organized advocates armed with study findings, who desire expanded public financing for services within their domains, be they affordable housing, economic development and job training, or expanded community mental health programs. Hard-pressed to decide which of these advocates will receive their primary attention, policy makers have often adopted an approach that spreads resources thinly among all the leading claimant groups, leading to an unfocused strategy (Rochefort & Cobb, 1994). At other times, such confusion may lead to inaction, with an issue languishing for years because the various stakeholders have differing views of what the issue is and of what options are acceptable.

Once an option is chosen, however, implementation should not be assumed. Implementation difficulties can result from lack of authority or capacity, lack of clarity in the original legislation, resistance from implementing agencies, competition among implementing agencies, lack of legislative oversight to assure that their intent is carried out, or any combination of the above.

Beatrice (1996) notes that implementation was never adequately addressed in the health care reform debate of 1993–94, especially the role that would have been required of the states. The states' role in health care has always been substantial. It has included protecting the public health and safety, providing health care services directly through state agencies and institutions, paying for health care services, licensing and training health care providers, and regulating providers and their activities in the health care marketplace. The massive reform options being considered might well have overwhelmed the operational capabilities of a number of states.

Although the absence of federal reform limits what states can accomplish, practically every state has made important changes in some part of their health care systems. Some states have developed purchase cooperatives to make care available and affordable to small businesses and uninsured individuals; some have expanded their Medicaid programs; many are using regulatory mechanisms to limit allowable insurance premium rate increases and setting rates for providers. Insurance market reforms have been implemented in dozens of states. States lack the financial resources, organizational capacity, and control over the health care system to implement comprehensive reform on their own. Even the states with the best track record on reform were only able to cover between one-fifth and one-third of the uninsured population through their reform efforts (Beatrice, 1996).

An excellent example of the policy process being played out at the state level may be found in Overman and Cahill's (1994) analysis of health data organizations (HDOs) in Colorado and Pennsylvania.

Information is essential to the success of the market-oriented health care policies that are presently being strongly pursued. Information on health costs and quality is collected and distributed by state governments through

HDOs to enhance competition and lower costs in the health industry and to improve consumer choice among alternatives. Also referred to as health care cost containment councils, HDOs were an innovation that swept through state governments in the middle and late 1980s. By 1993, 38 states had passed legislation creating HDOs, based on the premise that imperfect, inadequate, or nonexistent market information was at least partly to blame for a lack of competition and rising medical costs. Patient data, diagnosis, procedures, morbidity and mortality rates, discharge and financial information, and sometimes effectiveness and quality measures are collected, primarily from hospitals.

Analysis of the HDOs in Colorado and Pennsylvania showed that they were controlled by well-structured organizations or interest groups. HDOs were resisted by provider groups and their attempts to collect data thwarted. In Colorado, there were efforts to have the data provided by the hospital association and not by the state HDO. Yet the health industry saw HDOs as the least controlling of government policies and certainly as preferable to direct regulation of costs, profits, or services. In fact, the actual users of the information produced by HDOs have not been consumers but other players in the health industry (Overman & Cahill, 1994).

The policy lesson in this example is that HDOs became embedded in the same political and interest group politics that have marked the direct provision or regulation of health care in prior policy designs. In part, this was a problem in the drafting of the legislation and, in part, an implementation problem. Evaluation of the policy was equivocal, since rates of health care costs continued to rise. Perhaps the basic flaw was that the idea that drove the policy (that information would increase competitiveness), while not wrong, was incomplete. In addition, this example offers the lesson that information is always produced and interpreted by political and social institutions which, in this case, did not represent the public interest.

Other analysts describe the policy process in terms of learning, particularly within the context of an advocacy coalition or policy subsystem—those actors from a variety of public and private organizations, including researchers and journalists, who are actively concerned with a policy problem. The coalition shares a belief system—a set of basic values, causal assumptions, and problem perceptions. They share ideas, and have access to information, ideas, and positions outside the mainstream. Coalitions show coordinated activity over time as their ideas about what constitutes the problem and what to do about it change.

Learning occurs through dialogue and generally involves improving one's understanding of the state of important variables, or of logical and causal relationships. It may also involve crystallizing one's understanding of a position on the policy problem by responding to challenges to one's belief system (Bennett & Howlett, 1992; Sabatier, 1988). In order to inform others it is essential for players in the health policy field to have a body of research that supports their policy proposals or their proposal will frequently not be considered seriously.

The following example demonstrates how legislation originally proposed by a coalition (in this case, those with different "orphan diseases") to solve a problem later had unintended negative consequences for the same coalition.

The Orphan Drug Act, signed into law in 1983, was an attempt to stimulate development of drugs for rare diseases. It was based on the underlying assumption that orphan drugs were not profitable, so drug companies needed some protection or incentive to create them (Arno, Bonuck, & Davis, 1995). Drugs are "orphaned" because the potential market is considered too small and thus unprofitable to justify the research and development investment, because a product is not patentable, or because of liability concerns stemming from the nature of the target population (such as pregnant women or children). The Act provides 7 years of exclusive marketing rights to developers of organ drugs.

Certainly the Act can be viewed as a success if judged by the number of drugs designated as orphans. However, industry practices that serve to subvert the intent within the legal letter of the law, combined with extraordinary prices and larger sales generated as a result, have raised questions about need to amend the Act. One common industry practice is to apply for orphan drug designation for a narrow indication, knowing that a wide off-label market exists; less commonly, drug companies seek the designation for barely modified versions of existing orphans (Arno, Bonuck, & Davis, 1995).

In policy terms, Arno, Bonuck, and Davis's (1995) analysis questions the effectiveness of the Act as presently structured and also whether the marketing exclusivity incentive is needed. When Congress passed the Orphan Drug Act, the prospect that orphan drugs could become highly profitable was never seriously considered, so the Act presumes but does not require demonstration of limited profitability. Especially problematic is the fact that the government substantially participates in funding drug development, leading to a strong argument that the public deserves a return on its investment in the form of affordable drugs. Although policy options to alleviate these problems are available, these authors believe that the outcome of the 1994 congressional elections make substantial legislative change unlikely (Arno, Bonuck, & Davis, 1995).

Health policy is one domain of policy. Within this, as any domain, policies are often so closely interrelated that anyone intending to influence policy in one direction should always describe and analyze the interaction with other policies in the domain. Similarly, the consequences produced by one policy are increasingly likely to interfere with the working of other policies (Burstein, 1991). An example relating to health care is seen in the efforts to develop new programs to entice medical students to enter primary care. These efforts are undermined by the funding incentives for graduate medical education to hospitals through Medicare, which continue to make it more worthwhile for hospitals to train specialists.

All policies are developed using assumed causal relationships and effects that should follow from implementation of the policy. Policy-relevant research tests these relationships, either before the enactment of the policy or during evaluation of a policy that has been in place for awhile.

A third example of the policy process will demonstrate the potential repercussions stemming from a lack of knowledge of causal variables before a policy is enacted.

Welch, Wennberg, and Welch (1996) examined a key presumption under-girding Medicare's home health program. This program, which consists primarily of home visits by nurses and health aides, was conceived as a means to shorten length of stay in hospitals through transitional care. Because Medicare expenditures for home health care are growing exponentially, it is important to know whether the program is really a substitute for hospital costs. In 1980, the requirement that home visits be restricted to enrollees who had recently been hospitalized was eliminated, and home health began to be used more broadly. In the late 1980s, the Medicare manual for home health agencies was revised in response to litigation to ease restrictions on home care.

Using 1993 data from Medicare's National Claims History File, Welch, Wennberg, and Welch (1996) examined the temporal relationships between home visits and hospital discharge, as well as the number of months Medicare enrollees received home care. Seventy-eight percent of the visits either occurred more than a month after hospital discharge or were not associated with any inpatient care during the previous 6 months. Sixty-one percent of the visits were to enrollees who received home health care for 6 months or more. No evidence was found that home health care was substituted for hospital care, and there were dramatic geographical variations in use of these services. The authors conclude that home health visits are used primarily to provide long-term care and that there is a lack of consensus about their appropriate use. These results probably also reflect the impact of other policies, such as state Medicaid policy or nursing home and business practices (Welch, Wennberg, & Welch, 1996). These findings support the notion that this program is no longer being used for its original purpose and raise questions about how successful it is in reducing expenditures for other services.

■ CRACKS IN THE OLD PARADIGM

A single paradigm has guided U.S. health policy action for the last half century. It has assumed that health is determined primarily by the medical care provided. Very little weight has been given to the innumerable other factors known to contribute to health, including education, poverty, social well-being, and the environment. But despite advances in medical care, health outcomes are no longer improving, even with the application of a larger and larger percentage of the gross national product. The policy landscape is littered with examples of our efforts to improve health: both early attempts, which focused on health care delivery and improvement of access, as well as recent efforts, to improve health outcomes for specific populations and to change the mix of services to include more prevention. Once again, the United States and many other countries are at the point of what appears to be a major paradigm shift as they analyze the faults of the old paradigm and construct a new one.

The history of how the old paradigm formed is well documented for two of the major players—medicine (Starr, 1982) and hospitals (Stevens, 1989). In the world today, not all societies with scientifically advanced medical institutions have powerful medical professions. In the United States, however, physicians succeeded in shaping the basic organizational and financial structure of American medicine, hospitals, insurance, and other private institutions. They also succeeded in defining limits and proper forms of public health activities and other public investments in health care (Starr, 1982).

The growth of scientific knowledge made physicians more dependent on hospitals, which alone could afford the high costs of ever-more-sophisticated medical technology. Through this arrangement, technology was developed by research often paid for by public funds. It was then purchased by hospitals and made available to physicians free of charge in return for patient admissions without any restriction on physician fees to use the technology. In addition, the entire system of basic and specialty medical education, through which the knowledge and skills to use the technology were taught, became heavily subsidized by Medicare (public) funds. Similar public support was never extended to other health professions. All of this public aid to medicine did not, however, bring public control. Indeed, no coordinating authority among hospitals, public health, and medical practice was permitted to emerge because it would have threatened professional autonomy and control of the market (Starr, 1982).

The medical profession has actively sought licensing protection, some public health programs, public investment in hospitals, and research and use of state power to support the role of medicine in control of deviant behavior, as in involuntary confinement of the insane. All three of the major post–World War II health policy programs—medical research, the Veterans Administration system, and community hospital construction—showed a common pattern in respecting the sovereignty of the medical profession and local medical institutions. The concessions physicians and hospitals secured in the 1960s and 1970s for community mental health, Medicare, Medicaid and other public programs denied the government any leverage to control costs (Starr, 1982).

Economists have pinpointed the implementation of the Medicare program on July 1, 1966, and Medicaid on January 1, 1967, as the key dates after which Americans began outspending the rest of the world on health care. These two huge federal programs, without adequate controls, pumped so many resources into the U.S. health care system that it propelled forward the system's existing predisposition for a scientific and technological style of medicine (Drake, 1994).Thus, in order to gain the medical profession's acquiescence to passage of these programs, policy makers allowed physicians to dictate the conditions of their participation and to perpetuate and exaggerate the conditions already in existence in the private practice of medicine.

These conditions have continued, contributing considerably to the fiscal situation of health care today. A market dominated by any supplier group will soon reflect that group's wants and desires, not the consumer's. This was illustrated in the 1980s and 1990s when, despite the growing demand for expanded primary care services, the majority of newly graduated physicians continued to become specialists. Why? In part, because specialists have higher status and incomes than generalists. Whereas normally a labor market will work to reduce the earnings of categories of workers that are in excess supply, the health care market has not imposed such penalties on the oversupply of physician specialists. Why? Again, a partial answer is found in the continued proliferation of educational programs designed to turn out specialists. As noted earlier, these programs are subsidized by public funds; their students also provide an inexpensive labor pool to hospitals (Drake, 1994).

Indeed, there is historical evidence that the consumer's health care needs have never been well matched to the services the medical profession provided. By 1920, the assumption that the root problems impeding improvement of the public's health were, and would remain, the conquest of infection and treatment of acute, end stages of chronic illness was not accurate. In fact, moderate disability from chronic illness was more prevalent than infection or acute conditions even in 1920. This focus of medical care has meant that patients primarily receive care for chronic illnesses in their acute and end stages and not at other phases of their illnesses (Fox, 1993).

Patient education, symptom management, rehabilitation, and accommodation of homes and workplaces to the functional limitations of persons with disabling conditions have always received lower priority. Addressing these issues would require a very different distribution of the resources currently spent for health services. Most Americans have paid the costs of managing their own and their dependents' chronic illnesses out of current income, savings, and from uncompensated work of wives, mothers, and sisters. Rehabilitation and disability policy has never been effectively linked to health policy and has continued to have lower prestige (Fox, 1993).

This paradigm for health policy decision making, which remained in place for the 50 years between the 1920s and the late 1960s meant that the values and preferences of physicians determined what services were available and how health care was organized. Today, the transformation remains incomplete. In essence, what we have done in the name of public policy is to ration professional assistance in rehabilitation, clinical preventive and symptom management services, long-term care, and personal assistance with activities of daily living. We have done this by leaving much of the need for these services uncovered in public and private health insurance and by not giving these services priorities in subsidies for facilities, professional education, and research (Fox, 1993).

Such rationing has, in a sense, been unplanned rather than a deliberate result of health policy because decision makers assumed that decreasing expenditures for acute care services would leave people without emergency care when needed. Ironically, the services that were rationed were the very ones that could have prevented many emergencies and enhanced the independence and productivity of significant numbers of the population (Fox, 1993). It must be added that the excluded services were also those at which nursing is expert, thus reducing demand and, often equitable payment, for nursing services and nurses.

Stevens (1989) notes that hospitals, another major institution, have rarely tried to change the system in ways that would benefit the public, for instance, by inclusion of long-term care. Further, they have been dominated by physicians throughout most of this century.

The making of American national health policy has never been centralized, as it is in many other nations. Rather, it has been the result of negotiated consensus among shifting coalitions dominated by medicine and hospitals. Although centralized systems may also show favoritism toward particular groups, critics have concluded that our system of making policy contributed to the continuance of strong domination by medicine to the detriment of the public welfare.

Advanced Practice Nursing in the Old Paradigm

The recent history of advanced practice nursing provides an example of the impediments nursing has faced in the old paradigm. The historical pattern of medical dominance has been demonstrated most recently in the limiting of legal authority for advanced practice nurses (Safriet, 1992). Advanced practice nurses (APNs) have increased the public's access to basic health services in a wide variety of geographical and practice settings. In many rural and inner-city areas, they are the only providers available. Physician training costs are four to five times those for nurse practitioners (NPs), clinical specialists (CSs), nurse anesthetists (CRNAs) and certified nurse midwives (CNMs). Primary care physicians earn on average four times more than do NPs and CNMs, in part because of overvaluation of physician's services, which has resulted from their state-sanctioned monopoly and from the historically unregulated fee-for-service basis of their compensation.

Barriers to effective utilization of APNs include restrictive state provisions governing the scope of their practice and prescriptive authority. Safriet (1992) notes that any state that requires APN supervision by a physician has yielded its governmental power to one private individual (the supervising physician). It is a strange regulatory twist that prevents many APNs from getting paid directly as is the case with Medicaid, Medicare, and many state laws (they are paid through the physician). In addition, APNs frequently get paid less because of the type of provider they are, not related to the quality of the service they render. The restrictions on APN practice have more to do with protecting the competitive position of physicians than with the public health, and the barriers that have been erected create a legalized monopoly. This pattern should not be surprising.

Even in the face of long-standing problems of access that have not been ameliorated by various physician-oriented public policies, federal programs have often not been amended to directly reimburse APNs or other nonphysician providers. The nature of these practice restrictions, which tie NPs to physicians, make it difficult for nurses to settle in areas in which there is a shortage of physicians—the very areas where they could fill a need by providing access for an underserved public (Aiken & Salmon, 1994).

Other Health Issues in the Old Paradigm

The limitations of the medical paradigm can also be illustrated by looking at present policy on care of the aging (Estes, 1993). The dominant view, as reflected in public policy, is that the aged are a problem to society and that the aging process is one of biological, physiological, and cognitive decline and decay. In this view, old age is portrayed as a medical problem that can be alleviated through medical science. Physicians are placed in charge of the definition and treatment of old age as a disease. Consistent with this view, public policy supports the provision of individual acute care services and not of long-term and self-care services.

Probably the most disturbing construction of aging in the past decade is the contention that the nation's economic problems are caused by the elderly, causing the inevitability of rationing and intergenerational war. Estes (1993) notes that the present medical, national policy approach has supported the sustained development of a huge and highly profitable, largely private but substantially publicly funded, enterprise of largely medical facilities and services. The new paradigm should focus on aging within its social context and seek to ameliorate the as yet undetermined, but significant, amount of dependency which is preventable, modifiable, or reversible. Clearly, such an approach would require a change in social policies as well as a shift from the present treatment of functional debility and chronic illness with acute medical care to rehabilitation and policies to support family caregiving (Estes, 1993).

■ HOW THE NEW PARADIGM IS FORMING

A number of very basic assumptions of the old paradigm are changing dramatically, including the domination of treatment decision making by providers, the evaluation of care based on the values and preferences of providers, and the alignment of health care services to fit the beliefs and preferences of providers.

An ongoing example of the changed values undergirding the new paradigm are a series of political movements representing the interests of groups who believe that they have been ignored and/or mistreated under the old paradigm. These include the patient autonomy and women's movements.

Patient autonomy is one issue that deserves the support of nurses. The trend toward patient autonomy has been evolving since the 1960s, when informed consent really emerged as the legal and ethical embodiment of the new order. It is further evolving through such mechanisms as the Patient Self Determination Act and countless decisions by patients and their surrogates to limit care or to seek access to alternative health care they believe to be beneficial. The movement for patient autonomy becomes even more important in an era when the lack of knowledge of outcomes of care prescribed by physicians has become clear as has documentation of the phenomenon of supplier-induced demand.

The women's movement is now global. It focuses on reproductive self-determination including the right to sexual autonomy; safe, family centered, childbearing; increased resources for research and treatment of diseases that primarily affect women; affordable, effective, and humane health care; satisfaction of basic needs; a safe workplace; and freedom from violence. Hazards of some medical techniques and a fight for greater participation in reproductive research and development are a part of the movement's agenda.

At the heart of all feminist critiques of medicine is the recognition that women still lack power in defining health, the health professions, and health care institutions. Feminists identify misogynous implications in the sexual politics that are embedded in the conception of sickness and beliefs about appropriate care (Doyal, 1996). Recently, however, the women's movement has shown power in a number of new health policies, whose history is outlined below, including a women's health research agenda to correct a lack of funding for research on women's diseases, in the creation of available services for birthing, and in policy approaches to fetal abuse.

The policy origins of the current women's health research movement can be traced to a report on women's health issues by the Public Health Service in 1985. This document provided the "proof" in the form of a legitimate scientific report, that women's health activists, scientists, and members of Congress needed to push for further reform. In 1990 the Society for the Advancement of Women's Health Research was established by influential women in the health sciences to pursue a consensus research agenda for women's health and a media campaign to increase awareness of the problem. Much leadership came from the Congressional Caucus for Women's Issues, and from friends. A Government Accounting Office study revealed that the National Institutes of Health (NIH) did not have a system for monitoring its own policy about the number of funded studies involving male subjects only. In response, the 1992 NIH Revitalization Amendments permanently authorized the Office of Research on Women's Health at NIH (Auerbach & Figert, 1995).

The women's movement has also stimulated policy on provision of birthing services. With the closing of full-service hospitals, access to birthing services in many rural areas has become problematic. When the New York State Assembly addressed this issue, the policy options that were available to it reflected the influence of the women's movement. Three policy options were considered: promoting home births (for which there was judged to be low consumer and provider acceptance); reactivation of full-service obstetrical units at primary care hospitals (other attempts had not attracted sufficient volume); and freestanding birth centers. The state chose to implement a free-standing birthing service model. Legislation passed in 1994 allowed a network of rural providers to be licensed as a Central Service Facility governed by a community and provider board of trustees. A new category of hospital license, the primary care hospital, was codified to allow small rural hospitals that could no longer financially support full hospital services to be birthing centers. The model used in Western Europe, where 70 percent of births are attended by midwives with excellent outcomes, has encountered many barriers to implementation, including fierce medical resistance (Rosenthal, Ferrara, & Hesler, 1996).

A well-articulated example of the kind of gender bias that the women's movement addresses, may be found in the current debates about fetal abuse. The development of fetal abuse as a policy issue reflects a patriarchal stance, defining it as an issue that arises from negligence on the part of women. This very biased definition of the issue ignores the adverse birth outcomes caused by male behaviors such as battering and male substance abuse; it also ignores the consequences of societal conditions of poverty, which are more common to women. Instead, it assumes that mothers are primarily responsible for children. Such blaming of women without reference to any other causes was widely played out in the media during the ensuing policy debate, and supported as well by the medical and legal professions and the scientific community. The causal story fitted the historic gender biases of the institutions framing the problem (Schroedel & Peretz, 1994). Until and unless the issue is reframed with pressure from the women's movement, policy options will be limited and punitive to women.

Issues to be Addressed in the New Paradigm

A number of issues important to construction of the new paradigm remain unresolved. Perhaps the most basic is the ambivalence of a society that has never decided which of its citizens deserve access to health care in a formal way.

Related to this moral ambivalence is lack of clarity about the degree to which health care can be managed as a free market. In its purest form, a free market is based on the values of utilitarianism and concerned only about efficiency. Serious market failures are known to occur in health care. For example, an unregulated private insurance market suffers from adverse selection by consumers and risk selection by insurance companies, leaving no insurance coverage for the poor, the aged, and the disabled, and excess profit for the insurance companies. Certain states have required insurance plans to offer open enrollment periods and to charge a uniform premium rate (community rating), and federal legislation has recently been enacted. Past regulation of this issue has generally been ineffective because it can be circumvented by companies that use subtle methods to screen out high-risk individuals.

International experience with correcting market failures in clinical service markets includes price regulation and control of supply of the number of physicians and hospital beds. Price regulation of fees can be circumvented by providers who increase the volume of services by inducing demand. Global budgeting and capitation payment methods seem to be more effective means for price regulation. Alternatives designed to limit physician supply and hospital beds are now being considered. Certificate of need for expansion of hospital beds has had some limited success.

Ultimately, decisions about the structure of the health care sector rest on the social values a nation embraces—tradeoffs between equity, efficiency, and control of health costs. Centrally controlled health systems, such as Great Britain's, are introducing market forces and developing internal markets. All systems are struggling to achieve a useful balance between a free market and a centrally planned and regulated system (Hsiao, 1995).

Perhaps the largest threat to the construction of nursing practice in the new paradigm is the cavalier way in which its basic resource—its knowledge and human resources—are used. A recent Institute of Medicine (IOM) study undertaken to answer this very question found considerable literature devoted to the impact of registered nurses on hospital mortality rates, but a serious paucity of recent research on the definitive effects of structural measures, such as specific staffing ratios, on the quality of care when controlling for all other likely explanatory or confounding variables. The IOM panel conducting the study was shocked by the lack of current data relating to the status of hospital quality of care on a national basis, apart from information on indicators such as hospital-specific mortality rates. This vacuum meant that the committee was unable to draw any definitive conclusions or inferences about the relationship of nurse staffing to levels of quality of care (Wunderlich, Sloan, & Davis, 1996).

A subissue of this larger discussion is the appropriate use of unlicensed assistive personnel (UAPs). Despite the paucity of empirical evidence to determine the effect of increased numbers and types of UAPs on quality of care, patient satisfaction, cost, and efficiency, they appear to be used in greater proportions. A look at the research base shows that studies were frequently anecdotal in nature, conducted at a single institution, lacked comparison groups, and used instruments of untested reliability and validity, with small sample sizes. Yet untested delivery models incorporating UAPs are quickly taking shape without evidence to predict the effects on quality of patient care, patient and nurse satisfaction, and costs or productivity (Krapohl & Larson, 1996).

The use of UAPs is essentially an unregulated activity, since within broad limits employers are free to construct the staff mix for nursing services as they wish. It is an area in which positive effects from potential regulation (assurance of a certain level of nursing staff) could also have negative effects (use of these levels as a license to staff only to that level and eliminate any richer mixes). In the absence of a research base, policy makers are very reticent to challenge present practices. Therefore, a de facto policy develops as many institutions change their practices, and yet provider institutions are not required to monitor the effects of this change. In an era in which evidence-based medicine is increasingly necessary to justify payment for services, institutional policy should be required to meet at least as high a standard.

In general, health policy has not focused on conditions necessary for the population to access nursing care. It has remained caught within the medical model, considering questions about nursing to be subsidiary or not relevant to public policy, but rather confined to institutional practice. The task facing nursing in the new paradigm is to build on the public's move toward values more congruent with the nursing than with the medical model, demonstrating that nursing has the knowledge base to define causal models and develop services to alleviate patient and social problems.

The various policy examples described throughout this chapter profoundly affect services that patients can obtain and that nurses can provide. We are left to wonder, how would nursing have addressed these policy issues—their definition, the options available, their implementation, and the criteria by which their success would have been judged?

■ SUMMARY

Since policy creates the context for practice, it is essential that any profession be well positioned to define and influence policy that allows and facilitates delivery of its services to the public. Nurses who are patient care administrators have a special interest in the policies—such as nurse practice acts, laws governing insurance payments, and regulations affecting the services, monopolies, or other business controls—shaping organizations that deliver health services.

In the health sphere, medicine has clearly dominated and set the agenda throughout this century. Elements of this old paradigm are now being seriously challenged, and a new paradigm is evolving. Nursing must act in partnership and coalition with others in order to move the new paradigm to the forefront. The new paradigm champions efficiency but also challenges professional dominance over patient and health system definitions of the good. Still unresolved is a clear societal goal concerning the level of health of individuals. Within nursing, basic questions remain about how its workforce should be constituted and used. These questions need to be addressed in the context of nursing services with patients, their families, and communities; our future role in the promotion of self-caregiving; and the alignment of nursing's values with societal values and goals concerning health.

▪ BIOGRAPHICAL SKETCH

Barbara K. Redman received her BSN from South Dakota State University and her MEd in Nursing Education and PhD in Education from the University of Minnesota. She has held academic administrative positions in nursing at the University of Minnesota and University of Colorado and has also been a professor at both the University of Maryland and Johns Hopkins University. She has been a Scholar in Patient Education at the Veterans Administration and a fellow at Johns Hopkins University in health education, at Georgetown University in bioethics, and at Harvard University in medical ethics. Her scholarly areas of expertise are patient education and ethics. As Executive Director of the American Association of Colleges of Nursing and the American Nurses Association, she provided leadership in health policy issues of interest to the nursing profession. She has received honorary doctorates from Georgetown University and the University of Colorado. She is currently Dean and Professor at the University of Connecticut School of Nursing.

▪ SUGGESTED READINGS

Aiken, L.H., & Salmon, M.E. (1994). Health care workforce priorities: What nursing should do now. *Inquiry, 31,* 318–329. This is an excellent synthesis of what is known about the nursing workforce and how it is affected by employer actions on utilization of nurses, as well as by public policy.

Johnson, H., & Broder, D.S. (1996). *The system.* Boston: Little, Brown & Co. Written by political journalists, this book provides a detailed account of the 1994 effort at federal health care reform. It reveals the political motivations of various actors, as well as political and policy mistakes that contributed to the failed effort.

Ramsay, C. (Ed.). (1995). *U.S. health policy group.* Westport, CT: Greenwood Press. The book offers a good opportunity to understand the range of groups involved in health policy and their perspectives.

Safriet, B.J. (1992). Health care dollars and regulatory sense: The role of advanced practice nursing. *Yale Journal of Regulation, 9,* 417–488. Although recently published, Safriet's analysis of the policy barriers to advanced practice in nursing is already a classic.

▪ REFERENCES

Abbott, A. (1988). *The system of professions.* Chicago: University of Chicago Press.

Aiken, L.H., & Salmon, M.E. (1994). Health care workforce priorities: What nursing should do now. *Inquiry, 31,* 318–329.

American Nurses Association (1992). Nursing's agenda for health care reform. Washington, DC: Author.

Arno, P.S., Bonuck, K., & Davis, M. (1995). Rare diseases, drug development, and AIDS: The impact of the Orphan Drug Act. *The Milbank Quarterly, 73,* 231–251.

Auerbach, J.D., & Figert, A.E. (1995). Women's health research: Public policy and sociology. *Journal of Health and Social Behavior,* extra issue, 115–131.

Beatrice, D.F. (1996). States and health care reform: The importance of program implementation. In S.H. Altman & U.E. Reinhardt (Eds.), *Strategic choices for a changing health care system*. Chicago: Health Administration Press.

Bennett, C.J., & Howlett, M. (1992). The lessons of learning: Reconciling theories of policy learning and policy change. *Policy Sciences, 25,* 275–294.

Burstein, P. (1991). Policy domains: Organization, culture, and policy outcomes. *Annual Review of Sociology, 17,* 327–350.

Doyal, L. (1996). The politics of women's health: Setting a global agenda. *International Journal of Health Services, 26,* 47–765.

Drake, D.F. (1994). *Reforming the health care market: An interpretive economic history*. Washington, DC: Georgetown University Press.

Estes, C.L. (1993). The aging enterprise revisited. *The Gerontologist, 33,* 292–298.

Fox, D.M. (1993). *Power and illness*. Berkeley, CA: University of California Press.

Hsiao, W.C. (1995). Abnormal economics in the health sector. *Health Policy, 32,* 125–139.

Krapohl, G.L., & Larson, E. (1996). The impact of unlicensed assistive personnel on nursing care delivery. *Nursing Economics, 14,* 99–110.

Overman, E.S., & Cahill, A.G. (1994). Information, market government, and health policy: A study of health data organizations in the states. *Journal of Policy Analysis and Management, 13,* 435–453.

Rochefort, D.A., & Cobb, R.W. (1994). Problem definition: An emerging perspective. In D.A. Rochefort & R.W. Cobb (Eds.), *The politics of problem definition: Shaping the policy agenda*. Lawrence, KS: University Press of Kansas.

Rosenthal, T.C., Ferrara, E., & Hesler, E. (1996). Providing birthing services in rural health networks: Coping with change in New York State. *The Journal of Rural Health, 12,* 137–145.

Sabatier, P.A. (1988). An advocacy coalition framework of policy change and the role of policy-oriented learning therein. *Policy Sciences, 21,* 129–168.

Safriet, B.J. (1992). Health care dollars and regulatory sense: The role of advanced practice nursing. *Yale Journal on Regulation, 9,* 417–488.

Schroedel, J.R., & Peretz, P. (1994). A gender analysis of policy formation: The case of fetal abuse. *Journal of Health Politics, Policy and Law, 19,* 335–360.

Starr, P. (1982). *The social transformation of American medicine*. New York: Basic Books.

Stevens, R. (1989). *In sickness and in wealth: American hospitals in the twentieth century*. New York: Basic Books.

Welch, H.G., Wennberg, D.E., & Welch, W.P. (1996). The use of Medicare home health care services. *New England Journal of Medicine, 335,* 324–329.

Wunderlich, G., Sloan, F., & Davis, C. (Eds.). (1996). *Nursing staff in hospitals and nursing homes*. Washington, DC: National Academy Press.

APPLICATION 2–1   A Voice in the Wilderness: What Can I Do?

Nancy J. Sharp

Remember when you were young and your teachers asked you what you did on your vacation? Being a truthful little kid you would answer "nothing" and hope the teacher would go away.

Well, now you're an adult and a professional nurse—and I am asking, "What did you do over your vacation?" Your answer to me should be, "I met with Members of Congress (two Senators and one Representative) to describe the community's health care needs as I saw them and to tell them what nurses can do to meet those needs. Moreover, I asked my Members of Congress to help nurses find federal funding for a project designed to meet unmet health needs in the community through very cost-effective health services, using a wide array of health care professionals, including nurses in advanced practice."

■ EDUCATING YOUR COMMUNITY

Meeting with your Members of Congress should be *only one of the steps* in your strategic education plan to inform about and solicit support from community leaders for nursing's intentions to provide health care services in the community. There is a great deal of "WORK" to be done preparing for this challenge.

This material is adapted from an article that appeared in *Nursing Management, 25* (2), 29, 31, December 1994. Reprinted with permission from the December 1994 issue of Nursing Management, © Springhouse Corporation.

■ AND, WHAT EXACTLY IS THE WORK?

The work consists of *educating* everyone—your friends and family, your co-workers and neighbors, your child's teachers, your minister, priest, or rabbi, your local, state, and federal legislators—about what a nurse, particularly an advanced practice nurse (APN) is, and does. APN is a generic, umbrella term used for nurse practitioners (NPs), certified nurse midwives (CNMs), certified registered nurse anesthetists (CRNAs), and clinical nurse specialists (CNSs).

Describe the nurse and the nursing care provided by nurses. Use different examples to describe the various APNs' relationships with physicians in the various health care settings. Do not use nursing rhetoric or jargon; use common, plain, everyday English to describe the APNs and patient care situations.

■ ESPECIALLY, LEGISLATORS

Write or visit your legislators several times a year, so they become familiar with your name and face. Visit when they are home in the district. Invite them to your facility; ask them to give a speech; give them an award if they have done something good for your facility. Talk to them straight about the health care needs of the citizens in the home district—the poor, the elderly, the women and children, the minority populations. Be honest. Tell it like it is. Tell them about patients who need

APPLICATION 2–1 *Continued*

basic primary care and why they are not getting it.

Tell them what nurses in advanced practice could provide for these populations that no one else is providing. Describe what an ob/gyn nurse practitioner provides in a Medicaid women's health clinic. Describe what a psych/mental health clinical specialist provides in outpatient counseling. Describe what a nurse practitioner does in a migrant-worker rural health clinic. Describe what a certified nurse midwife provides in a birthing center.

■ BESIDES EDUCATING, WHAT CAN I DO?

A long list follows, and it is divided into several categories. It is important that you realize that you will have to take the initiative. No one can read your mind to tell if you are ready to get involved in advocacy activity, and no free information will come to you in your mailbox if you are not a dues-paying member of some nursing or public health association.

■ FIRST, LEARN TO NETWORK

- *Develop a core group of professional colleagues* with whom you share professional information. When you hear news of some aspect of health care reform that will have an impact on your nursing specialty, call others together over a cup of coffee to explore how you, your patients, and your colleagues will be affected.

- *Join a network group.* In Washington, D.C., we have a "Nurse in Washington Roundtable," which is a periodic dinner meeting with a Congressional or Administration speaker. For those of us who already are involved in networking, it does not matter who the speaker is or what we eat—the most important activity for the evening is networking with professional colleagues.

- *The Nurse's Directory of Capitol Connections* (Sharp Legislative Resources, 1997) is a networking directory listing over 500 nurses in health policy positions in the Washington, D.C., area and nationwide federal agencies. Use this directory to find a nurse in a department of the government that interests you. Call the nurse: inquire about the work, opportunities for internships, grant money available, and so on. Invite the nurse to lunch to get acquainted. The network grows. Call (301) 469-4997 for information.

■ SECOND, JOIN NURSING ORGANIZATIONS

- *The ideal* would be to join both your state nurses' association, which is part of the American Nurses Association, and your clinical nursing specialty association. There are numerous opportunities available for continuing education programs, journals and newslet-

APPLICATION 2–1   *Continued*

ters, updated standards of practice, liability insurance, and other benefits.

- *Volunteer to serve on the legislative committee*—either to learn the basics or to help guide the group in setting the agenda. When the group is going to the State Capitol, volunteer to drive; pick up the shy, timid folks; let them follow you around to see how you approach legislators, how you talk to them, what you tell them about nurses' work. When there is literature to distribute, testimony to write, testimony to present, or hearings to attend—again, *volunteer*.

■ THIRD, WRITE LETTERS TO THE EDITOR

- *Write to the editor* when you read something about a health care issue with which you either agree or disagree. State clearly that you are a nurse—"I am a nurse working in/at/for. . . . In response to your article on. . . . I believe. . . ." Sign your name with RN and whatever credentials you have.
- *Write editors* of newspapers, journals and newsletters, TV, and radio stations.

■ FOURTH, ATTEND PUBLIC POLICY WORKSHOPS

- *Attend* Lobby Day at the State Capitol when it is sponsored by nursing groups.

- *Attend* Lobby Days sponsored by other groups, such as the League of Women Voters, the parent teachers associations (PTAs), the American Association of Retired Persons (AARP), and other consumer groups in your hometown.
- *Attend* legislative workshops sponsored by Congressional Quarterly and the American Society of Association Executives in Washington, D.C.
- *Attend* public policy workshops sponsored by nursing associations, at both the state and national level.

■ FIFTH, ATTEND HEARINGS IN WASHINGTON, D.C., OR YOUR STATE CAPITOL

- *Here in Washington, D.C., it is so easy!* First, you buy the *Washington Post* and check the schedule in the box titled "Today in Congress," usually found around page A-4 or A-5. Then, hop on the METRO, the commuter rail system. Get off at the Union Station stop if you are going to a Senate hearing, or the Capitol South stop if you are going to a hearing on the House side. Find the right building, go through security, find the room, walk in, and sit down.
- *Observe the process.* See which Members of Congress are in attendance, who the witnesses testifying are, and who else is there observing. Observe the role of staff

APPLICATION 2–1 *Continued*

and the role of the leadership; note who is deferential to whom, and who is hostile to whom. Jot down what questions are asked, and what the body language says, too. Nurses are excellent observers because it is what we do each and every day—observe reactions to procedures, to good and bad news, to stress, and so on. There may be extra copies of the testimony on the press table for observers. If so, help yourself. Finally, if you and your nursing association colleague feel you should respond to the issue, the Congressional Record is open for 10 working days following a hearing. You can submit written testimony during that period. Introduce yourself to others sitting around you. They have interests similar to yours if they are attending this hearing.

■ FINALLY, READ!

- *Read* at least one national newspaper per day: *New York Times, Washington Post, Los Angeles Times.*
- Read legislative columns in: *Nursing Management, Nursing Economics, Nursing and Health Care, American Journal of Nursing.*
- Read legislative newsletters: *Legislative Network for Nurses, Capital Update, Medicine and Health, The American Nurse,* plus so many others. Check your library's political section.

■ SUGGESTED READINGS

Aiken, L., & Fagin, C. (1992). *Charting nursing's future. Agenda for the 1990s.* Philadelphia: Lippincott.

Auberdene, P., & Naisbett, J. (1992). *Megatrends for women.* New York: Villard.

deVries, C., & Vanderbilt, M. (1992). *The grassroots lobbying handbook: Empowering nurses through legislative and political action.* Washington, DC: American Nurses Association.

Feldstein, P. (1988). *The politics of health legislation.* Ann Arbor, MI: Health Administration Press Perspectives.

Goldwater, M., & Zusy, MJL. (1990). *Prescription for nurses effective political action.* St. Louis: Mosby.

Halvorson, G. (1994). *Strong medicine.* New York: Random House.

Harrington, C., & Estes, C.L. (1994). *Health policy and nursing crisis and reform in the US health care delivery system.* Boston: Jones & Bartlett.

Kalisch, B., & Kalisch, P. (1982). *The politics of nursing.* Philadelphia: Lippincott.

Kallowes, P. (Ed.). (1993). *Getting involved in health policy: A guide to action.* Aliso Viejo, CA: American Association of Critical Care Publications.

Mason, D., Talbott, S., & Leavitt, J. (1993). *Policy and politics for nurses: Action and change in the workplace, government, organizations and community.* Philadelphia: Lippincott.

O'Neill, T. (1994). *All politics is local.* New York: Random House.

Pick, M. (1993). *How to save your neighborhood, city or town.* San Francisco, CA: Sierra Club Books.

Redman, E. (1993). *The dance of legislation.* New York: Simon & Schuster.

Shames, K.H. (1993). *The Nightingale conspiracy: Nursing comes to power in the 21st century.* Montclair, NJ.: Enlightenment Press.

APPLICATION 2–1   *Continued*

Sharp, N. (1997). *The nurse's directory of Capitol connections* (4th ed.). Bethesda, MD: Sharp Legislative Resources.

Smith, H. (1989). *The power game*. New York: Ballantine Books.

Staff, P. (1994). *The logic of health reform*. New York: Penguin Books.

Satir, P. (1982). *The transformation of American medicine*. New York: Basic Books.

CASE 2–1 It's Politics, Not Policy . . . People!

Nancy J. Sharp

As the first session of the 104th Congress drew to an end, in the fall of 1995, we watched Senate and House Republican leaders conduct intense negotiations with recalcitrant Members of Congress over Medicare and Medicaid reforms. The historic budget and tax cut package created by this Congress would have major effects on the health care system. For weeks, speculation raged over whether the GOP-controlled Congress and the Clinton administration were headed for a "train wreck" over budget and tax priorities. In October 1995, House of Representatives' Speaker Newt Gingrich (R-GA) threatened to dump most of FY 96's budget in the President's lap on a take-it-or-leave-it basis. The following case explores the ways in which politics shaped policy in this debate over Medicare and Medicaid reform.

■ THE POLITICAL PROCESS IS NOT THE POLICY PROCESS

Faced with an impasse when moderate Republicans threatened to delay budget action in the Senate, Majority Leader Robert J. Dole (R-KS) and other GOP leaders agreed to a compromise that would preserve guaranteed coverage for

This material is adapted from an article that appeared in *Nursing Management, 26* (12), 18–19, 1995. Reprinted with permission from the 1995 issue of *Nursing Management,* © Springhouse Corporation.

the disabled. That provision had been added in a Senate Finance Committee to legislation overhauling Medicaid and Medicare as a concession to Senator John Chafee (R-RI), a moderate who had threatened to block the bill in Committee. But Dole and other committee Republicans sought informally to delete the provision after 24 Republican governors protested that it would saddle them with a new unfunded mandate.

As part of the compromise worked out in Dole's office, however, states would be allowed to define the disabilities that would qualify for coverage under Medicaid. "Now we'll see a battle in every state over who is covered," said Martha E. Ford of The Arc, a national advocate for the mentally challenged (Personal Communication, Oct. 1995). Every state legislature would be the next battleground for all persons concerned with health care issues.

■ AND THE AMA WINS AGAIN

In a major political coup for the Republicans, the American Medical Association (AMA) endorsed the Republican Medicare bill at a meeting in the Speaker's office, after Gingrich promised to work with the AMA to reduce proposed cuts in physician fees under Medicare. The powerful AMA had long praised the general structure of the Republican bill, but bitterly complained that formulas already in law and not fully corrected in this bill

CASE 2–1   *Continued*

would sharply reduce physician fees and discourage physicians from treating Medicare patients.

At a press conference the morning following the AMA endorsement, reporters asked whether physicians would get more in reimbursement than in the original version of the bill and Gingrich's aide Ed Kutler answered, "Yes." Kirk Johnson, AMA's general counsel, stated that physicians could end up getting "billions" more in payments. Kutler said the change likely would not be made until the bill was sent to the floor (Plainin & Devroy, 1995, p. A11).

The next day it was reported that AMA officials said Gingrich had agreed to changes that would avoid "billions" in fee reductions for physicians over the next 7 years, sparking Democratic charges of closed-door dealmaking. "The AMA took Gingrich's bribe of $3 billion to support a bill that rations health care for seniors," charged Rep. Portney "Pete" Star, (D-GA) (Rich & Planin, 1995, p. A6).

Republicans, rushing to control the damage from the October 11 statement, said that the changes in fees were justified and would be far less, more like $300 million to $400 million over 7 years, according to Rep. Bill Thomas (R-CA), Chair of the Ways and Means Medicare subcommittee. Finally, later that same day, AMA general counsel Kirk Johnson, who had used the term "billions" said, "There was no number agreed upon by the Speaker, only an assurance that absolute reductions in fees would be avoided. The existing House and Senate bills already corrected a significant part of the problem that in-

volved most of the 'billions' that were mentioned" (Rich & Planin, 1995, p. A6).

Finally, Spencer Rich reported in the *Washington Post* that there were clear winners on this Medicare deal. Physicians represented by the AMA, American Society of Internal Medicine (ASIM), and other groups appeared to have gained the longest list of new benefits. He went on to report that the private health insurance industry was also a big winner because insurers would be able to collect tens of billions of dollars in new premiums by selling policies to Medicare recipients. Rep. Bill Archer (R-TX), Chair of the House Ways and Means Committee, stated, "The policy changes made in our bill are good for all who depend on Medicare. The improve doctor–patient relationships and they are vital parts of improving health care delivery for all Americans" (Rich, 1995, p. A12).

■ THE "GOOD GUYS IN THE WHITE HATS" PROTEST

The American Nurses Association (ANA), the American College of Physicians (ACP), and the National Association of Public Hospitals (NAPH) came out in opposition to the Republican plans to cut Medicare and Medicaid. At their joint press conference, the groups stated that in weighing all of the elements of this bill, they believed the total package would be harmful to patients, nurses, physicians, hospitals, and the entire health care system.

Additionally, in a nationwide conference call that week, the ANA hosted a 50-person call with representatives from

CASE 2–1   *Continued*

ANA's Nursing Organization Liaison Forum (NOLF), ANA's Affiliate Organizations, and ANA's Lobbying Contracts to review the status of the pending Medicare legislation. All nursing organizational representatives on that conference call agreed to stand united in opposition to the Medicare cuts.

■ THE TALLY FOR ADVANCED PRACTICE NURSES

Antidiscrimination Language in Managed Care Plans

One little piece of the legislative action that had been pitched to the nursing advanced practice groups—the nurse practitioners (NPs), certified nurse midwives (CNMs), certified registered nurse anesthetists (CRNAs) and clinical nurse specialists (CNSs)—passed 25 to 24 at the House Commerce Committee's mark-up. That was Rep. Sherrod Brown's (D-OH) antidiscrimination amendment. This amendment prohibited discrimination against advanced practice nurses and other health professionals such as psychologists, occupational therapists, physical therapists, and others who are part of the "Advocates for Practitioner Equity Coalition" (APEC) fighting for provider status in the managed care environment. Unfortunately, this legislation did not survive the full House vote and was eliminated from the House reconciliation bill.

Nurse Practitioner Reimbursement in Medicare

Another piece of legislation that was still in the pipeline for NPs was Senators Tom Grassley's (R-IA) and Kent Conrad's (D-ND) amendment introduced earlier in the year as S.864, which was direct reimbursement to NPs and CNSs—in all geographical areas, all practice settings, and all specialties—under Medicare. Unfortunately, when it resurfaced in the reconciliation bill in fall of 1995, the CNSs had been removed, after a Congressional Budget Office (CBO) reported a large increase in cost projections to the Medicare program if the CNSs were left in the bill. The companion bill to S.864 in the House was HR 1750, introduced by Reps. Towns (D-PA) and Johnson (R-CT), and it did not survive the second round, so the House's version of the reconciliation package did not have any provisions for NP reimbursement in it at all.

As the House and Senate conferees met to make the bill ready for presentation to the President, this one little piece of legislation for NP reimbursement sat alone in the Senate version of the budget reconciliation bill. Well-connected nurse lobbyists in Washington gave it a 50:50 chance of surviving.

Nurse Practitioners in Medicaid

Since the entire Medicaid program was going to be entirely restructured into a block grant program, *all federal mandates would expire*. That meant that the Pediatric Nurse Practitioners (PNPs) and Family Nurse Practitioners (FNPs) who had previously been reimbursed for services under the Medicaid program would no longer be eligible for reimbursement under Medicaid. Additionally, some states

CASE 2–1   *Continued*

had opened up their Medicaid programs and reimbursed all other NPs, too. That was all gone now, and each state was left with the right to determine what health care programs it would offer and who would be reimbursed for services provided. The state legislatures would become the next battleground.

Nursing Education Act (NEA) Funding

The Appropriations Bill for Health and Human Services had not yet passed. It contained the money for the Nursing Education Act, which funded the Division of Nursing (DON), Health Resources and Services Administration (HRSA), in the Department of Health and Human Services (HHS), among other things. Without its passage, there was no money for continuing the NEA. There would be no money to fund traineeships for advanced practice nurse education or any other money to fund the many other programs administered by the DON. This battle was won by Congress later reappropriating the money at the 63 million dollar level. However, the war continues as the 1997 recommendation is for 7.7 million dollars.

As the battles continue, the nursing community and the nursing professional associations need to be stronger, more aggressive, more assertive, more focused and more united. Together, we can improve our nation's health care system.

■ BIOGRAPHICAL SKETCH

Nancy J. Sharp, MSN, RN, received her Diploma in Nursing from Augustana Hospital and her BSN from Augustana College in a combined program in Chicago, Illinois. She then worked as a nephrology nurse until receiving her MSN from Catholic University of America in Washington, D.C. Since then, Ms. Sharp has spent 17 years in clinical nursing and consulting in nephrology nursing with dialysis and kidney transplant patients. She served as President of the American Nephrology Nurses Association, marking her first step into association management. From there, she went on to serve 8 years as Director of Practice and Legislation for AWHONN, the organization for obstetric, gynecologic, and neonatal nurses in Washington, D.C., another position in association management.

Since 1982, Ms. Sharp has been busy building coalitions and networks by co-founding the *Legislative Network for Nurses,* a twice-monthly newsletter, co-directing the Nurses' Coalition for Legislative Action, directing 10 yearly "Nurse in Washington Internship" programs, and publishing *The Nurses' Directory of Capitol Connections,* which lists over 500 nurses involved in health policy development in Washington, D.C.

From 1993 to 1997, she held concurrent positions as Executive Vice President of the American College of Nurse Practitioners (ACNP) in Washington, D.C., and President of Sharp Legislative Resources, in Bethesda, Maryland. Ms. Sharp has also taught a graduate course in Health Policy for University of Miami, Florida, and has been a columnist on health policy for the journals *Nursing Management* (1991–1996) and *Nurse Practitioner Journal* (1996 to present).

CASE 2–1 *Continued*

■ SUGGESTED READINGS

White House. (1995, October 11). *Impact of the Republican budget cuts on rural America: A state-by-state analysis.* Washington, DC: White House.

■ REFERENCES

Personal Communication. (1995). October 17.

Planin, H., & Devroy, A. (1995). Leaders pledge full tax cuts by Senate GOP. *Washington Post,* October 11, A11.

Rich, S. (1995). AMA, internists, private insurers will be big winners under GOP Medicare bill. *Washington Post,* October 15, A12.

Rich S., & Planin, H. (1995). House committees back Medicare plan. *Washington Post,* October 12, A6.

Legal Aspects of Patient Care Administration

Marjorie Barter and Marva L. Furmidge

Patient care administrators need to be cognizant of four major areas of law: nursing practice, patient's rights, labor management, and employment laws and regulations, especially regarding professional workers. This chapter discusses the issues and current practices in each of these areas and alerts the nurse administrator to emerging issues.

The American legal system was largely founded on English law, and can be traced to the Roman Empire, which ruled Britain until the 5th century A.D. The sources of American law are: the Constitution; statutes passed by federal and state legislative bodies; judicial decisions, referred to as common or case law; and regulations that implement the intentions of statutes.

Regardless of source, most of the legal issues facing health care providers relate to contractual or civil law. This area of law addresses conduct between individuals and results in lawsuits, called torts, in civil courts. Criminal law, in contrast, deals with conduct harmful to society and is administered by the criminal justice system.

■ NURSING PRACTICE

The Nurse Practice Act

Each state regulates the practice of health professionals to protect the public from untrained or incompetent persons. States grant the right to use specified titles, and establish minimum qualifications, competencies, and standards of practice for health professionals. State legislatures delegate the interpretation and enforcement of laws defining the practice of nursing to state boards of nursing. The National Council of State Boards of Nursing administers the licensing examination (NCLEX) by all 50 states. Reciprocity for licensure regulations vary by state.

Nurse practice acts and common law define three types of nurses: licensed practical/vocational nurses (LPNs), registered nurses (RNs), and advanced practice nurses (APNs). APNs include nurse midwives, nurse practitioners, clinical specialists, and nurse anesthetists. More recently, boards of nursing have begun to develop language to regulate the use of unlicensed assistive personnel (Legislative Update, 1995; North Dakota Board of Nursing, 1994). Nurses have the broadest scope of practice of any health care provider except physicians. Most nursing practice acts recognize overlapping functions between RNs and physicians, particularly for APNs (Gilliam, 1994). The lack of uniformity in state nurse practice acts, particularly with regard to prescriptive authority, will be an ongoing source of regulatory and legal activity (Blouin & Brent, 1996).

New configurations of nursing personnel have generated significant discussion and concern about the liability of nurse managers for selection, assignment, delegation, and supervision of personnel. APNs, RNs, and LPNs are also concerned about their liability, based on their accountability for patient outcomes.

Assignment has been defined as the transfer of task and accountability for the outcome. The nurse manager has a legal duty to know what tasks are within the scope of practice of APNs, RNs, and LPNs and the competency of the assignee in the assigned task. If the nurse manager breaches the standard of care for either of those duties, she may be held to be negligent if harm results from the acts of the subordinate individuals. Otherwise, she is not liable.

Delegation is defined as transfer of task without transferring accountability. The RN can never delegate total patient care to a LPN or to an unlicensed person. The RN remains responsible for assessment, nursing diagnosis, planning, and evaluation of the patient's response to care. The RN may only be held liable if she or he was negligent in delegating the task or did not properly supervise the individual. The employer will be vicariously liable as long as the nurse and the unlicensed personnel were acting within the scope and course of their employment (Barter & Furmidge, 1994).

Nursing students are legally responsible for their own actions and liable for their own negligence. When nursing students perform nursing services that are customarily performed only by RNs, they will be held to the standard of care of the RN and be liable through the doctrine of "*holding self out*," alleging that one can do something that in reality one is not qualified to do. Consequently, if nursing students know they are inadequately prepared for a particular assignment or duty or need additional supervision, they must inform the person responsible for their assignment and request further information and supervision.

Faculty are legally liable for the students' assignments and for their reasonable and prudent supervision (Smith, 1996). Patients assigned to students are also assigned to RNs who continue to be accountable for patient outcomes and, thus, must also assess and evaluate patient care. The agency also continues to have corporate liability and must have a contractual agreement with the school. It is prudent to require assurance that the school has adequate liability insurance for the acts of students and faculty. This is especially problematic with community-based practice.

A standardized procedure is necessary when the function requires the nurse to perform procedures that require judgment based on medical knowledge beyond that which is usually possessed by a competent nurse in the area being considered. The standardized procedure must specify in writing: (1) the functions that the nurse may perform under specific circumstances; (2) any requirements that must be followed in performing that function; (3) the requisite education, experience, and training of the nurse performing the procedure; and (4) the methods for initial and continuing evaluation of the nurse's competence in performing the standardized procedure (Smith, 1996). Additionally, the nurse must be authorized by the agency, which must keep a list of qualified nurses. If a nurse without the authority of a standardized procedure performs acts that result in injury to a patient, a presumption of negligence may result against the nurse through application of the *holding self out* doctrine.

The licensing board in each state may place nurses on *probation,* or *suspend* or *revoke* their licenses. Situations that can lead to disciplinary action for nurses include criminal acts, use of controlled substances, mental incompetence, fraud and deceit, and unprofessional conduct (Fiesta, 1993).

Suspension is the temporary denial, and revocation is the permanent withdrawal, of a license to practice nursing. Nurses who are placed on probation may continue to practice, with provisions that may include special supervision and reporting to the board and testing for controlled substances. Most states have provisions for a nurse to petition the board for reinstatement of a revoked license after certain conditions have been met.

Liability and Malpractice

Legal liability, or accountability, generally follows control. As nurse managers gain additional responsibilities or control, they face increased risk of liability (Fiesta, 1993). They may be held liable along with the agency under the doctrine of corporate liability, or as an individual for professional malpractice or criminal acts.

The traditional legal principle of vicarious liability, or *respondeat superior,* holds that an employer is legally responsible for the wrongful acts of its employees. Courts generally hold that if the employee is practicing within the scope and course of his or her employment, and performs a negligent act, the employer is responsible for payment of claims. If a nurse acts beyond his or her scope of practice, or performs an intentionally harmful or criminal act, the agency is not responsible. The California Supreme Court, in a case called *Lisa M. v. Henry Mayo Newhall Memorial Hospital* (1995), extended this exemption from vicarious liability to sexual misconduct motivated by lust and not workplace responsibility even if the employee's duties include examining and touching patients (California Supreme Court Decision, 1996).

Health care agencies maintain professional liability insurance that covers negligent acts of their employees. In the rare instances of criminal or intentionally harmful behavior, the employee must seek his or her own legal assistance. Individual professional liability insurance generally will not provide legal counsel or pay claims until it has been determined that there is a claim naming the employee and that the employer will not defend that claim (Smith, 1996).

Hospitals and other health care agencies are increasingly being held accountable under the legal principle of corporate liability. An agency has a legal duty to provide appropriate facilities, meaning staff and equipment adequate to deliver the services offered and marketed to the public (Fiesta, 1994a). Corporate liability cases have thus far included staffing, equipment, security, safety and environmental issues, lack of policy formulation, and issues involving incompetent physicians (Fiesta, 1993). Agencies are now responsible for credentialing and recredentialing members of the medical staff, monitoring the competence of care delivered, and actively and affirmatively intervening on behalf of the patient when the care is substandard. This includes the emerging issue of the quality and quantity of staff to provide sufficient care (Fiesta, 1994b). It has been held that the Board of Trustees and management are responsible for not only what it does know, but also what it should know (Horty, 1993).

This knowledge is primarily gained from communication with its medical staff and employees, particularly nurses and nurse managers. The nurse's duty now extends to reporting incompetent, unethical, or illegal practice to the appropriate internal authority. A nurse manger's duty includes effective notification of the chief administrator when understaffing endangers patient welfare. An agency that ignores this information can be held liable for any adverse consequences from lack of remedial action. It should be stressed that clinical personnel must communicate in language clearly understandable to the lay management who will be receiving this information (Smith, 1996).

Agencies and nurse managers may be sued by patients for negligent hiring, negligent retention of incompetent or impaired employees, or the provision of negligent references concerning employees (Fiesta, 1994a). In addition, nurse managers' liability is increasing in nonmalpractice areas, such as employees' suits for wrongful termination of employment, discrimination, or sexual harassment.

Malpractice has been defined as any professional misconduct, unreasonable lack of skill or fidelity in professional or fiduciary duties, or illegal or immoral conduct. The law imposes greater legal burdens on nurses because of their greater, unique knowledge, training, and expertise. Thus, the nurse–patient relationship is legally based not on a contract but on a fiduciary duty (position of trust) and must meet the standard of care. Most malpractice actions brought against nurses usually involve negligence, but increasing numbers charge assault and battery, invasion of privacy, false imprisonment, fraud, deceit, or defamation (Smith, 1996).

Courts have recognized *standard of care* as requiring nurses to exercise the same degree of care and skill that a reasonably prudent nurse with similar training and experience performing professional duties would exercise under similar circumstances. A nurse's qualifications, experience, and education are always taken into consideration in determining whether a standard of care has been met.

In the past, standard of care was based on practices in the same or similar locality or community. Recently, national standards have been invoked, especially for specialized practice. Where there is more than one recognized standard of care for a diagnosis or treatment alternative, nurses are not negligent if, in exercising their best judgment, they select one of the approved standard methods that later turns out poorly.

Because malpractice involves matters outside general knowledge, these criteria must generally be established by an acceptable medical expert such as a nurse or a physician. This means that the patient must find an expert or demonstrate rule of *res ipsa loquitur*. This rule, meaning "the thing speaks for itself," requires three conditions: (1) that in the ordinary course of affairs, the accident would not have occurred if reasonable care had been used; (2) that the thing that caused the accident was under the exclusive control of the nurse; and (3) that the patient did not contribute to the occurrence of the accident. When the patient proves that these conditions exist, it is regarded in some states as circumstantial evidence of negligence, which judge or jury may accept or reject. In other states, it creates a presumption of negligence, which must be accepted (Smith, 1996).

Negligence by the nurse can be defined as: (1) the failure to do something that a reasonable nurse would do; or (2) the doing of something that a prudent and reasonable nurse would not do; or (3) the failure to exercise ordinary care under the circumstances; or (4) conduct that a reasonably prudent nurse should realize involved an unreasonable risk of invading a patient's interest; or (5) a failure to do an act that is necessary for the protection or assistance of a patient.

To establish negligence on the part of a nurse, a patient must provide evidence of the seven requirements listed in Table 3–1. The liability of nurses is reduced if they can show that the patient had contributory negligence, meaning conduct on the part of the patient that was a contributing cause to his or her own injuries (Fiesta, 1995).

In common law, patient's contributory negligence was an absolute and complete bar to any recovery for damages. Because this caused many harsh results, most states have adopted the doctrine of comparative negligence. Here, malpractice recovery places the economic loss on the parties in proportion to their fault. In a few states, patients can still recover a percentage of their damages even where their own negligence exceeds that of the defendant.

TABLE 3–1. Requirements to Prove Negligence in Court

1. The nurse had a "fiduciary" duty to provide nursing care to the individual.
2. The duty was breached by violation of the standard of care.
3. The breach of duty was not reasonable self-protection by the nurse in fear of danger.
4. Injury occurred that led to calculable harm.
5. The injury was caused by the breach of duty.
6. Contributory negligence by the injured individual was not present (this reduces but does not remove nurse liability).
7. The statute of limitations for the injury has not been exceeded.

Nurses are obligated to protect patients and the public from injury by other patients, health care staff members, and themselves. One responsibility is to assess a patient's hostile behavior for potential violence, act to protect the hostile patient and others from harm, document actions, and communicate the danger to other staff and management. At the managerial level, policies for training staff in violence control, maintaining records of violence competencies, and for a process of communication to warn others of danger should be actively implemented.

Another responsibility related to protection from harm is the continuous assurance that medical devices used in care are fully functional. According to the 1996 regulations of the Safe Medical Devices Act, this includes a broad range of items from drugs to cotton applicators. Nurse managers must see that staff are trained and supervised in proper use and storage, verifying function, documenting status, requesting repairs or replacements, tracking responses, and are aware that legal liability is based on knowledge not assignment of duty. Additionally, the Act requires reporting of injuries to the manufacturer and deaths to the manufacturer and Food and Drug Administration (FDA).

Defamation consists of the verbal or written communication about someone to another that injures that person's reputation. *Slander* is oral defamation; *libel* is written defamation. Slander is usually not actionable unless actual damage is proved by the plaintiff. Truth is a defense to suits for defamation.

The administration can reduce the probability of defamation between staff by establishing and implementing a policy and procedure for any caregiver to register complaints about the quantity or quality of patient service rendered by another (including physicians) in an objective, confidential, and effective fashion.

Employers have been sued for defamation by former staff members based on statements to prospective employers. The law, depending on the jurisdiction, extends a *qualified or absolute privilege* to such communications and there is no liability as long as the administrator was reporting what she believed was true without intending malice. All facilities should consider policies requiring a signed authorization for release of information before responding to inquiries (Cox v. Flight Safety International, 1995).

False imprisonment occurs when there is an intentional and unprivileged nonconsensual confinement of an individual. It is the unlawful restraint of an individual's personal liberty. A reasonable fear of force, rather than confinement itself, is all that is required. The tort of false imprisonment has been found in cases where patients have been detained in a hospital for failure to pay their bills, or when a patient who is not a danger to self or others was prevented from signing out against medical advice. Restraining a patient unnecessarily or with excessive or unnecessary force may constitute false imprisonment and possibly battery. Patient restraints are stringently regulated by state and federal agencies, so it is imperative that managers review policies regarding restraints for compliance.

Assault and battery are often mentioned together, but they have separate meanings. *Assault* is the unjustifiable attempt to touch another person or the threat to do so in such circumstances as to cause the other reasonably to believe that it will be carried out. *Battery* involves an intentional act that is harmful, or the offensive touching of another without that person's consent. Battery is unique in that it does not require actual injury as a result of the touching. Damage is presumed if the touching was without consent. Medical care and treatment without informed consent that involves the touching of another person has been held to constitute a battery. The lack of consent or privilege is an important part of the meaning of assault and battery. If a nurse goes beyond the limits to which a patient consented, the nurse may be liable (Smith, 1996).

Although less common, criminal actions generally involve murders of patients, or drug use. Frequently, deaths that are identified as murders involve ethical issues among the individual health care providers involved with caring for terminally ill patients. Other murders appear to be acts of a truly criminal individual, and are only discovered after a series of unexplained deaths occur. Also, nurses (generally male), have been found guilty of rape and other sexual inappropriate behavior involving patients (Fiesta, 1994a).

Under our system of law, patients who have suffered calculable, permanent harm from treatment by health care providers may sue to be made "whole" again economically. To that end, our courts award the victim monetary damages to compensate for the injury or suffering. There are three types of damages: nominal, compensatory, and punitive.

Occasionally, an injured person has suffered essentially no loss and the court acknowledges the injury or suffering with an award of *nominal damages*. If there is loss, there may be two types of awards. The first is *special damages* for reimbursement of actual economic loss such as physician, hospital, nursing, and assistive care fees; medicine; and loss of wages. These must be shown to be usual, customary, and reasonable charges that were actually incurred.

Additionally, *general damages* may be awarded for emotional injury including pain and suffering; indignation associated with the injury; mental anguish including anxiety, tension, and nervousness; grief; and other related symptoms or complaints. Their existence, severity, duration, and future impact must be established by expert testimony and considered to set monetary awards, within state mandated "caps."

On rare occasions when the defendant's conduct has been grossly negligent, willful, malicious, or with utter reckless disregard of the consequences of the acts, the courts will allow *punitive damages,* which may be fines or incarceration.

A basic concept of common law is to settle legal disputes within a period of time in a "civilized' manner. An alleged wrongdoer should not be held in legal jeopardy in perpetuity. The plaintiff must bring the complaint against the defendant within a state's legislatively prescribed period of time in the *statute of limitations*. If a lawsuit is not brought within the statutory period, the defendant may successfully have the lawsuit dismissed. Many medical negligence injuries are latent and are not discoverable by the patient for a significant period of time that may be beyond the statutory period. For this reason, almost all jurisdictions have adopted the "discovery" rule, which allows the statute of limitations to begin when the patient finds out, or should have found out, about the alleged negligence.

Medical Records

Medical records are crucial for treatment decisions and are important legal documents that may be recognized by courts as evidence to impugn a health care provider's professional activities. Nurses have a legal responsibility for accurate reporting and recording of patients' conditions, treatment, and responses to care. Entries must be timely, factual, relevant, pertinent, and material. The nurse must comply with professional standards and regulations, as well as the policies and procedures of the employer in maintaining complete and accurate documentation of all care rendered to the patient. Checklists and critical pathway flowsheets have replaced narrative charting in many organizations. Narrative explanation of inconsistencies in data found on flowsheets may avoid problems for health care professionals defending against future malpractice claims.

An RN is often asked to *countersign entries* in patient records for LPNs, unlicensed assistive personnel, and nursing students. If an RN's signature appears on the record and the RN does not have personal knowledge of the particular events, he or she should record this, explain his or her role clearly, and note that he or she read and approved the entry; then, in the event of litigation, the RN's role will not be misconstrued.

Altering of the medical record may result in disciplinary action by the nursing board and, in many states, may result in criminal penalties. Nothing should ever be added, deleted, substituted, or removed. Every health agency should have a written policy and protocol that specifies that an *erroneous chart entry* is never to be erased, obliterated, or destroyed. Rather, it is to be crossed through, labeled as erroneous, signed by the individual correcting the error with date and time, and retained in the record. Correct information is then entered.

Nurses have a duty to properly follow any physician's order unless it is patently erroneous; this is legally defined as illegible, incomplete, ambiguous, incorrect, or violating community standards of care or agency policy. The nurse must inform the physician when a medical order will not be implemented. If the physician persists in an order that violates community standards of care or internal policy, the nurse has a legal duty to *refuse the physician's order* and notify a supervisor. Prudent nurse administrators will establish and monitor chain-of-command procedures that facilitate the nurse reporting the problem through a supervisor to the appropriate medical administrator.

All *verbal orders,* including telephone orders, must be countersigned by the physician within the time frame indicated by regulation and/or agency policy. Legal liability may be reduced if telephone orders, especially questionable or high-risk orders, are received simultaneously by two nurses. Each nurse should then sign for receipt of the verbal order. No allied health practitioner should accept a verbal order that is not within that practitioner's legal scope of practice. Policies should be consistent with state licensing regulations and should clarify who may accept which verbal orders. For instance, respiratory therapists may administer certain medications via inhalants and, if state regulation permits, could receive verbal orders for these treatments.

Clerical personnel frequently *transcribe written physician orders,* which are then countersigned by an RN. Programs to train these clerical personnel and document ongoing competency in the transcription function should be in place to reduce liability exposure.

▪ PATIENT'S RIGHTS

Informed Consent/Refusal of Treatment

The adult patient, if mentally competent, should give written consent for routine care upon admission to the health care agency. This consent does not cover invasive procedures or procedures that are deemed to have considerable risks. The law in all states requires that the practitioner who will perform the treatment, usually the physician, obtain *informed consent* before complicated or nonroutine treatments. In the absence of that consent, the practitioner may be held liable in a civil lawsuit for battery, assault, and professional negligence. To give informed consent for treatment, the patient should be given sufficient information about the risks and benefits of the treatment and alternatives to treatment to make an informed choice. It is the practitioner's exclusive responsibility to convey the necessary information to the patient in language that the patient can understand at an appropriate time.

The responsibility of nursing and other staff is to verify that the appropriate signed consent form is present, and to notify the practitioner when a patient has questions or objections to treatment. Policies and procedures should clearly outline the responsibilities of physicians, APNs, nurses, and other staff regarding informed consent. Nurse midwives, nurse anesthetists, clinical specialists, and nurse practitioners, due to their expanded scope of practice, may have a greater duty to the patient in the informed consent process.

Patients may withdraw consent for treatment at any time, even if they have signed a valid consent form. A patient's refusal of treatment may involve an unwillingness to be resuscitated, a rejection of specific procedures, or an insistence on withdrawal of treatment. This is legally predicated on the right to privacy, which includes the right to control one's own body and to consent to treatment. Refusal of treatment should be documented in the patient record with a signed release form. If the patient refuses to sign a release form, this should also be documented in the patient record.

The Patient Self-Determination Health Act of 1990 requires that health care facilities, as a condition of participation in Medicare and Medicaid programs, inform patients, families, and employees of their legal rights under state law to direct their medical and nursing care, including the right to refuse treatment. The law requires that providers: (1) have written policies and procedures that inform individuals of their rights; (2) document whether or not patients have advance directives; (3) prohibit discrimination against individuals based on whether or not advanced directives exist; and (4) provide for education of staff and the community on issues concerning advanced directives. Advance directives may include *durable power of attorney, living wills,* or *health care proxies* (Pozgar, 1993).

Privacy is a patient's right to have peace of mind regarding the exposure and revelation of his or her body or depictions thereof to unauthorized persons. Confidentiality is the identical right to privacy of records. All patient care staff have a duty to protect the patient's right to privacy. However, the legal duty of confidentiality of information may be superseded by state laws that require reporting of conditions such as child or elder abuse or communicable diseases.

The relationship between the physician and the patient generally is protected as privileged communication in civil but not in criminal cases. Privileged communication is a statutory rule forbidding physicians from disclosing information learned in the course of treating a patient, unless the patient permits it. Because there is considerable variation as to whether nurses and all other health care providers can be made to disclose confidential patient information in court, it is prudent to assume that patient conversations might not be protected as privileged conversations unless the local laws are known (Hall, 1996).

The health care agency or individual practitioner has ownership of the records, and must comply with state law regarding access. In most states, the patient (or his or her representative) has a right to inspect the record while a patient, and may copy the record after discharge. Failure to provide record access, as required by law, may leave a health care provider liable for damages (Franklin Square Hospital v. Lubach, 1990). Records of individuals receiving treatment for drug and alcohol abuse have special protection under the Federal Drug Abuse and Treatment Act of 1972, and cannot be released without a court order (Pozgar, 1993). Policies with regard to record access by third-party payers, researchers, governmental agencies, and others should be developed.

All individuals, regardless of ability to pay, have a right to be medically screened and stabilized for emergency conditions in any Medicare-participating hospital or emergency facility under the Emergency Medical Treatment and Active Labor Act (1984). When patients refuse emergency care, they must be: (1) informed of risks and benefits of treatment, and (2) allowed to refuse treatment, in which case written informed consent of refusal should be obtained. Before the patient can be transferred, the condition must be stabilized within the capability of the emergency department, and the receiving agency must approve the transfer. Adequate documentation relating to all transfers and discharges from the emergency department should reduce hospital liability (Pozgar, 1993).

■ LABOR MANAGEMENT LAWS AND REGULATIONS

Types of Employment

Employee relations is one area of health care that is being particularly affected by health care reform. Workers may be hired in *traditional positions, "at will," by individual contract,* or work in your agency through an *outsourcing contract* and actually be an employee of another firm. It is important for nurse administrators to know and understand the type of employment of everyone delivering patient care, since the federal and state governments have enacted a variety of laws that regulate employment, compensation, and benefits of employees, depending on the type of employment relationship. Traditionally, human resources departments have handled employee–employer issues, but nurse administrators should also be aware of relevant laws and how they govern employees in health care agencies to avoid suits. The human resources department should be consulted on complex issues of leave, compensations, discipline, and termination (Leslie, 1992).

Employees may be employed "at will," under an individual employment contract, or under a labor agreement. Increasingly, all managers and more clinical nurses are employed "at will" in salaried positions. Theoretically, if employment is "at will," unless there is evidence of an express or implied contract of definite duration, either the employee or the employer may terminate employment at any time and for any reason, or for no reason at all. A large number of states have now made significant exceptions to the general right to terminate "at-will" employees (Simmons, 1995). For the most part, the courts have upheld an employer's ability to terminate "at will" as long as it does not transgress discrimination laws, other protective statutes, or the employer's express or implied contractual commitments (Duncan v. Children's National Medical Center, 1996).

Regarding employee claims of wrongful termination, the courts have ruled that employee handbooks become an implied contract. Therefore, if there is a stated grievance procedure, and it is not followed, the court is more likely to uphold a "wrongful discharge" claim. The courts have also ruled that a termination can be against public policy (Simmons, 1995).

Occasionally an employee may be employed under an individual employment contract, which will govern the terms of the employment. Generally, provisions will cover responsibilities, compensation, duration of employment, and conditions of termination. The Internal Revenue Service has strict guidelines as to who qualifies as an independent contractor and has increased surveillance in this area, particularly focusing on health care organizations. The consequence of violating the law is payment of back taxes and fees.

There may also be individuals working within a facility who are not employees of the organization, such as nurses employed by physician practices. Other individuals providing specialized services within an agency may be employees of a contractor for an outsourced department. Examples include pharmacy, medical records, housekeeping, dietary, emergency, and rehabilitation services. It is extremely important to be knowledgeable about the responsibilities involved in these relationships in the event that problems arise (Simmons, 1995).

The National Labor-Management Relationship Act

Labor organizations have become a significant factor in health care facility–employee relations. A number of different types of labor organizations are now recognized as collective bargaining representatives for groups of health care facility employees. These include: (1) craft unions, (2) industrial and governmental employee's unions, (3) professional associations, and (4) independent collective bargaining units.

The National Labor-Management Relationship Act (NLRA) consists of the National Labor Relations Act of 1935, the Taft-Hartley amendments of 1947, and the 1974 nonprofit Health Care Institution amendments. The 1974 amendments apply to any hospital, convalescent hospital, health maintenance organization, health clinic, nursing home, extended care facility, or other institution devoted to the care of sick, infirm, or aged persons. Government hospitals are explicitly exempted by the NLRA. The courts have interpreted this to apply only to health care institutions that are both owned and operated by federal, state, or local governments (Hardin, 1992).

The NLRA was enacted to eliminate industrial strife and establish the legal rights of employees, employers, and labor organizations. The Act protects the rights of employees to join or refrain from joining a labor organization and identifies their rights to bargain collectively through freely selected representatives. It also specifies the procedures for labor organization selection.

Section 7 of the Act ensures the right to "engage in other concerted activities for the purpose of collective bargaining or other mutual aid or protection." This phrase has a broad meaning relating to *organizing efforts* and can be applied to groups of employees who come to administrators to complain about wages, hours, or working conditions.

The NLRA is administered by the National Labor Relations Board (NLRB), a quasi-judicial agency. The NLRB cannot enforce its own decisions and must seek the assistance of the executive branch and court system to do so. The NLRB has two primary functions: to determine an employee's union representation status, and to resolve any labor–management dispute. Thus, the NLRB investigates and adjudicates all complaints of unfair labor practices. It also conducts and oversees the secret ballot elections among employees to determine whether they wish to be represented by any labor union, and if so, the choice of which organization (Hardin, 1992).

The process of labor organization recognition involves four major steps summarized in Table 3–2. To become the collective bargaining unit for a group of health workers, a labor organization must: (1) solicit interest through

TABLE 3–2. Process of Union Recognition

Organizing efforts
Solicitation
Distribution
Meetings
Showing of interest (30% of employees sign)
Petition
List
Union authorization cards
Bargaining unit determination
NLRB uses "Community of Interest"
States which positions are included
Union certification as exclusive bargaining agent for unit
Secret ballot elections for unionization and for selecting a union
Voluntary employee recognition
NLRB selection
Accretion

organizing efforts, (2) submit a petition demonstrating a *showing of interest* by 30 percent or more of the employees to ultimately be in the bargaining unit, (3) have the NLRB *determine* that the *bargaining unit* includes appropriate membership, and (4) be *certified* as the exclusive agent (Hardin, 1992).

Congress felt that a multiplicity or "proliferation of bargaining units" would cause administrative problems, including work stoppages and disruption of patient care. Thus, the NLRB *limits the number of bargaining units* using the community of interests criterion of: (1) similarity of skills, wages, hours, and working conditions; (2) collective bargaining history; and (3) desires of the employees. This usually results in one unit for professionals, including RNs and sometimes social workers and pharmacists, and another for nonprofessional nursing staff and other technicians, such as x-ray or laboratory staff.

The determination of boundaries for bargaining units has become a significant issue with the rapid mergers and acquisitions of health care facilities. The courts have held that the *single facility presumption* may preclude consolidation of employee bargaining units in multiple sites unless there is functional integration and a collective community of interests (California Pacific Medical Center v. NLRB, 1996).

A labor organization can become the *exclusive bargaining agent* through one of four different ways. The most common is by winning the secret ballot election conducted by the NLRB. Alternatively, an employer can voluntarily recognize a labor organization as the exclusive bargaining agent; this can constitute an unfair labor practice when other labor organizations are also seeking to represent the employees. A third way is by order of the NLRB. When the NLRB finds serious unfair labor practices, it has the authority to order the extraordinary remedy of recognition of a labor organization. A fourth way, termed *accretion,* is when a merger or acquisition involves one organization with a negotiated contract for a bargaining unit and one without; the employees in the site formally without representation are automatically covered by the preexisting contract. Accretion is increasingly being challenged, under the single facility presumption and community of interests standards.

The NLRA defines *supervisor* as:

> Any individual having authority, in the interest of the employer, to hire, transfer, suspend, lay off, recall, promote, discharge, assign, reward, or discipline other employees, or responsibly to direct them or to adjust their grievances, or effectively to recommend such action, if in connection with the foregoing, the exercise of such authority is not of a merely routine or clerical nature, but requires the use of independent judgment. (§ 152 [11], 61 Stat. 138, 29 U.S.C.)

The determination of supervisory status is extremely important as supervisors are expressly excluded from the protections and rights of "employees" under the NLRA. Practical effects of this exclusion on supervisors include: (1) their votes will not be counted in NRLB elections; (2) exclusion from bargaining units; (3) no protection by the unfair labor provisions of NRLA; (4) as legal agents of the employer, their actions may be judged to be unfair labor practices of the employer; and, (5) possible requirements by higher management to assist in lawfully opposing labor organizations. To prevent challenges, organizations need to thoroughly review the supervisory job descriptions to ensure actual duties and responsibilities are consistent with this status (Barnes, 1996).

The NLRB has long held that nurses and other health care professionals who direct other employees in patient care activities are typically not "supervisors" because their authority is exercised in the "interest of the patient" rather than in the "interest of the employer." In 1994, the United States Supreme Court (Court) rejected that distinction in its decisions entitled *NLRB v. Health Care and Retirement Corp.* In that case, the Court found the LPNs employed at a nursing facility were supervisors because they exercised ongoing direction over the work of lower-level employees (Furmidge & Barter, 1994).

After this decision, there was much confusion and uncertainty involved with labor organizing efforts for RNs and LPNs and existing RN and LPN bargaining units. In 1996, the NLRB, despite the Supreme Court's decision, reaffirmed in two decisions (Providence Hospital [charge nurses] and Ten Broeck Commons [LPNs]) its long-standing position that nurses were not supervisors, and made it clear that it would continue to find that most nurses and other health care professionals are making decisions according to professional norms and not management perogatives. It remains to be seen whether the NLRB's definition of supervisor will again be challenged in the court system.

Labor Contracts

Once a labor organization is recognized, management must bargain "in good faith" with that union to establish a labor contract. For first contracts, the parties are legally bound to: (1) meet at reasonable times to negotiate wages, hours, and other terms and conditions of employment in good faith, namely with an intent to reach an agreement; and (2) place into writing and execute a contract stipulating agreements when they are reached.

The NLRB looks at total conduct in the context of the bargaining relationship to justify bad faith bargaining charges. The NLRB carefully considers the number of meetings, the substantive nature of the meetings, the initiative of the employer in scheduling meetings, and the delays or cancellations of meetings. In making arrangements or sending documents and minutes, all parties should ensure that everything is sent by certified mail. Such documentation may be essential for defending against a charge of refusal to bargain.

The term *unfair labor practice* relates to any activity carried out directly or indirectly, by either the employer or by the labor organization, that violates the NLRA. Employer and labor activities that are unlawful are set forth in Section 8 of the Act. Employer unfair labor practices may be outlined as follows:

1. Interference, restraint, or coercion of employees in the exercise of their rights to join, not join, or form labor organizations.
2. Employer participation in, domination of, favoritism toward, or assistance to a labor organization.
3. Encouragement or discouragement of membership in labor organizations by discrimination in hire or in tenure, terms, or conditions of employment.
4. Discrimination against employees for filing charges or giving testimony under the Act.
5. Refusal to bargain collectively with the representative of the majority of the employees or the designated exclusive bargaining agent.
6. Refusal to bargain collectively concerning wages, hours, or terms and conditions of employment.
7. An employer may not refuse to provide statistical data to a labor organization for collective bargaining that does not invade the employees' right to privacy. This includes financial statements of its health and welfare, retirement, and pension funds (Hardin, 1992).

The NLRB mandates that the labor contract include wages, hours, and terms and conditions of employment. It is forbidden to contract for illegal employment practices or to insist that employees join a labor organization before they have been employed 30 days. Any other subject that both parties agree to bargain about is permissible including quality of work life issues. Once signed, a labor contract must be in effect for 12 months or more. The 1974 amendment to the Taft-Hartley Act specifies that a labor organization representing hospital workers must give 90 days' notice before terminating a labor agreement, while those in other industries need only give a 60-day notice. Conversely, an employer must give similar notice before locking employees out. This is due to the critical public health nature of the health care industry.

In all but the 21 states where it is illegal, an important point of negotiation in any new collective bargaining agreement is the *union security clause.* This clause states whether a contract (1) requires all employees to join and pay all dues and assessments (a closed shop), (2) requires only certain groups of employees to join, (3) imposes a service fee on all employees with optional membership, or (4) permits voluntary membership. The 21 states forbidding closed shops are generally called *right to work* states in that the laws protect employees' right to work if they refuse to join the labor organization (Hardin, 1992).

After negotiating a labor contract, management should spend no less care on its administration. Managerial rights that have been established at the bargaining table, sometimes at a high price, can be eroded or lost entirely through inattention. Of particular importance is the problem of discipline. Managers must be trained to administer discipline by the appropriate procedures under the contract. Grievances are formal written complaints by an employee or labor organization alleging a violation of the labor contract. Failure to follow guidelines may result in the finding of an unfair labor practice.

Work redesign has become a key issue and one of the biggest challenges in administering labor contracts. In September, 1994, the California Nurses Association filed a consumer-fraud lawsuit in an attempt to halt Alta Bates Medical Center's "patient-focused" work redesign, charging that it was really a profit-focused effort to slash care (Poole, 1996). Alta Bates was not the only California hospital undergoing restructuring, but with the hospital size, history, and prominent location, many commentators believe that it was chosen as a test case.

This is an example of the increased militancy of labor organizations when faced with the uncertain future presented by managed care. Nurse managers must know and understand the labor contract implications involved in work redesign and increased health care integration. They need to be prepared to work closely with staff and administration to balance the demands of upper management and patient care staff.

Only economic strikes and unfair labor practice strikes are legal. The *economic strike* is called by the labor organization in support of lack of progress in bargaining. A striker cannot be discharged, only replaced, for participating in an economic strike. An *unfair labor practice strike* is called in response to either the employer's unilateral actions on mandatory subjects of bargaining or the infrequency of the meetings. When the strike is over, the employer may be required to reinstate striking employees with their full rights and privileges if the employer is found to have committed the alleged unfair labor practice(s). The NLRB may seek legal recourse to fine labor organizations for illegal strikes called by themselves or employees.

The courts have ruled that *work actions* such as "working by the book," reporting sick, refusal to perform any task not in the job description, and mass resignations are not the equivalent of strikes and, therefore, are not governed by strike rules.

The 1974 health care amendments to the NLRA established special provisions for strikes in health care agencies when the parties are unable to resolve their problems. They must also report this situation to the Federal Mediation and Conciliation Service (FMCS), which *may* require *mediation* before any strike is deemed legal. If so, the FMCS will then appoint a Board of Inquiry to investigate the dispute, stipulate the facts discovered, and write recommendations that are advisory, not binding, to the involved parties. If no settlement is reached after the parties consider the recommendations and a required 10-day notice to the other party and FMCS has elapsed, there may be a lockout or strike. This notice requirement does not apply to strikes over unfair labor practices.

Like mediation, *binding arbitration* involves third-party intervention on unsettled issues in collective bargaining. The invocation of binding arbitration may be included in the contract or may be a mutual decision of the parties at the time of the dispute. An arbitrator holds a hearing on the issues in dispute and makes a decision that is binding to both parties. Disagreement by management or the labor organization may not result in a lockout or strike.

Decertification

When a labor organization receives NLRB certification, its majority status must be recognized for 1 year. Decertification petitions to withdraw from representation or change to another labor organization may not be filed until 60 days before the first anniversary of the contract. The petition must supply evidence that 30 percent or more of the employees desire a change. Acceptance of a petition will lead to a NRLB action to restart the certification process from the beginning.

■ EMPLOYMENT LAWS AND REGULATIONS

Workers' Compensation

Every state has some form of *workers' compensation* legislation that is designed to assure that employees will be compensated for losses due to accidental on-the-job injuries or employment-related illness. When the workers' compensation law applies, the employee is barred from suing the employer for the injury. The only way courts become involved is if there is an appeal concerning the decisions of the state official or agency administering the law.

In cases not routinely paid by the insurance carrier, the matter goes to a hearing before a state commission to determine questions of liability. Any injury caused by the job is covered. The key question is whether the condition arose out of or occurred in the course of employment. This definition is broad enough to cover the more common workplace injuries (occupational diseases, the cumulative effect of a working lifetime, even accidents that happen away from the normal workplace). Under workers' compensation laws, nurses have been compensated for disabilities arising from falls, assaults, pranks, heavy lifting, and infections contracted from patients.

Worker injuries and compensation may be administered by an Occupational Health Program, Risk Management Program, or human resources department (Herlick, 1996). Nurse managers should know internal policies and work with the appropriate department to meet legal specifications for notice to employer, claims filing, administration and settling of claims, and reporting of accidents by employers. Failure to follow these regulations may result in penalties and additional legal expenses.

Workplace safety is an area that is regulated by the laws of most states and by the federal OSHA laws. The Occupational Safety and Health Act of 1970 was enacted to "assure safe and healthful working conditions for working men and women." The statutes require the employer to take all reasonable steps that are necessary to protect life, safety, and the health of employees. It includes specific provisions regarding infectious patients, radiation, electrical equipment, and vaporous, flammable, or combustible liquids. The statute provides that when no federal standard has been established, state safety rules remain in effect. Health care institutions can be sanctioned for not providing a safe working environment for employees (Simmons, 1994).

In 1996, voluntary federal guidelines for preventing workplace violence were released. They emphasize a risk analysis of the worksite, the development of a program to address the risks, training and education of management and staff, and record keeping and evaluation of the program (OSHA, 1996).

Laws Regarding Discrimination

The federal government has enacted several laws to expand equal employment opportunities by prohibiting discrimination on various grounds, including sex, age, race, religion, handicap, pregnancy, or national origin. One of the few discrimination exceptions permits religious institutions to consider religion in relation to normal business operations as a criterion in their employment practices. These laws are enforced by the Equal Employment Opportunity Commission (EEOC). They cover hiring, assigning, leave, and retirement provisions (Simmons, 1995). There are also numerous state laws addressing equal employment opportunities. In hiring and assigning nursing personnel, the manager should abide by those federal and state laws that protect employees' civil rights.

Discriminatory treatment of pregnant women for all employment purposes was prohibited by the 1978 amendments to Title VII of the Federal Civil Rights Act of 1964. The Federal Employee Health Act (FEHA) developed provisions that require employers to provide unpaid leaves of absence of up to 4 months and reinstatement to former jobs (unless no longer available due to business necessity) to employees with pregnancy-related disabilities. This provision has been challenged as providing preferential treatment to pregnant workers, but has been upheld by the Supreme Court (Simmons, 1994). Some state's regulations regarding leaves differ from the federal regulations, leading to complex issues about the timing and length of the available leaves. It is imperative that nurse managers be knowledgeable about their institutions' compliance with local law.

Discriminatory compensation policies based on sex are prohibited by the Equal Pay Act. Equal work is defined as work requiring the same skill, effort, and responsibility that is performed under similar working conditions. In general, the courts require equal pay except when the employer has been able to prove actual differences in the work performed during a substantial portion of work time. The courts have adopted a case-by-case approach to the determination of whether work is equal (Simmons, 1995).

Employment discrimination may be found when: (1) work rules or employment practices are not applied in a consistent fashion; (2) an employment practice, such as a written employment test, has an adverse impact on minorities and cannot be justified as job related; and (3) minorities are in a disadvantageous position because of prior discriminatory practices. These conditions are all illegal.

The Americans with Disabilities Act (ADA), 42 U.S.C. Secs. 12101 *et. seq.,* prohibits an employer from discriminating against a qualified individual with a disability and requires reasonable accommodation to enable an individual to perform his or her duties. Under the ADA, the qualifications for being work-disabled are clearly defined. ADA also limits requirements for reasonable accommodation to employees qualified for a job's requirements (Simmons, 1994). The courts have been strict in interpreting the law regarding the showing of disability and the ability to perform job-related functions.

When hiring individuals, the ADA generally prohibits inquiries about medical conditions to protect the job applicant's privacy. The court has held that pre-employment inquiry is permissible when an applicant has a known disability, concerning (1) an applicant's ability to perform job-related functions, and (2) documentation from a doctor stating that the applicant has a disability and what functional limitation necessitates a reasonable accommodation (Grenier v. Cyanamid Plastics, Inc., 1996). This is an area of the law that is evolving, and special care must be taken in hiring and employing individuals with disabilities.

Civil Rights of Employees

The EEOC published final guidelines in 1980, affirming that *sexual harassment* in the workplace violates Title VII of the 1964 Federal Civil Rights Act. Under these guidelines, the employer can be liable for sexual harassment by co-workers, nonemployees, and supervisory and administrative staff. Employers will be considered absolutely responsible for sexually harassing acts against employees regardless of whether the specific acts complained of were authorized, sanctioned, or even forbidden by the employer and regardless of whether the employer knew or should have know of their occurrence.

Since the original guidelines were issued, courts have considered a multitude of sexual harassment cases, resulting in numerous decisions. The courts have defined two types of sexual harassment. The first is *quid pro quo,* in which an employee with the ability to affect another employee's terms of employment requires the subordinate to provide sexual favors or submit to sexual activity in order to be promoted or hired, or to avoid being fired or demoted. This is the type of activity that most individuals associate with sexual harassment (Simmons, 1994).

The second type is *hostile work environment* harassment, in which the complainant is subjected to unwelcome conduct that is sufficiently severe or pervasive to alter the conditions of employment and create an abusive work environment (Wilkinson, 1996). The hostile work environment is apparently much more prevalent, and more controversial to many individuals. It is also material to understand as a manager in a health care setting that sexual harassment complaints are not confined to male harassment of female subordinates. Cases are increasing in which the alleged harasser may be female, and some courts have declared that same-sex harassment is actionable (Sardinia v. Dellwood Foods, Inc., 1995).

It is extremely important that sexual harassment policies be actively and diligently enforced in a fair and sensitive manner, and that all complaints of sexual harassment be investigated. Still, the law requires an employer to diligently investigate and redress claims of sexual harassment to avoid liability. A New York case held that "[p]rompt and effective remedial action can be a complete defense to a claim for sexual harassment" (Wilkenson, 1996, p. 23). The law is still evolving in this area, so nurse managers should communicate closely with human resources managers if potential situations occur.

The Fair Labor Standards Act of 1938 (FLSA) establishes *minimum wages and maximum hours* of employment. The employees of all nonprofit and for-profit agencies are covered by this act. However, bona fide salaried executive, administrative, and professional employees are exempted. The current trend to changing nurse positions to professional salaried positions moves them to exempt status.

Most employers are required to pay overtime rates for work that exceeds 40 hours in 7 days. However, the law permits hospitals to enter into agreements with employees, establishing an alternative work period of 14 consecutive days, rather that the usual 7-day week. This does not relieve the hospital of the obligation to pay overtime rates for hours worked in excess of 8 hours in any one day, even if no more than 80 hours are worked during such a period (Simmons, 1994).

The federal Family Medical Leave Act of 1993 (FMLA) requires employers to provide up to 12 weeks of unpaid, job-protected leave within a 12 month period, with health insurance maintained during the leave, for eligible employees for specified family and medical reasons (Schneider & Grimaldi, 1996). The leave can be requested for care of the employee's child (birth or placement for adoption or foster care); care for a spouse, child, or parent who has a serious health condition; or for a serious health condition that makes the person unable to perform his or her job.

It important to understand that the definition of employer under FLSA is "any person acting directly or indirectly in the interest of an employer in relation to an employee" (20 U.S.C. § 203(d)). FLSA case law holds supervisors responsible for FLSA violations when they exercise control over the employee. In the FMLA, the definition of employer is quite similar to that of the FLSA, and the courts have used FLSA case law to hold that a supervisor, and a department manager, are individually liable under FMLA (Employee, 1996). This is significant because it is the employer's duty to determine entitlement of and notify eligible employees of their right to FMLA leave, and it is also the employer's responsibility to inform employees about the FMLA. Therefore, a nurse manager must not only know the policy, but also be able to recognize when employees are eligible for FMLA and inform them of their option.

■ EMERGING LEGAL ISSUES

There are several areas of interest to patient care administrators where the law is unsettled or increasingly under challenge. These areas are briefly mentioned to alert patient care administrators.

Work Redesign

Work redesign, as mentioned in the earlier labor discussion, has the greatest potential to impact future regulation by the federal or state government. The debate centers around the control of standards for cost-effectiveness and quality of patient care by clinician employees or managers and owners (Poole, 1996). This issue also has implications for nurse practice acts and their regulations, anti-trust regulation regarding merger and acquisition activity, and labor law regarding collective bargaining.

Privacy and Databases

Associated with the expansion of managed care, the mergers of agencies, and the general expansion of integrated care is the expansion of information technology to provide information about a patient across the continuum of care. The protection of patient privacy and confidentiality in this environment is an issue that remains unresolved (Fiesta, 1996). Policies and procedures adequate to protect patients must be current and sufficient (Rosenblum, 1995). Situations regarding limiting of access to private information, such as from provider to insurer; excessive system downtime, which may prevent access to records and delay timely provision of care; detecting the altering or destroying of records; and fraud or cover-ups through manipulating record systems are examples of evolving law and court challenges.

Drug Testing

Drug testing is being used by many hospitals both prior to employment and randomly "for cause" during employment. This civil rights issue faces periodic challenges. An employer's right to do drug testing has been upheld by the Supreme Court, and it is mandated in certain industries by federal or state regulations. A nurse manager should track the status of drug testing laws and agency compliance (Simmons, 1994).

Human Immunodeficiency Virus (HIV)

Three issues relating to pending and projected court cases related to HIV are of concern: anti-discrimination, privacy and confidentiality, and workplace safety. These issues have created legal dilemmas for patient care administrators who must consider the rights of both patients and staff. In one court case involving questions of anti-discrimination against an employee with HIV and patient safety, the court ruled that patient safety should prevail. Decisions are still being made on a case-by-case basis (Zachary, 1995).

Access to Care

More and more, consumers are calling for increased regulation regarding access to care in response to incentives to reduce care from capitated or global payment to providers. Utilization review decisions to approve or deny care are made by providers, such as a hospital or primary physician, or by purchasers of care, such as a third-party payor. Liability for utilization review decisions may depend on the particular arrangement for the review process (Fiesta, 1995). A liability decision will be influenced by a determination of whether the need for treatment was urgent, and whether the denial decision was concurrent or retrospective (Guanowsky, 1995).

Insurance Regulation

Currently, insurance companies are regulated primarily by state laws, but with the increased mergers and acquisitions many insurers are becoming national or even international purchasers of care. One initiative addressing this trend is a consumer demand for a federal "bill of rights" for health care targeting managed care.

Another related issue is the current "loophole" large employers are using to create health plans outside of state insurance regulation. The Employee Retirement Security Act of 1974 (ERISA) was enacted to protect employee pension and benefit plans, including health care benefits, from abuse. Recent court decisions have allowed employee benefit plans to be free of state insurance regulation of health financing. Claims for negligence based on utilization review decisions made by or on behalf of ERISA-qualified employee health benefit plans may be found not actionable by courts. The same exemption will not apply to individual practitioners directly delivering care (Brennan & Berwick, 1996). Challenges to the immunity provided to ERISA-qualified health plans will be an evolving area of legal and regulatory activity.

■ BIOGRAPHICAL SKETCHES

Marjorie Barter, EdD, RN, is an Associate Professor of Nursing at the University of San Francisco. She teaches Leadership and Management in the undergraduate and graduate programs and is currently chair of the curriculum committee. Her background includes management of home health and acute hospital programs. She obtained her BSN from California State University, her MSN from the University of California at San Francisco, and her EdD from the University of San Francisco. She is active in Sigma Theta Tau, ONE-C, and the National League for Nursing.

Marva L. Furmidge, JD, MS, RN, is the Director of Administrative Services/Managed Care at Columbia Palm Drive Hospital and Columbia Healdsburg General Hospital. Ms. Furmidge is responsible for human resources, managed care, physician and insurance contracting, risk management, and legal advice. Her previous experience includes home health administration, teaching, and private practice with a plaintiff litigation firm. She obtained her AA from Daytona Beach Community College, her BSN from Louisiana State University, her MSN from the University of California at San Francisco, and JD from the University of San Francisco. She is a member of the California State Bar, Sigma Theta Tau, and the National Health Lawyer's Association.

■ SUGGESTED READINGS

Janet Fiesta's column in *Nursing Management.*

Hall, J.K. (1996). *Nursing: Ethics and law.* Philadelphia: Saunders.

Horty, J. (1993). Responsibilities for the quality of patient care. *Action-Kit for Hospital Law,* Nov. 19.

Pozgar, G.D. (1993). *Legal aspects of health care administration* (5th ed. newsletter). Gaithersburg, MD: Aspen.

Wecht, C.H. (Ed.). (1994). *Legal medicine: 1994.* Salem, NH: Butterworth Legal Publishers.

■ REFERENCES

Barnes, J.G. (1996). NLRB rules that some nurses are employees, not supervisors, under Labor Relations Act. *HHRMAC News, June* (23), 1,11.

Barter, M., & Furmidge, M.L. (1994). Unlicensed assistive personnel: Issues related to delegation and supervision. *JONA, 24* (4), 36–40.

Blouin, A.S., & Brent, N.J. (1996). Collide or collaborate? Changing reimbursement and legal challenges facing advanced nurse practitioners and physicians. *JONA, 26* (4), 10–12.

Brennan, T.A., & Berwick, D.M. (1996). *New rules: Regulation, markets, and the quality of American health care*. San Francisco: Jossey-Bass.

California Pacific Medical Center v. National Labor Relations Board, 87 F.3d 304 (9th Cir. 1996).

California supreme court decision limits employer liability for employee misconduct. (1996). *Human Resource Bulletin, California Association of Hospitals and Health Systems, 88* (96), 5–6.

Cox v. Flight Safety International, No. 94–35308, (9th Cir. Nov. 19, 1995).

Duncan v. Children's National Medical Center, No. 95-CA9408 (D.C. Super. Ct. Feb. 29, 1996).

Emergency Medical Treatment Act. Consolidated omnibus budget reconciliation acts (COBRA), 42 U.S.C. § 13895 dd (1984, 1987, 1989, 1990).

Employees held individually liable under the FMLA. (1996) *Synergy,* Spring, 1–3.

Fiesta, J. (1993). Legal update for nurses—1992: Part III. *Nursing Management, 24* (3), 16–17.

Fiesta, J. (1994a). The evolving doctrine of corporate liability. *Nursing Management, 25* (3), 17–18.

Fiesta, J. (1994b). Staffing implications: A legal update. *Nursing Management, 25* (6), 34–35.

Fiesta, J. (1995). Legal update, 1994: Part III. *Nursing Management, 26* (4), 21.

Fiesta, J. (1996). Legal issues in the information age: Part 1. *Nursing Management, 27* (8), 15–17.

Franklin Square Hospital v. Lubach. 569, A.2d. 693 (Maryland, 1990).

Furmidge, M.L., & Barter, M. (1994). Supreme court decision affects bargaining rights of nurses. *JONA, 24* (7/8), 9–11.

Gilliam, J.W. (1994). A contemporary analysis of medicolegal concerns for physician assistants and nurse practitioners. In C.H. Wecht (Ed.), *Legal medicine: 1994* (pp. 133–180). Salem, NH: Butterworth Legal Publishers.

Grenier v. Cyanamid Plastics, Inc., 70 F.3d 667 (1st Cir. 1995).

Guanowsky, G.A. (1995). Liability in managed care for the health care provider. *Nursing Management, 26* (10), 24–25.

Hall, J.K. (1996). *Nursing: Ethics and law*. Philadelphia: Saunders.

Hardin, P. (1992). *The developing labor law* (3rd Ed.). Chicago: American Bar Association.

Herlick, S.D. (1996). *California workers' compensation handbook* (15th ed.). Charlottesville, VA: Michie, Parker Publications Division.

Horty, J. (1993). Responsibilities for the quality of patient care. *Action-Kit for Hospital Law,* Nov. 19.

Leslie, D.L. (1992). *Labor law* (3rd ed.). St. Paul, MN: West P.

Legislative update. (1995). *Kansas Nurse, 70* (4), 10.

Lisa M. v. Henry Mayo Newhall Memorial Hospital, 23 Cal. 4th 29 (1995).

North Dakota Board of Nursing. (1994). North Dakota Administrative Code, Title 54, Ch 54-07-05, Medication Assistant.

OSHA. (1996). *Guidelines for preventing workplace violence for health care and social service workers*. Washington, DC: U.S. Department of Labor.

Poole, W. (1996). Work redesign. *California Medicine,* March, 21–26.

Pozgar, G.D. (1993). *Legal aspects of health care administration* (5th ed.). Gaithersburg, MD: Aspen.

Rosenblum, J.B. (1995). Legal aspects of computerized records. In C.D. Wecht (Ed.), *Legal medicine: 1995* (pp. 205–225). Charlottesville, VA: Michie.

Sardinia v. Dellwood Foods, Inc., 69 Fair Empl. Prac. Cas. (BNA) 705 (S.D.N.Y. 1995).

Schneider, P.A., & Grimaldi, C. (1996). Avoiding the hidden pitfalls of the FMLA. *Human Resource Professional, March/April,* 26–29.

Simmons, R.J. (1994). *Employee handbook and personnel policies manual.* Van Nuys, CA: Castle Publications.

Simmons, R.J. (1995). *Employee discrimination and EEO practice manual* (4th ed.). Van Nuys, CA: Castle Publications.

Smith, J.W. (1996). *Hospital liability.* New York: Law Journal Seminars Press.

U.S. Chamber of Commerce. (1995). *Analysis of workers' compensation laws.* Washington, DC: Author.

Wilkinson, A.E. (1996). Lessons from 1995—Avoiding liability for sexual harassment. *Human Resource Professional, March/April,* 22–25.

Zachary, M.K. (1995). Balancing judicial interests in HIV cases: Part 1, Issues for nurse administrators. *JONA, 25* (10), 51–55.

APPLICATION 3–1 Managing Unionized Nurses

Mary Suzanne Hudec

■ ORGANIZING A UNION

Scenario

As the Nurse Executive of a 250-bed hospital, you have been made aware by your management staff that the State Nurses' Association (SNA) is campaigning to represent all the registered nurses as their collective bargaining agent. The SNA is distributing literature on the benefits and advantages of union representation. In addition, the SNA is attempting to obtain signatures for eligibility of a National Labor Relations Board (NLRB)-conducted election. The Health Care Administrative team (which includes nursing management) is concerned about its role. A meeting has been called to discuss management's responsibilities and to plan a course of action.

Discussion

Management must recognize that employees have the right to organize, as stated by the National Labor Relations Act (NLRA). Management must not obstruct organizing activities or exercise reprisals against employees involved. The following are recommendations for management during the campaign. Employing an attorney who is an expert in

This article was prepared on the author's personal time and was not part of her official responsibilities nor should it be attributed to the Department of Veterans Affairs.

labor law is very important. The lawyer should review all rules regarding employees and union organizing to ensure compliance with the law to avoid "unfair labor practices."

Recommendations

- Remember that the union is seeking to become the spokesperson for your employees, not an outside organization, a co-manager, or a threat to management.
- Dispel any personal biases toward unions in responding to organizing activities.
- Permit employees to campaign for a union as long as the activities do not interfere with the work of the organization. Solicitation is permissible in nonwork areas during nonwork times, including lunch hours and scheduled breaks. Pro-union propaganda, such as buttons and badges, is generally permissible unless it interferes with the agency's mission.
- Investigate the past history of the union to assess prior activities and practices.
- During the campaign and the election, management should maintain a fair and reasonable posture in dealing with issues of concern to employees.
- When questioned by employees regarding the union, always provide factual information.

APPLICATION 3–1 *Continued*

■ NEGOTIATING A CONTRACT

Scenario

Following the NLRB-conducted election, the SNA achieved certification and recognition as the nursing employee's exclusive representative. The union has presented management with a package of proposals for negotiation of a contract. As the Nurse Executive, you must plan a course of action.

Discussion

Management is obligated to negotiate. Because some initial negotiated contracts are in effect for years before they are opened for negotiation, management should seek an agreement that preserves management rights. The following are recommendations for management before and during negotiations.

Recommendations

- Review the NLRB union certification and become knowledgeable of basic NLRB tenets.
- Meet with the hospital's labor attorney to review all proposals. Use consultants as appropriate.
- Develop a negotiating team and team behaviors.
- Prepare for formal negotiations; do your homework.
- Obtain input from the grassroots of the organization so that management is aware of the issues. Be sensitive to all proposals.
- Analyze proposals beyond their language. What is the underlying issue? Are there other alternatives that the union may find acceptable?

- Anticipate demands that will be made. Review all past grievances and problems, especially problems or issues that have arisen in the last year.
- Establish priorities. On what items could management make concessions and on which is it necessary to hold the line?
- When developing management proposals, establish original proposals, and have fallback positions ready for use during negotiations.
- Bargain in good faith. Demonstrate a sincere intent to reach an agreement regardless of whether an impasse eventually develops.
- Maintain mutual respect between negotiating parties.
- Listen attentively and do not be intimidated.
- Refrain from use of resentment or anger. Objectivity is the most essential quality of a negotiator.
- Avoid flat rejections of union proposals. Be willing to compromise, however, do not make unattainable commitments.
- Specific details of the negotiation process are confidential and may not be shared outside of the proceedings. Relate only general information, otherwise, negotiations may be jeopardized.

■ CONTRACT ADMINISTRATION

Scenario

A nurse requests 3 weeks' vacation during the peak summer vacation period. The nurse manager denies the request,

APPLICATION 3–1 *Continued*

explaining that because of the number of requests for leave, only 2 weeks can be approved. The employee and the union steward meet with the nurse manager, alleging that the disapproval is in violation of a provision of the negotiated contract and past management practice. The employee threatens to file a grievance if the nurse manager does not approve the leave.

Discussion

Administering the contract is a responsibility of all levels of management. After the contract is signed, differences will exist on the content, meaning, and application of certain contract language. It is the middle manager and the first-line supervisor who interpret and apply the contract on a daily basis.

Contract administration is a dynamic activity, not a static body of cut-and-dried knowledge. Controversy is unavoidable.

Recommendations

- *Know* your contract; this includes all levels of management.
- Train the management staff to know the contract, especially on the intent of contract language, which may be deliberately ambiguous.
- Apply the contract fairly and consistently. A supervisor's actions or behaviors can establish contract interpretation or change the intent of the contract.
- Examine management's past practices before taking action.

- Review with managers what they can and cannot say or do. It is illegal to spy on union activities, make promises contingent on nonunion participation, and interrogate or threaten employees about union involvement.
- Read and interpret the contract fairly. Apply the contract in a firm and consistent manner.

■ UNFAIR LABOR PRACTICE
Scenario

The health care organization has been suffering from a financial crisis. Decreased admissions, reduced lengths of stay, and an increase in uncompensated care have resulted in the organization's inability to meet its financial goals. It has become necessary to eliminate 20 nursing positions. Management did not discuss these reductions with the union before issuing the layoff notices. Due to the failure of management to discuss these changes, the union filed an unfair labor practice charge.

Discussion

Management is ultimately responsible and accountable for the financial viability of the organization and, therefore, has the right to decide the number of employees required to accomplish the work. However, if there is to be a downsizing, the union has the right to be informed in advance and to negotiate the impact of these changes. An agenda of change that affects the bargaining unit employees must be communicated to the union officers. In

APPLICATION 3–1   *Continued*

this scenario, management violated a right of the union by failing to discuss the issue. This is in direct violation of one party's rights granted by labor relations law. Either party may be found guilty for failing to live up to its obligation.

Recommendations

- Establish, facilitate, and maintain effective relations with the bargaining unit.
- Communicate planned changes with the union, maintaining an accurate flow of information. This will allay fears and establish trust.
- Investigate immediately once an unfair labor practice has been filed.
- Examine the possibility of resolving an unfair labor practice charge informally.
- Admit the mistake at the onset if management is wrong. If management is in the right, however, do not be intimidated.
- Be willing to compromise. In many cases it is not important to prove who is wrong.
- Allow the union an opportunity to "save face." This may have long-range benefits.
- Work with the Director of Human Resources as a team.

■ GRIEVANCES

Scenario

On the night shift of a medical-surgical unit, there are two registered nurses (RNs) and one nursing assistant on duty.

The unit is very quiet and one of the RNs locks himself in the treatment room to sleep. The other RN, the charge nurse, is unaware of the nurse's actions. During the night, a patient develops respiratory distress and subsequently has a cardiac arrest and expires. A code has been called. The charge nurse, unable to locate the other RN, notifies the night supervisor of the incident. After a thorough investigation of the incident by management, the sleeping employee is fired. The union files a grievance on behalf of the employee. The union's position is that the nurse had been employed at the hospital for over 10 years and that the employee was denied the right to counseling concerning the sleeping incident.

Discussion

Most contracts specify that if both parties are unable to satisfactorily resolve a grievance through the grievance procedure, the process ends in binding arbitration. Management should examine each grievance very carefully at every step to determine whether settlement or resolution is more advisable than rejection of the grievance. A grievance should not automatically be considered as a threat to management's authority.

Winning or losing is not always the most important issue. The cost of personnel time to prepare for testimony, its effect on staff and patients, the potential long-term adverse effects on labor–management relationships, legal fees incurred, and the realization that the arbitrator's decision is binding should be

APPLICATION 3–1   *Continued*

examined and weighed by management. If management, however, is committed and confident of its position, it should proceed through arbitration.

Recommendations

- Place a high priority on resolving dissatisfaction of employees consistent with accomplishment of overall goals.
- Carry out the provisions of the contract and human resources policies consistently.
- All levels of management must know the labor contract and other policies.
- Act with deliberation, investigate carefully, and get all the facts. Be available and encourage a full discussion of the incident.
- Make a strong effort at the first-line management level to resolve grievances at the first step of the grievance procedure.
- Follow the steps of the grievance procedure exactly as outlined in the contract. Adhere to all time requirements, otherwise the outcome of the grievance may be jeopardized.
- Treat the union official as a professional. In preparing and presenting the grievance, the union official has equal status with the management official.
- Consider resolving the grievance before arbitration. If the grievance does go to arbitration, solidify management's position and remember that the arbitrator's decision is binding.

■ ATTITUDES AND RELATIONSHIPS

Scenario

As the Nurse Executive, you have formulated the following goals and objectives:

- To promote shared responsibility for planned change.
- To identify recurrent problems in patient care.
- To formulate/revise standards of care.
- To implement nursing service goals addressing clinical practice issues.

The goals are not being realized. You are considering approaches to attain these goals, but you are unsure of how to get union input.

Discussion

Management does not need to ask the union's approval for every administrative decision. However, sharing information at this point can be very helpful in advancing management's agenda. Informing union leaders of planned change before implementation opens an avenue for constructive suggestions to management and increases cooperation with employees. It is imperative, however, that union leaders acknowledge management's need for efficient and effective delivery of nursing services, otherwise, patient care ultimately suffers.

Recommendations

- Use the union as a vehicle for nurses' concerns.

APPLICATION 3–1 *Continued*

- Allow the union input on issues other than benefits and economic matters.
- Adopt a cooperative versus an adversarial role in allowing the union input into nursing practice issues and standards.
- Establish routine meetings with union leaders to address potential issues before they become a problem.

■ BIOGRAPHICAL SKETCH

Mary Suzanne Hudec is the Associate Director for Patient Services at the Washington, D.C., Veterans Affairs Medical Center. She began her VA career as a staff nurse, holding progressively more responsible positions in nursing administration at various VA medical centers before being selected as Chief, Nursing Service at the Dayton, Ohio VAMC. Ms. Hudec also served in active duty status with the U.S. Navy during the Vietnam War and was assigned to the hospital ship *U.S.S. Sanctuary*. Ms. Hudec has a BS in Nursing from the College of Mount St. Joseph, an MSN from the University of California at San Francisco, and is a past Board Member of the American Organization of Nurse Executives.

APPLICATION 3–2 Designing a Patient Care Risk Management System

George D. Velianoff and Diana K. Hobbs

Risk management is an interdisciplinary process designed to protect the financial assets of the organization and to maintain high-quality medical care. Risk management is responsible for the development of processes designed to reduce the causes and frequency of occurrences that have the potential to result in claims and lawsuits. When a potentially compensable event occurs, it is the responsibility of the risk manager to attempt to reduce the severity and impact of the financial loss.

Nurse administrators must be able to relate a corporate risk management program to daily patient care delivery. The nurse administrator must be knowledgeable and diligent in applying the risk management perspective to patient care issues. In collaboration with the risk manager, the nurse administrator must attempt to monitor and help reduce risk issues.

■ HEALTH CARE RISK MANAGEMENT

The nurse administrator needs to be aware of both state laws and Joint Commission for Accreditation of Health Care Organizations (JCAHO) requirements for hospital risk management programs. Each agency will design responsibilities of the risk management department to fit local needs. Regardless of design, nursing and risk management must work closely together to minimize financial loss from legal suits to the agency.

The American Society for Healthcare Risk Management (1989), in its position summary stated:

> The risk manager is responsible for the facility's risk management activities, which include coordinating insurance coverage and risk financing, managing claims against the facility, interfacing with defense legal counsel, administering the risk management program on a day-to-day basis, managing and analyzing risk management data, and conducting risk management educational programs and complying with JCAHO's risk management standards, all with the objective of controlling and minimizing loss to protect the assets of the facility.

In most agencies, risk management departments are responsible for a minimum of eight areas: (1) risk identification; (2) loss prevention and reduction, occurrence and incident reporting, and investigation; (3) insurance claims management; (4) coordinating legal defense, monitoring of medicolegal issues, and administering workers' compensation programs; (5) contract review to identify liability issues, including the review of warranties, service, and maintenance agreements; (6) risk management education of all employees and volunteers; (7) managing product recall and the requirements of the Safe Medical Devices Act; and (8) ensuring compliance with all federal, state, and local statutes and

APPLICATION 3–2 *Continued*

regulation, and accreditation standards. All of these areas interface with patient care administration.

■ RISK IDENTIFICATION

Gathering and analyzing information, while protecting it from improper disclosure, is essential to managing risk and achieving loss reduction. Information sources include: incident reports; patient comments and complaints; walk-through inspections; discussions with staff; reports from employee health, infection control, the safety committee, and department quality reviews. Nurses need to be aware of what information needs to be reported and the specific mechanisms to do so.

The traditional method of reporting adverse occurrences is the incident report. An incident report is filed whenever an event occurs that is not consistent with normal operating procedure, whether or not there is an injury. The risk manager then can decide whether follow-up is necessary. All members of the staff should be encouraged to complete an incident report when an unusual event occurs.

Typically, incidents are reported on a form with a checklist of most frequently occurring events making the task of reporting easy for the busy staff (see Table 3–3). Studies have shown that only 5 to 30 percent of adverse occurrences are identified on an incident report (Rakes, 1991). Reasons for this may include time constraints on staff, lax attitude or misunderstanding concerning in-

cident reports, and staff's misconception about the purpose of the incident report.

There is a common misconception that if an employee fills out an incident report, it will somehow adversely effect his or her merit rating or wind up in the employee's file. Therefore, staff education is of the utmost importance if the institution's reporting system is to be meaningful.

Incident reports are the primary source of information about medication errors. Overall medication prescribing errors by physicians number 3.13 per 1,000 orders. Of these errors 1.8 per 1,000 were considered significant (Lesar, 1990).

Accurate incident reporting greatly increases the efficiency of the risk manager. It is unrealistic, however, to believe that all adverse events will be reported. Today, computer database systems make data trending far more efficient and meaningful in protecting the financial assets of the institution. In addition, the introduction of continuous quality improvement (CQI) strategies has created indicator identification, review, and processes. Every department, including nursing, is required to show a CQI process (see Table 3–4).

The incident report is a confidential document and must be treated as such. However, the documents produced by the risk management program have the potential to become adverse evidence against the facility if used in a legal action. Some courts and legislatures have provided for immunity from discovery, protecting the confidentiality of risk management documents. This immunity will only be maintained if the facility treats the documents as "privileged." Copies of the re-

APPLICATION 3–2   *Continued*

TABLE 3–3. Data Abstract of Risk Management Indicators

INTRAVENOUS/BLOOD MEDICATION:

❏ Adverse reaction	❏ Medication missing	❏ Site problem
❏ Allergic reaction	❏ Mislabeled	❏ Transcription error
❏ Crossmatch problem	❏ Not available	❏ Tubing not changed
❏ Dispensing error	❏ Not documented	❏ Tubing pulled out/broken
❏ Flow rate/Too fast	❏ Omitted	❏ Wasted
❏ Flow rate/Too slow	❏ Out-of-sequence	❏ Wrong additive
❏ Given without order	❏ Outdated	❏ Wrong dosage
❏ Improper order	❏ Patient identification	❏ Wrong drug
❏ Incompatible additives	❏ Patient refusal	❏ Wrong solution/Type
❏ Incorrect route	❏ Patient took unprescribed medication	❏ Wrong time
❏ Infiltration	❏ Repeat administration	❏ Other _____
❏ Medication given before culture taken	❏ Repeated attempts to start	

TYPE OF INJURY (*Select the most serious*):

❏ Abrasion	❏ Electrical shock	❏ Phlebitis
❏ Amputation	❏ Excess blood loss	❏ Poisoning
❏ Anoxia/Respiratory distress	❏ External laceration	❏ Puncture wound
❏ Blister	❏ Fluid overload	❏ Rash/Hives
❏ Burn	❏ Fracture/Dislocation	❏ Retained foreign object
❏ Circulatory impairment	❏ Hematoma	❏ Sensory impairment
❏ Contracture	❏ Hyperthermia	❏ Skin tear
❏ Contusion	❏ Hypothermia	❏ Sprain/Strain
❏ Damaged teeth	❏ Infection	❏ Stillborn
❏ Decubitus	❏ Inflammation	❏ Wound disruption
❏ Deformity/Scar	❏ Internal laceration	❏ Not applicable
❏ Deterioration in condition	❏ Neurological deficit	❏ Unknown
❏ Edema/Swelling	❏ Perforation	❏ None
		❏ Other _____

SEVERITY OF INJURY:

❏ Minor	❏ Not applicable
❏ Moderate	❏ Unknown
❏ Serious	❏ None
❏ Death	

(continued)

TABLE 3–3. (continued)

FALLS:

❏ Bed
❏ Bedside commode
❏ Chair/Stretcher/Table
❏ Faint
❏ Fall/Slip
❏ Found on floor
❏ From toy
❏ Recreational activity
❏ Scales
❏ While ambulating
❏ Other

Check One:
❏ Attended
❏ Unattended

Surface Condition:
❏ Wet
❏ Dry

Activity Privileges (select one per medical order):
❏ Ambulate with assistance
❏ Ambulate without assistance
❏ Ambulate with device
❏ Bathroom privileges with assistance
❏ Bathroom privileges without assistance
❏ Bedrest
❏ Not specified
❏ Unlimited
❏ Up in chair/Wheelchair
❏ Other _____
_____

Bed Position:
❏ High
❏ Low

Siderails (indicate position at time of event, if applicable):
❏ None

Half Rails:
❏ 1 up
❏ 2 up
❏ 3 up
❏ 4 up

Full Rails:
❏ 1 up
❏ 2 up

Restraints (other than side rails):
❏ Yes
❏ No

Medicated past 4 hours:
❏ Yes
❏ No (if yes, check type of medication) _____

HIGH RISKS (*Select type event from other categories as appropriate*):

❏ 4th-degree laceration
❏ Anesthetic agent
❏ Apgar score <4; <7
❏ Change in diagnosis
❏ Complication of augmented labor
❏ Complication of forceps
❏ Complication of vacuum extractor
❏ Damaged organ or part of organ
❏ Delay in starting surgery
❏ Delivery cord blood <7.16

❏ Discharged without being seen by physician
❏ DOA within 7 days of discharge
❏ Extubation
❏ Held/Observed beyond hospital policy
❏ Intubation
❏ Meconium aspiration/Abnormal staining
❏ Neonatal complication
❏ Neonatal seizures
❏ Postpartum complication

❏ Precipitous delivery
❏ Pregnancy poststerilization
❏ Prolonged labor
❏ Return to delivery room
❏ Return to ER, same problem
❏ Return/Repeat surgery
❏ Sponge/Instrument/Sharp count
❏ Unattended delivery
❏ Unplanned removal of organ or part of organ
❏ Unrecognized CPD
❏ Other _____
_____

MISCELLANEOUS:

❏ Admission from outpatient unit
❏ Against medical advice
❏ Aspiration
❏ Assault/Violence
❏ Cardiac/Respiratory arrest
❏ Contraband
❏ Dissatisfied Patient/Family
❏ Elopement

❏ Excessive length of stay
❏ Fire
❏ In Bed—Other accident
❏ Misfiled chart form
❏ Needle/Sharp stick— Nonemployed
❏ Other accident while ambulating
❏ Property missing or damaged

❏ Readmission
❏ Self-inflicted injury
❏ Struck by object
❏ Third-party refusal/Denial
❏ Unplanned transfer to critical care
❏ Other _____
_____

APPLICATION 3–2 *Continued*

TABLE 3–4. QI Key Indicators: Nursing Key Indicators for Risk

DIMENSIONS	KEY INDICATORS	THRESHOLD	GOAL	QUARTERLY STATUS			
				1	2	3	4
Safety/Risk	Falls	Reduce falls with injury by 25% from 1995	No falls with injury				
	Medication errors	Each PERT report investigated and employee coached per policy	100%				
	Transcription errors	Each PERT report investigated and employee coached per policy	100%				
Patient/ Family Education	Patients will have discharge instruction sheets completed with signature of patient or significant other	90% compliance	95% compliance				

ports should never be made and the original should be forwarded to, and maintained in, the risk management office. If the report is reviewed by anyone other than the risk manager, all steps necessary to ensure the confidentiality and maintain any special legal status afforded under state law must be taken.

It is most important that an incident report not be made a part of the medical record. Further, the fact that an incident report was completed must not be mentioned in the medical record. This will negate the immunity.

Incident reports do not enjoy immunity in many states because they are regarded as being made in the normal course of business. Further, opponents of inadmissibility of incident reports are concerned about the inability of the patient/consumer to have access to the documents. It is felt that these documents contain important information regarding the competency of health care providers and hospitals and that discovery would aid the public in making informed decisions regarding health care. If there is no immunity in your jurisdiction, consult with hospital counsel for guidance on the best way to maintain confidentiality of reports.

■ ANALYSIS OF RISK

Risk analysis is the evaluation and classification of risk in terms of potential

APPLICATION 3–2 *Continued*

severity of loss. The analysis will allow the risk manager to set priorities. It is helpful to break risk into the following five classes when prioritizing: prevented risks, normally prevented risks, managed risks, unprevented risks, and unpreventable risks.

Prevented risks have the highest priority. These risks are to be avoided as their occurrence is far more costly than their prevention. Examples include operating on the wrong patient, allowing unqualified physicians to practice, and leaving a foreign object in the abdomen of a surgical patient. Policies and procedures need to be in place to avoid these situations. Risk management should adopt a zero tolerance policy toward this type of event.

Normally prevented risks encompass all types of negligence. This classification includes most negligent injuries and product liability actions. Although not always preventable, this class of risk can be greatly reduced with good prevention programs. Examples include patient falls, wound infections, and other medical complications. These risks are the basis for most medical malpractice claims.

Managed risks include instances in which a patient must prove a defendant owed a special duty to the plaintiff. The cost of prevention is only slightly greater than the cost of management. This category does not usually involve the delivery of patient care. Examples would be the care of patient's personal property.

Risks classified in the fourth category may not be fully preventable or the cost of their prevention may be higher than the occurrence. An example would

be the provision of high-risk services such as obstetrics. Some risks of providing the service are accepted and funded.

The last category of risk covers those that are deemed unmanageable. They come from forces that are beyond the control of the health care institution and are often referred to as "acts of God."

■ APPLICATION EXAMPLES

Example 1: Needle Sticks—"Normally Prevented Risk"

Every facility that deals with sharps has been confronted with issues related to employees being stuck with needles.

The ability for risk management to be involved when these incidents occur is crucial. The needle stick itself and a policy to deal with the individual receiving the stick are relatively easy to develop and utilize. It is the risk management component that really enlightens the issues of such a seemingly simple incident.

The risk management component emphasizes the disruption and issues created by careless disposal of sharps. For example, a nurse caring for a patient reaches under the covers to straighten the patient's leg and is stuck by a needle. No one is sure where the needle came from or why it was in the bed, and the patient was not on intravenous fluids or intramuscular medications. There is no blood in the syringe, but no one is sure if the blood on the tip of the needle is the employee's or from someone else. The employee is now thrown into a life-

APPLICATION 3–2   *Continued*

or-death scenario. Is the needle contaminated? Are there other transmittable organisms on the needle? Will he or she contract HIV? The wait to find out the answer will undoubtedly be very uncomfortable. Weeks pass before anyone knows and even then, there is no guarantee.

What may have seemed a simple mistake, a small oversight, has now disrupted not just the employee's life, but his or her entire family and work team. The unit staff is always haunted by the question, "What if it were me?"

Having appropriate incident reporting mechanisms is important. Having appropriate Human Resource policies and disciplinary processes is important. But an aggressive education program that incorporates a risk management perspective with case studies is crucial. Accurate reporting by staff and accurate record keeping by risk management will be most helpful in identifying any trends that may be developing. The identification will lead to corrective action, and the life of a fellow nurse, friend, and employee may be spared.

Example 2: Case Management— "Unprevented Risks"

Utilizing risk management in a case management process is advantageous. How often do you encounter patients who need to be transferred to subacute, long-term, or home care but cannot be moved to the most appropriate setting? This problem may occur when a family member or significant other is not available as a caregiver, the patient does not

have sufficient income or insurance, the case is too complex for the identified facility to accommodate, the facility lacks space, or the patient cannot care for himself or herself. In these cases, although social services, case managers, and discharge planners can do much to help the disposition and a financial counselor/expert may help with funding, it is the risk manager who can evaluate contractual issues, legal fine points such as guardianship, and overall risk/benefit analyses of the options available.

For example, should the hospital pay the patient's first 2 weeks in a long-term care facility if that facility will accept the patient now, rather than keeping the patient in the acute care setting for the 2 weeks? Or should the hospital risk the likelihood of being forced to keep the patient an additional 4 to 6 weeks with no reimbursement if the facility does not have a bed available in 2 weeks? In addition to the patient and financial risks associated with these options, what are the contractual risks? What about future issues or litigation? Remember, too, that the longer a person remains in the hospital, the more likely a patient injury will occur, thereby leading to increased risk, loss, and litigation.

Example 3: Credentialing

How can a risk management presence enhance the credentialing/recredentialing process? When patient issues arise or quality of care is suspect, a system to document, review, and track the issues is essential. With corporate liability and the potential litigation involved in

APPLICATION 3–2   *Continued*

credentialing practitioners, it is imperative to devise and maintain a system that reveals the pertinent information needed at the time of credentialing and reappointment. The credentialing process must be coordinated with the risk management plan and the quality management program.

■ CORRECTING THE RISK

Risk control involves loss-prevention techniques aimed at reducing the frequency and severity of losses. This is achieved mainly through staff education. Lack of education regarding risk management has been shown to be one of the major causes of loss. Staff should be made aware of common problems and ways to deal effectively with untoward events as they arise. A clear understanding of health care law and the duty imposed on health care workers has proven to be an effective management technique. Also, physician credentialing policies and departmental policies and procedures are proven loss-prevention strategies.

Risk funding involves transferring risk of loss due to an untoward event to a third party, such as an insurance company. Most health care risks are managed with a combination of the two strategies.

■ MONITORING AND EVALUATING

Information using data obtained through the many channels should be continuously monitored and trended. This information will show any changes in the frequency of occurrences and will give the risk manager continuous feedback on the effectiveness of programs.

Talking informally with the staff will provide a great amount of useful information. Often a 10-minute conversation with staff will give more insight into a problem than all of the incident reports received. Also, staff will often have a workable solution to the problem. It is the wise administrator who takes the time to listen to employees and involve them in setting policy and procedure.

■ RECOMMENDATIONS

ECRI, a nonprofit organization, offers the following recommended actions for risk managers.

1. Make use of as many types of information and communication sources as are available for identifying risk.
2. Ensure that the facility has an effective system of reporting hazards and adverse occurrences.
3. Ensure that the confidentiality of risk management documents is protected.
4. Ensure that there is a formal process of interaction and information sharing between quality assurance, medical records, utilization review, and risk management.
5. Use patient satisfaction surveys and grievances to gain insight into problems at the facility.
6. Establish a computerized database.

APPLICATION 3–2 *Continued*

7. Continuously monitor and evaluate the risk management program.

■ **BIOGRAPHICAL SKETCHES**

George D. Velianoff, a graduate of Bethesda Hospital School of Nursing and Indiana University, has held nurse manager and executive positions in various tertiary academic centers as well as primary community hospitals. He has also held adjunct clinical faculty positions guest lecturing and mentoring graduate nursing administration students. He has served on several boards and national committees, where he has been instrumental in advancing research-based professional practice. In his role as Nurse Executive, he has had administrative responsibility for risk management, legal services, and quality assurance/improvement departments and functions.

Diana K. Hobbs, after practicing nursing for 18 years, moved from clinical health care into health care law. She was employed by a Baltimore law firm as a nurse/paralegal in the medical malpractice/health policy department. Currently, Ms. Hobbs is employed as the Corporate Director of Risk Management and Legal Services and is a third-year law student. As Director of Risk Management, she is responsible for overseeing all aspects of risk management, including the hospitals, home health agency, and hospice agency. Her background in nursing and law has given her the ability to apply law to clinical health care.

■ **SUGGESTED READING**

Hospital Risk Control. (1992). *The role of the risk manager.* Plymouth Meeting, PA: Author.

Human Resources Division. (1989). *Health care: Initiatives in hospital risk management.* (U.S. General Accounting Office. Publication No. HRD-89-79). Washington, DC: U.S. Government Printing Office.

Joint Commission on Accreditation of Healthcare Organizations (JCAHO). (1991). *Accreditation manual for hospitals.* Oakbrook Terrace, IL: Author.

Korleski, D. (1991). *Developing a risk management policy manual.* Nashville, TN: American Society for Health Care Risk Management of the American Hospital Association. (On cassette.)

■ **REFERENCES**

American Society for Healthcare Risk Management. (1989). *Model risk manager job descriptions.* Chicago: Author.

Lesar, T.S. (1990). Medication prescribing errors in a teaching hospital. *Journal of the American Medical Association, 263* (17), 2329–2331.

Rakes, G.M. (1991). Risk management, safety management, and quality assurance. *Topics in Health Management, 59.*

Richards, E.P., & Rathbun, K. C. (1983). *Medical risk management.* Rockville, MD: Aspen Systems Corporation.

Cultural Diversity in the Workplace

Arlene J. Lowenstein

Immigration, both forced and voluntary, shaped the face of this nation. Each new wave of immigrants continues to add to the mosaic that created a world power in a relatively short time span. The strength of that mosaic is the ability to capitalize on new and different ideas. Its weakness is the clash between cultures that feeds prejudice and discriminatory behaviors. Cultural diversity has had and will continue to have an impact on the health care arena. Growing multicultural diversity of both patients and staff has multiplied opportunities for conflict and perceptions of prejudice and discrimination. The purpose of this chapter is to provide information to increase cultural sensitivity and provide resources for developing skills to work effectively in multicultural environments. A discussion of social change and related health care delivery issues will be followed by a review of theoretical issues and research in cultural diversity. Finally, strategies for managing cultural diversity will be presented.

■ SOCIAL CHANGE AFFECTING THE WORKPLACE

In the 1950s, assimilation was the preferred process for incorporating immigrants into American life. The United States was known as the "melting pot." It was expected that new immigrants would quickly learn the language and customs of their adopted land and disappear into the accepted fabric of American society. Assimilation worked for some members of European cultures who were primarily Caucasian. It was impossible for those whose skin color or appearance differed from those of the "ideal" American. Nor could it work for women confronted by the white, male-dominated power structure and defined gender roles of that time. Those citizens or aspiring citizens who were older or physically disabled also had difficulty melting into the American ideal.

Until the 1970s, education to prepare registered nurses was almost nonexistent for African Americans and other minorities, including men. Although a few Asian students were admitted to white schools, the few programs available to African Americans were segregated. This was not limited to the legally segregated south, but occurred in the north as well. Many of these schools had poor resources and limited learning opportunities (Carnegie, 1991; Hines, 1989; Lowenstein & Glanville, 1995). The poor primary and secondary schooling provided to African Americans affected their ability to complete registered nurse programs when they were eventually admitted. However, those students fought for their education and successfully overcame many barriers and challenges to become professional nurses. Most minority students interested in providing health care were directed towards less-skilled programs. A large number of African Americans working in health care today are still nursing assistants, technicians, and licensed practical nurses (LPNs); few have been able to climb the management ladder.

The 1960s and 1970s brought a cultural revolution to this country. Minorities and women began to assert their right to be different. The "Gray Panthers" advocated for older persons to be honored for their wisdom and utilized in the workplace, instead of being forcibly relegated to retirement. Handicapped persons began to be heard. The cultural revolution was sanctioned by our legal system. Laws were passed to ensure civil rights.

The Civil Rights Act of 1964 was a landmark ruling that outlawed segregation and promoted equal opportunity in employment. The law was strengthened by amendment in 1972. Women were empowered through the Equal Pay Act of 1963, which was specifically designed to disallow pay discrimination on the basis of gender. The Pregnancy Discrimination Act of 1978 allowed women to continue working throughout pregnancy, but also offered protection from hazardous working conditions without penalty. The worth of senior citizens was validated with the passage of the Age Discrimination Act of 1967. It took a bit longer for the physically disabled, but their political action saw fruit with the passage of the Americans with Disabilities Act of 1990 (ADA). These laws specifically disallow discrimination on the basis of sex, color, race, religion, pregnancy, national origin, age, or physical ability. The ADA mandates that a physical disability cannot be an issue in an employment decision if the individual is qualified or could be made qualified to do the job by a "reasonable accommodation" on the part of the employer (Cox, 1994).

These laws affect many areas of our society, including education, but they are especially relevant to the workplace. They provide regulatory guidelines for human resource decisions and are often used or threatened to be used in grievances or legal actions against employers. There is still debate about how much difference can be tolerated, as demonstrated in the controversies around English as a national language and the teaching of Ebonics. In addition, lesbian and gay advocates have not been as successful in gaining legal protection of alternative lifestyles, but they continue to challenge current laws. Although there has been progress toward improved race relations and increased opportunities for minorities, negative attitudes remain and discriminatory practices are still widespread (Feagin, 1991; Fredrickson, 1988).

Our society continues to change rapidly. Changing demographics include new immigration groups, maturing of the "baby boomers," exponential increases in the numbers of elderly, and minorities becoming the majority in some areas of the country. The United States ranks sixth in the number of Latinos/Hispanics in the world. Given their demographic characteristics, it is predicted that Latinos/Hispanics will shortly become the largest national ethnic/racial population in the United States (Molina & Aguirre-Molina, 1994).

During the years 1990 to 2010, the U.S. population is expected to grow by 42 million. Latinos/Hispanics will account for 47 percent of this increase, African Americans for 22 percent, and Asians and other people of color, 18 percent. The European American population is expected to account for only 13 percent of that growth (Loden & Rosener, 1991). It is important to note, however, that these population groups are not unidimensional groupings. There are many different cultures within each of these broad racial and ethnic groups. Mexican Americans may have different norms and values than Cubans and Puerto Ricans. The many Indian cultures of Latin America have had an influence on some Hispanic groups, but not all. The same is true of African Americans, and there are many different cultures within that broad rubric. Some Latinos identify themselves as Black, but persons from the Caribbean Islands have a very different culture than those whose historical origins are the African continent. In the same way, the culture of Haitians differs from that of Jamaicans or Black Puerto Ricans. Tribal differences in Africa also created different cultures in the Americas. Finally, many cultures have strong religious ties that overlay racial and ethnic identity. This is especially true in the European American population.

■ HEALTH CARE DELIVERY ISSUES

There are many challenges in making health care relevant to such a multicultural population. Commitment to their own cultural beliefs, values, and practices, which can include reliance on folk medicine and noncompliance with treatment programs designed by health professionals, has brought health care consumers into conflict with white, mainstream health professionals (Boyle & Andrews, 1995; Iturrino, 1992; Malone, 1993; Spector, 1996). In one study, nonwhite nursing assistants recognized more culturally based problems and had more disagreements with care for nonwhite patient populations than staff nurses and nurse managers (Lowenstein & Glanville, 1995). Although the nonwhite staff nurses and managers did not report as many problems as the nursing assistants, they did report more cultural prejudice than their white counterparts.

Cultural conflict can also occur when health care employees come from a wide variety of cultural backgrounds (Spangler, 1992). The composition of the health care workforce continues to change. For many years, historical circumstances, culture, and politics affected the employment of minorities in the health care industry, relegating them to lower pay and dead-end positions. In the 1980s and early 1990s, the health care workplace expanded, and new immigrants took their place at the bottom rung of the labor pool. They filled the unskilled labor positions needed in hospitals, long-term care facilities, and home care agencies, working alongside members of other minority groups (Svehla & Crosier, 1994). Conflict can occur among these low-status workers as new groups come in with different values and ideas than those already there. Competition for jobs can also increase tensions among minority groups.

It is not only the composition of nonprofessional staff that has changed. Methods to increase the registered nurse labor pool in an era of shortage resulted in recruitment and hiring of nurses trained in other countries (Jein & Harris, 1989). Foreign medical graduates were also recruited to fill positions in areas with physician shortages. Global travel and migration also affect the mix of health personnel. Increasingly, health professionals are multinational as well as multicultural. By 1990, one Los Angeles hospital reported that over 60 percent of its employees were minority group members (Burner, Cunningham, & Hatter, 1990), a trend that is increasing in many areas around the country.

Supervisor, employee, and patient responses to increasing cultural diversity have great potential for conflict, especially in the current era of restructuring and downsizing. Besides the possibility of culturally insensitive patient care, some health care consumers react poorly to being cared for by members of other racial or ethnic groups. Nonwhite nurses and nursing assistants have reported instances of racial slurs and prejudicial behaviors from their patients (Lowenstein & Glanville, 1995).

Professional and nonprofessional employees who hold different cultural and professional values may interpret managerial actions and decisions differently. Management decisions may be interpreted as favoritism for one race or another. These feelings may be expressed in different ways, from outright anger and verbal exchanges to silent resentment and lowered productivity. Negative racial attitudes and differing cultural expectations and values between employees of diverse cultural and educational backgrounds can result in underlying tensions between the groups. However, when well managed, diversity has also been shown to be a great strength for an organization (Cox, 1994; Fernandez, 1991; Jamieson & O'Mara, 1991; Loden & Rosener, 1991; Shea & Okada, 1992; Svehla & Crosier, 1994).

Research has shown that urban/suburban hospital executives report a more diverse workforce than rural hospitals, and diversity management programs have been concentrated in teaching hospitals (Wallace, Ermer, & Motshadi, 1996). However, it can be argued that although rural hospitals may em-

ploy a smaller number of culturally diverse groups, minorities are still represented, and often the nonprofessional level may be a largely minority population, whereas the professional staff is primarily white (Lowenstein &
Glanville, 1995). The importance of this staffing pattern is that administrators
have been shown to have a different perception of the workplace environment than that of their staff or patients, especially in regard to perceptions of
racial or cultural overtones in the environment (Cox, 1994; Lowenstein &
Glanville, 1995; Mays, 1995; Pinderhughes, 1996).

The challenge for nurses in patient care administration is twofold: first, to
ensure culturally relevant care for patients, and second, to capitalize on the
strengths of the workforce while reducing the potential for destructive conflict. When diversity can be tapped for creativity and new ways of problem
solving, a multicultural environment can be very rewarding for employees
and the organization, and productivity and efficiency can increase (Jamieson
& O'Mara, 1991; Loden & Rosener, 1994).

■ THEORETICAL ISSUES AND RESEARCH IN CULTURAL DIVERSITY

Group Identity

Social identity theory postulates that the concept of self is developed by a
combination of individual characteristics and by the various groups with
which one is affiliated (Ashforth & Mael, 1989). These group identities play a
part in how we define ourselves, but just as importantly, they influence how
others view us. Identification as a group member may be voluntary or involuntary. Socialization into accepted group norms, values, and behaviors can
occur for an individual member, but others outside a group may perceive a
stereotypical perception of all group members that does not accurately relate
to an individual group member. In actuality it is the combination of individual
and multigroup identities that makes each person unique (Cox, 1994). In
some ways, identification of group characteristics can be compared to probability theory. Each roll of the dice has its own probability, which is different
than the probabilities of outcome for a series of rolls. In the same way, although research may define group commonalities, each individual is unique,
and although that individual may belong to a group, he or she may adhere to
most, some, or none of the group's values, norms, and behaviors.

Groupings do not require formal organizational structures, such as those
found in religious orders, but may consist of informal similarities. Individuals
can define themselves through gender, racial/ethnic group, nationality, religion, friendship groups, employment groups, family groups, motherhood or
fatherhood, weight and height, wealth or poverty, student or worker (or
both), dog or cat owner, and so on. Nurse identity groups differ from physician identity groups and those two groups both differ from administration
identity groups. Each person defines herself or himself as belonging to many

different groups, both consciously and unconsciously. Cultural diversity as a term is most commonly used in relation to age, gender, racial/ethnic identity, physical disability, and lifestyle preferences. Socioeconomic class may also be considered within this category.

Cox (1994) used an interesting exercise to explore multigroup identifications. He asked his graduate students to sketch out a large circle as a pie chart of the group identity portion of their self-concept, answering the question "Who am I?" He requested that the pie be broken into sections in order of percentages of space occupied by their different group affiliations. There were major differences among students of different gender, race, and nationalities, often expressing common cultural traits. The Japanese student was the only one to identify a large percentage of himself as an employee. This is consistent with the well-known tendency for Japanese employees of large Japanese companies to have a high degree of company loyalty and identification. In the same exercise, race was more salient than gender for the African American respondent and gender more salient than race for the female respondent. The European American male indicated that the major determining factors of his self-concept were based on his individuality and not group identity, despite his understanding that this was an exercise to explore only the part of his self-concept that was reflective of group affiliation. Cox (1994) has found similar results in other European American men reflecting the emphasis on individuality as a strong cultural norm for this population. His research also demonstrates that European American men are often less aware of group identities than members of minority groups.

Cox (1994) theorizes that an individual's participation in an identity group occurs because of two factors, phenotype and culture. These factors are not mutually exclusive and, indeed, may operate simultaneously. Phenotype is based on physical and visible differences between groups. Assignment of a person to a phenotype group may not be voluntary. Others may identify and interact with them based on a phenotype characteristic regardless of how they think of themselves. Phenotype includes gender, skin color, and other physical characteristics, such as visible disabilities. Reactions to phenotype groups vary widely by individual, but certain patterns are more likely. For a long time, skin color was an important factor among African Americans and it continues to be so for many. Lighter skin traditionally denoted higher status within the wider community but had the opposite reaction in groups that stressed African American identity with phrases such as "black is beautiful." It has been documented that "whiter" racial and ethnic minorities report less racism than those whose appearance is less Euro-American (Fernandez, 1981). The same lighter–darker skin tone effects have been noted among Hispanics (Cox, 1994; Molina & Aguirre-Molina, 1994). Lesser status is associated with physical disabilities, obesity, and other physical differences. Women also report discrimination based on phenotype. Research in gender issues in the workplace has demonstrated that women applying for managerial positions who dressed in less feminine and more conservative, slightly masculine clothing were more likely to be hired (Jenkins & Atkins, 1990).

Cultural identity is based on sociocultural, as opposed to physical, distinctiveness. Members of cultural identity groups tend to share certain world views, norms, values, and goal priorities that distinguish one group from another. They may also share preferences for certain clothing, foods, music, art, and entertainment.

Two prominent approaches are used to describe racial/ethnic identity structures: stage of development models and acculturation models. These models describe the degree to which a person considers himself or herself to be a part of a specific racial/ethnic group, and how likely he or she is to interact with outsiders.

Stage of development models describe a linear process from lower to higher development of a culturally sensitive interaction pattern. Each stage is a "higher" level of identity formation than the previous one. However, as in any developmental hierarchy, many people are seen as not reaching the top level and remain somewhere lower on the continuum. Common themes among the various stage models are that individuals begin in a state of ignorance and total insensitivity; pass through several stages of struggle with identity, the individual's own as well as that of others; and finally reach a state transcending group identity, with the ability to be aware of and accept their own identity as well as that of others. At the highest level, there is also an interest in learning from members of other groups and an avoidance of prejudice (Cox, 1994).

Persons in the lowest stage often deny that racioethnic identity is relevant in interpersonal relations. They may be unaware or uncaring about how their actions affect others outside of their own cultural group. For many people this can be a conscious or unconscious way to avoid cultural issues that may be uncomfortable. Malone (1993) calls this the epidemic of color blindness, and notes that rewarding this behavior allows others to "become infected with the need to appear color-blind" (p. 23). She strongly contends that nurses in today's multicultural health care environment can no longer sustain this behavior and must develop models that successfully engage and manage cultural and racial differences in both patient care and in the development of managerial positions for minority nurses.

Increased awareness that racial/ethnic issues are affecting interpersonal interactions moves people toward the middle stage. In this stage, a person becomes aware of the negative effects of some behaviors on those who are different, realizes that many habitual behaviors are wrong, and recognizes a need for change. At the same time, the person feels unsure how to behave. Accompanying emotions may include anger, guilt, and confusion. As the women's movement grew, this reaction could be seen in men, as they tried to understand how their behavior harmed women and tried to define the new roles in society that they saw as being forced on them. This middle stage is an emotional time and a time when people are open to interventions to assist them in the transition to the next stage. Cultural diversity programs are often used both to increase awareness for those in early stages and to develop sensitivity and new behaviors regarding cultural issues for individuals in the middle stage.

By the final stage, the emotional turmoil and uncertainty of the middle stages have been worked through to a point where the individuals are fully aware of their identity, are comfortable with it, and will often seek opportunities to further examine the implications of group differences on human transactions as well as to actively combat prejudice and discrimination.

Acculturation models of culture identity measure the extent to which an individual identifies with the culture of his or her family of origin versus that of the majority or dominant group. They also seek to describe the mixture of cultural identities. Those who are multicultural are seen as most sensitive and interested in others' culture and perceptions. Spector's (1996) "heritage consistency" tool includes concepts important to cultural, ethnic, and religious background. It measures the extent to which people maintain their traditional heritage and the depth of that heritage, which includes the level of assimilation into the dominant U.S. culture. She advocates that nurses perform heritage assessments to enhance awareness of patient needs and potential patient responses to health care therapy and education that may conflict with deeply held cultural, religious, or ethnic values and ideas.

Much of the acculturation model research classifies individuals as monocultural majority, monocultural minority, or bicultural (Cox, 1994). Those individuals classified as belonging to the monocultural majority subscribe totally to the norms and value system of the cultural majority or dominant group. The majority culture in the United States is described as a Western European cultural system. Monocultural minority individuals demonstrate behaviors based on the norms and values of their minority group and reflect a minimum of assimilation to majority group norms. Examples of this group would include those from Amish or highly orthodox Jewish communities as well as immigrants who, although they have been in the United States for many years, may know only their native language and customs. Individuals who identify strongly with both the majority group culture and their minority group are said to be bicultural or multicultural.

Within the acculturation models is an awareness that few people are totally monocultural and each person belongs to many cultures. The Chinese American who speaks Chinese at home, has primarily Chinese friends, and teaches Chinese culture to her children with a strong sense of pride in Chinese history and culture may demonstrate one form of monocultural identification. On the other hand, to the degree that she works and has friendships with non-Chinese, encourages her children to be aware of American culture and history, adopts some of the majority views, and otherwise sees herself as Chinese, American, female, Christian, and a nurse, she is multicultural.

Some researchers consider all African Americans bicultural in the sense that there is a distinctive repertoire of standardized African American behaviors that are simultaneously present with behavioral patterns derived from the dominant culture. Socialization into both systems begins at an early age and continues throughout life, with both systems generally of equal importance in most individuals (Locke, 1992; Pinderhughes, 1996). The degree to which African Americans should be unique and the degree to which they should assimilate is controversial within this group. The Ebonics issue demonstrates some of the controversy involved in this area. Ebonics is a dialect of the English language spoken in many African American homes and neighborhoods. Some notable African Americans believe that teaching Ebonics as a subject in schools will provide recognition of heritage and uniqueness. Another group of notable African Americans believes it will slow acceptance into the mainstream culture and handicap the ability of those so taught to acquire high-status employment.

Cognitive dissonance may occur when a person's behavior is perceived as incongruent with cultural expectations (Cox, 1994; Locke, 1992). Consider the following example: A Vietnamese patient recognized a Vietnamese name on a nurse's nametag and began to speak to her in Vietnamese. In actuality, although this nurse's family background was Vietnamese, she had been born in the United States and did not speak the language or understand the culture very well. She and the patient had very conflicted feelings about this situation as they tried to communicate. In some instances, such feelings can turn into anger, hostility, or guilt.

Cultural Assessment and Cultural Norms

Cultural assessment research has provided tools to make health care more relevant to multicultural patients. The researchers agree that a helping professional's repertoire should include cultural adaptation of assessment, intervention, teaching, and evaluation skills. They vary, however, in the specific cultural elements they prescribe for use in performing a culturally sensitive assessment. Locke (1992), for instance, uses ten elements: degree of acculturation, poverty, history of oppression, language and the arts, racism and prejudice, sociopolitical factors, childrearing practices, religious practices, family structure, and values and attitudes. Giger and Davidhizar (1995) use six elements: communication, space, time, social organization, environmental control, and biological variation. Spector (1996) and Molina and Aguirre-Molina (1994) emphasize the importance of assessing the level of health beliefs and practices such as folk medicine and alternative therapies in every cultural assessment, as well as the role of family in patient care, and use of language and verbal meaning. Pinderhaus (1996) includes assessing how culture influences the power balance between provider and client, and the nature of provider's reactions to client empowerment. All of these authors, however, agree that helping professionals must recognize individual differences and balance those differences with the overall depth of cultural group identity in working with any patient.

Cox (1994) views knowledge of cultural assessment as promoting multi-cultural understanding in organizations. He identifies six areas of cultural differences in relation to gender, nationality, and racioethnic groups that are relevant to the workplace. These are: (1) space and time orientation, (2) leadership style orientation, (3) individualism versus collectivism, (4) competitive versus cooperative behavior, (5) locus of control, and (6) communication styles.

It has been reported that physical distance between persons conversing in public places varies widely and is affected by cultural norms (Hall, 1982). For instance, members of Arab cultures stand closer together than do those persons from Western societies. Standing, sitting close together, and physical touching during conversation are characteristic of many Latino-based cultures. Latinos favor and respond best to a congenial, personal manner and may respond better to a brief social conversation before beginning serious discussions (Molina & Aguirre-Molina, 1994). European Americans tend to prefer more distance. Moreover, there also are gender-related definitions of culturally appropriate distance. Violation of personal space norms creates psychological discomfort, and people may move to create the distance they are comfortable with. Persons from other cultures may interpret movement away from or up to them as rude behavior, and the stage can be set for interpersonal misunderstanding (Cox, 1994).

Other nonverbal behaviors are also culturally determined. When in conversation, cultural groups may differ in their degree of eye contact. European Americans may consider lack of eye contact an insult; but to some members of Asian cultures, not looking directly at the speaker is a sign of respect and making eye contact would signify an insult to the speaker (Cox, 1994).

Time orientations have been classified into linear–separable, circular, and procedural. Linear–separable time consists of past, present, and an infinite future. Time is seen as separable into quantifiable, discrete units, with fixed beginnings and endings. Circular time orientation involves repeated cycles of activities that focus on the past and present, rather than the future. Procedural time orientation treats time as irrelevant. Behavior is activity-driven and takes as much time as is needed for its completion. African American and Hispanic cultures report a more circular and procedural orientation than American culture (Asante & Asante, 1985; Cox, 1994; Molina & Aguirre-Molina, 1994). The description "CP (colored people) time," is used among African Americans to refer to culturally permissible lateness. It may be viewed as culturally normal to arrive late, and to treat starting and ending times with great flexibility (Cox, 1994). Languages have different concepts of time to reflect differing cultural origins.

Cultural and gender differences regarding preference for styles of leadership have also been described. Styles may be classified as task versus relationship and democratic versus autocratic. For some cultures, the primary emphasis among workers may be on relationships rather than task accomplishment. Task accomplishment is still valued, but it is achieved within a context in which rapport and relationships are addressed first or friendships may take precedence over institutional procedures. Research into Mexican culture has demonstrated a greater preference among workers for relationships, but that does not translate to a preference for democratic approaches. Mexican workers may expect a "boss" to give orders and not to be questioned, but those orders must be given with respect for the worker, regardless of where the worker stands on the hierarchy (Grossman & Taylor, 1995; Stephens & Greer, 1991). Many Asian cultures promote harmony and seek to avoid confrontation, whereas Western cultures tend to promote assertiveness. Thus, nurses from Asian cultures may not confront a supervisor or a physician, even when they disagree with the assignment or order; this may be difficult for an American nurse to understand (Jein & Harris 1989). Gender studies have confirmed that women are more relationship-oriented in their approach to work than men (Belenky et al., 1986). These issues can also surface in consumer responses to health care professionals.

Another distinction that is culturally based is the value of the individual versus the collective group (Bochner & Hesketh, 1994). Research has shown that the European American culture is high on the individualist scale, whereas the African American, Native American, Latino, and Asian cultures are more collectively oriented (Hofstede, 1984; Triandis, McCusker, & Hui, 1990).

People in individualistic societies emphasize values that may include autonomy, competitiveness, achievement, and self-sufficiency, whereas those from collectivistic cultures value interpersonal harmony, cooperation, and group solidarity. Collectivists are more likely to sacrifice personal interests for the attainment of group goals, and to be more satisfied with team-based rewards (Cox, 1994). However, gender differences complicate the scenario; women have been shown to be less competitive than men and to enter into helping behaviors more often (McClintock & Allison, 1989). Jein and Harris (1989) point out that nurse managers may find Asian nurses more cooperative and accepting of assignments than their American counterparts. However, the Asian nurse who perceives assignments as consistently unfair may choose to leave the position rather than confront the issue.

There is evidence that members of different culture groups differ in locus of control orientations (Cox, 1994). Americans tend to have a more internal locus of control, to believe that they themselves are the primary cause of events in their lives. On the other hand, fatalism, which includes a belief of predetermination of events and/or the control of events by God, may be found more often among members of some Arab, Asian, Latino, and African American cultures than in European cultures. However, some American fundamentalist religious groups may also share a fatalistic view.

Members of racial/ethnic minority groups may have a more external locus of control than majority group members because they are aware of how prejudice and discrimination reduce personal control. Cox (1994) found that women and members of low-power groups such as nursing assistants may also have a more external locus of control. One area where this concept is important is in the perception of advancement opportunities in the system. Cox notes that motivation and reward systems of U.S. organizations tend to be built on assumptions of an internal locus of control. However, some group members may not believe that individual achievement will lead to promotion. Furthermore, because of perceived discriminatory attitudes or behaviors, they may feel they have no chance for any reward under that system. Thus, they experience lower work motivation.

Communication styles have a major influence in interpersonal relationships. Tannen (1990) is well known for her research into gender differences in the use of language. Additionally, men and women may interpret the same words differently. Rich (1974) and Kochman (1983) found that African Americans and European Americans assigned different meanings to verbal and nonverbal behaviors, but were not aware of the differences. As a result, there were many miscommunications. Building on Kochman's work, Asante and Davis (1985) found that in addition to different cultural meanings, power position also mediated interpretation. In studying African American–white interactions, they found that what a white supervisor considered a request was more likely to be interpreted by African Americans as a demand. They also found differing concepts of persuasion and suggestion influenced employees' acceptance of task assignments.

Although some Asian cultures have communication styles that encourage shyness, modesty, deference, and reserve, other cultures such as African Americans encourage verbal attention seeking by self-assertion and expression of emotion. European Americans usually fall somewhere between both of these styles. Differing styles can create hostile feelings among work team members when some members feel that the style in use is inappropriate, based on the way they themselves would discuss an issue (Cox, 1994; Patterson & Smits, 1974).

The use of native languages by some employee groups may incite hostility and dissension among others outside that group. In actuality, many foreign-born persons are more comfortable using their own language and may not be aware of the effect on other staff. To reduce feelings of exclusion, some employers have required all employees to speak only English while at work. In most instances, this action has not decreased tension; in fact, tensions have been exacerbated. In addition, bilingual employees view forced compliance with English as a form of discrimination. As a result, court cases in this area are increasing (Fink, Robinson, & Wyld, 1996). In one court case, a hospital had restricted the Filipino nurses on the evening shift from speaking Tagalog, because the non-Filipino nurses contended that the behavior was disruptive and rude and they were being left out of the conversations (Dimaranan v. Pomona Valley Hospital, 1991). The case was decided in favor of the hospital. Fink and associates (1996) note that regardless of the legal permission to uphold the English-only rule, court cases are divisive and costly, and policies such as this should be used only as a last resort.

Stereotyping, Prejudice, and Discrimination

A stereotype can be characterized as "a fixed and distorted generalization made about all members of a particular group" (Loden & Rosener, 1991, p. 58). Many stereotypes come about through lack of contact between groups. Rooda (1996) found that white nurses who worked in settings with few African American patients had more biases about African Americans than did those working in settings with a large number of African American patients. Stereotypes of groups can be either positive or negative, but the main concept of distortion of reality holds. Stereotyping sets up expectation of behaviors. Persons who hold negative stereotypical ideas of a particular culture may still have positive feelings toward individual members of that culture. In those instances, their mindset functions to isolate the members from the stereotyped group behaviors, explaining that the person or persons they like behave differently than the overall group, and are not like the rest. On the other hand, positive stereotypes of a group can create conditions in which individual group members who are unable to function to the level of the stereotype can be ostracized (Kim, 1994).

Loden and Rosener (1991) note that the difference between stereotyping and prejudice is that prejudice involves judgments about specific cultural groups that reinforce a superiority/inferiority belief system. Stereotypes are then used to support and reinforce the prejudices. Discrimination refers to the actual negative behaviors that are shown to the out-group.

Cox (1994) notes that there are three sources from which prejudice and discrimination arise: intrapersonal factors, interpersonal factors, and societal reinforcement factors. Intrapersonal factors relate to certain personality types that have been shown to be more prone to prejudice and discrimination than others. One type is the authoritarian personality, which encompasses a constellation of several traits including less tolerance of minority groups, aggressiveness, power orientation, political conservatism, cynicism, and conforming to the prevailing authority structure. Another type is the person with low tolerance for ambiguity. Because cultural diversity creates uncertainty about expectations of human behavior, low tolerance persons feel threatened and are more likely to react negatively.

Interpersonal sources of prejudice include perceived physical attractiveness, communication proficiency, and effects from the history of intergroup relations (Cox, 1994). Prejudice against those who are physically unattractive or disabled takes many forms, including lower expectations in performance. Speech patterns such as stuttering, other regional dialects, African American dialects, or accented English may elicit negative prejudice and inhibit career promotion. Communication difficulties and/or prejudices may increase isolationism and separate groupings of employees.

Cox (1994) reports that a history of negative intergroup relationships has micro- and macro-effects that influence interpersonal feelings. Micro-effects refer to group identity-based experiences that we all have in our own personal histories that partly shape our attitudes toward other groups. These may include impressions of being excluded from an activity because of race or ethnicity. Because these personal experiences are numerous and vivid in minority group members, many are prejudiced against majority group members. Conversely, many majority group members are unaware of their own legacy of privilege and the personal histories of minority group members and are baffled and confused by negative initial interactions with minority group members.

The macro-effect refers to prejudicial feeling arising from significant intergroup historical events in which a given individual did or did not personally participate. Examples include African American feelings about segregation, Native American feelings about their ancestors being required to leave their tribal lands to move to reservations, or Japanese American responses to internment during World War II. For many persons in these groups, this sense of history has influenced their feelings about the majority group that they view as responsible for these events, even when the events happened long ago.

Prejudice is often reinforced by social forces (Cox, 1994). The way in which groups are portrayed in the media can be controversial. Portrayals of women often reinforce idealized models that are unattainable or undesirable for most women. The elderly and physically disabled are often ignored or presented using unflattering stereotypes. There has been much discussion about the failure of the educational system to provide appropriate information about Native Americans, African Americans, and other minorities in textbooks. Finally, despite legal prescriptions against various forms of discrimination, societal tolerance of sexual harassment and other prejudicial and discriminatory behaviors is alive and well.

■ MANAGING CULTURAL DIVERSITY

Much of the work in creating a climate that respects and uses cultural diversity for positive outcomes must be accomplished at the upper levels of management. The overall organizational climate and commitment of upper management is crucial to achieving this goal. Many organizations sponsor cultural diversity workshops as a singular method of reducing tensions and encouraging the valuing of diversity. Workshops in themselves cannot be effective without a strong context of policies, procedures, and accountability supported by the organizational management and clinicians. Too often, diversity departments are formed because they look good or seem the "right thing to do," but are then denied the resources and backup they need to do their job (Cox, 1994; Loden & Rosener, 1991; Svehla & Crosier 1994).

Diversity workshops focus on trying to reframe thinking and patterns of behavior. Sensitivity exercises are used to increase participants' awareness of minority members' feelings of exclusion and isolation. Although the impact may be felt at the time, the effects may soon wear off if opportunities are not provided to learn and practice new behaviors within the work environment. Because these workshops can also bring intense and damaging emotional issues to the surface, they need to be developed and run by experienced professionals in the field. Workshop organizers need to be able to deal with psychiatric emergencies that can occur because of repressed feelings and experiences. Another reaction by participants may be feelings of depression at the overwhelming scope of problems. However, competent workshop providers try to give participants a sense that changes do not happen overnight, and even small changes can be positive and make an impact (Cox, 1994).

Nurse administrators have a responsibility to provide leadership in moving the organization in the direction of valuing diversity, and to promote acceptance and understanding of cultural diversity for both patients and staff. Malone (1993) challenges nurses to "stand and deliver," and systematically address caring for culturally diverse racial groups. Nurses also need to raise cultural awareness in the health care workforce and to capitalize on new paradigms and ways of doing business that benefit from multiculturalism (Rooda, 1992). Nurses need to lead the fight for adequate resources for programs and educational materials that improve cultural communication. Nurse administrators need to move beyond the discomfort of addressing racial/ethnic issues and encourage dialogue and experimentation with different ideas to promote positive change.

Ensuring Culturally Sensitive Patient Care

The nurse administrator must set the tone for culturally sensitive care by ensuring that the staff is knowledgeable about cultural differences and has the resources to work comfortably with health care consumers (Habayeb, 1995). Poole and associates (1995) point out that cultural management of work teams is not usually an integral part of the education of health professionals. The staff should be mobilized to collect data about the cultural groups commonly represented in the unit and share this with new employees. Staff members also need to discuss personal definitions of respectful behavior among themselves. Identification of appropriate translator services should be developed and cultivated in advance of the need to ease communication. Minority group staff members, including nursing assistants, can be encouraged to discuss culturally relevant care issues from their perspective. Patient follow-up after discharge can also be used to elicit information that may improve care. Constituting a consumer focus group around cultural sensitivity issues is another method that may increase awareness and responsiveness (Leininger, 1991). Identification of resource people elsewhere within the agency can be helpful when used to reduce tensions and provide new ideas for care.

Nurse administrators must recognize the possibility of patient–staff conflict because of cultural differences. Procedures for dealing with patient discourtesies to multicultural staff and staff discourtesy to patients because of cultural differences should be thought through and developed before incidents occur. Staff need to participate in planning for this potential problem and problem solving how they will act when it occurs.

Managing Workforce Issues in Multicultural Environments

Managing workforce diversity is not easy and issues or conflicts may appear when least expected. Disputes may start small, but escalate quickly. A small number may move into the legal arena, a costly affair. Cultural and racial tensions may interfere with productivity and goal achievement, lower morale, and negatively affect patient care. Establishing a climate of trust and caring for employee needs can buffer these tensions. The nurse manager cannot do this alone, but must enlist the help of staff and upper administration. Appropriate outside consultation may be needed to provide unbiased feedback for help in problem assessment, assistance in increasing staff awareness of issues involved, and mobilization activities to address the tensions. Opportunities for a safe dialogue need to be available. Resources need to be available outside the unit to allow staff access to persons they can confide in and feel comfortable with without fear of retaliation. Recognizing and rewarding the positive effect differences can have on the work climate can have a positive effect on creativity. Establishing this climate may take time, and, given the individuality of employees, all employees may not be comfortable or willing to work in this way. Strong resistance behaviors that cannot be turned around can keep tensions alive and growing. However, including clear expectations in the job description, orientation, and disciplinary procedures will prompt those who are unwilling to work productively to leave.

Encouraging minority nurses to move into leadership positions can stimulate minority staff to aspire to promotion. Schmieding (1991) describes one approach that, over a period of 2 years, developed a minority nurse group to aid in retention of minorities and facilitate advancement. Groups such as this take time to develop and need continuous administrative support. They can backfire if they are begun without commitment, lowering morale and reducing trust instead.

A Model of Conflict

Managers who work together with employees of different backgrounds are often hampered by communication issues, insensitivity, and inadvertent misjudgments. Discussing racial or cultural conflict makes people uneasy. Persons seeking to address these issues may be concerned that they will be labeled as racist if the subject is brought up. Kavanagh and Kennedy (1992) note a pattern of avoidance and discomfort when issues regarding cultural diversity arise. However, these issues exist and will not go away easily. Learning how to facilitate discussions of racial/ethnic differences may provide managers and staff nurses with a tool to use in intervening.

The Lowenstein-Glanville conflict model presented in Figure 4–1 was developed to identify the factors shaping how minor disputes grow and escalate into major disputes. The goal is for managers to intervene early and abort the process. The model is based on the work of Felstiner and associates (1981), who described the transformation continuum of disputes moving to legal suits or labor grievances. The continuum begins with an unperceived injurious experience (UNPIE). When this changes to a perceived injurious experience (PIE), the injury is first named, then blame is placed. Blame is transformed into a claim, which may then go into legal or labor action if no redress is made.

In the Lowenstein-Glanville model, the transformation of UNPIEs into PIEs is influenced by individual characteristics, organizational climate, organizational rewards and punishments. Individual characteristics of age and experience contribute to the way in which an incident is perceived. Maturity and experience can temper an employee's view of an incident. Socioeconomic status, social position, and gender provide a framework for expectations of treatment in the workplace, based on societal and job norms. Experiences within an employee's lifestyle, which are related to socioeconomic base, gender, and cultural environment, also contribute to an individual's perception of the possibility of prejudice contributing to an incident. All of these interact to shape a person's perception and transform a UNPIE into a PIE or not.

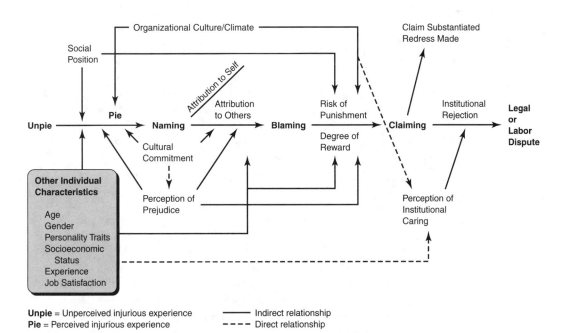

Unpie = Unperceived injurious experience
Pie = Perceived injurious experience

——— Indirect relationship
- - - - Direct relationship

FIGURE 4–1. Lowenstein–Glanville conflict model. *(Copyright Arlene Lowenstein, 1994. Used with permission.)*

Once the transformation to a PIE has occurred, the injury is named and the employees ascribe blame to themselves or to others. Individual characteristics, including social position, cultural commitment, and perception of prejudice continue to affect the course of attribution. Blaming one's self will most often end the process, whereas attribution to others may bring the grievance to the claiming stage. Social position, cultural commitment, and perception of prejudice also affect the transformation from blaming to claiming.

A person's social position in the organization will define her or his work, power, security, and who the person relates to on a regular basis. Those in higher positions are more likely to feel empowered to resolve the conflict and less likely to perceive prejudice against themselves. Cultural commitment is also of central importance. People vary widely in how consistent their cultural commitment is to their personal heritage. In the words of Spector, they may be "heritage inconsistent" (1996). Therefore, simply looking at race or culture does not provide enough information. This model reinforces the value of cultural assessment. Low cultural commitment reflects a lifestyle that is congruent with major elements of mainstream American culture. Likelihood to blame oneself is one cultural variable at play here; another is the value of assertion, confrontation, and individual justice.

Organizational culture and climate also influence the likelihood of the PIE moving to a claim. Organizational culture reflects the established formal and informal expected behaviors and the way grievances are handled within the work setting. This sets the framework against which employees can evaluate their own behavior and that of others in the workplace. Organizational climate also includes the employees' perceptions of organizational caring about employees based on observations of managers over time (Kahn, 1993).

An individual's perception of the risk of punishment or degree of reward enters the model at this point. Social position and employees' awareness of organizational climate influence that perception. If the organization substantiates a grievance and makes redress, the process will most likely end. When the organization rejects the claim, the perception of institutional caring may affect whether an employee continues the claim and the grievance transforms to a dispute requiring legal action or labor system mediation. Interventions along the way can reduce the risk of legal action.

Formal systems of appeal, ostensibly put into place to improve the processing of grievances have been found to function otherwise. Lewin (1987) found that employees who formally filed appeals and their managers were significantly more likely to quit, be fired, or have lower performance ratings and promotion rates than other employees. Miller and Sarat (1981) found that African Americans were at a distinct disadvantage for successful resolution of claims in relation to Whites, and that disadvantage was intensified in matters involving discrimination claims. This becomes more important when it is recognized that appeals are the major avenue in which minority group members, feeling a lack of power, may address conflict at work. Managers who desire the positive effects of diversity must try to avert formal claims and manage conflict earlier in the transformation process.

Conflict Interventions

Conflict may run the gamut from patent and obvious to hidden and festering (Kolb & Bartunek, 1992). Symptoms include: alienation, acceptance, denial, tension, distrust, annoyance, anger, verbal attacks, persistence, confrontation, and attempts at control (Rahim, 1985). Both ends of the spectrum can be destructive. Hidden conflict may result in low employee motivation and increasing anger. Situations can quickly turn nasty when culturally based conflict breaks out. People need time to back away from the emotions that are aroused. Although a commonly stated goal is "fairness" in conflict resolution, in reality there is no such thing as "fair." Each person has his or her own perception of what is fair, and they usually differ. Nurse managers should avoid stating this goal. Instead, they need to spend time trying to understand and reconcile each party's interest, to come out with a "win-win" situation. Ury and associates (1988) argue that reconciling interests is less costly than determining who is right, which in turn is less costly than determining who is more powerful.

Power plays are often used in cultural disputes through threats of lawsuit. Even though the majority-group member may have individual power in the setting, the minority member does have the power of law. Although it is sometimes necessary to seek redress by law, in most instances, disputes will not get that far, and managers should not allow themselves to be cowed by threats. The manager should redirect the claimant's energies by pointing out the disadvantages of seeking legal redress and the advantages of settlement with something for all to gain.

Some disputes may be best solved through use of a third party. Trained mediators may be able to view a dispute more objectively than fellow employees or managers and may provide a range of options for settlement. In many areas of the country, alternative dispute resolution is performed by trained volunteers at no cost to the individuals involved. Names of mediators can be obtained from many sources, including the local court system. Alternative dispute resolution may provide a way for all parties to get satisfaction, although there is also the risk of all parties being dissatisfied with the outcome.

The best way to treat conflict is to prevent it. This requires an institutional toleration for ambiguity with an emphasis on outcomes rather than sameness. Jamieson and O'Mara (1991) emphasize that managers must understand workforce differences due to cultural influences and need to move beyond the "one size fits all" model of management. Managers are challenged to look for ways to integrate—not assimilate—multicultural workers and to permit new ways of working. However, it is not enough to treat employees as individuals; the total organization must change, as well, to provide a climate that values difference.

In nursing, we have attempted to homogenize nurses into what are considered professional values, and to reward sameness and discourage and punish differences. We have begun to recognize diversity in patients, but as yet not in the nursing workforce. The nurse manager is in a pivotal position to identify, label, and deal with cultural differences and conflict resolution. Nurse managers must set the tone for their employees, but staff also have a responsibility to help their manager create a positive working climate. One method for doing this is to establish a comfortable climate for open discussion. Observe the current climate in meetings or interactions. Do staff feel free to discuss negative happenings and can they see and discuss positive ones? Do they feel that the climate is punitive? Do they feel administrative support for their ideas?

Communication patterns are often established through cultural conditioning. People from different cultures often use different methods and styles of communication to convey the same message (Loden & Rosener, 1991). Taking time to validate and clarify perceptions helps avoid the miscommunications that can so easily occur in multicultural environments. Too often people perceive things differently and are not willing to acknowledge that difference. A very common phrase found in conflict situations is "she/he should have known" just because "I know." Of course that is not possible. Stating and validating perceptions to another allows that person to recognize that you do not understand what he or she means. Clarifying helps bring agreement.

Persons from different cultural backgrounds may not view goals the same way. When recognized and facilitated, culturally diverse groups can work together to ensure similar goals and unit norms. Both individual and unit formal goals must be recognized and assisted to overlap. Individual goals must become congruent with organizational goals.

Finally, nurse managers must search for opportunities for staff to receive recognition, and find opportunities that can provide that recognition. Nursing assistants and LPNs have expertise in many areas. Recognizing what they do best and providing growth opportunities can be a major incentive, increasing perceptions of organizational caring, and reducing potential conflict situations. Finding each person's distinctive competence—what they do better than anyone else—and using it in the work situation also increases satisfaction and productivity. Valuing employees brings the best rewards to the employer.

■ BIOGRAPHICAL SKETCH

Arlene J. Lowenstein is a graduate of the diploma program of the Hospital of the University of Pennsylvania School of Nursing. She received a BSN from Fairleigh Dickinson University, a Masters in Nursing with a parent–child focus from New York University, and a PhD in Higher Education Administration from the University of Pittsburgh. In July 1996, Dr. Lowenstein became Professor and Director of the Graduate Program in Nursing, MGH Institute of Health Professions, in Boston. From 1985 to 1996, she was Professor and Chairperson for the Department of Nursing Administration at the Medical College of Georgia, in Augusta, Georgia. Previous administrative experience included serving as Director of Nursing at University of Kentucky Medical Center, in Lexington, Kentucky, and as Acting Director of Nursing at the Peter Bent Brigham Hospital, in Boston. Her research areas include racial and class conflict in the health care workplace; a study of relationships between nursing assistants, staff nurses, and nurse managers; hospital and community nurses' perception of discharge planning; and women with HIV/AIDS. She has published extensively.

■ SUGGESTED READINGS

Burner, O.Y., Cunningham P., & Hattar H.S. (1990). Managing a multicultural nurse staff in a multicultural environment. *Journal of Nursing Administration, 20* (6), 30–34.

Grossman, D., & Taylor, R. (1995). Cultural diversity on the unit. *American Journal of Nursing, 95* (2), 64–67.

Kolb, D.M., & Bartunek, J.M. (Eds.). (1992). *Hidden conflict in organizations: Uncovering behind-the-scenes disputes.* Newbury Park, CA: Sage.

Lowenstein, A.J. (1990). *Racial segregation and nursing education in Georgia: The Lamar experience.* Galveston, TX: Proceedings of the Conference of the American Association of History of Nursing, October.

Lowenstein, A.J., & Glanville, C. (1995). Cultural diversity and conflict in the health care workplace. *Nursing Economics, 13* (4), 203–209.

Malone, B. (1993). Caring for culturally diverse racial groups: An administrative matter. *Nursing Administration Quarterly, 17* (2), 21–29.

Poole, V., Giger, J, & Davidhizar, R. (1995). Delegating to multicultural teams. *Nursing Management, 26* (8), 33–34.

■ REFERENCES

Asante, M.K., & Asante, K.W. (Eds.). (1985). *African culture.* Westport, CT: Greenwood.

Asante, M., & Davis A. (1985). Black and white communication: Analyzing workplace encounters. *Journal of Black Studies, 16* (1), 77–93.

Ashforth, B., & Mael, F. (1989). Social identity theory and the organization. *Academy of Management Review, 14* (1), 20–39.

Belenky, M.F., Clinchy, B.M., Goldberger, N.R., & Tarule, J.M. (1986). *Women's ways of knowing.* New York: Basic Books.

Bochner, S., & Hesketh, B. (1994). Power distance, individualism/collectivism, and job-related attitudes in a culturally diverse work group. *Journal of Cross-Cultural Psychology, 25* (2), 233–257.

Boyle, J., & Andrews, M.M. (1995). *Transcultural concepts in nursing* (2nd ed.). Phiadelphia: Lippincott.

Burner, O.Y., Cunningham, P., & Hattar, H.S. (1990). Managing a multicultural nurse staff in a multicultural environment. *Journal of Nursing Administration, 20* (6), 30–34.

Carnegie, M.E. (1991). *The path we tread: Blacks in nursing, 1854–1984* (2nd ed.). New York: National League for Nursing.

Cox, T. (1994). *Cultural diversity in organizations: Theories, research & practice.* San Francisco: Berrett-Koehler.

Dimaranan v. Pomona Valley Hospital, 57 FEP Cases 315. (C. D. Cal. 1991).

Feagin, J.R. (1991). The continuing significance of race: Antiblack discrimination in public places. *American Sociological Review, 56,* 101–116.

Felstiner, W.L.F., Abel, R.L., & Sarat, A. (1981). The emergence and transformation of disputes: Naming, blaming, claiming. *Law and Society Review, 15* (3–4), 631–654.

Fernandez, J.P. (1981). *Racism and sexism in corporate life: Changing values in American business.* Lexington, MA: Lexington Books.

Fernandez, J.P. (1991). *Managing a diverse workforce.* Lexington, MA: Lexington Books.

Fink, R.L., Robinson, R.K., & Wyld, D.C. (1996). Balancing fair employment considerations in a multicultural and multilingual healthcare workforce. *Hospital & Health Services Administration, 41* (4), 473–483.

Fredrickson, G.M. (1988). *The arrogance of race: Historical perspectives on slavery, racism, and social inequality.* Middletown, CT: Wesleyan University Press.

Giger, J.N., & Davidhizar, R.E. (1995). *Transcultural nursing assessment and interventions* (2nd ed.). St. Louis: Mosby.

Grossman, D., & Taylor, R. (1995). Cultural diversity on the unit. *American Journal of Nursing, 95* (2), 64–67.

Habayeb, G.L. (1995). Cultural diversity: A nursing concept not yet reliably defined. *Nursing Outlook, 43* (5), 224–227.

Hall, E.T. (1982). *The hidden dimension.* New York: Doubleday.

Hines, D.C. (1989). *Black women in white: Racial conflict and cooperation in the nursing profession 1890—1950.* Bloomington, IN: Indiana University Press.

Hofstede, G. (1984). The cultural relativity of the quality of life concept. *Academy of Management Review 9,* 389–398.

Iturrino, H.E. (1992). *Hispanic diabetic elders: Self care behaviors and explanatory models.* Unpublished doctoral dissertation, University of Iowa.

Jamieson, D., & O'Mara, J. (1991). *Managing workforce 2000: Gaining the diversity advantage.* San Francisco: Jossey-Bass.

Jein, R.F., & Harris, B.L. (1989). Cross-cultural conflict: The American nurse manager and a culturally mixed staff. *Journal of the New York State Nurses Association, 20* (2), 16–20.

Jenkins, M.C., & Atkins, T.V. (1990). Perceptions of acceptable dress by corporate and noncorporate recruiters. *Journal of Human Behavior and Learning, 7* (1), 38–46.

Kahn, W.A. (1993). Caring for the caregivers. Patterns of organizational caregiving. *Administrative Science Quarterly, 38* (2), 539–563.

Kavanagh, K.H., & Kennedy, P.H. (1992). *Promoting cultural diversity.* Newbury Park, CA: Sage.

Kim, P.S. (Fall, 1994). Myths and realities of the model minority. *The Public Manager,* 31–35.

Kochman, T. (1983). *Black and white cultural styles in conflict.* Urbana, IL: University of Illinois Press.

Kolb, D.M., & Bartunek, J.M. (Eds.). (1992). *Hidden conflict in organizations: Uncovering behind-the-scenes disputes.* Newbury Park, CA: Sage.

Lewin, D. (1987). Dispute resolution in the nonunion firm. *Journal of Conflict Resolution, 31* (3), 465–502.

Leininger, M.M. (1991). Becoming aware of types of health practitioners and cultural imposition. *Journal of Transcultural Nursing, 2* (2), 32–39.

Locke, D.C. (1992). *Increasing multicultural understanding: A comprehensive model.* Newbury Park, CA: Sage.

Loden, M., & Rosener, J.B. (1991). *Workforce America! Managing employee diversity as a vital resource.* Burr Ridge, IL: Irwin.

Lowenstein, A.J., & Glanville, C. (1995). Cultural diversity and conflict in the health care workplace. *Nursing Economics, 13* (4), 203–209.

Malone, B. (1993). Caring for culturally diverse racial groups: An administrative matter. *Nursing Administration Quarterly, 17* (2), 21–29.

Mays, V.M. (1995). Black women, work, stress, and perceived discrimination: The focused support group model as an intervention for stress reduction. *Cultural Diversity and Mental Health, 1* (1), 52–65.

McClintock, C.G., & Allison, S.T. (1989). Social value orientation and helping behavior. *Journal of Applied Social Psychology, 19* (4), 353–362.

Miller, R.E., & Sarat, A. (1981). Grievances, claims, and disputes: Assessing the adversary culture. *Law & Society Review, 15* (3–4), 525–565.

Molina, C.W., & Aguirre-Molina, M. (1994). *Latino health in the US: A growing challenge.* Washington, DC: American Public Health Association.

Patterson, D.L., & Smits, S. (1974). Communication bias in black–white groups. *The Journal of Psychology, 88,* 9–25.

Pinderhughes, E. (1996). Developing theory as a personal response to systemic entrapment. *Cultural Diversity and Mental Health, 2* (3), 157–169.

Poole, V., Giger, J., & Davidhizar, R. (1995). Delegating to multicultural teams. *Nursing Management, 26* (8), 33–34.

Rahim, M.A. (1985). A strategy for managing conflict in complex organizations. *Human Relations, 38* (1), 81–89.

Rich, A.L. (1974). *Interracial communication.* New York: Harper & Row.

Rooda, L.A. (1992). The development of a conceptual model for multicultural nursing. *Journal of Holistic Nursing, 10* (4), 337–347.

Rooda, L.A. (1996). Attitudes of nurses toward culturally diverse patients: An examination of the Social Contact Theory. *Journal of Black Nursing, 6* (1), 48–56.

Schmeiding, N.J. (1991). A novel approach to recruitment, retention, and advancement of minority nurses in a health care organization. *Nursing Administration Quarterly, 15* (14), 69–76.

Shea, S., & Okada, R. (1992). Benefiting from workforce diversity. *Healthcare Forum Journal, 35* (1), 23–24, 26.

Spangler, (1992). Transcultural nursing care values and caregiving practices of Phillipine-American nurses. *Journal of Transcultural Nursing, 4* (2), 28–37.

Spector, R.E. (1996). *Cultural diversity in health and illness* (4th ed.). Stamford, CT: Appleton & Lange.

Stephens, G.K., & Greer, C.R. (1995). Doing business in Mexico: Understanding cultural differences. *Organizational Dynamics, 24* (1), 39–55.

Svehla, T.A., & Crosier, G.C. (1994). *Managing the mosaic.* Chicago: American Hospital Association.

Tannen, D. (1990). *You just don't understand: Women and men in conversation.* New York: William Morrow.

Triandis, H.C., McCusker, C., & Hui, C.H. (1990). Multi-method probes of individualism–collectivism. *Journal of Personality and Social Psychology, 59,* 1006–1020.

Ury, W.L., Brett, J.M., & Goldberg. (1988). *Getting disputes resolved: Designing systems to cut the costs of conflict.* San Francisco: Jossey-Bass.

Wallace, P.E., Jr., Ermer, C.M., & Motshabi, D.N. (1996). Managing diversity: A senior management perspective. *Hospital & Health Services Administration, 41* (1), 91–104.

CASE 4–1 A Workplace of Difference

Anne Dickinson Cohen

This is a particularly challenging time to be involved in health care, not only because of the way that care is delivered, but also because of the diversity of the consumers and providers of health care services. The demographics of the United States are changing. These trends were first widely discussed in the "Workforce 2000" report. In 1987, the Center for Immigration Studies and the Hudson Institute released this study of the predicted composition of the American workforce by the year 2000. After reviewing birthrates, immigration rates, and early retirement plans, a number of projections were made. In the year 2000, White males will make up 33 percent of the American workforce. Two-thirds of our workforce will be women and people of color. In addition, people of color, women, and immigrants will make up more than five-sixths of the net additions to the workforce between 1987 and the year 2000. White males will account for only 15 percent of new entrants into the U.S. workforce during this time.

These exact statistics have been revised and challenged by a number of sources; however, the trends remain constant. The Non-Hispanic White population is declining, while the populations of what used to be called "minority" groups such as Hispanic, Asian, Black, and American Indian populations are increasing.

Given these statistics, corporations will be challenged to create environments in which all employees can grow and prosper. Diversity training will not just be "the nice thing to do"; being able to work in a multicultural environment will be a distinct job skill.

Recently, issues on cultural diversity have been receiving increasing media coverage, in the news as well as on prime-time television. Hate crimes and bias incidents are on the increase throughout America. However, the employees of Beth Israel Medical Center in New York City are at an advantage in dealing with such issues because of the "A Workplace of Difference" program—a full-day workshop designed to educate and sensitize staff to issues of employee and patient diversity.

Early in 1991, the administration of Beth Israel looked at incidents that were occurring in the immediate environment of New York City. The administration wanted to be proactive in dealing with such incidents before they began to occur within the organization. Beth Israel has an extremely diverse staff and patient population. Although it is important not to generalize or stereotype individuals based on their heritage, cultural differences do have an impact on the workplace. Many of us have been educated with the concept of America as a "melting pot"—a place where all cultural characteristics were added to a huge pot and stirred up to become a singular American culture. This homogeneous culture has not developed—differences do exist, and if they are ignored, job satisfaction and productivity are decreased.

CASE 4-1 *Continued*

The result of this investigation was a collaboration with the Anti-Defamation League (ADL) of B'nai B'rith to present the ADL program, "A Workplace of Difference" at Beth Israel. All employees, including top management, were required to attend this dynamic program, and over 3,500 have done so since April 1991. The program is now a part of the new employees' orientation, to promote at the onset of employment that Beth Israel is a diverse workplace, and that discrimination is not an acceptable behavior in our work environment. Evaluations have been excellent; in fact, word of mouth has been so positive that employees have requested to attend.

Initially, six employees from Nursing Education and Human Resources were trained by the ADL to present the program at Beth Israel. Two instructors, who were as diverse as possible, were paired for each program. Class size has ranged anywhere from 10 to 100 participants, with an ideal class size of 20 to 30 to encourage as much participation as possible. Initially the program was designed to address issues of employee diversity, but early on it was recognized that these same concepts apply to how we treat the patients as well.

■ **PROGRAM GOALS AND CONTENT**

The basic concept of the program is that everyone seeks out what is comfortable and familiar to them—the "taste of home syndrome." There is nothing wrong with this, but if you have enough information about others, especially those you work with every day, you can expand your "taste of home." The goals for program participants are to:

- Increase awareness of one's own attitudes and beliefs about culture.
- Critically examine stereotypes and assumptions.
- Appreciate commonalities among different cultures.
- Identify enriching aspects of diversity in the workplace.

The program employs a number of exercises and videos to accomplish these goals. Usually, people will sit with someone they know, so the first exercise involves participants moving around and changing seats based on birth dates. They are now ready for small group discussion.

Another exercise is called "four questions." Each person is asked to describe his or her own heritage in four words. Participants then identify one important experience in their life that made them think about themselves in those terms, one positive thing about being that kind of person, and one difficult or embarrassing thing. Listing all the various descriptors of the group demonstrates the rich diversity of the small group of people in the class. Discussion of the positive and negative life experiences makes participants aware of seeing beyond limiting and inaccurate stereotypes in order to understand the individual.

The group is then given a cultural self-knowledge exam to assess knowledge of prominent people from a variety of cultural and religious backgrounds. Most participants are surprised to dis-

CASE 4–1 *Continued*

cover how little they know about people from cultures other than their own. The exercise becomes very easy with input from the entire group, illustrating the importance of group resources and being responsible for your expanding your own knowledge base.

The morning session ends with a very powerful film of an exercise first performed on schoolchildren, then repeated on adults. It demonstrates the potential in each of us to be both victims and perpetrators of prejudice. Discussion after the film reveals many issues, such as the fact that prejudice is a learned behavior, and that people tend to live up or down to others' expectations of them. All of these issues have great implications for the work environment.

The afternoon session involves watching a series of short video vignettes. Among the participants, some will view the videos as portraying outright discrimination; others will not be so sure. The discussion is always lively and demonstrates how stereotypes and assumptions can influence behavior. The program ends with each participant developing an action plan as to how he or she will use the material learned during the day in the work environment.

■ CASE STUDIES

Probably the most valuable part of the program is the personal stories shared by participants. There are always a few people who state at the beginning of the class that they do not understand the need for such a program; that it is simply better not to talk about these issues. By the end of the program, after listening to the experience of various colleagues, all have become more sensitive. Consider the following scenarios:

- A preceptor is working with a new nurse educated in the Philippines, who seems very quiet and never has any questions. Whenever the preceptor explains a new procedure or policy, the orientee nods her head, but will not make eye contact. The preceptor begins to rush through her explanations, assuming that the orientee either knows the information, or else is not interested. Soon the preceptor stops explaining how things are done.

- One Saturday, on a busy med-surg unit, the charge nurse becomes annoyed with her elderly, Orthodox Jewish patient. The previous day, the patient had no trouble using the call light and bed controls. Today, she will not use her call light and continuously calls out for the nurse to adjust the head of her bed. The nurse asks the patient not to call out but to use her call light, but the patient insists that she cannot. The nurse is frustrated—she feels that the patient just wants special attention.

- A nurse feels that some of the Hasidic Jewish fathers in the nursery do not trust her clinical skills. When she arrives with a new baby and tries to hand it to the fa-

CASE 4–1 *Continued*

ther, he asks her to place it on the bed. Only then will he pick the infant up. He will not take the baby directly from the nurse. Once she attempted to shake a father's hand in congratulations, but he looked at her outstretched hand and shook his head. The nurse felt rejected and confused.

- An Asian nurse, new to the country, is giving out medications with her preceptor. The preceptor observes that while the orientee's technical skills are excellent, she does not give any education about the medications. One patient refuses his medications, and the orientee says, "Just take it, your doctor ordered it, so it is good for you." Afterwards, the preceptor discusses the importance of patient education and patient rights. When a similar experience occurs a week later, the preceptor tells the head nurse that the orientee is clinically competent, but not a patient advocate.

- An instructor prepares to administer a CPR exam to a group of licensed practical nurses (LPNs) who have just arrived from Russia. After asking them to separate their seats, she distributes the test. Within 5 minutes, she hears them talking and looking at each others' answer sheets. The instructor is surprised and reminds them to keep their eyes on their own paper. Within minutes, the same thing occurs. The instructor angrily collects the papers, tells

them that cheating is not permitted, and sends the LPNs back to their units. The students seem confused.

Each of these scenarios represents a situation that can prove challenging for any nurse. The employees of Beth Israel are better prepared to deal with issues of cultural differences because situations such as these are discussed during the workshop. For instance, in certain Asian cultures it is considered a sign of disrespect to look an authority figure, such as the preceptor or educator, directly in the eye. It is also considered rude to question an authority figure, which might cause them embarrassment or "loss of face." People from Asian cultures are also not likely to be assertive; their culture emphasizes group harmony, not speaking up. In the American society, if someone does not look you in the eye or ask questions, you are likely to assume that he or she is disinterested, bored, or even untrustworthy. These cultural differences can easily lead to misunderstandings, especially on a busy unit.

The concepts of patient education and patient rights are alien in certain cultures—some Asian cultures even believe that it is a burden on patients to give them decision-making power. An Asian nurse may not realize the importance an American nurse will place on these issues. Additional classes on these topics may be necessary.

In the Hasidic Jewish culture, cultural and religious beliefs prohibit a man from touching women other than immediate

CASE 4–1 *Continued*

family. All orthodox Jews consider Saturday a holy day when they cannot do certain things—such as use any electrical appliances. A nurse who does not have this information may personalize an orthodox patient's actions, or just assume that the patient is being unfriendly or even difficult.

In some parts of Russia, tests are usually taken as a group. Discussion and debate is encouraged to learn new information. Also, to many Russians, handshaking and smiling are considered to be signs of frivolity and immaturity. The instructor who starts a class this way, or the nurse who greets a patient this way, may not be taken seriously.

■ STRATEGIES FOR NURSES

During the workshop, nurses learn strategies to deal with diversity issues. First, it is important for each of us to examine our own attitudes and stereotypes, and whether they affect our behavior. Most of us have been guilty of this at one time or another. Prejudice is a learned response, and it is up to each one of us to change our own behavior. To help prevent yourself from acting in this manner, start by asking a trusted friend or colleague to point out to you when you act on unfair assumptions—you may not even realize you are doing it. If you have made a foolish assumption, do not ignore it; apologize and offer explanations whenever possible. This leaves a person's dignity intact.

Second, do not ignore prejudice or stereotyping when it arises. Many of us are afraid of the tension surrounding these issues, but if you do not say anything, you send the message that you are in agreement with such behavior. Tension may be unavoidable, and some of these issues will not disappear without a struggle. Use the following guidelines to respond to others you feel have offended you:

- Speak to the person privately.
- Do not respond by attacking with an equally offensive comment.
- Assume that the person was not trying to offend you.
- Start off by telling the person why you value his or her relationship.
- Then explain why the comment or action bothered you.
- Do not preach or try to make the person feel guilty; make your point and then move onto other things.
- Finally, practice the diversity skills of asking questions and giving answers.

Following these guidelines will let other people know how you feel, without attacking them. We can all stand to learn more about ourselves and the people we work with on a daily basis. Ask your colleagues and patients about their cultural and religious beliefs, and tell them about yours. Only by discussing, explaining, understanding, and forgiving incidents will attitudes and behavior change.

■ BENEFITS OF DIVERSITY TRAINING

There are many benefits in successfully working with people of various cultures and beliefs. These include opportunities

CASE 4–1 *Continued*

for increased innovation and ideas, and enhanced recruitment and retention of skilled workers. Employees and patients both experience increased satisfaction and empowerment when their environment values and respects differences.

Although a one-day workshop is an important first step, Beth Israel continues to seek innovative initiatives to improve employee understanding of cultural traditions. Special grand rounds have been held on a variety of cultures; the Beatrice Renfield Division of Nursing Education and Research has planned joint training programs with the Chinatown Manpower Project for Asian health care workers; and in 1995, the Nursing Department made cultural awareness the focus for Nurse Recognition week.

In seeking numerous ways to understand diversity, Beth Israel Medical Center is rising to the challenge of an increasingly multicultural society. It is an organization that values diversity and is committed to creating an environment where all patients and employees, regardless of race, gender, religion, or sexual orientation, can grow and succeed.

■ BIOGRAPHICAL SKETCH

Anne Dickinson Cohen is the Acting Director and Staff Development Coordinator at Beth Israel Medical Center in New York City. She coordinates the activities of the 16 professional and support staff of the Beatrice Renfield Division of Nursing Education and Research. Most recently, she coordinated the staff education for the hospital reengineering initiative. First at NYU Medical Center, then at BI, she held progressively responsible positions in medicine, the operating room, and ambulatory surgery before becoming a nurse education specialist. Ms. Dickinson Cohen has a BS in Nursing from College of Mount St. Vincent in Riverdale, New York, and an MA in Nursing Administration from New York University. Her professional activities include national and regional presentations on managing cultural diversity and serving on the Continuing Education Review Team and other activities for the New York State Nurses Association. She is also certified by ANCC in Continuing Education and Staff Development.

■ SUGGESTED READING

Briehn, J. (1996). Creating an organizational climate for multiculturalism. *Health Care Supervisor, 14* (4), 11–18.

Baldonado, A. (1996). Transcending the barriers of cultural diversity in health care. *Journal of Cultural Diversity, 3* (1), 20–22.

Giger, J.N., & Davidhizar, R.E. (1995). *Transcultural nursing: Assessment and Intervention.* (2nd ed.). St. Louis: Mosby.

Hudson Institute for Labor Relations (1987). *Workforce 2000.* New York: Author.

Kavanagh, K.H., & Kennedy, P.H. (1992). *Promoting cultural diversity.* Newbury Park, CA: Sage.

Leininger, M. (1989). Transcultural nursing: Quo vadis: (where goeth the field?). *Journal of Transcultural Nursing, 1* (1), 33–45.

Locke, D.C. (1992). *Increasing multicultural understanding: A comprehensive model.* Newbury Park, CA: Sage.

Stewart, B. (1991). A staff development workshop on cultural diversity. *Journal of Nursing Staff Development, 7* (4), 190–194.

CASE 4–2 Feminist Management at a Community Health Center

Katrina H. Clark and Elizabeth Magenheimer

The Fair Haven Community Health Center is a 25-year-old community health center that serves the residents of an inner-city neighborhood in New Haven, Connecticut. Over the years, the Center has developed and implemented certain practices and policies that challenge the traditional male-dominated hierarchical medical models of health care delivery and management. We have identified three qualities that embody our philosophy of health care management: *education, empowerment,* and *nurturing.* We continually are challenged to structure and adapt our philosophy to create a model that promotes both quality patient care and a healthy and sane work environment.

The Center began as an alternative institution, inspired by the early 1970s dream of community people and health care providers working together to make health care accessible and affordable in an inner-city, low-income neighborhood. For many Americans, the early 1970s were a time of anti-war, anti-institution, and anti-establishment sentiment. The founders of the Fair Haven Center shared the ideals of the anti-establishment movement, but quickly found that it was one thing to demand that "health care is a right, not a privilege" and quite another to be confronted with the reality of providing those services.

Free clinics, alternative institutions, and neighborhood health centers sprang up by the hundreds throughout the country in the 1970s. Professionals worked with community people to bring health care into inner-city neighborhoods. By the mid 1970s, many of these institutions were forced to close when caught in the squeeze between patient care, economic survival, and their refusal to comply with bureaucratic demands of public funding.

The Fair Haven Community Health Center is an exception to that pattern. The Center also began as an alternative to city hospital clinics and the associated long waits, high costs, and fragmented, culturally alienating care. The Center initiated services by offering care to individuals with episodic problems. Over time new services were added as families began requesting ongoing care for their family planning, prenatal care, well-child care, hospital care, and chronic problems such as hypertension, diabetes, and arthritis. The Center developed a system of primary care providers, whom the patients could trust and know, long before the concept of the gatekeeper was created. Fair Haven health care providers began to look beyond episodic care to the life situations that influenced their patients' health, such as housing and welfare assistance. They came to realize it was more effective to get heat in an apartment than to continue to treat a variety of respiratory complaints.

The Center wanted to grow and change to meet the demands of the community and to provide continuity of care. We decided that we could hire

CASE 4–2 *Continued*

clinicians and increase our services without losing the sensitivity to patients that our dedicated volunteer physicians, nurses, and other workers provided. We accepted the challenge of increased paperwork, fiscal responsibilities, and intrusive governmental regulations and forms, while maintaining our values. We needed the autonomy of our own building, and the financial security of both public monies and third-party reimbursement.

The Center staff and Board of Directors creatively developed strategies that would allow the Center to survive and grow. The Center negotiated and became a model practice site for the Yale School of Nursing faculty and student nurse practitioners and midwives to provide comprehensive family-centered primary care. We applied for grants and state contracts to begin our prenatal and hypertension programs to meet community health needs. Our volunteer physicians helped us to find specialists in the private sector who would see our patients on referral. We successfully worked with our Health Systems Planning Agency to get our community designated as a Health Professional Shortage Area so that Fair Haven could apply for National Health Service Corps Scholars. We lobbied the General Assembly of the State of Connecticut to buy us a building. Hard work, hustle, having fun, taking risks, and sharing our vision of what we wanted to become have been the driving forces.

From an original $5,000 budget and 1,000 visits in a rented storefront and a local elementary school in 1971 the Center now, 25 years later, has an operating budget of over $4 million with 45,000 visits a year and our own building. The building is centrally located and community based so that the majority of patients can walk to the Center. We also operate three satellite clinics: one at an elderly housing complex and two school-based clinics. We offer comprehensive primary care services, with someone on call 24 hours a day, plus an array of educational support programs such as the Women, Infants and Children (WIC) Nutrition Program, childbirth preparation, diabetes and asthma support, HIV counseling, and outreach and referral services.

The Center currently has a staff of over 80 salaried employees, including 24 direct primary care providers (physicians, nurse practitioners, and nurse midwives). It is supported by federal, state, city, and private grants, which constitute 40 percent of the budget; the other 60 percent is generated through Medicaid, Medicare, private insurance, and patient fees, which are charged on a sliding fee scale. Since 1995, the Center has been dealing with the state's mandated managed care program for Medicaid recipients. This and other changes in the private sector, including Medicare patients moving into managed care and health maintenance organizations (HMOs), have created new financial and management challenges.

Within the context of these major changes, we feel even more committed to maintaining our management philosophy in order to retain our level of quality care and quality staff. For many professionals who work at the Center, salaries are lower than what they might be in a

CASE 4–2 *Continued*

more traditional institution; the social and economic problems that confront our patients are also more frustrating. However, the rewards of caring for whole families as primary care providers, of working where people function as a team and respect one another's opinions, and of knowing that the direct care provided is complemented by social service and community outreach and education activities all compensate for the costs.

■ **EDUCATION**

The importance of education permeates all levels of the Center: for professionals, for support staff, and for patients. Our emphasis on the importance of ongoing education, both formal and informal, constantly reminds team members that they can learn from each other. For example, professionals are often unaware of the cultural differences that stand as barriers to good patient care. When a pediatrician recommends to a Puerto Rican mother whose child has croup, that she open the windows at night to let in the cool, moist air, the pediatrician loses all credibility because the mother believes the night air is dangerous. The Center neighborhood worker helps to bridge the cultural gap by educating both the physician and the patient, helping to create a plan of care that is acceptable to the patient and will help the child. The Center strives to promote an environment that allows people to admit mistakes and improve; to trust others,

learn to give and take criticism, and help people to grow.

Formal education is encouraged through traditional continuing medical education for professionals plus release-time and tuition support for all staff members to take outside courses or work toward a college degree. Staff members are encouraged to use new skills within the organization. For example, one of our social service counselors started with us as a lab technician and is now, after 5 years, completing her Masters in Family Counseling. She is able to use her new skills and training with our patients.

The benefits of education and training go beyond the employee to the entire organization as people assume additional responsibilities and have more confidence in their work; they perform better at their jobs. Often it takes more time to teach a person new skills rather than hire someone who is already skilled. However, we feel this policy is part of our commitment to the community and to diversity. Our entry-level employees are usually local women, without a high school diploma or technical training, who are single heads of households. They bring knowledge of the community, their beliefs, perspectives, language, and problems. We train them as clerks, outreach workers, and receptionists.

Another aspect of education within the Center is formal in-service education. On a rotating basis, the clinicians present grand rounds to each other every Friday morning. This may be a literature review of a timely issue discussed by a

CASE 4–2 *Continued*

guest speaker, or a discussion of internal productivity, schedules, or clinical protocols. For 1 hour every 2 weeks, the entire staff meets for a general in-service session, which may involve a representative from an outside agency or one of our own clinicians presenting a medical topic such as asthma, hepatitis, or breast cancer screening. The better understanding the support staff has of the importance of what we do as a health center, the more effectively they will be able to communicate that to patients.

Over the past 7 years, the Center has developed an innovative program for allowing clinicians to exchange a clinical session for an education or administrative session. Examples of some of the projects that clinicians have undertaken include: an internist and a nurse practitioner developing diabetes protocols and education modules for patients; a pediatrician instituting an early literacy program, called Reach Out and Read; a developmental pediatrician providing support and training for child care providers; a midwife offering stress reduction and meditation techniques to patients and staff.

■ EMPOWERMENT

This element relates to empowering staff, community, and patients. For example, when a triage nurse returns a call for a prescription refill or a medical assistant takes the temperature of a 1-month-old infant, each contact is treated as an opportunity to empower patients to take more control over their own health care. As a result, the elderly patient understands how to take her pills with meals and the young parent learns to read her child's temperature. The entire staff understands that teaching and empowerment are essential for patients to gain control of their lives.

Participative decision making, consensual theory, quality circles, continuous quality management, and self-management are all terms that are currently popular. The Center has advocated these concepts for years. In putting them into operation, we have not erased the hierarchical conflict that exists in any institution, but we have found ways to minimize the stratification and medical task superiority. One example is that managers and clinical providers perform "lower level" support tasks that increase their appreciation and respect for the skills involved. Administrative staff take turns staffing the front desk, which gives them a better insight into why problems occur and allows a better understanding of how to work toward solutions.

On occasion, clinicians have complained that phone messages were not accurate or appropriate. A solution was to have clinicians attempt to answer phones; after that, they not only appreciated how difficult and stressful a task it was, but also developed improved systems for how to take messages, how to respond faster, and how to educate patients about their role in presenting accurate information. The receptionists on an ongoing basis evaluate their own messages for completeness and accuracy to improve their skills. A positive self-reinforcing cycle is created when people

CASE 4–2 *Continued*

see that they can have an impact, develop an ability to think about and formulate ways to improve the Center, and are allowed to share the power. It is a slower way to resolve problems, but it seems to reduce the number of problems overall.

The work environment supports cooperation by communicating the importance of each job to the overall functioning of the Center. An important role of the manager is to show how a job fits into the whole—and how a job well-done benefits everyone. Although the Center does have supervisors, we emphasize that no one is working for an individual boss; rather, everyone is working for a common purpose. This is supported by developing ad hoc work groups to evaluate and assess a specific issue (such as reasons for no-show rates, lost files, etc.) and by encouraging suggestions and participation through regular staff meetings.

The most significant factor is the 25-year-old policy that the Center does not have any patient appointments on Friday mornings and reserves that time for rounds, flow meetings, ad hoc task groups, in-service education, and staff meetings. The "flow meetings" deal with specific issues such as billing, the elderly, adolescents, prenatal patients, and telephone/appointments. These meetings are designed to deal in depth with and make decisions and recommendations about specific topics or problems by including the people who are most directly affected by them. Participants include all the staff members involved in that particular topic or problem. Re-

cently, we became aware that our productivity had declined at our Satellite Clinic for the Elderly. The entire staff, including physicians, nurses, social worker, receptionist, and administrators, met to discuss the issues and came up with solutions that have reversed the decline. Some of the solutions require compromises on various staff members' parts, but with everyone involved there has been less resistance to the changes and more participation.

The entire staff meets every other Friday for a staff meeting. The Chair and Recorder of the minutes rotate through the staff to foster leadership skills in everyone. The Chair of the meeting must call the meeting to order, read the previous minutes, solicit reports and recommendations from all flow groups, and go around the room inviting each staff member to speak if he or she has anything to say. Individual issues may range from "who didn't turn off the microscope" to a report on an outside meeting or an event, to a personal event in someone's life. At times we question the cost and loss of productivity by closing Friday mornings, but we continue to conclude that it is a wise investment that saves us later costs of poor communication, power struggles, and a poorly informed staff.

Another formal extension of empowerment is the role of the Board of Directors, both in the decision-making process and with the staff. Staff representatives serve on each of the Board's committees, and one is an elected member of the Board of Directors. The Board is extremely respectful of staff ideas and

CASE 4–2 *Continued*

makes a point of soliciting staff's recommendations on important clinic issues that will affect their jobs and patient care. Nearly 75 percent of the Board members are either patients of the Center or live in the community. Their recommendations, concerns, and power have a direct consequence on their health care and on their neighbors.

■ NURTURING

Nurturing is the ability to create an environment that is comfortable both physically and organizationally. In the past, women managers and administrators often felt that they could not promote traditionally defined female qualities such as nurturing, family support, and mutual respect for fear of being called poor administrators. Much of that has changed with mandated policies affecting family and medical leaves, and sexual harassment. By instituting flex time, job sharing, and liberal maternity and paternity leaves, we have been able to be sensitive to the whole employee—which positively contributes to employee retention, productivity, and morale.

The Center recognizes the importance of allowing for flexibility in employees' schedules to accommodate personal and family responsibilities. We have a commitment to helping people resolve the conflicts of combining a career and a family. We have not been able to offer day care on site, but are lenient about children coming to work in emergencies when they are sick or if there is no childcare. All staff—men and

women, single or married—are allowed to define their schedules within reason (trading 12-hour days for 4 day weeks, working part-time, or working extra evening sessions if baby sitting is a problem) and to align schedules with school, day care, or breast-feeding. We have been able to recruit and retain excellent clinical staff by allowing job sharing, which requires people working together to cover clinic sessions and meet personal needs.

The staff turnover at the Center is comparatively low when compared with other nonprofit agencies. There are 10 staff members who have celebrated over 20 years with the Center, and another five who have over 10 years. This is reinforced by activities that foster strong intra-staff relationships and friendships. The Center holds an annual holiday party and a summer picnic that includes staff and their families. Monthly potluck birthday lunches are an integral part of work life. This includes the staff relaxing, celebrating together, and sharing cross-cultural foods.

Nurturing is also provided by the comfort of the Center facility—which we want to make warm and inviting for staff and patients. The Center facility itself consists of three converted and connected buildings that are cheerful and welcoming. The buildings stand as an attractive anchor on the main street of an area that is trying to renovate itself after the emigration of many residents during the 1980s left many buildings abandoned. In the waiting room, we have a reading corner for the young patients, and we encourage them to take home

CASE 4–2 *Continued*

the slightly used books that they have been reading. (The books have been contributed by local suburban schools, boy scout troops, and friends.)

■ FEMINIST ADMINISTRATION

In discussing administration at the Fair Haven Community Health Center, we have reviewed the organizational practices and structures that encourage education, empowerment, and creation of a supportive and nurturing environment. One may ask, how is this feminist? Theoretically, there is nothing exclusively female in such management practices. Encouraging quality is not exclusively female—but it takes courage and desire for a manager to break traditional hierarchical rules and expectations.

We believe women managers have a challenge and a responsibility to use the traditional female qualities that we possess by virtue of our social and cultural roles to create a productive working environment that encourages a team approach in working toward a common goal. We hope men managers will also embrace these qualities and improve not only the quality of work life, but also the health care delivered in their organizations.

■ BIOGRAPHICAL SKETCHES

Katrina H. Clark has been director of the Fair Haven Community Health Center for more than 20 years. After graduating from Cornell University in 1967 as a history major, she joined the Peace Corps and served in Colombia for 2 years. The Peace Corps experience awakened an interest in health care, and she attended the Yale School of Public Health, receiving a Masters in Public Health in 1971. She held several positions at the Yale Medical School before joining the Fair Haven Health Center. Ms. Clark has had a faculty appointment as a lecturer at the Yale School of Public Health since 1980. She has served on numerous community boards and has received several awards for her service to the community, including the YWCA's Outstanding Woman of the Year Award, the Peace Corps' 25th Anniversary Sargeant Shriver Award, and an honorary Doctorate of Humane Letters from Albertus Magnus College.

Elizabeth Magenheimer has been a family nurse practitioner at the Fair Haven Community Health Center since 1976. She received her Masters in Community Health Nursing from the Yale School of Nursing in 1976 and is certified as a family nurse practitioner and a nurse midwife. She received her BSN from Villanova University, then worked as a public health nurse with the United Farm Workers in California and as a coronary care nurse in a community hospital in New York before beginning her graduate education. Upon completion of her graduate degree, Ms. Mangenheimer held positions as a family nurse practitioner and certified nurse midwife. In 1992, she was licensed as an Advanced Practice Registered Nurse (APRN) by the State of Connecticut. She has dealt with a wide range of medical and social problems in her diverse clini-

CASE 4–2 *Continued*

cal practice. She is a lecturer at the Yale School of Nursing, precepts nurse practitioner students, and treats students at the Albertus Magnus College Health Services. Currently, in conjunction with her clinical practice, she is the Director of Nursing at the Fair Haven Health Center. In 1995, she was awarded the Outstanding Nursing Alumni Award from Villanova University.

TWO

Organizational Strategies

Managing Change in Health Care Organizations

Joyce E. Johnson and Molly Billingsley

Change is certain, progress is not.

Hillary Rodham Clinton
First Lady of the United States
August 27, 1996

It is a new era in health care. If there is one word that characterizes the health care industry in the past 30 years, it is change. Whether defined as a transformation, conversion, or alteration in form, state, nature, or content, change has been constant. This has never been seen more dramatically than in the tumultuous years since the introduction of Medicare's prospective payment system ushered in the beginning of contemporary health care reform. Driven by a myriad of economic and societal forces, this tidal wave of change has not been a phenomenon exclusive to the health care landscape.

Throughout business, industry, and virtually all organizations, leaders have struggled to guide their organizations through the revolutionary changes of the last two decades. More than merely a faster pace of business, this new era called for what Hammer and Champy (1993) termed the reinvention of business in which:

> Managers need to abandon the organizational and operational principles and procedures they are now using and create entirely new ones. The new organizations won't look much like today's corporations, and the way in

which they buy, make, sell and deliver products and services will be very different. Business reengineering means starting over, starting from scratch. (p. 2)

The successful businesses in the future would be those that transformed themselves into learning organizations, defined by Senge (1990) as "the organizations where people continually expand their capacity to create the results they truly desire, where new and expansive patterns of thinking are nurtured, where collective aspiration is set free, and where people are continually learning how to learn together." (p. 3)

Unlike the ancient Greeks who believed that tampering with the basic character of things was disastrous, modern business leaders believe that such change is an opportunity to bend fate to their own ends. Deliberate change reorients relationships and responsibilities, and also creates conditions that make such changes possible (Kanter, Stein, & Jick, 1992).

In this chapter, we will discuss large-scale organizational change rather than routine or incremental change. We begin with a summary of the major transformations in today's health care industry, followed by a review of theoretical concepts that are helpful for understanding the process of change, a pragmatic guide for change to assist nurse leaders, and two case studies of health care organizations in which nurses have played leading roles in successful institutional change. The chapter concludes with our thoughts about nurses not only as caregivers, but as change agents in the creation of the next century's health care system.

■ THE CHANGED WORLD OF HEALTH CARE

For more than 20 years, changes in the U.S. health care industry have stimulated an enormous literature on the industry's modern transformation. Beyond the scope of this chapter, the literature has documented not only the extensive regulatory, reimbursement, and structural changes in health care, but also the industry's uneven course of adaptation and the impact of change on the health care professions. A new lexicon with such terms such as competition, capitation, case management, cost-effectiveness, and co-payments has evolved as well.

Within the last 5 years, organizational change has continued to dominate the health care literature (Billingsley, 1991; Bolton, et al., 1992; Cauthorne & Tracy, 1992; Greene, 1992; Hancock & Bezold, 1994; Issel & Anderson, 1996; Johnson, 1995b; McKibbin, 1995; Newland, 1994; Rosenfield, 1990; Solovy, 1995; Taft & Stearns, 1991). The following major trends and transformations in health care can be identified:

- *Cost management rather than revenue management.* Driven by the runaway costs of hospital care in the technology age, health care legislation, and new reimbursement policies, the emphasis in hospital management has shifted from generating revenue to controlling costs. Resistance from third-party payors to rising costs brought an end to unlimited hospital services. Reduced revenues forced hospitals to operate on business principles. In reality, this powerful force redefined health care as a business; to survive, hospitals had to redesign the way they operated.

- *A new emphasis on wellness combined with shorter hospital stays.* Doing business in the new health care environment needed to reflect not only a renewed emphasis on wellness, prevention, and early interventions by primary care providers, but also the tightly regulated reality of shorter hospital stays. These changes sparked the massive downsizing of acute care facilities, the closing and/or merging of some hospitals, and the creation of more innovative ways to provide acute, post-discharge, and preventive health care across a spectrum of settings—including hospitals, clinics, private offices, home care, and community health centers.

- *Service orientation.* Hospitals that in previous eras enjoyed secure, unthreatened monopolies on patient care were now driven to compete in an intensely competitive marketplace in which patients and payors, rather than physicians, select the service site. Given the number of hospitals that have excellent clinical facilities, integrated services, and cost controls, the selection decision is increasingly made based on an institution's reputation for service and hospitality. Hospitals slowly began to understand the need for a service orientation and started looking to the world of business for guidance.

- *Responsiveness to consumer demands.* The new service orientation in health care drove hospitals to recognize the diversity among consumers. This resulted in the development of specific marketing approaches and programs to meet targeted needs within the different segments. A simultaneous trend among all consumers is increasing sophistication as they have grown more knowledgeable, discerning, and outspoken about health care. Physicians, who traditionally were rarely questioned, must now respond to inquiries about the rationales for their decisions and to demands for more holistic and higher quality health care. Recent public outcry about overregulation in health care and the decline in the quality of care, as illustrated by "in-and-out" obstetrical care, are examples of consumer demands at the policy level.

- *Public–private partnerships.* Executives from traditional public hospitals have increasingly looked to partnerships in the private sector as a means of survival in the new age of health care. Such strategic alliances offer some distinct advantages, such as greater flexibility in designing employee compensation packages, more opportunities for joint ventures with physician groups, and less public business operations.

- *The move toward systems thinking.* New organizational realities have broken down traditional, internal territorial boundaries; formed new team working relationships; and changed perceptions of the importance of professional autonomy within health care systems. These realities have stimulated a renewed awareness of interdependence and expanded interest in systems thinking, the means for organizations to learn from feedback within their interdependent parts and continuously improve (Senge, 1990). In successful health care organizations today, employees at all levels understand the goals and vision of their institution, the value of teamwork, and their personal roles in directly ensuring their institution's success.

- *Refocusing professional education.* Professional schools and licensing agencies have begun to see the critical need to significantly revise both curricula and state practice acts for all the health professions in ways that reflect the changing health care marketplace. Curricula must now include not only state-of-the-art science, but also a greater emphasis on interdisciplinary patient care, organizational change, team building, integration of technology in health care, and innovative ways of delivering patient care. The health professions are also grappling with supply-and-demand projections that predict a surplus of specialty physicians, acute care nurses, and even pharmacists at the turn of the century and high demand for community-based family physicians, nurse case managers, and home care specialists. Changes in education for allied health workers include new curricula for community health workers and consolidation of many categories into multiskilled workers (Johnson, 1995a) who can work wherever they are needed within the health care system.

As Thomas said in 1993, "these changes have permanently changed the character of the health care system. Any one of these developments by itself would have shaken the industry, so it is no wonder that health care is still reeling from a decade that changed its world forever" (p. 16). Adapting to these realities requires systemic and personal change, and the type of strong leadership necessary for a major shift in the corporate culture of today's hospitals.

■ THEORETICAL PERSPECTIVES ON CHANGE

Lewin's Ice Cube Metaphor

Kurt Lewin is generally regarded as the pioneer in the study of planned change and his model is the acknowledged "gold standard." It is through participating in change that consultant and organizational members realize the truth of Lewin's observations (Rothwell, Sullivan, & McLean, 1995). Lewin used an ice cube metaphor to conceptualize change as a process in which organizations move through three stages:

Unfreezing → Moving → Refreezing

According to Lewin, this movement was facilitated by group process and open feedback in which new norms were developed and new roles were re-designed and accepted by the group. The simple, linear quality of Lewin's model had and continues to have appeal for managers, although critics such as Kanter and her associates (1992) suggest that organizations are never truly frozen and that a concept based on linear stages does not reflect current real-ity in today's more chaotic organizational life.

Force-field analysis, a tool developed by Lewin (1951, 1958), is a staple in the repertoire of leaders and management consultants who are exploring the prospects for change within organizations. Lewin's central theory sug-gested that stability among elements in a social system was maintained by balancing opposing forces. Change would only occur when a shift in either direction disrupted this balance. Force-field analysis involves the identifica-tion of *driving forces,* factors that move participants and actions in the direc-tion of a planned change, and *restraining forces,* which increase the likeli-hood of resistance to change. Force-field analysis provides a useful framework for data gathering that, according to Brager and Holloway (1978, 1992) incorporates data from the individual, group, and organizational levels, and also addresses the dynamics of stability and change.

Shewhart's PDCA Cycle

Another classic change model that has endured the test of time is Thomas Shewhart's four-stage model, which dates back to 1924. As illustrated in Fig-ure 5–1 and popularized through Deming's work on continuous improve-ment, this four-stage cycle reflects the iterative process in which organizations reflect on their needs for change, and then plan (*P*), implement by doing (*D*), check (*C*) and monitor effects and act (*A*) to continually evaluate the impact of those change efforts.

Real Time Strategic Change

A more recent addition to the theory menu, this approach focuses on bring-ing about changes in the character and performance of very large organiza-tions. As defined by Jacobs (1994), real time refers to:

> . . . the simultaneous planning and implementation of individual, group and organization-wide changes. Participants in large group gatherings experi-ence, experiment with, refine and institutionalize these new ways of doing business in the events themselves and continue to do so over time as they respond to an ever-changing environment. (p. 21)

This large-scale approach involves large numbers of individuals working together in one room over a 3-day period, using a specific process and a vari-ety of technologies. Proponents of real time strategic change through large-

Cycles of Transformation Efforts

Though no hard and fast rules exist, there seems to be adequate testimony and experience to roughly describe the first "cycles of transformation" for a typical organization. We have chosen "cycles of transformation" as the descriptive phrase because transformation is an iterative process and the Shewhart cycle is an elegant model. Each iteration of the cycle includes:

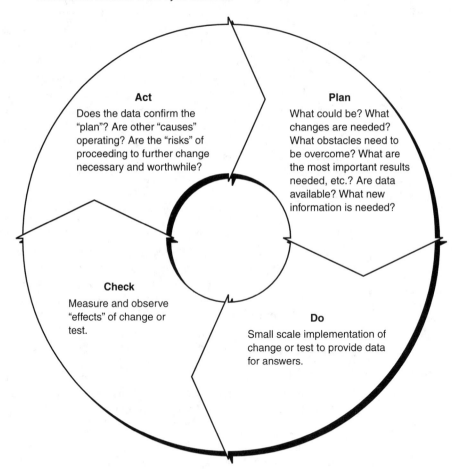

Act
Does the data confirm the "plan"? Are other "causes" operating? Are the "risks" of proceeding to further change necessary and worthwhile?

Plan
What could be? What changes are needed? What obstacles need to be overcome? What are the most important results needed, etc.? Are data available? What new information is needed?

Check
Measure and observe "effects" of change or test.

Do
Small scale implementation of change or test to provide data for answers.

FIGURE 5–1. Shewhart's PDCA cycle. *(Reprinted with permission from Schultz, L. & Parker, B. (1988). Visioning the future. In G. McLean & S. DeVogel (Eds.)* The role of organization development in quality management and productivity improvement: Theory-to-practice monograph *(pp. 47–67). Alexandria, VA: American Society for Training and Development, p. 53.)*

scale interventions base their work on the simple, enduring change formula credited to David Gleicher (Beckhard & Harris, 1987):

$$\text{Dissatisfaction} \times \text{Vision} \times \text{First steps} > \text{Resistance to change}$$

The resistance to change is only overcome in large organizations when there is agreement among a critical mass of people on: (1) dissatisfaction with the status quo, (2) a clearly articulated vision with possibilities for the future, and (3) concrete steps that can be taken to realize that vision. This creates a multiplicative effect that moves change forward.

Proponents suggest that real time strategic change is preferable to sequential, traditional change models in the kind of information available to the people involved, how commitment is gained, the scope of commitment, how change occurs, people's perspectives of change, the pace and nature of change, and the kind of changes made (see Table 5–1 for comparisons). Although there is a paucity of research data supporting claims of success, anecdotal data suggest that this approach, when carefully implemented with the assistance of expert consultants, has significant potential.

"Big Three" Model of Change

Kanter and her associates (1992) have proposed a change model that includes three interconnected aspects of organizations: organizational forces, types of change, and action roles involved in managing the change. This "big three" model includes:

- *Three types of organizational forces:* The *environment,* the organizational *life cycle,* and *politics* involving power and control issues.
- *Three types of change:* Changes in organizational *identity* defined through its products, business, or ownership; *coordination* changes; and changes in *control* in environments involving "makeover through takeover."
- *Three action roles:* the *change strategists* who create the organization's new direction; the *change implementors* who execute and manage the hands-on change effort; and the *change recipients* who are directly affected by it.

Kanter and associates (1992) suggest that understanding all three dimensions of the "big three" model is critical for mastering change. The interactions of these elements illustrate the complexity of organizational change; the rich opportunities for successful, sustained, planned change efforts; and the many possibilities for failure, as well.

▪ PRAGMATIC CHANGE GUIDE

Managing change involves 11 steps in a spiral process in which the end leads to a new beginning. These steps are summarized in Table 5–2 and discussed in the following sections.

TABLE 5–1. Real Time Strategic Change vs. Traditional Change

ASPECTS OF ORGANIZATION CHANGE EFFORTS	COMMON CHANGE APPROACHES AND RESULTS	REAL TIME STRATEGIC CHANGE APPROACH AND RESULTS
The kind of information available to people involved	A small group's narrow, fragmented views of reality form the basis of information they use to plan changes that others will be charged with implementing in the rest of the organization	A large group's broad, whole picture views of reality form the basis of information everyone uses to plan and implement change across the entire organization
How buy-in, commitment, and ownership is gained	Through a campaign waged by a small group of people promoting their strategies, plans, and recommendations to the rest of the organization's total change effort	As a natural by-product of involving people in the process of change
The scope of people's buy-in, commitment, and ownership	People feel and are responsible for only their part of the organization's total change effort	People feel and are responsible for the total organization's total change effort
How change occurs	Sequentially, initiated in different parts of an organization at different times	Simultaneously, initiated in the whole organization at the same time
People's perspectives of change	Change is viewed as a disruption to people doing their "real work"	Change is viewed as an integral component of people's "real work"
The pace of change and the nature of change	Change occurs at a slow pace and in pockets of an organization; planning and implementation are distinct phases	Change occurs at a fast pace and in real time throughout an organization; planning and implementation are inseparable
The kind of changes made	Either substantial changes are made in part of an organization or limited changes are made across an entire organization	Substantial changes are made across an entire organization

Reprinted with permission of Jacobs, R. W. (1994). Real time strategic change. San Francisco: Berrett-Koehler.

Step 1: Learn From the Experiences of Others

Health care organizations can draw valuable lessons from the well-documented experience of organizational transformations in other industries. Hundreds of case studies of successful transformations to meet the demands of changing times have been reported. Janov (1994) refers to these cases as "inventive organizations" that constantly encourage experimentation, chal-

TABLE 5–2. The Steps in a Pragmatic Guide to Managing Change

1. Learn from the experiences of others.
2. Analyze the perceived need for change within your organization.
3. Create a vision for your organization.
4. Define goals.
5. Identify and support a strong leader.
6. Enlist commitment, involvement, and political support.
7. Identify specific, measurable objectives for success.
8. Create a detailed, timed action plan for implementation.
9. Assess and realign the organizational structure.
10. Communicate, communicate, communicate.
11. Institutionalize change.

lenge their basic business assumptions, enhance their ability to imagine, and change their business through well-planned change efforts that are aligned with the organization's structure, policies, and practice.

Lessons from American business suggest that changes that endure in these types of organizations share eight common characteristics (O'Toole, 1995). They are:

- *Built on the unique strengths and values of the corporation.* Values grow out of experience and evolve over time; they are not created by fiat. This is similar to Peters and Waterman's (1982) finding that truly excellent companies know what business they are in and what their values are.
- *Not imposed by top management.* Reinforcing Lewin's conclusions about the essential value of group participation from all levels of the organization, this characteristic suggests that successful change efforts openly involve diverse people from all levels of the organization.
- *Supported both philosophically and materially by the organization's top management.* Top managers must be committed to the effort, provide the required resources, and be personally committed to changing their own behavior as well.
- *Holistic and based on systems thinking.* The interdependence within organizations requires seeing the whole system and its parts, and then changing all parts of the organization. This is why Senge (1990) advocates seeing interrelationships, rather than linear cause and effect, and processes of change over time, rather than snapshots.
- *Planned.* Successful change projects incorporate meticulous long-term planning that includes informing all members of an organization about the whole process, and then breaking the process down into small, clearly defined, manageable action steps.

- *Designed to change the "guts" of the organization.* This involves changing access to information, power relationships, and reward systems in meaningful ways.
- *Designed from the stakeholders' perspective.* An external view as seen by the customer must be the guiding force for the direction of the change.
- *Ongoing.* Criticisms of Lewin's change model focus on this critical point. Since organizations are dynamic and not static, change must be integrated and institutionalized as a continuing process.

Step 2: Analyze the Perceived Need for Change Within Your Organization

An effective change effort requires preliminary analysis not only of the organization's strengths and weaknesses, but also of the potential impact of any proposed changes on the organization (Nadler & Tushman, 1989). Table 5–3 demonstrates the type of data generated by the use of force-field analysis in the Strengthening Hospital Nursing Program to summarize the forces influencing large-scale change (Taft & Stearns, 1991). This program quickly pointed out that nursing is not independent of the organization, and that strengthening nursing involved strengthening the entire hospital. Key organizational factors identified by the researchers were environment, resources, history, and strategy. This project also highlighted the importance of a catalyst for change and a climate conducive for making large-scale changes.

An important component of this stage is leadership to convince others of the need for change, what Gilmartin (1994) calls making a compelling case. This involves convincing large numbers of people about the limitations of maintaining the status quo, and then rallying diverse constituencies around the cause.

Step 3: Create a Vision for Your Organization

Business strategists agree that creating a vision must begin early in a successful change effort. Father Theodore Hesburgh, former president of Notre Dame University, is reported to have said:

> The very essence of leadership is that you have a vision. It's got to be a vision you articulate clearly and forcefully on every occasion. You can't blow an uncertain trumpet. (Gilmartin, 1994, p. 144)

Senge (1990) echoed this sentiment with his emphasis on shared vision as the vital force in learning organizations. Shared vision is not merely an idea, but a force with impressive power to create a sense of commonality that permeates the organization and gives coherence to diverse activities. He goes on to propose that companies that have dramatically changed our way of life, such as

TABLE 5–3. A Force-Field Analysis of Factors Influencing Large Scale Change in Hospitals

ENVIRONMENT	RESOURCES	HISTORY	STRATEGY
Hindering Forces[a]			
• Unpredictability in environment • Poor competitive position • Hostile or threatening legal or regulatory climate • High demand on organization that exceeds organizational resources	• Declining, threatened, or insufficient resources for growth or maintenance of status quo (e.g., finances) • Shortages of critical trained personnel • Limited or inflexible facilities • Specific to nursing: antiquated licensing laws and entry into practice standards	• Negative hospital image • Past history of poor relationships among the health professionals • Long-standing paternalistic health care culture • Professional organization's traditional resistance to change	• Multiple organizational agendas • Short-term priorities • Absence of shared core values
Facilitating Forces[a]			
• Outside impetus to change—catalyst • Clarity of focus on one or more particular issue(s) in the industry	• Funding and viability for creating change • Adequate/flexible facilities • Favorable cost-benefit analysis of change • Excellent consultants • Specific to nursing: support from a school of nursing, presence of a partnership; well-educated nurses	• Positive hospital image • Recognizing and acknowledging the failure of past approaches • Recognizing a need to improve	• An organizational commitment to quality • An organizational commitment to patient care • Specific to nursing: a hospital strategy that recognizes nurses as key to the accomplishment of the mission

[a]Facilitating or hindering forces were identified in an open-ended question by respondents in the study. Many of these may have *both* positive and negative effects, however, so there is no clear dichotomy between hindering and facilitating forces, as the chart implies.
Source: Hospital Leaders' Questionnaire, Strengthening Hospital Nursing Program Evaluation. Reprinted with permission: Taft, S. H., & Stearns, J. E. (1991). Organizational change toward a nursing agenda. Journal of Nursing Administration, 21, 12–21.

Ford, AT&T, and Apple, would not have been possible without shared vision and common identity among diverse people at all levels in these companies.

Developing a clear, powerful vision is also critical for health care institutions considering large-scale change efforts. As in other organizations, this process involves strategic thinking, education, and data gathering to not only generate needed information, but also build both individual and organizational understanding and acceptance of the change. Employees at all levels of the health care hierarchy should be given the opportunity to articulate their goals for the agency in the years ahead as well as the changes they believe would be needed to accomplish these goals. This collective vision for the institution can then serve as the foundation for specific individual and collective actions, and the standard for an organization's direction that must be met by advocates of change (Gilmartin, 1994).

Step 4: Define Goals

Goals should chart the future of the organization, be congruent with the organization's mission and strategic plan, use resources wisely, and create minimal conflict within the organization. In a 5-year organizational change project at Cedars-Sinai Medical Center, the major goals focused on high standards and a shared desire to improve the institution's ability to admit, care for, and discharge patients in an efficient, effective, and caring manner. The needs assessment phase of this project identified five specific goals:

1. Foster change as an integral part of the strategic plan, focusing on the new executive leadership's vision for health service delivery that is a societal force for health.
2. Develop new approaches to change in which individuals from all disciplines and departments work together to improve patient care.
3. Streamline internal operational systems to admit, care for, and discharge patients in an efficient, effective, and caring manner.
4. Develop, implement, and evaluate a Patient Focused Care Delivery Model, supported by expanded collaboration with colleagues and universities.
5. Forge ties to the community to attract individuals into the health care profession and educate the community through a positive media presence.

The goals enhanced the project's potential for attracting support from organizational members, as well as financial support (Bolton et al., 1992).

Step 5: Identify and Support a Strong Leader

Although experts agree that strong leadership is key to the success of large-scale change efforts, there is no consensus on the definition of great leadership. Defining and describing leadership has been the focus of an extensive amount of research, as well as speculation. McWhinney (1992) found more than a dozen distinct styles of leadership and an extensive variety of classification schemes for leadership.

There is general agreement that, as advocates for change, leaders play a key role in creating the vision, motivating employees to support the change, and crafting a reward system that supports behaviors that are congruent with the new vision. This requires not only exquisite communication skills but also time spent in daily coaching and nurturing of project work groups and individuals (Bolton et al., 1992). Leaders need to be champions who generate enthusiasm, lobby the political system for resources and support, and stay closely involved in the change process (Cauthorne & Tracy, 1992). These actions build credibility, integrity, and trust, which are essential attributes of good leaders (Janov, 1994).

As the debate about leadership continues, it is safe to say that leaders are vital to the change enterprise and are special individuals with the courage to create, motivate, and move organizations forward.

Step 6: Enlist Commitment, Involvement, and Political Support

Although business experts have many theories about leadership, they do agree that leadership alone cannot bring about large-scale change. A broad base of support is needed. Support, commitment, and buy-in is needed from all stakeholders who may be affected by the change, and if not committed to it may become powerful obstructions. This includes the institution's medical staff, board of directors, nursing staff, ancillary hospital departments, and external stakeholders such as the community, vendors, or financiers (Kanter, 1983; Newland, 1994). Encouraging meaningful involvement early in and throughout the change process can diminish the type of resentment and obstructive behavior seen in individuals who are handed work decisions for which they had no input or active involvement.

Step 7: Identify Specific, Measurable Objectives for Success

A critical step in the early stages of a change process is designing specific measurable objectives that can assess the endeavor's success. This detailed, often time-consuming work provides specific answers to the questions: What are the results of our collective efforts? How will we know if we are successful? What measures of validation will we use?

A common mistake in writing objectives involves using vague or general terminology that cannot be easily measured or provide the type of feedback needed to maintain the ongoing effort. Studies of successful large-scale change projects have shown that precise, measurable objectives; regular data collection; and systematic review and discussion of indices of change are essential for measuring success, making mid-course corrections, and motivating employees along the way.

Step 8: Create a Detailed, Timed Action Plan for Implementation

For each major change effort, the organization needs a blueprint for change. A plan is needed that specifies the timetable for everything that needs to be done—from the preliminary meetings to individual assignments—detailing the myriad of activities involved in the daily challenges of managing a change project. In addition to laying out the road map, such detailed interactive planning also helps to reinforce the goals of the effort, promote teamwork, and reduce the natural anxiety that occurs along the way (Beckhard & Harris, 1987).

Step 9: Assess and Realign the Organizational Structure

Senge (1990) has written forcefully about the importance of assessing and re-aligning structures in organizations:

> Structures of which we are unaware hold us prisoners. Conversely, learning to see the structures within which we operate begins a process of freeing ourselves from previously unseen forces and ultimately mastering the ability to work with them and change them. (p. 94)

The development of enabling structures can help to facilitate the change process. These diverse structures may involve, but are not limited to, such areas as reward systems, training programs, and communication patterns, or more symbolic areas such as institutional signage, names, logos, and physical space (Kanter, Stein, & Jick, 1992). External as well as internal organization development consultants often play an important role in assisting organizations in the process of assessing and redesigning structures and processes that support the transformed organization.

Step 10: Communicate, Communicate, Communicate

In 1988, Beer advised that involvement, communication, and disclosure can be potent tools for overcoming resistance and giving employees a personal stake in large-scale change. Since that time, numerous reports on change projects have stated that communication, from the initial announcement of the change, and keeping lines of communication open are both difficult and critical to success.

According to Hammer and Champy (1993), business leaders have learned from experience that they always underestimate how much communicating they must do. Kanter and associates (1992) cite the case of Jack Welsh of General Electric, who has been extremely successful at communication across various layers of his company. "Real communication takes countless hours of eyeball to eyeball, back and forth," they quote Welch as saying. "It means more listening than talking . . . It is human beings coming to see and accept things through a constant interactive process aimed at consensus" (p. 389).

Direct, frequent communication works to offset the type of misperceptions and rumors that ferment within an organization in which massive changes are taking place. For example, nurse researchers at Cedars-Sinai Medical Center found that formal newsletters, progress reports to committees, and press coverage simply could not keep up with changing hospital events. Weekly informal news bulletins, which could be quickly produced and disseminated, were then used as a more effective way to keep the hospital staff updated about current events and issues. The project team also found that using a more indirect, train-the-trainer strategy to deliver information from top management was not as effective as direct, personal communication from

the leadership (Bolton et al., 1992). Effective dialogue, with exchanges between all constituencies, must include expressions of perceptions and active
listening (Ashkenas & Jick, 1990). Dialogue helps the group go beyond any
one individual's understanding and gain new insights (Senge, 1990). This
type of exchange can be structured through forums that bring stakeholders
together in discussions in which reactions, underlying assumptions, and de-
fensive routines can be revealed and overcome (Arygris, 1993; Kanter, Stein,
& Jick, 1993). Lewin's beliefs about the key role of participation in the change
process are as true today as they were 30 years ago.

Step 11: Institutionalize Change

This final step overlaps with beginning anew and repeating the cycle. Often,
as one change is institutionalized, the need for another arises or a refinement
learned from the experience of others emerges as an important challenge.
Before moving on, it is important to step back, celebrate the value of the
hard-won change, and invest in seeing it institutionalized in policies, procedures, and the routines that guarantee it becomes a part of "how work is
done here."

Hammer and Champy (1993) estimate that 50 to 70 percent of organizations that begin a reengineering effort do not achieve the intended results.
Common errors include:

- Trying to "fix" a process instead of changing it.
- A focus on areas other than business processes.
- An exclusive focus on process redesign to the exclusion of other fac-
  tors such as management systems or job redesign.
- A lack of attention to people's values and beliefs.
- Being willing to "settle" for minor results.
- Quitting too early.
- Trying to make reengineering happen from the bottom up.
- Allowing existing norms in corporate culture to prevent major change.
- Choosing the wrong leader.
- Pulling back when there is resistance to change.
- Taking too long to complete the change process.

■ CHANGING TO A SERVICE CULTURE AT AN URBAN TERTIARY CARE CENTER: A CASE EXAMPLE*

The Washington Hospital Center (WHC) is a 907-bed tertiary care facility that
is the largest not-for-profit hospital in the metropolitan area. In 1992, the Vice
President for Nursing was appointed to an expanded position of Senior Vice

---

*Case adapted from Johnson, J.E. and Billingsley, M. (In Press.) Reengineering the Corporate Culture. *Nursing and Health Care: Perspectives and Community*.

President, Patient Care Services Division, which included responsibility for formerly unrelated departments such as clinical nursing, facilities management and construction, biomedical engineering, protective services, pastoral care, nutrition services, telecommunications, environmental services, patients and guest services, human resources, and materials management. Over a year's time, these departments reengineered their collective approach to customer service, and developed a working identity as a cohesive team. These efforts sparked a major initiative that ultimately shifted the corporate culture of this 4500-person health care institution to a customer service orientation.

Beginning initially with the division's 250 managers and supervisors, the initiative consisted of a variety of exercises, events, and clarifications of behavioral expectations designed to:

- Heighten awareness of personal expectations as internal consumers of service.
- Broaden insights into the functions and challenges of other departments.
- Enable managers from different areas to socialize and discuss common concerns.
- Establish explicit behavioral norms between leaders, staff members, and patients.
- Establish new ways of helping each other provide better, more efficient hospital services.

Throughout the 3-year large-scale change process, customer satisfaction was assessed regularly through more than 3000 patient interviews per year. Patient satisfaction with nursing care, physician care, housekeeping, security, and registration procedures improved steadily.

As the customer service initiative and systematic data collection at WHC continue, the initiative has expanded to additional areas of hospital service. The WHC experience illustrates that, without the use of an external consultant and with broad support and involvement within their hospital community, nurse executives can assist the agency to align actual employee behavior with the mission, thereby providing significant rewards to both patients and hospital staff (Johnson, 1995c).

■ REDESIGNING PATIENT CARE DELIVERY SYSTEMS AT A COMMUNITY HOSPITAL: A CASE EXAMPLE

Since 1990, John C. Lincoln Hospital, a 236-bed community hospital, in Phoenix, Arizona, has been managing a change process that involved "sweeping" changes that affected every department and area in the hospital. Initially, the changes were implemented on a pilot unit; they were then expanded to the rest of the agency. The goal was to find and implement creative ways to deliver patient care that more effectively utilized the hospital's professional staff and lowered costs.

Several key factors were seen as critical for the project's early success. First, the hospital's corporate culture was supportive of change. There was a high degree of trust and credibility between the managers and staff, and the long-term staff were committed to the hospital's success. Second, Lincoln's CEO expressed support for the project and demonstrated that support by engaging in ongoing dialogue with the nurse managers, other managers, and staff.

The top nurse executive designated a full-time project director to be the primary change implementor on a 36-bed surgical pilot unit. The project director led the staff through a series of design and implementation stages. Initially, management and staff worked for 6 weeks to analyze the hospital experience from the patient's perspective and to design 17 recommendations for reconfiguring patient-centered care. Measurable and feasible outcomes were also identified. The second major task involved designing job descriptions and functions for new work roles for both licensed and nonlicensed staff. In the third step of the process, an implementation team—consisting of nursing staff from the pilot unit and employees from support services—focused their attention for 4 months on logistical and implementation issues. This team, along with the unit manager, then interviewed and selected the staff who would work in the pilot unit.

This redesign of patient care was implemented without the use of external consultants. Ongoing evaluation included quality of care indexes, financial measures, and customer satisfaction. Preliminary data showed positive trends on the quality of care and degree of satisfaction perceived by both patients and staff.

The change process was supported by a clear, well-defined vision, a group of highly placed champions, a culture that supported innovation and risk taking, and most of all, extensive participation by employees. Of all the factors contributing to success, the decision to encourage and insist on employee participation was the most powerful in creating a positive organizational change (Cauthorne & Tracy 1992).

■ NURSES AS CHANGE AGENTS: AN EXPANDING ROLE

As hospitals move through these changing times, they are increasingly calling upon nurse executives to assume the roles of Vice President for Patient Services (VPPS) and Chief Operating Officer (COO) in small and large hospitals throughout the United States. These nurse executives have assumed new and broader responsibilities, which evolved with institutional downsizing.

In a recent survey co-sponsored by The Association of Nurse Executives (AONE), nurse COOs were managing an average annual budget of $48 million, approximately one-third of the mean hospital budget of $145 million (Witt/Kieffer et al., 1994). Nurse COOs reported assuming the responsibility for a huge variety of new departments, programs, and services. In addition to nursing services, these varied operations include the management of all hospital facilities, construction, waste removal, infection control, housekeeping, food service, pharmacy, human resources, risk management, quality assurance programs, and medical records; as well as services provided by biomedical engineering, telecommunications, and security.

The Association of Nursing Executives has identified three major factors responsible for this shift in roles: the change from "nursing services" to patient care, the redesign of patient care, and the competitive pressures to produce "seamless" care at the bedside (Beyers, 1995). Patient-focused work transformation, according to Kathy Vestal, national director of Work Transformation Services for Hay Management Consultants, stresses creating more efficient, cost-effective work processes that benefit patients and employees (Newland, 1994).

Unlike most traditional hospital administrators, nursing executives bring a unique executive perspective. No one else has comparable experience in hands-on direct patient care. Perhaps more than anyone involved in hospital care, nurses understand the linkages and sensitive balance between the needs of the organization and the delivery of patient care. As the primary caregivers and advocates for patients, nurses naturally function from a perceptual framework in which patient care is central. From their long experience in operating from a limited power base, nurses are also comfortable with working in teams, resolving conflicts, and building consensus.

Hospitals have recognized that nurse VPPSs and COOs bring a patient orientation as well as a business perspective to diverse, interdependent operations that either directly or indirectly influence patient care. In addition to traditional management functions, these nurse executives also assume three additional roles not typically viewed as the responsibilities of nurses: politician, negotiator, and change agent.

In the political realm, these nurse executives interact with physicians, the hospital board of trustees, credentialing organizations, and a variety of diverse individuals and organizations from the community the hospital serves. As one of the hospital's negotiators, the nurse VPPS or COO conducts hospital business with a variety of labor unions, vendors, attorneys and other representatives from the legal system, members of the hospital's institutional review board, and in recent years, representatives from managed care groups.

In their expanded roles, nurse executives have the skills and the organizational opportunities to design and execute the types of large-scale organizational development projects needed to bring about a major paradigm shift in a health care institution's corporate culture. Thus, nurse leaders today are and will continue to be working as change agents within their institutions as the transformation of our health care system continues.

In her 1983 book *The Change Masters,* Rosabeth Moss Kanter said:

Change masters are literally the *right* people in the *right* place at the *right* time. The right people are the ones with the ideas that move beyond the organization's established practice, ideas they can form into visions. The right places are the integrative environments that support innovation, encourage the building of coalitions and teams to support and implement visions. The right times are those moments in the flow of organizational history when it is possible to reconstruct reality on the basis of accumulated innovations to shape a more productive future. Change efforts have to mobilize people around what is yet unknown. Change masters have to operate integratively, bringing other people in, bridging multiple realities, and reconceptualizing activities to take account of the new, shared reality. (p. 306)

As illustrated in the case studies presented earlier in this chapter and numerous other reports in the literature, nurse leaders are increasingly directing successful, institution-wide change efforts in their hospitals. Nurses may work as *change strategists*—by sensing the needs in hospitals, deciding what can be done, and then sparking the energy to make it happen—and as *change implementors* who manage the day-to-day process and details of change.

As they work in either of these roles, nurses undoubtedly confront multiple transitions, incomplete transitions, uncertain future states, and slow transitions over long periods of time (Nadler & Tushman, 1989). These challenges put a leader's skills to a new test. As one change agent said, "How are you supposed to change the tires on a car when it's going 60 miles an hour?" (Kanter, Stein, & Jick, 1992, p. 361)

Repeated admonitions from the community of futurists suggest two important thoughts. First, if there is anything that is certain, it is that change will be a constant in our lives in the years ahead. According to Alexander and D'Aunno (1990), change is especially likely to continue in health care institutions, which are hybrid technical and institutional environments filled with inherent conflict, instability, and incomplete institutionalization. Although the health care system of the next century, say the futurists, will incorporate many of the characteristics we see evolving in the current system, it will continue to evolve with the changing times and will be shaped by human decisions and action (Greene, 1992; Hancock & Bezold, 1994).

Second, change agent skills will become increasingly important for nurses both at the bedside and in administrative or executive roles. For the nursing profession, this fact has significant implications. Florence Nightingale's definition of a "trained nurse" did not include skills in organization development and organizational change. Yet, in our health care systems of today and tomorrow, opportunities abound for nurses to be involved in the management of change within their institutions. It is a new era in health care. It is a clarion call for the nursing profession not just to be involved, but to meet this challenge with energy and determination to prepare nurses to possess the knowledge, skills, and vision to see that change keeps the benefit of the patient as the center of our work.

■ BIOGRAPHICAL SKETCHES

Joyce E. Johnson received her diploma in nursing from South Side Hospital School of Nursing in Pittsburgh, her baccalaureate in nursing from Boston College, and her masters and doctoral degrees from Catholic University. She was a Johnson and Johnson fellow at the Wharton School, University of Pennsylvania. She has held multiple clinical, supervisory, and management positions in acute care agencies. She is currently Senior Vice President of Nursing and Patient Care Services at the Washington Hospital Center in Washington, D.C.

Dr. Johnson is a professor of nursing at Catholic University of America, Washington, DC. She lectures throughout the country and has published numerous articles on management. She has published books on bedside computers and business plans for nursing, the latter of which received the *American Journal of Nursing's* "Book of the Year" award. She is on editorial boards of several nursing periodicals and is the publisher and founder of *NursingConnections,* the first nationally refereed scholarly journal to be published from a practice setting.

Dr. Johnson is active in a number of national health care and nursing organizations. Since 1995, she has been a fellow in the American Academy of Nursing and was the 1997 recipient of the American Organization of Nurse Executives' Baxter Award for Quality Innovations in Patient Care.

Molly Billingsley is currently Administrative Director of Nursing and Patient Care Services at the Washington Hospital Center in Washington, D.C., a position she has held for 11 years. Prior to that, Dr. Billingsley spent 12 years teaching at the baccalaureate and masters level in colleges of nursing at George Mason University, Simmons College, and the University of Massachusetts at Lowell. Clinically her practice has been as a pediatric and adult nurse practitioner with a specialty in Adolescent Health Care. She was co-founder and senior nurse practitioner for 8 years at the Teen Health Service in Lowell, Massachusetts. She formerly held positions as Associate Editor and Research Editor of *The Nurse Practitioner: The Journal of Primary Health Care,* and for the past 10 years has been Editor-in-Chief of *NursingConnections;* both are scholarly journals in nursing. She has written over 50 articles and book chapters in the field of clinical and contemporary issues in nursing and health care. Dr. Billingsley's original degree in nursing is from the University of Virginia; she subsequently earned masters degrees from the University of Virginia and George Mason, and a doctoral degree from Boston University.

■ SUGGESTED READINGS

Argyris, C. (1993). *Knowledge for action: A guide to overcoming barriers to organizational change.* San Francisco: Jossey-Bass.

Issel, L.M., & Anderson, R.A. (1996). Taking charge: Managing six transformations in healthcare delivery. *Nursing Economics, 14,* 78–85.

Johnson, J.E. Quarterly column in *NursingConnections.*
Mick, S.S., et al. (Eds.). *Innovation in healthcare delivery.* San Francisco: Jossey-Bass.
Nadler, D., & Tushman, M. (1989). Organizational framebending: Principles for managing reorientation. *Academy of Management Executive, 3,* 194–202.

■ REFERENCES

Alexander, J.A., & D'Aunno, T.A. (1990). Transformation of institutional environments: Perspectives on the corporatization of U.S. health care. In S.S. Mick et al. (Eds.), *Innovation in health care delivery.* San Francisco: Jossey-Bass.
Argyris, C. (1993). *Knowledge for action: A guide to overcoming barriers to organizational change.* San Francisco: Jossey-Bass.
Ashkenas, R., & Jick, T. (1990). Organizational dialogue. (Working paper.)
Beckard, R., & Harris, R. (1987). *Organizational transitions.* Reading, MA: Addison-Wesley.
Beyers, M. (1995). The changing world of nurse administrative practice. *Journal of Nursing Administration, 25,* 5–6.
Billingsley, M.C. (1991). Hard times all around. *NursingConnections, 4,* 12–14.
Bolton, L.B., Aydin, C., Popolow, G., & Ramseyer, J. (1992). Ten steps for managing organizational change. *Journal of Nursing Administration, 22,* 14–20.
Brager, G., & Holloway, S. (1978). *Changing human service organizations: Politics and practice.* New York: Free Press.
Brager, G., & Holloway, S. (1992). Assessing prospects for organizational change: The uses of force field analysis. *Administration in Social Work, 16,* 15–28.
Cauthorne, C., & Tracy, T. (1992). Organizational change from the "Mom and Pop" perspective. *Journal of Nursing Administration, 22,* 1–64.
Gilmartin, J.J. (1994). Responding to health care reform: How managed care providers can manage major change overload. *Medical Interface, 7,* 143–146.
Greene, J. (1992). Systems geared up for coming reforms. *Modern Healthcare, 23,* 25.
Hammer, M., & Champy, J. (1993). *Reengineering the corporation.* New York: Harper-Collins.
Hancock, T., & Bezold, C. (1994). Possible futures, preferable futures. *Healthcare Forum, 37,* 23–29.
Issel, L.M., & Anderson, R.A. (1996). Taking charge: Managing six transformations in healthcare delivery. *Nursing Economics, 14,* 78–85.
Jacobs, R.W. (1994). *Real time strategic change.* San Francisco: Berrett-Koehler.
Janov, J. (1994). *The inventive organization: Hope and daring at work.* San Francisco: Jossey-Bass.
Johnson, J.E. (1995a). Meeting patient needs through multi-skilling. *NursingConnections, 8,* 1–2.
Johnson, J.E. (1995b). Satisfaction belongs in the health care equation. *NursingConnections, 8,* (4), 1–3.
Johnson, J.E. (1995c). Changing the corporate culture: How nursing leadership can prevent the hospital bus from going to Abilene. (Unpublished manuscript.)
Johnson, J.E., & Billinglsey, M. (In press.) Reengineering the corporate culture. *Nursing and Health Care: Perspectives on Community.*
Kanter, R.M. (1983). *The change masters.* New York: Simon & Schuster.

Kanter, R.M., Stein, B.A., & Jick, T.D. (1992). The challenge of organizational change. New York: The Free Press.

Lewin, K. (1951). *Field theory in social science*. New York: Harper & Row.

Lewin, K. (1958). Group decision and social change. In E. Maccoby, T. Newcomb, & E. Hartley (Eds.), *Readings in social psychology*. New York: Holt & Co.

McKibbin, S. (1995). The paradox of change. *Hospitals and Health Networks, 69,* 40–42.

McWhinney, W. (1992). *Paths of change: Strategic choices for organizations and society*. Newbury Park: Sage.

Nadler, D., & Tushman, M. (1989). Organizational framebending: Principles for managing reorientation. *Academy of Management Executives, 3,* 194–202.

Newland, A. (1994). Old habits die hard. *Management, 41,* 28.

O'Toole, J. (1995). *Leading change: Overcoming the ideology of comfort and the tyranny of custom*. San Francisco: Jossey-Bass.

Peters, T., & Waterman (1982). *In search of excellence*. New York: Harper & Row.

Rosenfield, R. (1990). Hospital turnarounds—thinking strategically. *Healthcare Executive, 5,* 28–29.

Rothwell, W.J., Sullivan, R., & McLean, G.N. (1995). *Practicing organization development: A guide for consultants*. San Diego, CA: Pfeiffer.

Senge, P. (1990). *The fifth discipline*. New York: Doubleday.

Solovy, A. (1995). Predicting the unpredictable. *Hospitals and Health Networks, 69,* 26–29.

Taft, S.H., & Stearns, J.E. (1991). Organizational change toward a nursing agenda. *Journal of Nursing Administration, 21,* 12–21.

Thomas, R.K. (1993). *Health care consumers in the 1990s*. Ithaca, NY: American Demographics Books.

Witt/Keiffer, Ford, Hadelman, and Lloyd. (1995). *Senior nurse executives in transition: New roles and new challenges*. Oakbrook, IL: Author.

CASE 5–1 The Human Side of Change: Transition to Teams

Barbara Balik and Ethel Muchlinski

"I thought you said working as a team would help us provide better patient care? Well, you're wrong." The retreat for staff on the newly redesigned surgical patient care department was off to a roaring start. The staff, known for excellence in care and professionalism in interactions before the redesign and movement to teams, were extremely frustrated and voiced their anger over the team concept. The leadership team and team facilitators listened and agreed. Something was not right about this "team thing."

Does this example sound familiar? In this era of rapid redesign internally, and mergers, alliances, and interactions related to managed care externally, nurse leaders are grappling with new forms of working relationships. Teams have emerged as a significant vehicle to address the growing complexity in health care. Transformation of care relationships from individualistic models to those based on teams demands different leadership skills and facilitation techniques. Most leaders find this transition a daunting challenge. The case study that follows examines two patient care departments and their different paths in advancing the use of teams. These examples illuminate a framework and tools that leaders can use to facilitate and manage such change.

■ WHY TEAMS?

To clearly understand the direction they have chosen, leaders must have a grounding in the changes affecting health care delivery and the strategic implications of choosing a team approach to caregiving. Teams are not simply another way of assigning work groups or leaders; rather, they are a fundamental commitment to interdependency to address the complexity in the health care environment. Coile (1993), a health care futurist, has described the changes in health care organizations and the rationale for the shift from systems based on individuals to teams as the means of providing services.

> In third wave organizations, cross-functional teams will become the dominant work unit of the twenty-first century health care organization. Teams will replace individuals because they can better manage complexity, provide more flexibility in use of individual skills and expertise, and allow an organization to make cost-effective use of its "human capital." . . . Teams will actively reconfigure ideas, people, processes, and resources. (p. 1)

This significant change in how people work together challenges many of the traditional structures and norms in health care organizations. The development of

CASE 5–1 *Continued*

teams offers a way of exploring the changes.

Cross-functional teams are a way of working together that is based on the concept of a small group of people who come together to provide services or to accomplish a project and who are interdependent in accomplishing this work. A definition from Katzenbach and Smith (1993), adapted by Manion (1996), identifies a team as:

> . . . a small number of consistent people committed to a relevant shared purpose, with common performance goals, complementary and overlapping skills, and a common approach to their work. Team members hold themselves mutually accountable for the team's results or outcomes. (p. 6)

The services described can involve care provided to an individual or to the systems that support the care. Teams usually include individuals who come from different educational, professional, and work backgrounds. Often, the members' only commonality is that they are all involved in health care.

As Coile (1993) indicates, the direction in which health care is moving is a shift from systems based on the current style of individual service delivery to systems based on cross-functional team service delivery. Unlike the traditional structures and roles, the new relationships and structures for teams reflect interdependency to meet the dual demands of increased customization of service and lower costs.

The framework utilized by the leaders in the case study that follows is derived from William Bridges's book, *Managing Transitions* (1991). The change theory grounding of many leaders is based on concepts of unfreezing and refreezing, change agents, resistance to change, and overcoming change barriers. This traditional description of change speaks to the *external* aspects of change. Planned change processes (Table 5–4) are essential for the development of teams. But they are not enough. Traditional thinking about change is focused on the external environment. Bridges addresses transitions; that is, the *internal* individual experience. His model offers a framework for viewing transitions that coordinates rapid changes with the "people side" of transformation. Focusing on changes and neglecting transitions are what resulted in

TABLE 5–4. Planned Change Process

1. The need is established and communicated.
2. The change announced is perceived as an effective solution.
3. The impact of the change is identified and communicated.
4. Those affected are involved in the change process.
5. The details of implementation of the plan are understood.

Adapted from Bridges (1991).

CASE 5–1 *Continued*

the angry staff retreat described in the opening scenario. As we will see, a combination of external and internal models of change can provide leaders with a more effective, integrated approach.

■ BACKGROUND

United Hospital, part of the Allina Health System, is a 500-bed, private, nonprofit hospital located in St. Paul, Minnesota. In 1993, with a mature and aggressive managed care environment, a strong history and commitment to continual improvement of service and quality, and a facility that needed remodeling, the organization began a complete redesign of core processes, organizational structure, leadership, and facilities through a patient-focused care (PFC) redesign (Table 5–5). Bridges's (1991) model was identified early in the redesign process as a supportive tool. United's transition to a team structure provides a rich case study illustration and illuminates the application of Bridges's framework for transitions in a health care setting. The lessons learned at United highlight the continuing develop-

ment of the application of the model. Learning about systems change and use of the model is ongoing and often involves retracing our steps to better comprehend what aspects of the theory were not applied. However, the descriptions of the changes in the two care centers that follow illustrate the insights gained by leaders and staff in the journey so far through these transitions.

The Surgical Center

The staff of United's Surgical Center had seen many changes: they had relocated and redesigned their care environment, their work processes, and their organizational structure to support the patient-focused care philosophy. Changes to the organizational structure emphasized the move from individual to team accountability.

Leaders within the Surgical Center wanted to prepare and equip both staff and themselves for the change to teams. Changes were minimized where possible by assigning staff to teams based on their current schedule, work appointment, and weekend schedule, while still maintaining

---

TABLE 5–5. Patient-focused Care: The Change Process

1. Define patient needs and group patients according to care and service needs.
2. Redesign work processes to create efficiency, eliminate redundancy, and promote continuity for the patient.
3. Create and modify work roles to support the redesigned process.
4. Redesign the facility to support patient needs and new work processes.
5. Assign staff to the patient care unit where services are provided (pharmacy, housekeeping, respiratory care, etc.).
6. Expect and support shared and team decision making at the point of care.

CASE 5–1 *Continued*

the appropriate skill mix. The goal was to have a small group (ideally six to ten people) who worked consistently together. This would allow the caregivers to function as a team, develop trust, communicate effectively, and learn from each other. Small team size is important because "large numbers of people have trouble interacting constructively as a group and agreeing on actions to take" (Katzenbach & Smith, 1993, p. 45).

Retreat days for each of the teams focused on preparation for working together in new and different ways. The goal of the retreats was to help staff:

- Describe why the change to teams was important—to reduce fragmentation of care, introduce a new skill mix, and manage the increased complexity of care by involving staff in decisions.
- Understand the three stages of personal transition that Bridges (1991) described: endings, neutral zone, and beginnings (Table 5–6). Staff identified personal strategies to help them through the change and manage their personal transitions to teams in a redesigned work environment.

- Understand the diversity of their team by using a tool that described work styles.
- Establish group and behavioral norms.
- Describe the changing roles and responsibilities.
- Assess current team functioning by completing a team assessment tool (Table 5–7).

At the end of the first retreat, the staff had what can best be described as "guarded optimism" about the plan for teams. They saw some opportunity to make their work easier but also saw barriers; most adapted a "wait and see" attitude.

To support the surgical staff in their move towards teams, leaders used several strategies. In the earliest stages of team development, leaders helped the staff articulate and clarify roles, establish team purpose and goals, and encourage open and honest dialogue with each other.

Teams quickly and predictably moved into the "state of confusion," which Orsburn and associates (1990) identify as the second stage of team de-

---

TABLE 5–6. Bridges (1991) Model For Transition

Transitions: The psychological (and internal) process people go through to come to terms with a new situation.

Steps in the transition process:
1. Endings: Letting go of the old and the current reality.
2. Neutral zone: The gap between what is and what will become.
3. New beginning: Making a commitment to be and do something new.

CASE 5–1 *Continued*

TABLE 5–7. Team Assessment Tool

Team Name: _____   Date: _____

Please respond to each statement about your team as it exists now. Your responses will be combined with others from your team to identify developmental, educational, and retreat opportunities. Complete the assessment by rating each item according to the legend below:

> 5 = Almost everyone (80–100% of team)
> 4 = Many (60–80% of team)
> 3 = Some (40–60% of team)
> 2 = Few (20%–40% of team)
> 1 = Almost no one (<20% of team)

Purpose and Goals: *To what extent do team members:*
_____1. Describe the mission and purpose of our work to others.
_____2. Know who the customers are and focus the work on meeting customers' needs.
_____3. Have clear and common goals for our work.
_____4. Support the strategic direction of United Hospital and Allina Corporation.
_____5. Understand how our work makes a meaningful contribution to outcomes.

Roles and Responsibilities: *To what extent do team members:*
_____1. Understand their roles and accountabilities.
_____2. Remain flexible in their roles and not let rigid hierarchy get in the way.
_____3. Accept diversity in work styles and encourage others to use their strengths.
_____4. Delegate work in the same way.
_____5. Distribute work fairly among all team members.
_____6. Understand lines and levels of authority.
_____7. Accept responsibility for actions and decisions rather than making excuses.
_____8. Know what the team norms are and understand what is expected by other team members.
_____9. Demonstrate commitment to each other and the team.

Interdisciplinary Teaming: *To what extent do team members:*
_____1. Understand the work and licensure requirements of other disciplines.
_____2. Value the contributions individuals make from other disciplines.
_____3. Work collaboratively (in partnership) with other disciplines to meet patient needs.

Change and Transition: *To what extent do team members:*
_____1. Understand the purpose of the moving toward a team environment.
_____2. Have a clear picture of the intended outcome of our team.
_____3. Understand the plan being followed to implement teams.
_____4. Know the part each person plays in developing a team.
_____5. Understand the emotions that happen during a time of change.
_____6. Realize that change is a constant in the work setting.

(continued)

CASE 5–1 *Continued*

TABLE 5–7. (continued)

Legend

5 = Almost everyone (80–100% of team)
4 = Many (60–80% of team)
3 = Some (40–60% of team)
2 = Few (20%–40% of team)
1 = Almost no one (< 20% of team)

Communication: *To what extent do team members:*

_____1.   Listen and try to understand the other person's point of view.
_____2.   Ask for what they want from others.
_____3.   Know how to influence decisions made on the unit.
_____4.   Create an environment of openness and trust.
_____5.   Use respectful and honest communication with one another.
_____6.   Respect confidentiality of employees and patients.
_____7.   Confront disruptive issues that face the group.
_____8.   Offer to help without being asked.
_____9.   Use direct communication with each other to resolve conflict.

Shared Leadership and Learning: *To what extent do team members:*

_____1.   Assume responsibility for teaching other team members how to do something.
_____2.   Express enthusiasm and support to each other.
_____3.   Receive feedback, both positive and constructive, from other team members.
_____4.   Acknowledge and learn from mistakes.
_____5.   Periodically review our quality outcomes and make changes as needed.
_____6.   Seek information and knowledge from others on our team.
_____7.   Encourage leadership from whomever has the skills or knowledge needed at a particular time.
_____8.   Feel accountable for orienting new employees.
_____9.   Readily share information with others on the team.

Overall, this team, as it exists today, works together effectively: (please circle)

Strongly Disagree   Disagree   Agree   Strongly Agree

Comments: _____
_____
_____
_____
_____
_____

CASE 5–1   *Continued*

velopment. This state can be likened to "something like a rainy first night of a child's camping trip, when the temperature drops, the wind howls and the tent leaks. Regret, frustration, hostility, dread—one fierce emotion after another—chill the high spirits of team members and leaders like an unexpected north wind" (Orsburn et al., 1990, p. 92). In this stage, the leaders needed to provide increased attention to the teams and allow and encourage team members to find the solution, but they also needed to be directive and remove barriers as the members struggled through this stage.

At the second retreat, about 4 months after the teams were implemented, the emotions described in the opening scenario surfaced. The feelings about the team experiment had changed dramatically. The staff were extremely frustrated and expressed anger over the team concept. They had difficulty seeing how they could have continuity with their patients and with their team members; so many variables had inhibited their ability to work consistently with the same six to ten people. And if they could not work consistently with each other, then it surely meant that they could not be a team. Their focus was on the *structure* of their teams, not the *essence* or real purpose of teams. The structure of teams was emphasized by leaders as a means to facilitate the development of teams. Embedded in the development of teams and team structure was attention to the essence or purpose, but the focus on structure overshadowed the core essence of team behavior and outcomes.

In this instance, both members and leaders were having difficulty moving from a traditional to a team organization because they were focused on the wrong things. We had been focusing on structure, since barriers to team function in the structure could sabotage any individual's best efforts at teamwork, and the available literature emphasized the importance of structure. Leaders needed to help provide a focus for staff and an environment where teams could be realized. Eventually, the frustration of leaders led to the realization that what was missing from their team-building efforts was a clear articulation of what Bridges (1991) describes as the "four P's" of teams. By shifting the focus to the four P's, the leaders realized, the entire department could understand the move towards teams and the impact it would have on each person and his or her work. Bridges's framework would not be just another new management fad based on theory, but instead a blueprint for helping staff and leaders through their personal transitions. Here is how the leaders applied the four P's of teams to the Surgical Center's situation:

1. *Purpose.* Answering several questions established the purpose behind the idea of teams. What was the problem that teams were trying to resolve? Were the external environmental changes really a problem? How would teams help to fix this problem?
2. *Picture.* According to Bridges (1991), this refers to how the outcome will look and feel. He ex-

CASE 5–1 *Continued*

plains that people will need to experience this imaginatively before they can give their hearts to it. Questions focused on: How would teams look within the Center? How would change of shift report happen? How would decisions be made throughout the shift? How would the team communicate?

3. *Plan.* A step-by-step plan is a key component in developing a work group. Articulation of the steps necessary to implement teams and establishment of a means to overcome barriers to teams was required. How would it start? When would team members know which team they were on? How would this be decided? How would performance issues be resolved? What if there was conflict between members that could not be resolved? How long would the changes to teams take? Bridges (1991) offers this comment: "The existence of the plan sends a message: somebody is looking after us, taking our needs seriously, and watching out so we don't get lost along the way" (p. 59).

4. *Part to Play.* Staff would need a clear idea of their role on the team and how they could contribute to making teams work. They needed help to articulate the importance of making a personal decision to join and commit to this team. Commitment could not be legislated or demanded from team members.

As leaders looked at the development of the surgical team, they realized that time had been spent on Picture and Part to Play in the retreats, but that the Purpose and Plan had not been articulated. It was not until leaders did this and clarified the purpose around *essence* of teams or the spirit and intent of teams, not the *structure,* that the staff could move forward in their transition. Their eager sharing of this learning helped other leaders to build on their experiences and gain from them.

The Oncology Center

When the next patient-focused care redesign was implemented, in the Oncology Center, leaders focused on articulating the Four P's for the team. They looked systematically at each of the Four P's and identified them for staff (see Table 5–8). This accomplished several things:

- It provided a clarity about the purpose. The purpose was *not* to create a small "structure" of people who consistently worked together. This was an outcome measure that would occur if certain system barriers to teams could be overcome. Rather, the purpose or *essence* of teams was to create an environment where people could communicate directly and respectfully with each other, continually learn from each other, and rely on a multidisciplinary approach to solve problems and enhance patient care.

CASE 5–1 *Continued*

TABLE 5–8. High Performing Teams at United Hospital

What is the **purpose** of teams?
- Improve outcomes of care.
- Increase satisfaction of patient and employees.
- Establish mutual accountability for patient outcomes.
- Establish interdependencies of care.
- Increase communication among caregivers from all disciplines.
- Value contributions from all team members.
- Provide consistency with whom I work.

What will teams look like on our unit? How do I **picture** the future?
- Seventy percent (70%) of the time I will work with the same people (RNs, LPNs, and patient care associates) and report off to the same people.
- I will meet with my team at the change of shift for a team meeting and have a *dialogue* that includes: progress in meeting patient or work outcomes, what the work is for our shift to meet those outcomes, and how we will divide the work between us.
- I will feel, over time, that our team is "clicking." We will understand each other's work styles, we will hold each other accountable, we will continually learn from each other, and we will communicate openly in a safe environment. We will also have fun working together.
- I will see our team as part of the whole team of our Center that focuses on a whole experience of care for our patients.
- We will understand and appreciate other roles and disciplines. We will take advantage of our similarities and our differences to accomplish positive patient outcomes.

What is my **part to play** on these teams?
- Make a personal decision to belong to a team.
- Focus on support to each other, accept diversity, and challenge each other.
- Ask questions to clarify roles, responsibilities, and relationships.
- Celebrate successes, however small.
- Focus on long-term results and goals.
- Be patient, realizing that the chaos of moving into a team environment is a natural and temporary part of every transition.
- Be part of the solution when problems are identified.

How will we get there? What is our **plan**?
- Name the teams and team members.
- Meet with the teams in a workshop or retreat setting to establish an identity, roles and responsibilities, and group norms.
- Attend education sessions to prepare us for the transition to teams and patient-focused care.
- Redefine change of shift report, which would provide opportunity for dialogue and division of the work and achieve the best use of resources with the best outcomes for the patient.

From Muchlinski, Krotz, Wasserman, 1996, United Hospital, St. Paul, Minnesota

CASE 5–1 *Continued*

- It honored the past. Leaders acknowledged that teamwork was already found in the current setting and that the teams would be built on that fine base.
- It helped develop more specific ideas and agreement within the leadership team about the purpose, picture, and plan for getting to teams. This provided the staff with adequate clarity and offered a grounding of understanding so they could formulate questions, identify areas of confusion and, finally, clarify and define their part in the team.

As the Oncology Center implemented its redesign changes, application of Bridges's Four P's supported and nurtured leaders and staff alike. It allowed members to focus on managing the personal transitions through the process of endings, neutral zone, and new beginnings identified by Bridges. In addition, it provided a framework or grounding as issues or questions about implementation arose.

Lessons for Leaders

Use of the Four P's model at United Hospital provided an important foundation for leaders in facilitating the transition to teams. A variety of team and patient-focused tools provided a further base for incorporation of team skills (see Table 5–9).

The magnitude of changes and transitions facing today's health care leaders are not for the faint of heart or the impatient. The transition to teams at United is founded on the belief that the use of cross-functional teams, as described by

Coile (1993), is a robust strategy—one that will enable caregivers to meet the growing complexity of care in a variety of environmental or market changes. Successful multidisciplinary teams will be a hallmark of success in any thriving health care organization.

The ability to keep one's eye on the long-term goal while respectfully accompanying people through the transition is a key leadership capability. Leaders facilitate an environment conducive to transition when they create a belief in the individual's capacity to change, support the development of transition skills, and enable people to shape the future together. Patience and persistence are essential in this work.

Leadership for transitions assumes excellence in other key leadership skills. A model for transitions will not overcome a lack of core competencies by leaders. Key among those skills is grounding in:

- Empowerment of others.
- Skillful facilitation.
- Effective removal or reframing of barriers (because some barriers cannot be removed).
- Shared decision making.
- Diligent follow-through.
- Willingness to address tough interpersonal and performance issues respectfully and directly.

One colleague asked, "Is it really necessary to do all of this process? Can't we just get on with it?" The experience of leaders and staff at United Hospital is that you can "just get on with it"—*and* you still have to do this type of process. Rushing through or missing key compo-

CASE 5–1 *Continued*

TABLE 5–9. Development Tools Used to Clarify and Facilitate the Continual Improvement of Different Components of Teams

1. **Purpose and Goals**
   Customer service education
   Identification of patient/family expectations
   Goal setting
   Development of team vision

2. **Roles and Responsibilities**
   Review of position requirements
   Development of team norms
   Personal style inventory
   Delegation education
   Levels of decision-making authority
   Approaches to team decision making
   Development of commitment statements
   Leading effective meetings

3. **Interdisciplinary Teaming Strategies**
   Exercise: What is my primary work?
   What other work can I do to help others?
   What do we need from others to be successful?

4. **Change and Transitions Strategies**
   Managing Change education
   Four P's articulation
   Business of Healthcare education
   Review of financial and patient care data (review of the problems patient-focused care and teams were designed to address)
   Leadership development

5. **Communications**
   Communication and Conflict in the Workplace education
   Confidentiality education
   Communication and conflict role playing
   Decision-making education
   Learning partners
   Performance development plan

6. **Shared Leadership and Learning**
   Problem-solving activity
   Tools for giving constructive feedback
   Critical thinking development

From Krotz, Muchlinski, & Wasserman (1996).

CASE 5–1 *Continued*

nents takes more time in the long run. Just ask the surgical leaders and staff. Acceleration of the overall change comes when leaders and staff understand the transition process and use strategies that facilitate its progress.

The move to interdependent, flexible teams that can create a caring community of service, respond and adapt to changing patient needs, and achieve superb quality outcomes is new ground for health care organizations. While leaders can draw to some degree on previously developed skills, they also face the daunting challenge of learning new skills while acting as facilitators of the change. The juggling act is difficult for any leader, but the long-term gains are satisfying. Frameworks can act as supportive guides to facilitate learning as leaders move through these changes. In the end, it is the ability of leaders to engage in dialogue, identify assumptions, and learn with each other and with staff teams that is the essence of team skills and at the heart of leadership.

■ BIOGRAPHICAL SKETCHES

Barbara Balik received her BSN from Marycrest College in Davenport, Iowa, her MS in Maternal-Child Nursing from the University of Minnesota at Minneapolis, and is currently a doctoral student at the University of St. Thomas in St. Paul, Minnesota. As the Patient Care Vice President at United Hospital in St. Paul, she has facilitated major redesign and other change activities to assure cross-functional team development in managed care environments. Through extensive publications and presentations, she has shared her experiences in consumer and employee empowerment, collaboration, trends in managed care, and development of quality improvement cultures. Ms. Balik is active in several national professional organizations and has received the Sigma Theta Tau, Zeta Chapter Leadership Award and the Minnesota Nurses Association State Service Award.

Ethel Muchlinski received her BSN from the College of St. Benedict in St. Joseph, Minnesota and her MSN in Maternal-Child Health and Nursing Education from the University of Minnesota. She has developed organizational change strategies in many of the positions she has held and currently leads the Education Department and the Organizational Development work at United Hospital. Recognized as a leader in team development and change, she frequently consults on facilitation of organizational change in health care settings. She has developed and implemented team assessment tools used to improve team processes and has created a template for team meetings of direct care providers when communicating about patients at the change of shift.

■ REFERENCES

Bridges, W. (1991). *Managing transitions.* Reading, MA: Addison-Wesley.

Coile, R. (1993). Third-wave organizations: Cross-functional teams and workplace democracy increase productivity and satisfaction. *Hospital Strategy Report, 5* (8), 1–8.

CASE 5–1 *Continued*

Katzenbach, J., & Smith, D. (1993). *The wisdom of teams*. Boston: Harvard Business School Press.

Krotz, S., Muchlinski, E., & Wasserman, A. (1996). *Team development assessment survey*. St. Paul, MN: United Hospital.

Manion, J., Lorimer, W., & Leander, W. (1996). *Team-based health care organizations: Blueprint for success*. Gaithersburg, MD: Aspen.

Orsburn, J., Moran, L., Musselwhite, E., & Zenger, J. (1990). *Self-directed work teams: The new American challenge*. New York: Irwin.

CASE 5–2 Strategic Implementation: A 10-Year Retrospective on Opening a Continuing Care Retirement Center

Alice Story Biache

This case reviews the actual *implementation* of health care services at Goodwin House West and my observations as to the efficacy of the original strategic planning efforts that were described in the first edition of this book. Also included are lessons learned and how they are being applied to current strategic planning undertaken with regard to the $35 million renovation and expansion of a second facility, the original, three-decade-old Goodwin House, as well as refurbishment and renovation of Goodwin House West itself. The format is to reprint the original case study with minor updates; retrospective reflections are indented and set off by the heading, "Comment."

Goodwin House is a nonprofit Continuing Care Retirement Community (CCRC) in Alexandria, Virginia, under the sponsorship of the Episcopal Diocese. It has, since its inception 29 years ago, provided an alternative style of retirement living for persons over 65 years of age. Included in this style of living is the provision of services not readily available when living in the traditional "community," e.g., meals served three times each day, housekeeping services, assistance with insurance claims, and a full scope of health services. These health services range from wellness programs for the independent, ambulatory population to 24-hour nursing care for persons who are frail or acutely ill.

By 1980, Goodwin House was reaping the benefits of an excellent reputation—a 5-year waiting list of applicants. The Board decided to build an additional facility to meet existing and future needs. It was also decided that sound strategic planning and policy formation had to be used to ensure success of this large venture.

A review of the literature in hospital health care administration revealed that this segment of the economy was many years behind the corporate segment in developing strategic management and strategic planning for policy and management benefits. Strategic management recognizes that "the rational process of planning is only a component of a much more complex sociodynamic process which brings about strategic change" (Buller & Timpson, 1986, p. 8). emphasize that the critical ingredient of successful strategy formulation does not necessarily lead to a successful strategy implementation.

■ **GUIDING FRAMEWORK**

This edition will use the updated McKinsey 7-S framework (Waterman, 1982, Waterman, 1987) to illustrate how the Administration developed a strategic plan and proceeded to implement it for nursing services for its new facility, Goodwin House West. Waterman's revised definitions appear in italicized

CASE 5–2 *Continued*

print for reference in the following discussion. The 7-S framework includes: strategy, symbolic behavior, structure, systems, staff, shared values, and skills (see Figure 5–2).

Strategy

Strategy, narrowly defined, is an organization's plan for allocating resources and achieving sustainable competitive advantage.

From the moment that Goodwin House West became a possibility, the President of the Corporation included the members of the nursing staff in the planning development process. This strategy assured involvement and subsequently a feeling of the staff being vested in the project. Such a strategic approach was felt at the initial City Council meeting when approval for the land

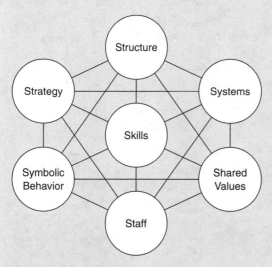

Figure 5–2. The McKinsey 7-S framework. *(Waterman, 1982.)*

use was being sought and continued throughout the implementation of building plans. Nurses were valued throughout the strategic planning process.

- *Item:* The architect consulted countless hours with the Director of Nursing, and she, in turn with her staff, to determine such things as the best location on the nursing care unit for clean linen, for utility rooms, and features the nurses' station should contain. These plans had to fall within state regulations and space constraints of the building design.

Comment. Although the design of the health care unit was felt to be state-of-the-art 9 years ago, within 2 years the design was obsolete. New models were emerging. The long-term care field was moving away from the hospital model of long corridors flanked by patient/resident rooms. There was a movement toward a more home-like atmosphere with a cluster or pod design and away from the sterile institutional look. Plans are now underway to use this approach to completely renovate the area at Goodwin House West and also when expanding and renovating the original Goodwin House facility. The traditional central nurses station will be eliminated and a substation will be built on each wing. Smaller communal dining rooms will be created, as well as home-like lounges. The patient call system will be noiseless, except for a soft sound from the caregiver's beeper.

CASE 5–2 *Continued*

Could the planning have been improved? Perhaps if more design research had been done around the country, the pod model could have been found. Also, this example points out that extensive study and research for a building project should be done (not only in the United States, but in other countries, as well) before the architect puts pen to paper.

- *Item:* It had long been a dream of the nursing staff that a protected outdoor garden be available for those individuals residing on the nursing care unit. This would add an important dimension to their lives, enabling persons to walk off excess energy, provide a place where those who gain satisfaction from tending flowers could do so, and where the sunshine could be enjoyed. The design of the building precluded the possibility of such a garden being built on the ground floor so the architect created a roof garden extending out from the units that filled the stated needs.

Comment: Other building requirements necessitated that the rooftop garden have a southwestern exposure. As a result, the residents do not wish to use the space due to the glare and heat from the afternoon sun. In addition, there appears to be a reluctance on the part of those individuals with a dementia diagnosis to walk there at all. It may be sense of fear of not being on the ground level. The answer may have been to initially build an overhang using structural supports on the southwest side and also put in lattice work to give a greater enclosed feeling.

- *Item:* In creating bathing areas for those residing on the units, the president of Goodwin House, Inc., requested that several manufacturers bring bathtub and shower products to the facility. Then, members of the nursing staff stood in the showers; stepped over and sat in tubs; sat in the chair that raised a person up, over, and down into a whirlpool bath; and tested the grab bars on the walls to determine the best location. The architect also worked with the nursing staff on the placement of the whirlpool tubs to be certain there would be adequate workspace for the wheelchair, resident, and employee to maneuver easily.

Comment: This planning proved to be very effective for residents and patients. In our renovation and refurbishment plans, hand sinks will also be surrounded by vanities so that an adequate placement of toiletry items can be accomplished. The goal is to make each task as simple as possible to promote independence for the resident.

- *Item:* The selection of beds was an issue that involved many opinions. Several manufacturers were invited to bring their products so that the nursing staff could com-

CASE 5–2 *Continued*

pare their features. After months of deliberating, a model was selected that the nursing staff felt would protect the caregiver from possible back injury, provide the most comfort for the patient, and fall within budgetary guidelines.

Comment: This approach has worked well. The beds have proven to function adequately, and have been durable and relatively maintenance free.

- *Item:* In designing the placement of the oxygen and suction wall outlets, the electrical engineer worked in consultation with the nursing staff. The staff held the view that these outlets should be at eye level and in close proximity to the bed so that they would be easily visible. To allow for the differences in staff height, an average was taken to determine the ideal placement. This electrical outlet approach held true for wall sockets, as well. Instead of placing them at baseboard level as is done in many private homes, it was a staff decision that 18 inches from the floor would provide easier access, not only on the nursing unit but also in the residential apartment setting. A most important aspect of this decision was the idea of minimizing bending and thereby reducing back injury.

Comment: The approach of protecting the caregiver, as well as the resident, should be an integral part

of any design planning. Staff and residents alike have appreciated the placement heights of the outlets.

- *Item:* A significant component of the health care service at Goodwin House and one that continued at Goodwin House West is the Health Care Center and Clinic. This area serves those persons living independently in their apartments. Staff members were asked to assist in the designing of the clinic space to ensure smooth traffic flow, privacy, convenience of equipment for the practitioner, and easy accessibility for the resident. Based on staff opinions, the equipment, such as examination tables, cabinets, sinks, and lights drawn in the architect's plans, were selected and installed.

Comment: Office space has proven to be too limited to efficiently house and handle medical records and to provide space for expansion programs such as home care and additional physician consulting areas. Plans for growth should play an important role in the design of such a health care center and clinic. These improvements are being implemented in the further renovation of both Goodwin House and Goodwin House West.

- *Item:* It had been the observation of many staff members that the use of the traditional bathtub in the independent living apartment

CASE 5–2 *Continued*

is very difficult for older persons to use. The height precludes easy access into the bathtub for arthritic persons and, once seated, it is very difficult to pull oneself to a standing position. It was, therefore, decided to create two options for the resident moving into Goodwin House West; one would be a shower with a molded seat built into its frame and the other, a bathtub with a reduced side height of 14 inches. Also included in the bathroom design were faucets that would not require wrist action; a feature the staff felt would be helpful for those with limited hand movement.

Comment: These plans proved to be beneficial to all residents.

Symbolic Behavior (formerly termed *Style*)

Waterman believes that symbolic behavior is the tangible evidence of what management considers important by the way it collectively spends time and attention (i.e., its style). It is not what management says that is important; it is the way management behaves.

A large measure of the success of Goodwin House lies in the leadership style of its management. The administration attempts to demonstrate, by example, a nonpatronizing attitude toward the residents and a "do-with," not "do-for," approach when working with them. This genuine concern for each resident extends to the resident's family as well.

This special kind of care becomes very personalized over time and such an approach is expected of every employee of the organization.

The concern for others is very evident and extends to employees. Great care is taken in knowing persons by name, recognizing accomplishments, soliciting opinions, and using positive reinforcement. It is felt that these factors of style or symbolic behavior contribute greatly to the success of the organization.

Comment: With a new administration, this philosophy has expanded to an even greater extent. Total quality management (TQM) with its tenet of always putting the customer (resident/patient) first, is now a continuing driving force behind services given. The benefits of using TQM have been even greater in terms of customer satisfaction.

Structure

This includes the organization chart, job descriptions, and the ways of showing who reports to whom and how tasks are divided and integrated.

As with the original Goodwin House, Goodwin House West provided full services. The organizational chart of the new site was a replica of the existing organization. Because the site of the new facility was within one mile of the older building, a single management team for both facilities was used. Savings were passed on to the residents.

CASE 5–2 *Continued*

In addition, the management of two facilities under one administration had the very important advantage of minimizing any sense of competition while maintaining uniform quality. Each administrator had an office in each building and traveled between the two, as needed. Although each facility had its own nursing staff, the PRN pool served both.

> **Comment:** Within a few years, the Goodwin House West staff and residents alike began to feel the growing pains of identity and independence. That process of separation has continued with all departments with the exception of health care and its ancillary services, which is scheduled for the near future. Only time will tell whether there will be benefits of this separation of Goodwin House and Goodwin House West.

Systems

The formal and informal processes and flow within an organization. How things get done from day-to-day. Everything from systems to service delivery, accounting, quality control, and performance measurement.

Because all health care services offered at each site (nursing, physical speech and occupation therapies, medical records, pharmacy, home care, and medical claims) have not separated, the two health care staffs continue jointly to meet on a bi-weekly basis. Thus, consistency of management and communication, both formal and informal, is assured.

> **Comment:** The systems for medical accounting and quality control will continue to be directed from the central office, thereby assuring constancy of policies and procedures in both facilities.

Staff

The people in an organization, their demographic characteristics, their experience, education, and training. The fit between the positions and jobs that need to be done and the skills of the people who fill those positions.

In examining the Staff "S" in the Goodwin House organization, one must think of the terms "vested" and "commitment." The majority of the management staff had been with Goodwin House since its inception 20 years before Goodwin House West opened. Their roles and responsibilities expanded to that of corporate staff and they had oversight of the new project. Many of the hourly employees had 10 to 15 years of service with the organization. A nucleus of "old" employees was transferred to Goodwin House West and new employees worked first at Goodwin House to learn the philosophy and management expectations before transferring to Goodwin House West.

> **Comment:** This approach for the staffing of the new facility worked well. Goodwin House West was established on a sound footing with employee leaders experienced in working within the organization. However, at times, this created a weakness at Goodwin

CASE 5–2 *Continued*

House where these individuals had been drawn from. This all occurred during the nursing shortage of the late 1980s!

The staff strategy, which was implemented to retain new employees, was a continuation of the existing program including: (1) a built-in career ladder program for all positions that encourages higher education, (2) tuition reimbursement for higher degrees, (3) sending staff to continuing education classes within and outside the organization, (4) financial rewards for RN Certification in gerontology by the American Nurses Association, and (5) scheduling of work hours to allow for college attendance and personal needs. Several nurse assistants have earned their Licensed Practical Nurse or Registered Nurse degrees and have been promoted.

Thus, despite the fact that national health care appears to be going in the direction of having care delivered to the patient by an individual who has the least amount of education to do so, Goodwin House, Inc., is standing firm in its beliefs that those most educated in caregiving provide the highest quality of care.

Shared Values

What the organization stands for—stated and implied, good and bad. What an organization is proud of or would like to be proud of. Shared values go beyond simple goal statements but might well include them.

As can be seen in the previous discussion, the philosophy of the Goodwin House, Inc., administration is to filter down its style and values to each employee. This aspect of treating each employee as important enough to solicit his or her opinion and incorporating these opinions into the design implementation of Goodwin House West, provides greater assurance for success in meeting the "shared value" goal.

Comment: To further emphasize just how important this shared value "S" is to the organization, a company pledge was created one year ago by "employees-for-employees." Each employee has a pledge card and understands that shared values are vital for the teams to function. Yearly evaluations include how well the employee practices the tenets stated on the card, which are all connected with resident/patient service.

Quarterly, all-employee meetings are held to share and reinforce the values of the organization. Breakfasts are held for the night staff with the president and nursing administration so that they will feel a strong sense of inclusion and sharing of values.

Skills

In the center of Waterman's current 7-S framework is the dependent variable, skills. His idea is that an organization as a whole will be skilled at something to the

CASE 5–2 *Continued*

degree that the other six sibilants support that skill.

> **Comment:** The skills that Goodwin House, Inc., has had for 29 years are in the provision of housing and services for those over 65 years of age. What has changed dramatically in the last 9 years is the competitive marketplace. The organization has been a leader in the field and now, with competition from other providers at an all time high, new techniques and skills must be and are being learned to enable staff to "work smarter with less" and still provide optimal customer/resident satisfaction.

■ BIOGRAPHICAL SKETCH

Alice Story Biache, MSN, RNC, LNHA, has focused most of her professional career on planning and implementing care for the elderly. As Director of Staff Development, she developed facility-wide training programs for staff at Goodwin House. In addition, Ms. Biache has served as Director of Nursing and was Senior Vice President of Professional Services at Goodwin House. Goodwin House, Inc., is a non-profit, continuing-care retirement community in Alexandria, Virginia. She has served on the Governor's Task Force for designing the required curriculum for Nurse Assistants who wished to work in Virginia and served on the Ethics Committee for the American Association of Homes and Services for the Aging. She continues to teach aspects of gerontology on a regular basis for the Continuing Education Program at the University of Virginia. Ms. Biache has published in several journals and serves on the Advisory Boards of nursing programs in area universities as well as the Alzheimers Association.

■ REFERENCES

Buller, F., & Timpson, L. (1986). The strategic management of hospitals: Toward an integrative approach. *Health Care Management Reviews, 11* (2), 7–13.

Waterman, R. (1982). The seven elements of strategic fit. *Journal of Business Strategy, 2,* Winter, 333–339.

Waterman, R. (1987). *The renewal factor— How the best get and keep the competitive edge.* New York: Bantam Books, 57.

6

Marketing in the New Health Care Environment

James W. Harvey

Fundamental to market-driven strategy is adapting to environment change (Day, 1990). Certainly change poses a threat to any organization's ability to create value for clients and successfully compete against new rivals and new practices. Since 1990, health care in the United States has undergone unprecedented regulatory, competitive, and scientific change. New medical knowledge, delivery restructuring, system redesign, new forms of competition, regulatory reform, and a new health care consumer have combined to affect the health care industry in a manner that has been aptly described as "breathtaking" (Auerbach, 1996).

This chapter reviews the current issues in U.S. health care that represent the challenges and opportunities for marketing decision making. The discussion is organized into six sections covering current issues in health care, marketing in health care management, the role of marketing in strategic planning, the importance of social marketing, essentials of writing a marketing plan, and professional services recruitment and retention.

■ CURRENT ISSUES IN HEALTH CARE

Changes Since 1990

The paramount change in the U.S. health care environment arguably is the move from a fragmented fee-for-service structure to the beginnings of an integrated system of managed care in order to slow the growth of spending and to control the widespread variability in quality. Even without passage of federal health care reform legislation in 1993, the health care market is responding to cost-control pressures by becoming more integrated and business-driven.

This is illustrated by how the number of Medicare managed care programs more than tripled between 1983 and 1991 (Weiss, 1995), with the number of all Americans receiving care in health maintenance organizations (HMOs) predicted to reach 56 million by 1995 (Bartling, 1995). Yet it is the *implications* of this transformation that is driving the new environment for health care marketing decision making, not the least of which is a "new" force in reshaping the industry: America's employers (Lifson & Dandalides, 1996; Troy, 1995).

A major influence on health care delivery that had been considered unthinkable 5 years ago is the ability of American business to secure cost and service concessions from health care providers. Coincidentally, American employers saw actual drops in their health care costs during 1993 and 1994 after two decades in which costs outpaced inflation (Appleby, 1995). Employers and individual consumers are also increasingly asking for measurement of medical outcome quality (Addleman, 1995).

Another "unthinkable change" has been the move to capitation payment. Capitation sets a per capita payment that an organization is paid to provide a client enrollee with a defined package of services. The underlying rationale for capitation is to change incentives from "providing more" to providing both high quality and exceptional efficiency (Fromberg, 1996). A critical capability for organizations to negotiate realistic capitation agreements is an information system that reliably tracks costs, population needs, and outcomes.

Ever since the introduction of prospective payment in the 1980s the length of stay in hospitals has been steadily dropping. Advances in technology have also reduced the invasiveness of many procedures, moving them from delivery within hospitals to ambulatory care. Capitation, by creating incentives for more efficiency, feeds the trend to reduced length of stay. One potential risk associated with the capitation approach to managed care is that delivery systems will reduce utilization of care too much, resulting in vital medical procedures or observations by qualified health care professionals being omitted ("How Good," 1996). One counterbalancing factor is that providers typically purchase insurance to cover the financial risk between capitation payment and the cost of services provided (Grimaldi, 1995).

The rapidity of change is creating fear and discomfort among the public and many providers that cost containment and effective care are out of balance. One result is a demand for health policy to regulate the underprovision of health care. An example is the legislation passed to require hospitals to offer mothers and newborns a 48-hour length of stay (Ginzinger, 1996). Another health policy concern is the shrinking number of Americans with health care insurance coverage due to underemployment, chronic health care conditions, and social welfare reform (Curtin, 1996). Continuing initiatives are expected.

The New Health Care Consumer

Several studies underscore the emergence of a new health care consumer. Individuals are taking a more proactive approach to their own health care, seeking out information, and adjusting their lifestyles to improve their health, including diet and nutrition, sleeping habits, and smoking secession ("Individuals Gathering," 1995). In a shift of values, Americans are moving away from the idea of health as the absence of disease and the result of medical intervention to a broader definition that includes both personal responsibility and quality of life, with self-care and prevention key watchwords ("What Creates Health?", 1995). One objective of medical self-care is to avoid unnecessary service.

A market response to this trend is continued growth in products for in-home diagnostics, such as blood sampling kits for HIV testing (Conlan, 1995). Another response has been the change from prescription-only to over-the-counter and direct-to-consumer promotion of some prescription drugs. One outcome is the pharmacist increasingly assuming the role of provider (Cardinale, 1995). At least one study has validated the reduced health care costs to insurers of this change; however, this study did not investigate the effect on adverse consequences to the patient (Gurwitz, McLaughlin, & Fish, 1995). This self-care trend is an opportunity for nurses to be sources of referral and help in guiding people to optimize their health and to be more responsible for managing their own health risks (Joel, 1995).

Another example of a market-driven response to this new consumer is health care CD-ROMs and access to the internet for personal computers. This type of software gives users quick access to medical information as well as guidelines for long-term well-being, diet, nutrition, and exercise. The overall objective of such software is to help users become better consumers of medical care and better-informed managers of their own health (Tucker, 1996).

Convenient access to health care information is an important engine that is driving the self-care trend. For example, during the second half of 1996, the sixth most frequently accessed web site in America is the National Institutes of Health (http://www.nih.gov/). Another market option is choosing an insurance plan using a website such as *Healtheon* (http://www.healtheon.com). Healtheon's first services include automated enrollment and management of members' health plans, and descriptions to help users evaluate and enroll in specific benefit plans (e.g., medical, dental, vision, life, disability insurance), evaluate costs and payment options, and provide personal health information resources in an interactive format.

Changes in Provider Structure and Strategy

Hospitals across the United States are undergoing profound changes that, in the next century, could transform patient care and the traditional role of the hospital in the community (Olmos, 1996). Managed care has forced hospitals to overhaul operations by emphasizing outpatient services, purchasing primary care physician groups, expanding home care, downsizing patient beds, and merging to reduce costs and expand services. For instance, home health care is predicted to grow at 15 percent a year through the end of the decade (Palmeri, 1995).

Subacute care has emerged to fill the gap between acute and long-term care for the individual who has had an acute illness, injury, or aggravated disease process. It is delivered either in a hospital or skilled nursing facility immediately after or instead of acute care, and it rarely includes high-technology monitoring or diagnostic procedures.

These changes to integrate health care delivery are driven by a goal to increase productivity through synergy. An analysis of recent data highlighted that integrated delivery systems require significant capital investment and that the wiser strategy may be to avoid asset-based integration in favor of *virtual* integration (Coile, 1995). This approach emphasizes patient-management agreements, partnerships with suppliers and other providers of complementary services, provider incentives, and investment in information systems, rather than facilities and in-house services.

Another trend in health care is disease management, also called care management. The emergence of disease management stems from the recognition that chronic medical conditions affect 40 percent of the population, cause 80 percent of all illnesses ("DM Critical," 1995), and usually involve continuing education, a multidisciplinary team approach that includes family members and significant others (Hurt, 1995). The increased use of pharmacists and nurses as contact points in care management is consistent with their perceived credibility.

Technology is being used to support provider strategies for improving patient care, controlling costs, and gaining a competitive edge—not just for operational support (Trainer, 1995). For example, since 1987, the UCLA/Kaiser Permanente Therapeutic Learning software program has assisted 14,000 patients to cope with stress using a user-friendly point-and-click approach (Berlin, 1995).

Technology may soon restore the "house call" by data being transported online (Blanton & Balch, 1995; Rosner, 1996). A recent survey reported that consumers are more accepting of health information, including advice about treatment received through a telephone or on-line service, even if it means giving up a face-to-face visit with a care provider ("Health Care," 1996).

The Metamorphosis of the Modern Physician

A reality for physicians today is that they are losing status and income level in an economy where clients are unwilling to pay ever-increasing fees for service (Adelman, 1996). In addition, more than half of medical school graduates currently pursue training in lower-paying generalist fields such as family practice, internal medicine, and pediatrics; an indication that tomorrow's physicians are responding to the new demands for more primary care physicians and fewer specialists ("Business Bulletin," 1996).

An additional change in service provision affecting physicians is the decrease in independent practice with an accompanying rise in physician hospital organizations (PHOs) and physician organizations (POs) (Kleiman, 1995).

The Short-term Future of Health Care

Oliver (1996) predicts that the next 10 years will see hospitals closing, physicians quitting their specialties, HMOs merging, and traditional indemnity health insurance becoming virtually extinct. However, hospital survivors will grow and a few will dominate the market. Integrated systems that own their own facilities will suffer since it will continue to be cheaper to buy services "just in time."

Accountability will receive increased attention by providers, recipients, and policymakers alike (Burke, 1995). The Health Plan Employer Data Information Set (HEDIS) developed by the National Committee for Quality Assurance (NCQA) is the primary standard-setting initiative for managed health care. The objective of this tracking system is to assist employers and consumers in choosing health plans based on quality of care and value (Borfitz, 1995). *Consumer Reports* has developed a consumer-focused venue for increasing health care client awareness of the importance of HEDIS data ("How Good," 1996).

■ MARKETING HEALTH CARE

Management and Marketing

The essence of marketing is the analysis, planning, and control of exchanges in order to develop and hold relationships with priority clients, suppliers, partners, and relevant publics, such as employers, other health care providers, and the media. Figure 6–1 presents examples of the types of publics with whom health care organizations have exchange relationships. Future marketing should produce more collaboration among insurers and providers, prevention efforts, and targeting of specific types of consumers (Jaklevic, 1995b).

Central to the practice of marketing is understanding the reasons for transactions between organizations and patients, which are the underpinnings of strategy development. For example, in exchange for needed health services, patients give agencies a guarantee of payment and positive recommendations to friends based on satisfaction. Moreover, health care includes many other exchanges between suppliers, boards of directors, volunteers, regulatory agencies, donors, management, insurance carriers, the media, social activists, and providers. Observers see the tangible manifestations of a health care strategy, such as expansion of a hospital wing, an advertisement on television, or a direct mail newsletter. What one cannot see are the marketing processes that led to these tangible results.

To many people, marketing is advertising, promotion, and sales. Some health care administrators view marketing as a stop-gap measure; a way to improve their short-term revenues through advertising tactics. However,

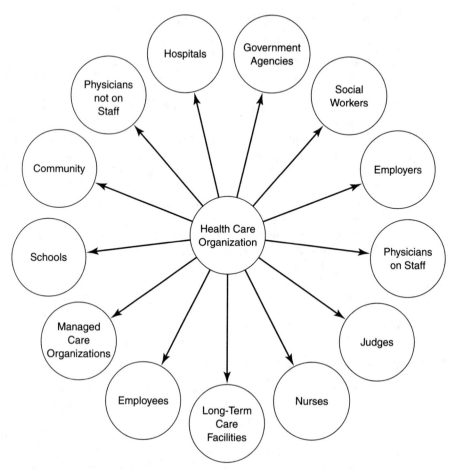

FIGURE 6–1. Complexity of health care markets. *(From Berkowitz, E.N. [1966].* Essentials of health care marketing. *Gaithersburg, MD: Aspen.)*

savvy administrators with a comprehensive understanding of marketing, seek long-term solutions by directing the development, planning, and control of the traditional "four P's" of marketing—(a) *products and services,* (b) *price,* (c) *place* (distribution and location), and (d) *promotion*—toward client satisfaction. Using market research to identify client needs, serving those needs, understanding competitive and environmental dynamics, and developing strategies within the organization's mission and objectives, collectively represent the underpinnings of a *market-driven* health care organization.

Alternative orientations for health care organizations illustrate the importance of being market driven. *Product driven* organizations depend on managers or other "experts" to define client needs. *Production-driven* organizations identify the primary task of managers as assuring production and distribution efficiency while assuming the market will purchase what is produced. Organizations that are *sales-driven* seek to persuade possible customers to purchase their existing products and services. In contrast, managers in market-driven organizations use an exchange perspective. Success is determined by market dynamics; the match of needs of segments of the market identified by research to the organization's mission, objectives, environmental concerns, and competitive advantage.

Uniqueness of Service Marketing

Services possess five basic differences that underscore the uniqueness of marketing intangible offerings. These differences explain, in part, the considerable difficulty of some health care board members from packaged goods industries in transferring their knowledge of marketing to health care. The five differences are:

- *Intangibility:* Services are actions, not objects; they cannot be seen, felt, tasted, or touched.
- *Heterogeneity:* Services are performances that vary according to the characteristics and situations of *both* the provider and the service recipient.
- *Simultaneous Production and Consumption:* Whereas goods are produced first, then sold and finally consumed, services are sold first and then simultaneously produced and consumed.
- *Perishability:* Services cannot be saved, stored, resold, or returned.

The intangible nature of service offerings, the inseparability of provider and recipient, the inability to store exchanges, the local nature of the market, and the provider's role as inextricably determinant of consumer satisfaction are unique issues encountered by all service providers. Decision making when purchasing health care is also quite different from that involved in choosing packaged goods. In choosing health care there is a higher risk in making a wrong choice and a lack of essential information for a wise choice due to the need being an uncommon life event requiring technology in which patients lack the expertise to evaluate. Health care is also unique in that, especially for emergency or highly specialized health problems, client options are often restricted, with the choice of service being made by providers who act as gatekeepers.

In searching for the best marketing strategies, health care managers are frequently encouraged to think in terms of packaging, brands, brand managers, product lines, and loss leaders. This is a mistake to translate a packaged goods mentality to health care service marketing. Better insight into strategy development is afforded to health care planners by comparing their needs to the success or failure of strategies used by other local-service marketers outside of health care, such as banks or hotels.

Characteristics of the Market-Driven Organization

Whether your organization is market driven may be assessed using the questions listed below:

- Where is marketing within the organizational structure?
- Are target markets well defined and their needs understood?
- Is strategy development based on provider/market relationships?
- Are strategic objectives measurable, explicit, and do they specify a timetable?
- Does the organization have a distinct market identity?
- Are services seen as solutions to patients' problems?
- Are location, layout, and convenience seen as key to provider choice?
- Are prices based on value to customers?
- Is promotion understood as playing a limited, specific role in overall strategy?

Ethics of Marketing Health Care

Many professionals argue that marketing health care is unethical; others point out that marketing has increased sensitivity to consumer needs and desires, increased awareness of services, and has neither sacrificed industry standards nor client trust (Bloom, 1984). The American Marketing Association's Academy for Health Services Marketing has developed a set of professional ethics for health care marketing professionals, which encourages them to: (1) respect the primacy of patient and customer welfare; (2) ensure the competitiveness of their organization; (3) provide communications that inform and persuade but do not deceive; (4) compare competitive offerings in ways that are fair and can be substantiated; (5) never enter relationships that constitute a conflict with existing client interests; (6) respect the privacy and confidentiality of patient, customer, and client relationships; and (7) be vigilant in encouraging the application of these standards ("Ethics for Emerging Field," 1985).

More recent discussions of ethics issues in health care marketing reveal several of the challenges posed in the new era of managed care, including pricing and allocating scarce specialty resources; developing new fee-for-service health "products" for the wealthy, such as plastic surgery procedures; and promoting internal referrals that are not in the patient's best interest. Wicks (1995) examines urgent problems and proposes that bioethics can also serve as a useful guide for business ethics.

■ ROLE OF MARKETING IN STRATEGIC PLANNING

After a decade of downsizing and reengineering, suddenly strategic planning, the idea of "pondering the future of markets and competitors," is back in vogue (Byrne, 1996, p. 46). A strategic plan consists of four sets of related decisions, usually performed by top-level administration: (1) defining the business, (2) determining the mission or role of the business, (3) formulating functional strategies, and (4) budgeting.

The marketing division often contributes to this effort by providing an analysis of external factors offering opportunities and threats, and a consumer analysis, including customer satisfaction and market segmentation, followed by a competitor analysis. A second contribution is a review of internal strengths and weaknesses through self-assessment. Together, these actions are often referred to as a SWOT (*s*trengths, *w*eaknesses, *o*pportunities, and *t*hreats).

In 1993, a 390-bed acute care hospital in the intensely competitive and managed care-oriented Minneapolis-St. Paul market initiated a strategic plan. That planning process began by separating the local market into its several constituent segments and continued by collecting and analyzing data to assess the fit between the markets, its affiliated physicians, and managed care payors. The results of that planning process showed hospital administrators that a redefinition of the mission was needed—future success meant becoming a regional provider of a continuum of ambulatory to inpatient health services rather than remaining primarily an inpatient facility. Strategies were then developed to reach this goal (Allen & Weber, 1995). This case illustrates how marketing supports strategic planning through: (1) competitor analysis; (2) consumer analysis, including client satisfaction and market segmentation; (3) self-assessment; and (4) strategy development. The first three topics use market research to gather data. Strategies can only be as good as the quality of the data collected and the analysis performed.

Competitor Analysis

Competition arises from both direct and indirect sources. Direct competition stems from other health care institutions, using similar methods (Jensen, 1986). Indirect competition, often neglected in strategic analysis, comes from prospective clients choosing industries and technologies other than mainstream health care. Figure 6–2 illustrates the many possible alternative approaches to health care as they are perceived by consumers to provide care along the dimensions of the benefits of transactions costs (convenience) and degree of specialization. Services and devices that are located in close proximity to each other in this figure are thought of as near substitutes by consumers, as they are seen as possessing similar combinations of desired benefits. Brainstorming is often useful in identifying alternatives.

Consumer Analysis

Physicians have long been recognized as hospital customers, based on their gatekeeping status. Now they are increasingly potential partners in joint ventures. For example, Abbey and Treash (1995) found that physicians join PHOs to improve contracting positions with managed care organizations,

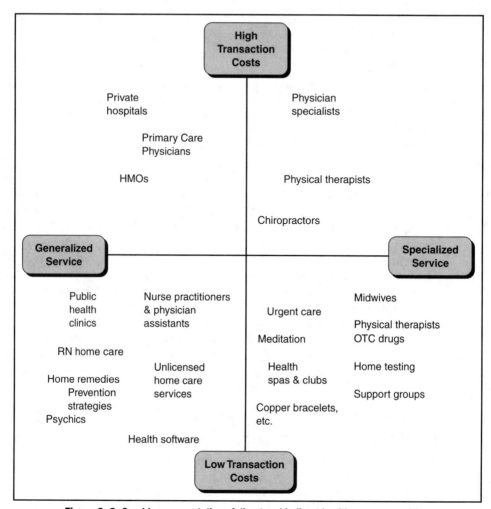

Figure 6–2. Graphic representation of direct and indirect health care competition.

facilitate collaborative efforts among physicians, and enhance their abilities to accept and manage capitation.

The second customer to be considered is the payors. Managed care contracts, indemnity providers, and health maintenance organizations all have referral potential of differing sizes, demographics, and predominant health care needs. They also have financial health indicators and past payment practices as factors to consider when making contracts.

Two methods to employ in analyzing the needs and exchanges of the final consumer are market segmentation and consumer satisfaction. Recall that the ultimate goal of a marketing program is "attract and retain." Therefore *patient satisfaction* is a crucial indicator of successful marketing (Courts, 1995).

Although Americans generally report high levels of satisfaction with their health care services, some researchers question the sensitivity of the questionnaires (Alt, 1995). To address the skepticism raised by high levels of patient satisfaction, the National Committee for Quality Assurance has developed a standardized survey to make results comparable from plan to plan (Morrissey, 1995).

An important adjunct to patient compliments are complaints, which also provide valuable insight into patient motivation. For example, Murray (1995) found that most patient concerns stem from being kept waiting; providers speaking at, not to the patient; inability to reach someone at the office; appearance of the office; and office hours that accommodate evening appointment. Practices that scored better in meeting these concerns led to increased referrals. Strasser and associates (1995) found that hospital inpatients gave higher satisfaction ratings for their medical care and services than did their family members and friends. This group can also be influential in future utilization.

Identifying discrete subgroups within the market for health care services and responding appropriately to differences in their health care needs and preferences represents one of the most effective approaches to marketing. This process of identification is called *market segmentation*. Market segment analysis assists health care organizations to (1) better understand that they serve multiple sets of clients who possess different wants and needs, and (2) deliver services that are congruent with these diverse values and desires.

Kurtenbach and Warmoth (1995) propose that the key factors in understanding market differences in order to plan strategically are age, sex, and race differences; socioeconomic uniqueness; epidemiological trends; lifestyle and environmental changes; and employer demographics. Haley (1985) disagrees because these elements are based on arbitrary categories of descriptive factors. They do not reveal why people choose a service, only the characteristics of users and nonusers. This lack of causality is the basis for the relatively poor performance of demographic segmentation in predicting future behavior, such as receptivity to persuasive communication and product/service changes.

To address the lack of causality inherent in segmentation strategies, many organizations have turned to the use of *benefit segmentation*. Defining markets on the basis of homogeneous preferences for attributes or benefits of services is believed to assist in prescribing actions to improve satisfaction. For instance, in examining preventive health care behavior, John and Miaoulis (1992) identified segments of people he called health seekers, followers, "band-aiders," "do not bug me" types, hypochondriacs, and self-sufficient people. Focusing on hospitals, Finn and Lamb (1986) found patients whose primary expectations while in the hospital varied from "take care of me" to "cure me," "pamper me," and "explain to me." Strategies to address these expectations would have to include methods to identify individual expectations.

Self-Assessment

Self-assessment of internal organizational strengths and weaknesses, indicators of resources, effectiveness of activities, constituency and support groups, and market position is also essential.

One of the best known methods for internal assessment is service portfolio analysis, originally developed by the Boston Consulting Group. Each service is classified into one of four categories, as defined by two dimensions: First, the relative share of the market already captured by each service (high/low), and second, the prospects for growth of that market (high/low). The rationale for this fourfold typology is concern for current performance (market share) and prospects for the future (market growth). Market share provides the organization with cash through sales of the service, whereas market growth absorbs cash, necessitated by adding facilities, staff, and supplies to meet increased levels of activity. The four areas are labeled "cash cows" (they should be "milked" for their revenues, but no investment for growth is indicated), "question marks" (they generate low revenues, but potential growth may or may not indicate investment), "dogs" (they generate poor revenues and growth potential, and should be divested), and "stars" (high revenues fund their high growth potential, hence they are shining stars).

For example, a hospital may be a local leader in delivering babies (high share), but because of the aging of the nearby population, the potential future growth rate is low (low growth). This service is a "cash cow"; the hospital will want to hold its market share position and maintain quality, but not expand capacity.

Although service portfolio analysis fails to consider long-term community needs, image value, services required for the public good that are unprofitable (e.g., indigent care) or other subjective criteria, portfolio thinking does encourage administrators to evaluate the financial contribution of each service in relation to the organization's overall offering of services. An expanded portfolio analysis could be used more comprehensively to compare the services a health care organization offers.

Another technique used for this in health care administration is Importance-Performance-Awareness (IPA) mapping (Graf, Hemmasi, & Strong, 1996). This methodology provides insights into the organization's strategic strengths and weaknesses. By comparing the profile of importance, performance, and consumer awareness of each service provided, management can better set priorities for changes in allocation of resources such as promotion and services to monitor or consider discontinuing.

Strategy Development

Strategic plans must also include strategies for promoting services. Rynne (1995) states convincingly that the best approach to strategy development is to apply the fundamentals of marketing. There are five steps to this approach:

trace how the purchase decision is made, interpret the process in terms of consumer benefits, reinvent the product and configure the marketing mix to mirror the consumer benefits, clarify the system's identity, and integrate a communications campaign that is consistent with the overall strategy.

In the context of managed care, Firshein (1996) identifies several such strategies. These approaches point to the value of focusing on local market needs, being willing to partner with purchasers, competing on strategies other than price, emphasizing an educational component in the marketing plan, and emphasizing differences. Discussing a "grand strategy" approach, Goh and Pritula (1996) note that in the past decade managed care organizations have gained market shares by information management, attractive local markets, alternative settings for specialty care, and hospital consolidation.

The final set of strategies chosen results in what marketing experts refer to as *positioning*. An organization seeks to have a market position that is distinct and positive in the minds of its consumers (Church, 1996; Goldberg, 1995). Administrators seeking to position their facilities need to ask themselves: (1) what do we stand for? (2) what are the objectives of our marketing plan? (3) how can we highlight our strengths? (4) what type of client mix is desired? and (5) what is our competition doing? On the basis of research and insight into questions such as these, a market position that maximizes the organization's strengths and minimizes its limitations is adopted. Adapting Porter's (1985) model for positioning opportunities, Autrey and Thomas (1986) show how health care providers can build differential advantage using any mix of three basic strategies: (1) cost leadership—offering the lowest price; (2) differentiation—creating uniqueness by technology, equipment, staff, services, or quality offered; and (3) focus—concentrating on a particular type of client. Underlying a strong position is the recognition that an institution cannot successfully be all things to all parts of the market.

■ APPLYING SOCIAL MARKETING TO HEALTH CARE

Social marketing is the 25-year-old discipline that applies the marketing technologies developed in the commercial sector to the solution of social problems for which the bottom line is promoting behavior change (Andreasen, 1995). Successful applications of social marketing to tourism, performing arts audience development, substance abuse, seat belt use, mental health, condom use, blood pressure, aggressive driving, smoking cessation, and heart disease are commonly reported (Andreasen, 1994; Kotler & Roberto, 1989; Kotler & Zaltman, 1971; Lefebvre & Flora, 1988).

In health care, social marketing is especially applicable to health practices and behavioral changes that improve health. Breastfeeding is an excellent example. Oglethorpe (1995) notes that there is a worldwide decline in the incidence and duration of breastfeeding, despite universally recognized benefits to both mother and child. When infant feeding method is examined as a social marketing issue, one examines it (1) in the context of an exchange transaction; (2) as the first complex consumption decision that is made for a child; (3) in a sociocultural context; (4) as a policy issue affecting the health care system, the workplace, and the law; and (5) as a methodological challenge to marketing and consumer behavior researchers. Factors such as being a good parent, bonding, having a healthy child, convenience, love, enjoyment, immunity transmission, emotional contact, no bottles, natural nutrition, physical contact, mother–baby relationship, and child mental health were emphasized by a sample of reactions from breastfeeding mothers.

Strategies are developed using these key principles of social marketing: (1) the final objective is to influence the behavior of a target market; (2) programs must be cost-effective; (3) all strategies start with the customer; (4) intervention involves all four Ps of marketing strategy (products/services, price, place, promotion); (5) market research is essential to the design, testing, and evaluation of programs; (6) markets are always segmented; and (7) target behaviors compete with comfortable alternatives.

■ ESSENTIALS OF WRITING A MARKETING PLAN

The strategic plan defines goals for the organization and the strategies executives have chosen to achieve them. The annual marketing plan outlines strategies to achieve strategic goals. According to Hedden (1996), the steps in a marketing plan are:

1. Analyze the organization and its environment, including company objectives and industry trends.
2. Analyze the market, including key targets, client knowledge, and competition.
3. Develop a marketing strategy that links clients to organizational capabilities.
4. Develop and support staff to enable them to achieve stated objectives.
5. Project revenue and expenses.
6. Identify the pitfalls and prepare for contingencies.
7. Track key indicators to see if the plan is working.

Conklin (1994) recommends that annual marketing plans be written in three parts: one for activities targeted at traditional payers, another targeting managed care, and the third to identify strategies that work for both.

Communication tools to reach the external environment are vital to marketing success. Promotion of health care may include advertising, personal selling, and public relations.

Advertising

The 1995 National Hospital Marketers' Survey reported that advertising expenditures for hospitals and health systems climbed for the second straight year in 1994, but total marketing expenditures declined slightly. National advertising expenditures were $856 million, up 11.4 percent from 1993. Growth in marketing expenditures has come from larger hospitals and systems. The typical 300-bed facility spent about 8 times what a hospital with fewer than 100 beds spent on marketing (Jaklevic, 1995a), with conditions favoring a continued increase in expenditures (Weisend, 1995). Clow (1995) argues that to remain profitable, health care providers are turning to marketing—and primarily advertising—as a means of gaining new patients.

The push for name recognition through advertising in a market-driven environment is responsible for dramatic increases in hospital marketing costs during the last decade. A key new element in health care advertising is the introduction of direct-to-consumer advertising of prescription drugs. The goal is primarily to encourage individuals to seek additional information about the product. People who have a positive attitude toward this type of advertising reported having additional discussions with either a friend or pharmacist rather than a physician (Williams & Hensel, 1995).

Typical of the themes and appeals of broad-market advertising are: (1) the services offered; (2) the technology available; (3) physician referral for prospective clients; (4) geographical appeal and local accessibility; (5) satellite locations that underscore accessibility and community involvement; (6) cost/quality, especially cost-reduction with a reason, such as ambulatory surgery; and (7) image—"feel good" advertisements. Although consumers are becoming more active participants in their health care decisions, making them receptive to direct-to-consumer advertising, they are growing increasingly cynical and skeptical of such approaches (Hodnett, 1995).

Advertising is an extremely powerful and effective method of achieving organizational goals. There are, however, also examples of successful marketing campaigns in which advertising played a minimal role, and advertising budgets do not have to be large to achieve marketing objectives. For example, suppliers and providers can cooperate to develop wellness health fairs that benefit all participants and attract only individuals who are interested. The size of the promotional budget is not the only key to success. An advertising budget contains inherent waste; by the nature of its broad-scope character, it reaches many irrelevant groups, as well as the consumers who represent the primary objective of the communication. However, the "shotgun" feature of advertising is beneficial when the character of the target audience is somewhat unclear or when the goal is to create image and positioning beliefs for the general community, using general interest media, such as newspapers, radio, television, and magazines. Furthermore, much advertising can be targeted to specific populations through careful choice of media, such as newsletters sent to specifically desirable groups and specialty magazines with clearly identified readers.

Thornton (1995) notes the many advantages of direct mail, particularly its low level of waste—because the user can precisely target specific consumer groups by preselecting exactly who will receive mailed information. Also, direct mail recipients are more likely to read and respond to messages received through the mail than to other forms of paid advertising because there is generally less advertising clutter in direct mail and direct mail is a less threatening form of advertising.

Personal Selling

Many administrators perform personal selling functions by visiting important customers, such as physicians, other referral agents, community leaders, insurance executives, and suppliers. These visits are important opportunities for administrators to explain current initiatives, outline future plans, and provide symposia on current issues facing the health care industry. Brochures that highlight available staff and services, as well as business cards and other promotional literature, are usually left with the potential customer for future reference. Such marketing visits are becoming an increasingly common expectation of health care administrators. In a major shift driven by health care reform, promotion of health care has evolved from an emphasis on advertising to the current increase in personal selling. Along with public relations and planning research, sales is becoming a significant part of the marketing function of health care organizations. For a profile of personal selling in the health care industry, see Bowers, Powers, and Spencer (1994).

Public Relations

Confusion often exists as to the differences among personal selling, advertising, and public relations. Personal selling and advertising are techniques that have narrowly defined objectives, ultimately designed to stimulate the demand of a target group. Public relations, on the other hand, involves techniques that are used to encourage broad community support. These techniques are designed to educate, inform, introduce, and create favorable images of the organization, either directly or indirectly, and include means such as institutional advertising, publicity, and personal appearances.

Among the public relations techniques developed to influence more directly community attitudes toward health care organizations are speeches made by staff, open houses, and seminars to introduce the community to available services and programs. Often, however, the role of public relations is to deal with bad news. High-profile instances of medical errors that raise questions about the public's trust in physicians and hospitals are the true test of an organization's public affairs prowess. Hegarty (1995) cautions that to help restore the public trust, organizations must be more vigilant in guarding against human error, recognize that medical mistakes can happen anywhere, speak more openly about the limitations—as well as the successes—of medicine, and work harder to put better information in the hands of consumers and community-wide opinion leaders.

■ PROFESSIONAL SERVICES RECRUITMENT AND RETENTION

Health services was the 14th fastest growing "well paid" industry in 1996, growing at 3.3 percent, creating over 9.4 million new jobs in the first quarter with an average salary of over $34,000 (Dobrzynski, 1996). Health care is also predicted to account for 16 percent of the economy by the year 2000, with starting salaries for registered nurses averaging $36,000 (Auerbach, 1996).

Despite the positive outlook for industry growth, Curtin (1995) notes a shift in job security. As the nation moves to managed care, an estimated one-third to one-half of all hospitals will close their doors. Hospitals and physicians who are not part of a network are unlikely to survive. The future will see hospitals change their skill mixes and nurse/patient ratios, develop subacute services, and search for the least costly way to deliver care to patients—all of which will affect staffing levels. The long-term job prospects for nurses look good, but experience and education will become more important in determining staff income.

Nurses who are willing to try new things, learn new ways, and work in multidisciplinary teams will find opportunities opening up to them. Responses to the new health care environment include staff redesign that has led to increased productivity, and patient and staff satisfaction (Gould, Thompson, Rakel, & Jensen 1996). Koester, et al. (1995) assert that the new approaches to leadership for frontline health care providers will emphasize (1) job knowledge and performance, (2) continuing professional progress, (3) initiative in professional performance areas, (4) credibility and dependability, and (5) cooperation and interpersonal skills.

More recently, Lamm (1996) concurs that staff restructuring is underway, stating that a massive change in the numbers, types, and skills of health professionals will occur. The numbers and roles of nurse practitioners, physician assistants, certified nurse midwives, and other allied professionals will increase. The distribution of nurses by employer will change. The numbers and types of unlicensed health personnel will increase. Nurses will increasingly work within interdisciplinary teams for patient care, rather than teams of nursing personnel. Trends indicate a lower ratio of registered nurses to patients and the closure of many hospitals as care increasingly is provided on an ambulatory basis or with shorter length of stay. Some authors are expressing concern that these changes are leading to a decrease in the quality of patient care (Dowling, 1996).

Another challenge to traditional employment is the growing practice of outsourcing—using temporary nurses to balance out staffing requirements. Outsourcing concerns many people because it spells a loss of control. Nurse managers need to know that the direct cost of outsourced personnel may be higher than if care had been performed by in-house personnel. Furthermore, the outsourcing vendor may not know the particular enterprise as well as an internal employee (Simpson, 1995a, 1995b, 1996).

These trends suggest how nurses should present themselves to the market. Nurses should not plan for lifetime employment in one institution. They also need to learn interview and resume writing skills. Nurse resumes should emphasize skills and functional capabilities gained rather than just chronological years of experience within acute care specialties. Nurses need to proactively seek to transfer acute care skills and expertise to new settings such as ambulatory surgery, case management, insurance utilization review, and home care.

Health care managers recruiting and retaining nurses need to emphasize the temporal nature of positions during times of rapid change and restructuring and assist nurses to creatively imagine how they fit into new configurations of care. Often, nurses need to increase their visibility and sell others on why they should be considered for a nontraditional position or why a service would be enhanced by including a nurse position. In managed care environments, new ambulatory care services are often envisioned by physicians and health care management and the potential contribution of nurses is overlooked and not designed into the system.

■ BIOGRAPHICAL SKETCH

James W. Harvey is Associate Professor of Marketing in the School of Business at George Mason University, Fairfax, Virginia. He received his PhD in Business Administration from Penn State University and is active in strategic planning and marketing management for both profit and not-for-profit organizations. Dr. Harvey has participated in over 100 marketing studies, task forces, consultancies, and executive development seminars for managers of profit and not-for-profit organizations, including Department of the Interior, Bureau of Land Management; Department of Health and Human Services; Fairfax County Park Authority; Federal Trade Commission; Graydon Manor Psychiatric Hospital; Internal Revenue Service; Kodak; National Academy for Voluntarism; National Glass Association; National Institutes of Health; and United Way of America. Dr. Harvey has also published over 30 works in journals, proceedings of professional associations, and books of readings.

■ SUGGESTED READINGS

Andreasen, A.R. (1995). *Marketing social change: Changing behavior to promote health, social development, and the environment*. San Francisco: Jossey-Bass.

Berkowitz, E.N. (1996). *Essentials of health care marketing*. Gaithersburg, MD: Aspen.

Clark, B., & Boissoneau, R. (1995). Strategic planning and the health care supervisor. *Health Care Supervisor, 14*, (2), 1–10.

Lindgren, J.H. & Shimp, T.A. (1996). *Marketing: An interactive learning system.* Fort Worth: Dryden

McAlexander, J.H., Kaldenburg, D.O. & Koenig, H.F. (1994). Service quality measurement. *Journal of Health Care Marketing, 14* (3), 34–40.

Zeithaml, V.A. & Bitner, M.J. (1996). *Services marketing.* New York: McGraw-Hill.

■ REFERENCES

Abbey, F.B., & Treash, K.M. (1995). Reasons providers form PHOs. *Healthcare Financial Management, 49* (8), 38–48.

Addleman, R.B. (1995). Value-driven healthcare. *Healthcare Forum, 38* (6), 46–50.

Adelman, S.H. (1996). 'Off the pedestal' is a fine place for physicians to be. *American Medical News, 39* (6), 20.

Allen, D.W., & Weber, D. (1995). Ambulatory care planning for a hospital. *Health Care Strategic Management, 13* (2), 17–20.

Alt, S.J. (1995). Patient satisfaction rates are too high. *Health Care Strategic Management, 13* (8), 2–3.

Andreasen, A.R. (1994). Social marketing: Definition and domain. *Journal of Marketing and Public Policy,* Spring 108–114.

Andreasen, A.R. (1995). *Marketing social change: Changing behavior to promote health, social development, and the environment.* San Francisco: Jossey-Bass.

Appleby, C. (1995). Health care's new heavyweights. *Hospitals & Health Networks, 69* (9), 26–34.

Auerbach, S. (1996). Falling health care employment could hurt economy, experts warn. *Washington Post,* July 24, D1–2.

Autrey, P., & Thomas, D. (1986). Competitive strategy in the hospital industry. *Health Care Management Review, 11* (1), 7–14.

Bartling, A.C. (1995). Trends in managed care. *Healthcare Executive, 10* (2), 6–11.

Berlin, L. (1995). Cybertherapy? *Forbes* Oct. 9, ASAP Supplement, 158–162.

Blanton, T., & Balch, D.C. (1995). Telemedicine. *Futurist, 29* (5), 14–17.

Bloom, P.N. (1984). Effective marketing for professional services. *Harvard Business Review, 62* (5), 102–110.

Borfitz, D. (1995). Are you ready for the new grading system? *Medical Economics, 72* (16), 151–166.

Bowers, M.R., Powers, T.L., & Spercer, P.D. (1994). Characteristics of the salesforce in the US health-care service industry. *Journal of Services Marketing, 8* (4), 36–49.

Burke, G. (1995). Health care delivery in the 21st century—Part II. *Health Systems Review, 28* (2), 36–40.

Business bulletin: What's up with docs? (1996). *The Wall Street Journal,* April 4, A, p. 1.

Byrne, J.A. (1996). Strategic Planning. *BusinessWeek,* August 26, 46–52.

Cardinale, V. (1995). New realities. *Drug Topics, 139* (10), 63–65.

Church, L. (1996). Positioning hospital-based home care agencies for managed care. *Healthcare Financial Management, 50* (2), 28–32.

Clow, K.E. (1995). Advertising health care services. *Journal of Health Care Marketing, 15* (2), 9.

Coile, R.C., Jr. (1995). Assessing healthcare market trends and capital needs: 1996–2000. *Healthcare Financial Management, 49* (8), 60–65.

Conklin, M. (1994). Marketing must make integration transition. *Health Care Strategic Management, 12* (10), 15.

Conlan, M.F. (1995). FDA open to home test kits for detecting HIV virus. *Drug Topics, 139* (6), 60.

Courts, N.F. (1995). Steps to a patient satisfaction survey. *Nursing Management, 26* (9), 64OO–64PP.

Curtin, L.L. (1995). Job security: Is nothing sacred anymore? *Nursing Management, 26* (7), 7–9.

Curtin, L.L. (1996). The abandonment of the patient. *Nursing Management, 27* (2), 7–8.

DM critical to continued success of managed care (1995). *Employee Benefit Plan Review, 50* (6), 26.

Day, G.S. (1990). *Market driven strategy: Processes for creating value.* New York: The Free Press.

Dobrzysnki, J.H. (1996). The new jobs: A growing number are good ones. *New York Times,* July 21, Money and Business, D1, 10ff.

Dowling, K. (1996). Ask the patient with the tubes how expendable nurses are. *The Los Angeles Times,* April 17, B1, 9.

Ethics for emerging field. (1985). *Marketing News,* June 7, 20–21.

Finn, D.W., & Lamb, C.W., Jr. (1986). Hospital benefit segmentation. *Journal of Health Care Marketing, 6* (4), 26–33.

Firshein, J. (1996). 20 strategies for marketing your managed care plan. *Healthcare Executive, 11* (1), 15–17.

Fromberg, R. (1996). Capitation is coming. *Healthcare Executive, 11* (1), 4–9.

Ginzinger, B. (1996). The revolt against the one-day stay. *Health Care Strategic Management, 14* (1), 6–7.

Goh, Y., & Pritula, M. (1996). The new value creators in healthcare. *McKinsey Quarterly,* (1), 193–198.

Goldberg, A. (1995). Product positioning isn't dead yet. *Medical Marketing & Media, 30* (7), 112–114.

Gould, R., Thompson, R., Rakel, B., & Jensen, J. (1996). Redesigning the RN and NA roles. *Nursing Management, 27* (2), 37–41.

Graf, L., Hemmasi, M., & Strong, K.C. (1996). Strategic analysis for resource allocation decisions in health care organizations. *Journal of Managerial Issues, 8* (1), 92–107.

Grimaldi, P.L. (1995). Capitation savvy a must. *Nursing Management, 26* (2), 33–34.

Gurwitz, J.H., McLaughlin, T.J., & Fish, L.S. (1995). The effect of an Rx-to-OTC switch on medication prescribing patterns and utilization of physician services: The case of vaginal antifungal products. *Health Services Research, 30* (5), 672–685.

Haley, R.I. (1985). *Developing effective communications strategy.* New York: Wiley.

Healthcare on the information superhighway. (1996). *Information Today, 13* (1), 24.

Hedden, C.R. (1996). Getting started. *Marketing Tools,* Jan./Feb., 58–65.

Hegarty, S.J. (1995). Restoring public trust. *Hospitals & Health Networks, 69* (13), 50.

Hodnett, J. (1995). Targeting consumers. *Medical Marketing & Media, 30* (11), 90–95.

How good is your health plan? (1996). *Consumer Reports, 61* (8), 28–42.

Hurt, L.W. (1995). Care management. *Nursing Management, 26* (11), 27–33.

Individuals gathering more information about personal health. (1995). *Health Management Technology, 16 (7), 47.*

Jaklevic, M.C. (1995a). Hospitals' advertising spending up 11.4%. *Modern Healthcare, 25* (14), 56.

Jaklevic, M.C. (1995b). Marketing will resurface, but with fresh approach. *Modern Healthcare, 25* (1), 44.

Jensen, J. (1986). Healthcare alternatives. *American Demographics, 8,* 36–38.

John, J., & Miaoulis, G. (1992). A model for understanding benefit segmentation in preventive health care. *Health Care Management Review, 17* (2), 24–25.

Joel, L.A. (1995). Expanding paradigms of self-care. *American Journal of Nursing, 95* (8), 7.

Kleiman, M.A. (1995). Provider integrating: PO versus PHO. *Healthcare Financial Management, 49* (6), 22–24.

Koester, J., Nunley, J.A., Higgins, E.G., Laarkamp, C.M., & Baker, J. (1995). A nursing career leadership program. *Nursing Management, 26* (9), 84–88.

Kotler, P., & Roberto, E.L. (1989). *Social marketing: Strategies for changing public behavior.* New York: The Free Press.

Kotler P., & Zaltman, G. (1971). Social marketing: An approach to planned social change. *Journal of Marketing, 35,* 3–12.

Kurtenbach, J., & Warmoth, T. (1995). Strategic planning futurists need to be capitation-specific and epidemiological. *Health Care Strategic Management, 13* (9), 8–11.

Lamm, R.D. (1996). The coming dislocation in the health professions. *Healthcare Forum, 39* (1), 58–62.

Lefebvre, R.C., & Flora, J.A. (1988). Social marketing and public health intervention. *Health Education Quarterly, 15* (3), 299–315.

Lifson, A., & Dandalides, P. (1996). American health care: The journey from cottage industry to the twenty-first century. *Compensation & Benefits Management, 12* (1), 36–44.

Morrisey, J. (1995). New NCQA survey seeks standardization. *Modern Healthcare,* 25(31), 16.

Murray, D. (1995). Turn patient complaints into patient pleasers. *Medical Economics, 72* (12), 74–82.

Oglethorpe, J.E. (1995). Infant feeding as a social marketing issue: A review. *Journal of Consumer Policy, 18* (2/3), 293–314.

Oliver, S. (1996). Doctor downsizing. *Forbes, 157* (2), 104–106.

Olmos, D.R. (1996). Hospitals reinvent themselves. *Los Angeles Times,* Jan. 11, A, p. 1.

Palmeri, C. (1995). Drip bags in the living room. *Forbes, 155* (11), 154–156.

Porter, M.E. (1985). *Competitive advantage.* New York: The Free Press,

Rosner, H. (1996). Patients as consumers. *Brandweek,* Jan 15, *37* (3), 17–20.

Rynne, T.J. (1995). Bringing an integrated system to market. *Healthcare Forum, 38* (6), 52–59.

Simpson, R.L. (1995a). Outsourcing: Should nursing care? *Nursing Management, 26* (4), 22–24.

Simpson, R.L. (1995b). Reengineering: Embracing technology to improve patient care. *Nursing Management, 26* (1), 31–33.

Simpson, R.L. (1996). Will the Internet supplant community health networks? *Nursing Management, 27* (2), 20–23.

Strasser, S., Schweikhart, S., Welch, G.E. II, & Burge, J.C. (1995). Satisfaction with medical care. *Journal of Health Care Marketing, 15* (3), 34–44.

Thornton, P.M. (1995). Direct mail: The darling of marketing. *Nursing Homes, 44* (8), 32–33.

Trainer, T. (1995). Listening to your customers. *Informationweek,* Sep 18, (545), 236.

Troy, T.N. (1995). That was then . . . this is now. *Managed Healthcare, 5* (12), 18–20.

Tucker, M.J. (1996). "Doc-in-the-box" discs and the market for health-oriented consumer CD-ROM. *CD-ROM Professional, 9* (1), 48–56.

Weisend, T. (1995). Critical conditions spur ads. *Adweek* (New England Ed.), Nov 27, 1995, *32* (48), 5.

Weiss, B. (1995). Managed care: There's no stopping it now. *Medical Economics, 72* (5), 26–43.

What creates health? (1995). *Healthcare Forum, 38* (3), 89–90.

Wicks, A.C. (1995). The business ethics movement: Where are we headed and what can we learn from our colleagues in bioethics? *Business Ethics Quarterly, 5* (3), 603–620.

Williams, J.R., & Hensel, P.J. (1995). Direct-to-consumer advertising of prescription drugs. *Journal of Health Care Marketing, 15* (1), 35–41.

CASE 6–1 Initiating Marketing in a County Health Department

Joanne M. Jorgenson

Here we were—six of us—attending a 2-day workshop on marketing. We are members of the management team of an official health agency whose services were primarily focused on preventive care to a cross section of a large suburban community. We wondered why we were devoting precious time to learning about a corporate business activity. We did not need to increase our service demand, and we had little choice in the products we offered. Two days later, we returned to our agency, excited, enthusiastic, and committed to sharing what we had learned with anyone who would listen! Publics—features—target—benefits—product promotion—marketing. Words applicable to public health! Internal marketing versus external marketing? Could marketing be used to work smarter rather than harder? We agreed staff could not work much harder; service demand already exceeded service supply; resources were limited. We envisioned no new resources. How could we "market" what we had learned to our supervisors, to our co-workers?

Aware that marketing endeavors must have support from the top, we agreed that our first task was to gain total administrative support. Using our newly learned marketing principles, we decided the key to a successful presentation rested on the "benefits package." To convince the Agency and Divisional Directors that investing in marketing would bring valuable benefits, we incorporated the values, beliefs, and preferences of administration into a marketing proposal. Our first endeavor was a success! A marketing steering committee was authorized to begin the process of incorporating marketing principles into our service activities.

The second task was more difficult—to "market" marketing to our co-workers. We realized that this was a formidable task. For services, we needed to follow all the steps of marketing; no shortcuts could be taken, the timetable could not be rushed.

Our first endeavor would be to present marketing concepts to the staff. It was not feasible or practical to present a 2-day workshop to all staff. So, how could it be abbreviated without losing any essential content? How could we present the information in a way that would make sense to the nursing service staff?

"Packaging the product in the target's terms," one of the nine steps in marketing, was the key. We would use what was already familiar—the nursing process (identify, assess, plan, intervene)—as the cornerstone process.

■ PHASE I. INTRODUCTION OF MARKETING: "TO MARKET, TO MARKET"

The "Marketing Team," as the steering committee became known, took their workshop on the road—to staff in each of the five field offices. A 1½-hour workshop on the steps in marketing using the

CASE: 6–1 *Continued*

nursing process framework was presented (Table 6–1). We emphasized marketing strategies used in the business world, making the marketing terms real and recognizable to staff.

The objective of phase I was to increase the awareness of staff regarding the marketing steps and their results. Success would be evaluated by the degree to which staff could mentally apply what they had learned to their own activities over the following 2 months. The time frame for phase I—from our original workshop to the completion of the final field office presentation—was 3 months.

■ **PHASE II. APPLICATION OF MARKETING PRINCIPLES IN THE WORK SETTING: "100% OF 10%"**

Two months after completion of Phase I, the "Team" met again with staff in each field setting. The meetings were informal. We gathered information and responses from staff regarding their ideas and reactions to using marketing concepts in the work setting. Suggestions were solicited from the staff regarding marketing techniques that could help them feel better about their work. Many ideas were implemented during the course of this phase; these included procurement of personalized calling cards for each staff person, agency sponsorship to attend courses on development of audiovisual aids, and initiation of a staff newsletter. A spark had been ignited within our staff—the interest, enthusiasm, and excitement of the workshop possibilities caught on!

Keeping in mind a marketing concept that it is better to reach "100% of 10% rather than 10% of 100%," we requested that interested staff volunteer to serve on agency-wide, program-based marketing committees. Our agency already had a matrix structure with staff assigned by service area in each geographically defined office. Each service area was, in marketing terms, a product line: adult health, maternal/child health, and school health. The charge of each marketing committee was to identify a service problem and develop a market plan, using the nine steps of marketing learned in the workshops.

Throughout Phase II, which lasted approximately 1 year, staff in each office were involved in creating, implementing, and evaluating a marketing plan. In doing assessments of target populations, they learned where to find demographic survey data, and to supplement it with interviews and surveys they designed. The nurses gathered general information about their target population, validated with clients the definition of the service problem, and solicited their solutions. This often led to fresh perspectives on old problems. For example, the maternal/child health committee identified as a service problem the fact that less than 25 percent of maternity patients entered prenatal care in the first trimester. In profiling the community and defining who came to clinic, they realized that many clients had received initial pregnancy tests from service providers external to the agency, and had not been promptly referred or informed of the available community services. The solution was to develop and implement a

TABLE 6–1. Marketing Framework

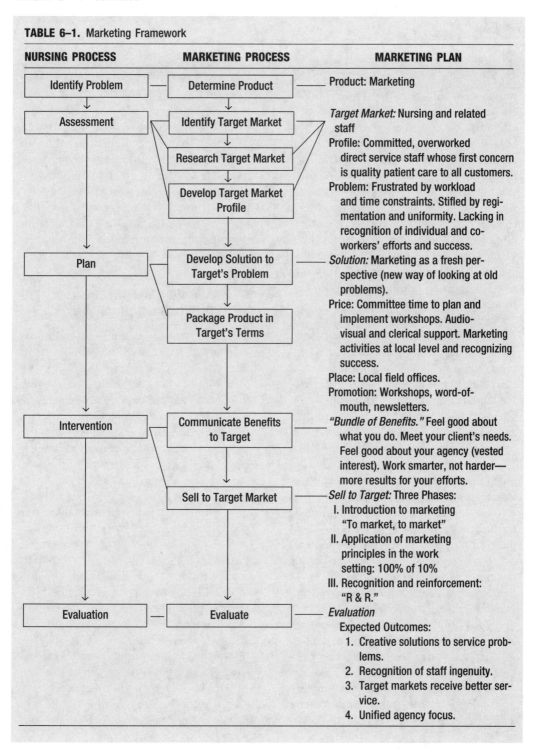

NURSING PROCESS	MARKETING PROCESS	MARKETING PLAN
Identify Problem	Determine Product	Product: Marketing
Assessment	Identify Target Market	*Target Market:* Nursing and related staff
	Research Target Market	Profile: Committed, overworked direct service staff whose first concern is quality patient care to all customers.
	Develop Target Market Profile	Problem: Frustrated by workload and time constraints. Stifled by regimentation and uniformity. Lacking in recognition of individual and coworkers' efforts and success.
Plan	Develop Solution to Target's Problem	*Solution:* Marketing as a fresh perspective (new way of looking at old problems).
	Package Product in Target's Terms	Price: Committee time to plan and implement workshops. Audiovisual and clerical support. Marketing activities at local level and recognizing success.
		Place: Local field offices.
		Promotion: Workshops, word-of-mouth, newsletters.
Intervention	Communicate Benefits to Target	*"Bundle of Benefits."* Feel good about what you do. Meet your client's needs. Feel good about your agency (vested interest). Work smarter, not harder—more results for your efforts.
	Sell to Target Market	*Sell to Target:* Three Phases: I. Introduction to marketing "To market, to market" II. Application of marketing principles in the work setting: 100% of 10% III. Recognition and reinforcement: "R & R."
Evaluation	Evaluate	*Evaluation* Expected Outcomes: 1. Creative solutions to service problems. 2. Recognition of staff ingenuity. 3. Target markets receive better service. 4. Unified agency focus.

CASE: 6–1 *Continued*

plan by which these external service providers would each be visited to discuss available community maternity services; in addition, the agency would increase emphasis internally on follow-up of all women who tested positive for pregnancy in our own services. The result of this endeavor increased maternity service registration and improved first trimester utilization of service to almost 40 percent. Without the use of the marketing approach, we probably would still be focusing on internal efforts and not recognizing the impact of uninformed external service providers.

As work proceeded in each office, the marketing committees met to discuss problems, keep up momentum, share information, and build their knowledge of marketing. One agency-wide problem—inadequate brochures depicting services—was identified. The committees agreed to assume this additional task and revise and develop new brochures that would be better marketing tools. This enabled them to get "first-hand experience" at using promotion and advertising.

The marketing steering committee continued to meet on a monthly basis during phase II. The committee focused on ways to assist the three marketing committees develop additional tools for their use, coordinate efforts to avoid duplication, and determine ways to secure necessary funding or material resources. The steering committee also functioned as a liaison with other management/administration staff within the agency. Workshops were provided for sanitarians, administrative staff, support staff, and other specialty service units.

At the end of 1 year, the marketing perspective was becoming a part of our everyday business. Marketing terms became commonplace—"What's the B.O.B. (bundle of benefits)?" frequently followed requests for action from peers or management. New services, procedures, and policies were presented to staff using a marketing format; that is, product, benefits, features that enhanced acceptance, understanding, and implementation.

■ PHASE III. REINFORCEMENT AND RECOGNITION: "R & R"

Reinforcement—building on knowledge—and recognition of efforts, constitutes the ongoing phase III. We introduced basic marketing ideas; we now felt the need for more expertise. The steering committee developed and presented a proposal to secure a consultant within the existing budget. With authorization, the consultant was hired who originally tapped the imagination of the steering committee 18 months previously in the 2-day workshop. He helped analyze our product: service; he helped us to emphasize that when the product is service, providers of the service are an integral part of the product. The consultant also helped us to look objectively at our progress, recognize our limitations, and develop a long-range plan. With his assistance we chose "agency image" as our focus. The first stage was another round of workshops in each field office given by the consultant on our new marketing plan.

The total agency is now involved in marketing endeavors. A community edu-

CASE: 6-1   *Continued*

cation committee, comprised of representatives of all divisions of the agency, has been established. The image of the agency is the focus of this group, and how to project it positively to our various "publics." Development of an agency logo and slogan is in progress.

The initial marketing plan implemented by the six excited, enthusiastic nursing management staff was a success! Integration and internalization of marketing concepts was accomplished, on a much wider basis than originally envisioned. Marketing has become an integral component of our agency:

- A marketing module is included in the orientation of all new employees.
- Community assessments are now routinely done before initiating changes in service delivery.
- Clients are now surveyed regarding satisfaction with our services and ideas for improvement.
- Agency brochures are continually critiqued as marketing tools.
- "Bundle of benefits" are identified for various services by staff initiative.
- Marketing activities are included in the pay for performance standards.
- An agency newsletter with reporters in each field office keeps marketing efforts visible and provides recognition for creativity.

"Word of mouth," one of the best promotion techniques, became real as the requests came in from other parts of the state: would we be willing to share with other jurisdictions what we were doing with our staff? The "Team" went on the road! Workshops were presented in six areas of the state. The enthusiasm was contagious; health department staff learned that marketing not only benefits the client and the agency, but it also adds an element of fun to work as it allows creativity and ingenuity to flow freely.

The marketing process received official recognition by the local government in the form of the highest award given to a public employee—the Health On-thank Award—when the Steering Committee Chairman was nominated and selected as a recipient. The award was accepted on behalf of the staff involved.

We began with six managerial staff having an interest in incorporating marketing techniques into a large suburban health department. After attending a workshop where we learned basic marketing ideas, we had to "sell" the need for marketing to our superiors, peers, and staff. We developed a market plan to be implemented in three phases over a minimum of a 3-year period (Table 6–2):

- Phase I: Introduction to staff marketing principles
- Phase II: Application of marketing principles to work activities
- Phase III: Reinforcement and expansion of marketing principles to total agency

We envision that the consultant obtained in phase III will provide periodic guidance and assistance indefinitely as the administrative staff identify areas of need.

CASE: 6–1 *Continued*

TABLE 6–2. Marketing Begins With Me: Phases and Tasks

	TASKS	RESPONSIBLE PARTY	TIME FRAME
Phase I: Introduction of marketing principles: "To market, to market"	1. Proposal to Health Officer 2. Design and schedule workshops for field staff 3. Conduct workshops and allow 2 months for integration of ideas	Steering Committee	3 months
Phase II: Application of marketing principles in the work setting: "100% of 10%"	1. Meet with field office to gather information and level of integration achieved 2. Implement suggestions from staff 3. Appoint marketing committees for each program area 4. Marketing committees develop and implement a market plan to solve mutually identified service problem; involves program peers in process 5. Conduct workshops for other divisions within agency	Steering Committee Steering Committee Interested Staff Steering Committee	12 months
Phase III: Reinforcement and recognition: "R & R"	1. Secure consultant to add depth, evaluation, and agency-wide coordination/focus 2. Establish community education committee 3. Recognition—activities, staff, successes, and failures	Steering Committee Division Directors All via newsletters, awards, articles, etc.	Ongoing

JoAnne M. Jorgenson is currently Director of Patient Care Services with the Fairfax County Health Department in Fairfax, Virginia. A graduate of South Dakota State University and the University of Minnesota School of Public Health, she has held a variety of positions in public health nursing during her career. She is a member of the Virginia Nurses Association and the American Nurses Association, holding offices on the local and state level. In addition to membership in the American Public Health Association and Sigma Theta Tau, she is Secretary of the Virginia Public Health Nurse Leaders.

CASE 6–2 Integrating Marketing into the Psychiatric Clinical Specialist's Job Responsibilities

Carol A. Patney

Perhaps the single most difficult challenge facing a service delivery group is to maintain the quality of care, meet community needs, and ensure that, economically, the practitioner or organization remains in the black. Additionally, in investor-owned organizations, stockholders seek a prospectus that indicates a considerable return on investment.

Marketing departments and strategic planning are vital to health care organizations wishing to remain viable and profitable in the 21st century. Health care administrators, as well as individual clinicians, must learn a new language and become conversant with terms such as market penetration, market segmentation, and relative market share. Marketing is the responsibility of every employee within a health care organization, from the C.E.O. down to the laundry technician. Thus, nurses have a marketing responsibility not only to the organization in which they practice, but to the nursing profession as a whole. This is not a new role, but rather an old emphasis cloaked in a new language.

Nurses have promoted products when they have assured patients that Tylenol would ease their discomfort, Triaminic would relieve nasal congestion, and Metamucil would ensure regularity. They have professionally endorsed providers when they recommended Physician A instead of Physician B to friends or family. One nurses' association, aware of the power professional endorsement can carry, recently received compensation for endorsing one brand of disposable diaper on national television while also increasing public awareness of their nursing specialty. Pause for just a moment to ponder the diversified roles that nurses can assume in promoting health care delivery and other products. Possibilities are almost limitless.

The purpose of this case application is to present one example of how marketing principles were applied by nurses. Marketing and business terminology are used throughout in an effort to assist the reader in becoming more comfortable with these terms.

Certain conditions must exist in an organization before it is ready for a marketing program. The organization must define its mission and goals, develop an appropriate strategy to reach these goals, build an appropriate organizational structure that will carry out this strategy, and equip the organization with effective systems of information, planning, control, and rewards to get the job done (Kotler, 1984). All successful health care organizations have these conditions.

In addition, the successful organization also contains the following four soft strengths:

1. *Style*. The employees share a common style of behaving and thinking (Kotler, 1984). Success-

CASE: 6–2 *Continued*

ful companies exhibit a distinct and widely shared culture that fits its strategy (Deal & Kennedy, 1988).

2. An appropriate mix of *skills,* which is needed to carry out the company's strategy.
3. *Staffing.* The company has hired able people and has put them in the right jobs to exercise their talents.
4. *Shared values.* The employers share the same guiding values and goals as the organization.

Today, these soft strengths are becoming more identifiable in the health care field.

An investor-owned psychiatric hospital in a large urban, metropolitan tri-state area decided to improve its reputation in the community by providing some new *product* (service) that could be made available to all community members regardless of economic status, and would simultaneously be economically beneficial to the hospital. It was hoped that increased visibility and a demonstration of concern for community problems would increase the hospital's *market share.*

The Vice President for Nursing (VPN) and Director of Marketing (DOM), as part of the strategic planning management group, were charged to identify a product that would meet community needs, to create a marketing plan for this product, and then to present their plan for top management approval. The VPN convened key nurses and the DOM to brainstorm. This VPN was quite progressive; she had been introducing market-

ing concepts to her staff for some time. Many of the nurses already realized the importance of these concepts to the hospital and their profession.

The first meeting began with a statement of the task. Next the group reviewed the mission statement, goals, and objectives of the hospital. The group agreed on the following summary: This is a private, free-standing psychiatric hospital that provides quality psychiatric care to members of the community who meet admission criteria. The hospital's *business domain* consists of those individuals who (1) have a psychiatric illness not responsive to outpatient treatment, and (2) are free from medical disorders warranting care in a general hospital setting. All DSM-IV diagnostic categories can be treated at this facility. The organization's main goal is to provide quality psychiatric care, remain profitable, show continued growth, see market-share improvement, have the ability to diversify, and remain innovative in the health care industry.

The group identified the hospital's *distinctive competency* as the psychiatric care delivered across all psychiatric diagnoses. The DOM agreed and translated the nurses' product-oriented definition of what they did into a consumer-oriented definition; that is, they offered the best hope in the area to individuals with problems. The DOM also summed up the hospital's mission more succinctly: To improve service to customers and to increase return on investments.

One of the nurses noted that "individuals living in the suburbs are reluctant to come into the city for treatment, espe-

CASE: 6–2 *Continued*

cially since they know very little about the hospital." Another nurse added, "very few people really know anything about mental illness or mental health." A third observed that "people are afraid to go into a 'shrink's' office." After several minutes of discussion the VPN offered an idea. The group expanded this idea to include nurses offering emergency evaluations that were convenient and required no appointment.

The group continued to brainstorm. Nurse therapists could perform several functions: (1) they could provide community education programs with no fee, as a community service sponsored by the hospital; and (2) patients seen by nurses could be evaluated for short-term crises intervention and, if needed, referred to physicians affiliated with the hospital for longer term treatment, or referred directly for inpatient treatment in a hospital.

The hospital would provide both education and psychiatric treatment in the suburbs and nurse therapists would be the link between the hospital and the community. Nurses would be the staff for this service as they would be less threatening, holistically oriented, and less costly. This idea was presented to top management and was accepted. The green light was given for step two, the *marketing plan*. The *marketing management* process put into action consisted of analyzing market opportunities, researching and selecting target markets, developing marketing strategies, planning marketing tactics, and implementing and controlling the marketing effort (Kotler, 1984).

A *target market* was selected from an analysis of demographic data provided by the state health departments, county offices of Research and Statistics, and hospital admission demographics. County A was identified as having a high incidence of drug abuse, a well-insured population with few admissions into our private psychiatric hospital. *Full market coverage* would be given to County A: the full spectrum of services offered by the hospital would be promoted, as well as a new service cluster, crisis evaluation and referral and education.

A *marketing strategy* was formulated for the new service cluster. Marketing strategy consists of making decisions on the business' marketing expenditures and marketing allocations in relation to expected environmental and competitive conditions (Kotler, 1984). This is accomplished through the "four P's" of marketing—*product, price, place, and promotion*.

A master's prepared psychiatric nurse therapist would staff one suburban evaluation and education office. Secretarial support and phone coverage would be provided at the main hospital. *Pricing* included no charge for evaluation, a sliding scale for short-term follow-up, and no fees for the indigent. Revenues generated by the hospital admissions from this service were planned to offset the costs of the nurse's salary, office supplies, lowered outpatient revenues due to indigent care, and sliding scale fees. A private psychiatrist offered a site (*place*) at no cost in exchange for the appropriate referrals of patients to his practice. The site for the office was

CASE: 6–2 *Continued*

convenient to public transportation and centrally located. *Promotion* for this product (service) consisted of local newspaper advertisements and a press release, interviews by the nurse therapist on radio and television programs, and personal appearances with selected target groups in the community (Table 6–3). These target groups were local suburban private practices of psychiatrists and family physicians, occupational health nurses, and employee assistance counselors in local businesses. The nurse, in addition to raising awareness of the evaluation and educational services, would also mention treatment programs at the private psychiatric hospital.

The marketing plan was presented by the DOM to top management and implementation of the first suburban evaluation and education office was approved. Gatekeepers were identified and the promotion activities directed toward them. We decided that face-to-face contacts would be more productive than just phone calls or letters. A schedule was devised for the number of community contacts expected for the nurse therapist each month (Table 6–4). Over time, the number of expected visits decreased. It was assumed that as outreach efforts were successful, time spent speaking and making calls would decrease. A quarterly reporting form was devised to report the progress and productivity of the office (Table 6–5) to the supervisor. The hospital agreed to fund this experiment for 1 year.

Initially the nurse staffing this service was not comfortable with a marketing role but over time and when results

of marketing contacts began to pay off in referrals she became more comfortable. This pay-off did not occur immediately; it took 4 months before results could be seen. The nurse did not become discouraged, however, as she believed in her product and received support from her supervisor.

The first two quarterly reports were promising. Feedback from the community about the presence of the service was positive and encouraging. A consumer survey conducted by the hospital marketing department compared with a similar survey done before this "experiment" showed a significant increase in consumer recognition of the psychiatric hospital. The third quarter report indicated at least eight direct admissions through this service and eight indirect admissions. The final (or first annual) report of the first year showed a total of 12 direct admissions and 14 indirect admissions. Referrals for admission from Employee Assistance Programs (EAPs), guidance counselors, and emergency rooms (target groups for the nurse therapist to market) were up by 65 percent. The revenues generated by these admissions far offset the expenditures for the project. As a result, the management group decided to open at least three more suburban offices. Many people, including other professionals, began to see nursing in a new light.

Just as major corporations must understand and effectively use marketing, the nursing profession must seize this time to move to the forefront with innovations in the delivery of care. The future of the profession depends on deci-

TABLE 6–3. First-year Marketing Plan

TYPE OF MARKETING EFFORT	1ST QUARTER	2ND, 3RD, AND 4TH QUARTERS	RESULTS
Personal Contact Nurse Therapist	Marketing visits to physicians, businesses, and other target groups to be interspaced with patient appointment times.	Number of visits to each group will be formulated with supervisor and marketing.	1st Qtr.—0 Admit. 2nd Qtr.—3 Admit. 3rd Qtr.—3 Admit. 4th Qtr.—4 Admit. 1st Yr. Tot. = 10 Admit.
Education	Open luncheon conference for each target group. To be set up by Marketing Representative and Nurse Therapist. Three luncheons in 1st Qtr.	Educational workshops for identified group; 2–3 presentations per quarter to be set up by either Marketing Representative or Nurse Therapist and staffed by both.	
Media Print PIW Inkblot	News blurb with location and directions to new office and additional information as determined by Marketing. News item will be placed by marketing.	Each quarter, update on offices with relevant articles provided by nursing staff. Marketing will review article and place in Inkblot.	
Yellow Pages	Marketing to place ad as early as possible and to include small maps if not cost prohibitive.		

(continued)

TABLE 6-3. (Continued)

TYPE OF MARKETING EFFORT	1ST QUARTER	2ND, 3RD, AND 4TH QUARTERS	RESULTS
Introductory Letter and Brochures	Letter prepared by nurse to be mailed with brochure to all Mental Health Professionals and Groups, along with nonpsychiatric M.D.s in defined geographical area that office will service. To be sent during first month of operation by marketing.	Direct mailing each month of newsletter to group identified in 1st Qtr. Mailing list will be expanded by appropriate referral names as supplied by institute personnel. Nurse will provide newsletter, marketing will do mailing.	
Radio: Talk Shows	Marketing will target station that specifically serves defined geographical area. Nurse for that office and Nurse Administrator will do shows.	One show per quarter by nurse. Marketing will set up time and station. Special attention should be directed toward holiday seasons and summer months.	
	One paid ad at local station.	Repeat one each quarter if first airing is successful.	
Press Release:	Press release at least 8 times by marketing. Paid ad 1 per week first month and then 2 per month in local publications.	Press release—4 per quarter	
	Bus and metro ads, marketing will assume responsibility for this.		
Research	Information Base: Develop list of M.D.'s offices and Health Care Agencies for each catchment area.	Update regularly.	

Used with permission of The Psychiatric Institute of Washington, D.C.

CASE: 6–2 *Continued*

TABLE 6–4. Target Population and Contact Frequency

First Quarter

Week		1	2	3	4	5	6	7	8	9	10	11	12
Phone Calls to Community		40	30	25	20	20	15	15	15	15	10	10	10
Physician contact	Personal Contact	3	3	3	3	3	3	3	3	2	2	2	2
Community contact		2	3	3	2	2	2	2	2	2	2	2	2
EAPs		3	3	2	2	2	2	1	1	1	1	1	1

Second Quarter

Week		13	14	15	16	17	18	19	20	21	22	23	24
to Community		10	10	10	10	10	10	10	10	10	10	10	10
Physician contact	Personal Contact	2	2	2	2	2	2	2	2	2	2	2	2
Community contact		2	2	2	2	2	2	1	1	1	1	1	1
EAPs		1	1	1	1	1	1	1	1	1	1	1	1

Third Quarter

Week		25	26	27	28	29	30	31	32	33	34	35	36
Phone Calls to Community		8	8	8	8	8	8	8	8	8	8	8	8
Physician contact	Personal Contact	2	2	2	2	2	2	2	2	2	2	2	2
Community contact		1	1	1	1	1	1	1	1	1	1	1	1
EAPs		1	1	1	1	1	1	1	1	1	1	1	1

Fourth Quarter

Week		37	38	39	40	41	42	43	44	45	46	47	48
Phone Calls to Community		8	8	8	8	8	8	8	8	8	8	8	8
Physician contact	Personal Contact	2	2	2	2	2	2	2	2	2	2	2	2
Community contact		1	1	1	1	1	1	1	1	1	1	1	1
EAPs		1	1	1	1	1	1	1	1	1	1	1	1

EAP = Employee Assistance Program.
Used with permission of The Psychiatric Institute of Washington, D.C.

TABLE 6–5. Quarterly Report

To: Nursing Administrator of Outpatient Services
From: Nurse Therapist's Name
Subject: Quarterly Progress Report for: _____ Crisis Center Covering _____
        to _____.

QUARTERLY REPORT OUTLINE

This report documents the progress of the _____ Crisis Center during the _____ quarter of operation from _____ to _____. Included you will find information related to four primary areas: (1) marketing; (2) clinical service; (3) finances; and (4) conclusions and directions for the future.

MARKETING

Summary paragraph (Report on follow-up of needs identified in previous report)
Referral Development Record

Date of Contact	Name of Organization	Contact Person	Outcome

Source of referral information for clients admitted to Crisis Center between _____ and _____.

Name of Referral Source   # Referred

Name of Referral Source	# Referred

Summary comments related to statistical significance of marketing information (i.e., number of referrals (percentage of referrals) from various referral sources; percentage of referrals resulting from nurse therapist's marketing, E.A.P. referrals, Hopeline, etc.)

CLINICAL SERVICES

Summary to clinical statistics for _____ quarter and year to date

	MONTH	MONTH	MONTH
Number of patients admitted			
Number of patients discharged			
Number patients followed end of month			
Phone consults:			
A.M.			
P.M.			

(continued)

TABLE 6–5. (continued)

Summary to clinical statistics for _____ quarter and year to date

	MONTH	MONTH	MONTH
Hospitalizations:			
P.I.			
Other			
Outpatient Disposition:			
(Name of group assoc. with C.C. office)			
M.P.G.			
Community			
D.A.A.			
D.I.			
D.S.C.			

Summary paragraph explaining any special circumstances related to clinical statistics (i.e., R.P.I.—refused, no medical back-up times 1 week so centers closed to new admits, etc.)

_____

_____

_____

Summary paragraph addressing percentage of admissions to C.C. admitted to P.I., referred to community, seen in C.C.I.S., etc.

_____

_____

_____

Demographic data on clients admitted to Crisis Center during the quarter.

Sex:

    Female   _____

    Male   _____

Race

    White   _____

    Black   _____

    Oriental   _____

    Hispanic   _____

    Other   _____

Age:

    13–18   _____

    19–25   _____

    26–35   _____

    36–45   _____

    46–55   _____

(*continued*)

CASE: 6–2 *Continued*

TABLE 6–5. (continued)

Age:

    55–65 _____

    65–75 _____

Marital Status:

    Single _____

    Married _____

    Separated _____

    Divorced _____

    Widowed _____

Chief Complaint:

    Chemical Dependency—Self _____

    Chemical Dependency—Family Member _____

    Depression/Chemical Dependency/Stress _____

    Depression/Co-Alcoholic _____

    Family Violence _____

    Grief _____

    Multiple Stresses/Personal Crisis _____

    Developmental Crisis _____

    Marital Dysfunction _____

    Family Dysfunction _____

    Adolescent Behavior Problems _____

    Affective Disorder _____

    Anxiety _____

    Sex Offence _____

    Other _____

Summary paragraph(s) addressing any pertinent clinical issues:

_____

_____

_____

FINANCES

Insurance coverage of clients seen in the Crisis Center during quarter.

No coverage _____

Has insurance but doesn't know name of company _____

Alphabetical listing of insurance companies _____ number patients involved by Co.

    1. _____

    2. _____

    3. _____

(*continued*)

CASE: 6–2 *Continued*

TABLE 6–5. (continued)

Summary paragraph(s) commenting on percentage of patients admitted to Crisis Center with insurance, percentage of insured patients with inpatient/outpatient mental health coverage, employers providing insurance benefits with poor mental health coverage.

_____

_____

_____

Income generated by the _____ Crisis Center during

_____

quarter.

     Hospitalizations at P.I. $ _____

     Crisis Center visits—evaluations only $ _____

     Crisis Center visits—brief treatment $ _____ plus

                                          _____

     Total revenue generated by _____ $ _____

     Crisis Center _____

Summary paragraph(s) reporting number of hospital patient days or particular unit at per diem rate; also comments on numbers of hospitalizations and cost of hospitalizations resulting from nurse therapists' marketing efforts, E.A.P.s, Hopeline, etc.

_____

_____

_____

CONCLUSIONS AND DIRECTIONS FOR THE FUTURE

Summary paragraph(s) highlighting pertinent issues presented in report. Comment on progress of Crisis Center from your perspective. Identify any clinical, marketing, administrative concerns that need to be/will be addressed in our next quarter. (list)

_____

_____

_____

cc: President/Medical Director
      Administrator
      Director of Patient Services

Used with the permission of The Psychiatric Institute of Washington, D.C.

CASE: 6–2 *Continued*

sions made today. Those who desire to lead in nursing must become experts, not only in clinical care, but also in all aspects of management and corporate operations.

■ BIOGRAPHICAL SKETCH

Carol A. Patney received her basic nursing education at the Mercy Hospital School of Nursing in Wilkes Barre, Pennsylvania. She then earned her BSN from College Misericordia in Dallas, Pennsylvania, and her MSN in Mental Health Nursing from the University of Pennsylvania. On completion of graduate work, Ms. Patney joined the U.S. Army, where she designed and functioned in the role of Psychiatric Liaison Nurse. For her performance of duty at Walter Reed Army Medical Center she was awarded the Meritorious Service Medal (the peacetime equivalent of the Bronze Star). On leaving the military Ms. Patney worked for the Psychiatric Institute of America, first in Norfolk, Virginia, and then Washington, D.C. She functioned in positions of increasing administrative responsibility, including development of the Crisis Service that is illustrated in this case. For this work, she was awarded the Distinguished Service Award by the D.C. Hospital Association. Since coming to the Washington metropolitan area, Ms. Patney has completed a certificate in Nursing Administration at George Mason University, Fairfax, Virginia, and is currently a doctoral candidate in Nursing at the University of Virginia, Charlottesville, Virginia. She is also certified by the American Nurses Association as a clinical specialist in psychiatric nursing. She is currently Director of Quality Management and Education and Mental Health at Health Management Strategies in Alexandria, Virginia.

■ REFERENCES

Deal, T., & Kennedy, A. (1988). *Corporate cultures: The rites and rituals of corporate life.* Reading, MA: Addison-Wesley.

Kotler, P. (1984). *Marketing management.* Englewood Cliffs, NJ: Prentice-Hall.

What's Your Niche?
Starting a New Venture

Belinda E. Puetz and Karen J. Kelly Thomas

Starting a new venture can be an exciting and enduring enterprise or it can be frightening and full of excess risk. This chapter discusses how to develop an idea into a nursing business or an intrapreneurial change in a way that will help manage the risk and retain the excitement of starting something new. New ventures begin with ideas, some good and some bad. Generating ideas for new ventures and niche formation will be described in this chapter as well as the strategic thinking process of developing a business plan.

Money is important to any venture, but may not be necessary in large quantities to develop the idea and business plan. Not all good ventures generate revenue, but any venture attempted must at least pay for itself. Strategic thinking and planning are at the core of any sound business venture; business planning models are included for the purpose of informing the reader of the systematic process used to plan a business venture. Costing, benefits, and forecasting will be presented in the development of a model business plan for a private consultation practice. Other ideas for new ventures will be integrated into each section, all of which can be used as a basis for a model business plan.

Ventures are about risk, experimenting, and investment. Ventures are also about hard work, creativity, and innovation. Following these guidelines and thinking clearly about the purpose and goals of a new service or product will help the nurse administrator with an entrepreneurial spirit start a new venture.

■ THE IDEA

Idea development has been investigated within the context of neuroscience, thinking, creativity, and knowledge development. How do people get ideas? Ornstein (1984), in his seminal work about the architecture of the brain, says getting new ideas is a cortical activity, and probably occurs on the surface of the cerebrum. He further acknowledges that the cortex is like an executive branch of the brain, responsible for making decisions and judgments on all the information coming into it. Turning down the logical, linear left hemisphere and allowing the right brain to play out its natural, kaleidoscopic nature enhances idea generation.

Although how ideas and creativity happen is still a puzzle, Rubenfeld and Scheffer (1995) suggest that new ideas and creativity comprise a specific mode of thinking that is unique and individual. Idea generation and creativity can be learned. Brookfield (1993) believes that developing alternative ways of thinking produces creativity. Brainstorming, envisioning alternative futures, developing preferred scenarios, futures invention, and aesthetic triggers are suggested alternative thinking activities to tap into creativity and idea generation. An idea can be generated alone or in a group by starting the creativity process with words like "transpose," "invert," "flatten," "stretch," "substitute," "by-pass," "separate," and many others.

Henry and associates (1989) discuss ideonomy as a useful concept in delineating new knowledge. They suggest the notion of spinning and combining ideas using a computer program to systematically generate new ideas. By listing a series of words associated with terms such as nursing and management, new two-word descriptions are generated and new analogies are formed. An example of a new analog from the terms nursing and management is technological caring. Using these principles of spinning and combining terms, new word matches can serve as the basis for a different perspective and perhaps generate new venture ideas.

Drucker (1985) proposed, in his book titled *Innovation and Entrepreneurship: Practice and Principles,* that innovation is the specific tool of entrepreneurs. It is the means by which they exploit change as an opportunity for a different business or a different service. He posits that innovation and idea generation can be learned and practiced as a discipline. According to Drucker, systematic innovation means monitoring seven sources for innovative opportunity. They include:

- *The unexpected*—the unexpected success, the unexpected failure, the unexpected outside event.
- *The incongruity*—between reality as it actually is and reality as it is assumed to be or as it "ought to be."
- *Innovation based on process need.*
- *Changes in industry structure or market structure* that catch everyone unaware.
- *Demographic* (population) *changes.*
- *Changes in perception, mood, and meaning.*
- *New knowledge,* both scientific and nonscientific (p. 35).

Drucker lists these sources in descending order of reliability and predictability and calls for careful analysis of each of the overlapping sources of innovative opportunity.

A common thread throughout the literature on ideas is the belief that ideas are nurtured. The notion of the "Ah-ha!" experience is described by those considered to have had great ideas as more like an "ah-ah-ah-ah-ha-ha . . . ah-h . . ." experience. The period of time some people have nurtured ideas is sometimes years longer than is useful to starting a new venture and generating revenue. And some who nurture an idea never get to a point at which they want to take action. Nonetheless, nurturing and articulating an idea through the process of developing a business plan is a worthwhile exercise for those serious about starting a new venture. In addition, a focus on the hard reality of the business aspects of any new venture is requisite for developing any idea into an actual venture.

It is not uncommon for individuals interested in starting a new venture to have a mental list of many worthwhile ideas that could serve as the basis for a new venture. The key is to consider many different solutions to problems and pursue one as a new venture. Though new ventures are often the result of many ideas considered and discarded, one idea used as the underpinning theme to the venture will help articulate, communicate, and develop the idea into a business plan. This central idea or theme is called a niche.

■ CREATING A NICHE

A market niche is the unique selling point or specialization of a business venture. Florence Nightingale had a niche. In addition to hygiene, she was known for taking health care to the place where it was needed, including the front lines of war and other frontiers. Niches for new ventures often grow out of changes in lifestyle and consumer preferences. Technological continuities and discontinuities can also create a niche for a new venture. Taking high-technology care to new frontiers, given advances in equipment size and ease of operator use, is a potential niche. Creating a "high-touch" emphasis within a high-technology environment may also serve as a market niche for a new venture. Innovation in where, how, and who provides nursing care and other clinical services may also serve as the niche. Telehealth services, using available communication technologies such as cellular phones, video conferencing, and the Internet's World Wide Web, also provide many opportunities for a unique niche and a new venture.

Niche characteristics have been defined (Dalgic & Leeuw, 1994) as markets that have:

- Sufficient size to be potentially profitable.
- No real competitors, or markets that have been ignored by others.
- Growth potential.
- Sufficient purchasing ability.
- A need for special treatment.
- Customer goodwill.
- Opportunities for the entrance company to exercise superior competence.

Kotler (1991) also advises that niche markets are relatively small initially, although they might grow to become large markets.

Even the management of understandings can serve as a niche. Brown (1995) describes the political processes through which legitimacy was sought for a large information technology system by its sponsors and key supporters. This case study research design was conducted within an interpretive perspective while the investigator was immersed in the stream of organizational events. This experience, the inquiry process, and the resulting ethnographic account yielded data that could be used as a niche for new ventures by the organization or the investigator, depending on what types of agreements were made in the contracting or agreement stage of any such inquiry. Nurses involved in innovative programs and projects should consider the experience, the inquiry and development process, and the resulting outcome as potential niches for a related new venture.

Providing telehealth services through new media is an important idea that is generating many ventures from a variety of health care service systems. One large Midwest university system provides an interactive decision-making program on-line to participants in its health maintenance organization (HMO) to help patients make care choices in five major disease categories. Use of the technology and marketing it as a benefit to members of the health plan blends technology and access to information for decision making in a way that enhances the services of the system and benefits patients and providers. The market niche of the system, that of rapid access to information for decision making, is also enhanced and expanded.

Weber (1994) demonstrated that defining market niche too broadly is a pervasive problem deterring most industrial product firms from developing effective marketing and strategic plans. Drawing on applications to over 10 companies, he suggests a narrow, purchase influence-based delineation of target niches. A new venture created within a complex health care services system will have a greater chance for success if the unique selling point or specialized service is limited and narrow. Dalgic and Leeuw (1994) encourage niche marketing for those who want to remain healthy survivors in a highly competitive environment. They further suggest niche marketing is a creative process used to carve out a small part of the market whose needs are not fulfilled. Customizing and specializing along market, customer, product, or marketing mix lines creates the opportunity for a company to match the unique needs of a selected and targeted group of clients or patients.

■ CHARACTERISTICS OF ENTREPRENEURS AND INTRAPRENEURS

Taking an idea and attempting to get others to believe in the value of the idea takes certain characteristics. They include an entrepreneurial or intrapreneurial spirit, willingness to work hard and take risks, and a tenacious and unremitting belief in the value of the idea.

Intrapreneuring was first described by Pinchot (1985), who helped many business leaders understand how to generate new ideas, market niches, and new revenue streams within existing companies by creating opportunities for individuals with the spirit and characteristics of entrepreneurs. Intrapreneurs also need team-building skills and a firm grasp of business and marketplace realities. Pinchot describes intrapreneurs as those employees who:

- Want freedom and access to corporate resources.
- Are goal-oriented and self-motivated.
- Respond to corporate rewards and recognition.
- Possess an urgency to meet self-imposed and corporate timetables.
- Get their hands dirty, can delegate, but also do whatever needs to be done.
- Are self-confident and courageous.
- Like moderate risk.

Like entrepreneurs, intrapreneurs do their own market research and intuitive market evaluation. They usually do not value traditional status symbols; rather, intrapreneurs treasure symbols of freedom. Similarly, entrepreneurs and intrapreneurs are adept at getting others to agree to a vision or idea. Both have the essential characteristic of a *doer*.

Entrepreneurial spirit is a temperament that enjoys the adventure and risk associated with new ideas and changing processes. Zoghlin (1991) describes a plethora of entrepreneurial options for executives wanting to make a transition to a different work arrangement. Included are:

- Consulting.
- Spin-offs such as franchises, licensing deals, or distributorships.
- Equity arrangements in which a salary is received along with partial ownership of a venture.
- Buying an existing business.
- Starting from scratch as a corporation, sole proprietorship, or partnership.

Advantages and disadvantages exist for each option, and the nurse executive with an idea is served well by an examination of the various options.

Money is also associated with the entrepreneurial spirit, but it does not necessarily mean actual money, rather a belief in the ability to place value on ideas. Drucker (1985) advises that entrepreneurs must learn to practice systematic innovation within the context of a business strategy. Change and progress always provide opportunities to offer new and different products and services. Drucker postulates that "systematic innovation consists in the purposeful and organized search for changes, and in the systematic analysis of the opportunities such changes might offer for economic or social innovation" (p. 35). As previously mentioned, there are seven sources of purposeful innovation listed by Drucker in descending order of reliability and predictability. Each innovation calls for careful analysis of each of the overlapping sources of innovative opportunity for the entrepreneur or intrapreneur.

A willingness to work hard is basic to the work ethic of most entrepreneurs, along with a desire for flexible work hours. The hard work of continuous problem solving is evident among entrepreneurs as unpredictable opportunities present themselves. The continuous investigation of choices is a necessary part of any venture; these choices create the work. Belief in the value of the idea is the certainty that the idea has merit. The idea may be for a product or service. The ability to define the value of the product or service idea in dollars is another requisite characteristic for the entrepreneur or intrapreneur proposing a new venture.

An overwhelming majority of new ventures fail. Although statistics vary, an estimated 50 percent of new businesses go under within 2 years and fewer than 10 percent are left after 5 years (Lasher, 1994). Some of the reasons include poor choice of venture type, location, lack of knowledge, failure to get professional advice, insufficient planning and research, insufficient capital, inadequate costing and pricing practices, and poor management. Starting a new venture is like a juggling act—the individual planning and operating the new venture must keep many balls in the air at the same time. The savvy administrator has experience with this juggling act and is comfortable with the ambiguity and risk-taking associated with starting a new venture.

Flanagan (1993) listed more than a dozen entrepreneurial or intrapreneurial options for nurses, including health promotion, health risk management, disability management, geriatric case management, home infusion therapy, home care management of special populations, nursing clinics, consulting, and a diabetes resource center, among others (p. 14). She further describes characteristics of an independent enterpriser as including friendliness, enthusiasm, sincerity, industriousness, vigor, perseverance, positive attitude, responsibility, decisiveness, and self-discipline. Although these characteristics are common among nurses, a careful assessment of these personal characteristics and answers to reality-based questions are steps in the strategic planning process.

Entrepreneurs also enjoy the characteristics of an active imagination, creativity, and confidence. These characteristics serve the entrepreneur well for certain aspects of a new venture, but a balance of other characteristics is also required. Few individuals can do all things well. Professional help in the form of advice or staff can provide the balance. Every venture requires professional help. Accountants, lawyers, bankers, and insurance agents may all be consulted or retained to provide balanced advice for all aspects of the business during the planning and operation of a new venture.

The complexity and associated risks of the venture prescribe the amount and kind of help needed. For example, designing and planning a colposcopy service for underserved women will require the assistance of state and local health department staff, financial staff, and social services. Health care organization staff from pathology, records, admitting, and information services will likely be required. Building engineers and other regulatory bodies may also be involved. The venture planner should begin to list the help required to adequately research the plan during the early stages of plan development. For example, suppose the niche for the proposed new colposcopy service is rapid, simplified access focused on helping the patient access and move through the procedure with one stop (rather than the usual several stops at admitting, examination and testing, financial counseling, and others). The manner in which all the identified parties interact and interrelate is defined by the niche. Innovation will be required to change traditional thinking and work patterns to accomplish the purpose of the new venture within the niche identified.

Intrapreneurs who work in established companies often do so because the corporate culture is one that recognizes the need to create an environment in which people are given freedom to accomplish a mutual goal in a nontraditional way using innovative strategies and unusual techniques. As a concept, intrapreneuring attempts to describe a traditional business environment that supports and allows the entrepreneurial spirit to thrive within the structure of an established business. The story of Art Fry's many-year experiment with 3M as he developed the "glue that would not stick" for Post-it Notes is commonly used to illustrate the return on investment for companies willing to allow creative and imaginative employees to develop their ideas. Fry's basic need was to create a bookmark that would stick to but not damage the page of his church hymnal. His intrapreneurial characteristics included a willingness to use corporate funds, proprietary corporate technology, as well as existing manufacturing facilities and marketing channels. He tried out his idea in many different departments and when he met with resistance, he used machines himself to develop the adhesive or conducted his own market research. Fry believed in his idea and the economic viability of notes and markers that could be repositioned. He was right.

The environment in health care organizations today lends itself particularly well to the individual who is willing to take some risk and negotiate starting a new venture. Though it may take several years of long hours, hard work, financial sacrifice, and stress, the entrepreneurial spirit can thrive. Good health, high energy, and a sound business plan are needed.

■ STRATEGIC BUSINESS THINKING

Business planning is an essential and integral component of any new venture. The process of developing a business plan reduces to paper the development of the idea, explains the venture's goals and methods for others, and serves as the outcome of strategic business thinking. The business plan creates the opportunity to articulate details required for endorsement, support, or financial backing. Lasher (1994) describes four kinds of planning associated with the development of a business plan. They are:

- Strategic planning.
- Operational planning.
- Budgeting.
- Forecasting.

Each of these activities will be examined in the context of starting a new venture. The amount of detail recorded as a result of these planning activities is determined by the number and kind of readers. For example, a business plan developed for a private consultation practice run from a home office with limited risk may generate a page or two of ideas and financial projections to cover expenses only. A business plan written to propose or support a new service line, such as an outpatient chemotherapy service, will require more detail. Lasher (1994) also describes the "three M's" of business planning—market, management, and money. They are a useful reminders of the essentials.

Strategic Planning

Strategic planning is an activity that involves gathering masses of data for analysis to predict what a business will do over a certain period of time, usually about 5 years. Mintzberg (1994) recently refined his notion of strategic planning based on his continuing research of organizations and management. Strategic planning models in use today do not adequately communicate the dynamic nature required to bring products and services to the market fast. Speed is a significant element in the development of new ventures. Though time is required to think through and plan adequately, the tension of speed should always be an element of the process. Mintzberg proposes a new way of strategic planning that he calls "strategic thinking and strategic acting"; this is part of line management's role. He believes strategic planning is an oxymoron and that planners should be more concerned with finding emerging strategies and feeding important information often overlooked by line managers involved in the strategy planning process. Nurse managers interested in creating a new venture will benefit from connecting to organizational planners for data and thinking of the whole picture during the development of the business plan.

A modified strategic decision-making process originally proposed by Wheelen and Hunger (1986) is proposed to assist the intrapreneur or entrepreneur and guide the dynamic strategic thinking and planning process that is requisite for new ventures and initiatives in today's health care market. These steps, with questions to guide the process, are modified below for the nurse intrapreneur interested in starting a new business within or separate from an existing organization. They include:

1. *Evaluate current performance results.* What is the "business" of the idea or venture? What quantitative indicators are available to show that the business or service has been provided? What qualitative indi-

cators are available regarding the performance of the new product or service?

2. *Examine current mission.* Does the written and practiced philosophy support innovation and an entrepreneurial approach? What message is projected through the philosophy that may serve as a basis for an internal new venture? Is it necessary to create a new philosophy in order to support an internal venture? Is a separate and distinct mission and separate entity required for the venture? Is there a similar existing program or service that is like the one under consideration? What are the goals or objectives of the existing program or service that might be used to develop the new idea? What strategies are used to help consumers understand how and when to use the existing services? What are the internal policies regarding new ventures and innovation?

3. *Review strategic managers.* Who are the internal and external organizational players important to the idea or venture? Are there other key individuals who should be involved in the development of the idea into a strategic plan?

4. *Scan the external environment.* What other new services or product lines are offered by the organization and by others in the region? What are the economic trends affecting the organization? What are the organization's most dominant and important capabilities, skills, and relationships? What are the strengths and limitations of the organization as it relates to innovation and intrapreneuring? What information is available regarding the service area and people in the community or catchment area?

5. *Scan the internal environment.* How do those in the present organizational work unit feel about who they are and what they deliver as a unit within the present structure? What will a new venture mean to their workloads? How will it affect productivity in established services presently offered through the defined work unit? Will a new and separate work unit need to be defined and dedicated to the new venture or will it be part of an already established assignment?

6. *Select strategic factors from strengths and limitations.* How can commitment to the new venture be achieved? What marketing strategies are needed? What can be done to improve the return on investment for an established program or service within the context of a new venture?

7. *Select strategic factors from threats and opportunities.* What opportunities exist in the environment to help accomplish the development of the idea and new venture? What are the potential threats to the venture? What other new services related to the new venture will also be needed? What other related services or programs might be generated as a result of the new venture?

8. *Analyze strategic factors.* What share of the market is desired? How should the new venture be cultivated so it is synchronized with other

organizational imperatives? If a separate entity should be created, how will it co-exist with and complement the established organization? If a reporting structure is needed, what will it look like? How will the communication line be held open?

9. *Revise mission and objectives.* With the above data aggregated and analyzed, what changes need to occur to create an environment for intrapreneuring? Considering the culture, status, and goals of the present organization, how will the new venture fit into the defined strategic initiatives? What changes will need to be made internally to support an intrapreneurial effort?

10. *Formulate a plan.* Of all the things that can be done, and given the data available, what are all the alternatives that should guide the development of the business plan? Is the plan based on realistic assumptions and accurate information? Is the plan internally consistent with the data? Will the strategy create economic or political value within acceptable risk limits?

The sense of urgency is also an integral part of this planning process. Although the steps in the strategic thinking process may seem a long and drawn out way to develop a simple idea, the complexity of the idea will dictate the depth and breadth of this exploration of the possibilities and realities. The sense of urgency is communicated through the business plan and the testimonies of key individuals who believe with the intrapreneur or entrepreneur that the opportunity described as a new venture is time limited. These questions are helpful to the intrapreneur or entrepreneur considering a new venture within an established service or product setting. Much of the data collected is used to complete the business plan.

The use of strategic planning during the development of the business plan helps the entrepreneur or intrapreneur develop the mission and strategy of the venture. Broad, sweeping issues are considered and desires to be "first in the field" or "the largest provider" of a service are often integrated into the plan development. Details of how to offer a service, product, or program are included in the operational, budgeting, and forecasting aspects of the plan. The strategy required for the product or service and the market that exists for it now and in the future are the most important considerations in drafting the business plan.

Operational Planning

Operational planning involves translating business ideas into concrete, short-term projections, usually for about a year (Lasher, 1994). Although more detailed than strategic planning, operational planning is still not highly detailed. During the operational planning phase, discussions take place about how much will be sold, to whom, and at what prices. Depending on the nature of the venture, labor, materials, and equipment, and what they will cost are also determined. Short-term goals and revenue targets are set along with quotas and product or service development milestones. Unlike the strategic plan, which uses primarily words to describe the strategy, an even mix of numbers and words are used to describe the operational plan.

Budgeting

Budgeting is the same process used in other areas of nursing administration. It is the process of making accurate financial projections over a relatively short term, usually about 6 months or a year. Budgeting attempts to determine exactly how much money will flow in and out of the venture and fixes responsibility on selected people to make it happen. A proposed budget often serves as the basis for funding an intrapreneurial effort. In the case of an entrepreneurial effort, the budget serves as the basis for loan or venture capital applications. References listed at the close of this chapter provide ample detail for the nurse in need of budget preparation information.

Forecasting

Forecasting is an attempt to predict, based on limited data, where the venture or strategic business unit will be in a month or a year. If forecasts yield undesirable results, short-term actions may be taken, such as increasing the amount of services or product or reducing staff. Forecasting is important in relation to cash requirements. If a new venture or business is to pay its bills and make payroll, an accurate picture of the cash expected to flow in and out over 6 months to a year is essential. Relationships with financial sources such as banks may need to be established specifically to keep a new venture running until collections catch up with disbursements.

An Integrated Process

The business planning process includes the aspects, steps, and phases mentioned above. If placed on a time continuum of long- to short-term, the long-term end would start with strategic planning, followed by operations, budgeting, and forecasting at the short-term end. Strategic planning is more conceptual, and forecasting is detailed and numerical.

Innovation and entrepreneuring within an existing structure or institution requires the executive team to free its best performers for the challenges of innovation. As Drucker (1985) indicates, "[f]irst, the organization must be receptive to innovation and perceive change as an opportunity rather than a threat" (p. 150). Some systematic appraisal or measure of the organization's performance as entrepreneur and innovator is also required to determine if the environment will support a new venture. This may be the first and only question a nurse executive need ask to help make the personal decision to attempt a new venture as an intrapreneur or an entrepreneur. Specific, and usually different, policies and procedures are usually required for new venture structures, staffing, managing, compensation, incentives, and rewards.

■ THE BUSINESS PLAN

Translating an idea into a successful business requires an organizing framework. Such a framework can be found in the traditional business plan. A business plan provides a road map to allow entrepreneurs to decide where they are going and also permits them to know when they have arrived at the desired destination.

Gumpert (1990) defines a business plan as "a document that convincingly demonstrates that your business can sell enough of its product or services so as to make a satisfactory profit and be attractive to potential backers" (p. 6). This view of a business plan as a sales tool encourages the entrepreneur to "sell" the business to potential backers, potential partners, potential employees, and, perhaps most importantly, to himself or herself. The enthusiasm the novice entrepreneur feels about his or her idea for a business will be reflected in the business plan and, thus, will sell others on the business as well.

Although many businesses have grown and prospered without a business plan, the reasons to write one are compelling enough to encourage the new entrepreneur to undertake the task. The current marketplace, in which nurses are moving into entrepreneurial ventures in droves, and business arenas characterized by competition rather than cooperation or collaboration, are two such reasons.

Assistance with developing a business plan is available from a variety of sources: Books abound that guarantee the reader the ability to write a successful business plan. Several are cited in this chapter. Computer software packages also offer a means to developing a business plan (but see a cautionary note below). Small Business Development Centers affiliated with colleges and universities offer assistance, as does the Small Business Administration, and the Service Corps of Retired Executives (SCORE), both of which can be found in the telephone directory.

Although the entrepreneur should take advantage of the assistance available, it is important for the entrepreneur to write the business plan and not rely on others to do it. The reason for this is simple: No one will know or understand the business better than its owner.

There are a variety of approaches to writing a business plan, and no one best way. However, the novice entrepreneur should avoid a "boilerplate" approach in which information about the company is forced into a standardized template. Such a standardized presentation may not showcase the business appropriately. Computer software packages that rely on this boilerplate approach should not be used.

A business plan is useful in allowing the business owner, and others, to take an objective, critical, unemotional view of a business. The business plan also can be used as an operating tool to manage the business or guide it toward success.

Business plans are particularly useful in three areas of a business:

- In a start-up venture to obtain financing.
- When additional financing is needed.
- For new activities within a business.

Other uses for a business plan, as outlined by Gumpert (1990), are:

- Arranging strategic alliances between companies.
- Obtaining large contracts.
- Attracting key employees.
- Completing mergers and acquisitions (p. 9).

Key points to consider when writing a business plan are conveying the energy and excitement of the business, stressing what makes the business unique, and being as honest about negative aspects of the business as about positive ones. Care should be taken not to disparage others in the field, particularly when describing the competition for the entrepreneur's products or services (Puetz & Shinn, 1997).

Writing the Business Plan

Writing the business plan is time consuming and may best be scheduled over a period of several weeks. A draft form of the plan should be reviewed by colleagues not directly associated with the business and revisions made based on their suggestions before the plan is accepted as final. It may be necessary to have several revisions before the plan is deemed acceptable, but at all draft stages it should be reviewed by individuals outside of the business.

The business plan should not be an excessively lengthy document. About 12 to 15 pages should be adequate for a start-up venture. An older, more established business may require a longer business plan because of its history. Strive for completeness and conciseness.

A business plan must contain at a minimum:

- Cover page.
- Table of contents.
- Executive summary.
- Description of the company.
- The target market.
- The product/service.
- Marketing strategies.
- Finances (Gumpert, 1990; Lasher, 1994; Vogel & Doleysh, 1994).

Each of these sections is described in detail on the following pages and then applied in an abbreviated format to the venture described in this chapter, starting a consulting business in continuing education in nursing. See Appendix 1 for a sample business plan.

Cover Page

The cover page of the business plan should contain the name of the company, its business address, telephone number, and the owner's name. Include zip codes with addresses and area codes with telephone numbers. Gumpert (1990) stresses the importance of not overlooking the need for a cover page, since a banker is unlikely to look up a company's telephone number in order to discuss financing (and attention to detail is an important characteristic of a successful entrepreneur). Gumpert (1990) further advises that the cover page contain a number prominently displayed if copies of the plan are distributed to individuals in a bank, for example. The return of the copies of the plan can be tracked by the number on the cover page.

Table of Contents

A table of contents is necessary for the reader's convenience in turning to areas of particular interest. Number all of the pages of the business plan (including the appendices, if any) and reflect the page numbers on the table of contents.

Executive Summary

An executive summary encapsulates the contents of the business plan for the reader. The executive summary should stress the most important components of the business plan: the target market, current and future services, and financing needs (Vogel & Doleysh, 1994). Then, using the table of contents, the reader can explore sections of interest in depth.

The executive summary should convey the priorities on which the business is focused and be written in a way that entices the reader to want to explore the business plan in more detail. An individual who works in public relations or journalism may be of assistance in developing an enthusiastic, energetic executive summary.

Gumpert (1990) suggests writing the executive summary before the business plan is written as a way of guiding the writing of the plan, then rewriting it after the plan has been written. This approach should lead to a better final product because the revision of the executive summary takes place over an extended period of time, with the writer in different phases of the process and holding different perspectives in each phase.

Description of the Company

The purpose of this section is to describe what the business is, how it will be run, and why the business will be successful (Bangs, 1982). The company description should include how the business was started, its current status, and future projections. If the company is a start-up venture, information about how the idea evolved should be included. The principal owners or operators should be described in this section. Include information such as educational background, experience in the field, accomplishments, and abilities. The emphasis in these descriptions must be "real life business accomplishments" (Gumpert, 1990, p. 66) that allow the reader to ascertain what the individuals involved have done successfully in the past and then to draw inferences about what the individuals involved are likely to do in the future. A résumé, curriculum vitae (CV), or a biographical sketch of the principals can be included as an appendix, but this should not be relied upon to be the only description of the individuals involved in the business. If the company is composed of more than one principal, job descriptions for all of the individuals involved should be included in the appendices. All of the human resources in the business, whether paid or volunteer, should be included in this section.

The Target Market

This section includes information on the company's clients, both current and potential, the competition, and marketing efforts that have been implemented or are contemplated. Describe the target market in detail: List what is known about characteristics of potential clients and estimate the extent to which they will avail themselves of the company's services. Try to predict the extent to which the target market will be reached in 1 year, 3 years, and 5 years (Vogel & Doleysh, 1994). Evidence to substantiate claims about the potential market must be included in this section or, if extensive, added as an appendix.

The description of competitors should include information about size, services offered, profitability (if known), strengths, and weaknesses. Care should be taken not to make disparaging remarks about competitors (Shenson & Wilson, 1993). The entrepreneur should objectively describe the products and services offered by competitors and compare them with what will be offered by the entrepreneur without making a judgment about the value of either product or service.

The Product/Service

This section of the business plan should clearly and specifically identify what the company has to offer clients. In the case of a product, such as a continuing education workshop, for example, the course outline and marketing materials provide evidence of the nature of the product and can be placed in the appendices.

It is more difficult to describe a service such as consultation on accreditation or evaluation. The description of the offered service should be reviewed for clarity by individuals not related to the company before being included in the business plan to ensure it can be understood by those not involved in the business. Aspects that make the product unique or more valuable to clients than competitors' similar products should be described in this section.

Marketing Strategies

This section contains a description of how the entrepreneur intends to reach consumers in the target market and convert them into clients. Marketing strategies can include indirect approaches such as publishing and presentations, and direct approaches such as direct mail and cold calls (Metzger, 1993). Samples of promotional materials can be used to illustrate marketing strategies. Plans for marketing activities should be detailed so that readers know that the entrepreneur not only knows the target market but also knows how best to reach it.

Finances

In this section, a complete financial picture of the company must be presented. Sources of financing should be described. If the company has been in business for a while, past results as well as future projections should be included. This section is accompanied by "cash flow projections, profit-and-loss statements, and balance sheets" (Gumpert, 1990, p. 20).

■ PREPARING THE BUSINESS PLAN

The appearance of the business plan is equally as important as the content. Individuals' responses to the business plan—and the business it represents—are influenced by how the plan is organized and how it looks. Therefore, care should be taken in writing the business plan.

Start by writing all of the sections, then putting them aside for a time before reading them. Revisions should be made after this initial reading. Once the material is revised, it should be reviewed by individuals who are not involved in the business and who will have an objective viewpoint about the plan. Individuals such as accountants, attorneys, and similar professionals are better choices for reviewers than family members or close friends. In the event that the plan reflects content that is better known to colleagues, such as nursing professionals, by all means ask them to review the draft of the plan.

The plan should be produced in an easily readable format. A word-processing program will allow the writer to make changes and revisions while keeping the original version intact. Use a font size of 12 or 14 for ease in reading. A sans serif font (such as Ariel) is easier to read than a serif font such as Times Roman in which characters can touch or appear to run together. Avoid techniques such as underlining or bold for emphasis. Also avoid exclamation marks.

If using a word-processing program, spell check the document several times. If the program has a grammar-checking feature, use it to assess the extent to which common errors, such as using passive voice, appear in the plan and correct them when possible. Assess the reading level of the document as well. Aim for a level of eighth grade.

When complete, read the plan carefully for typographical errors. If possible, ask someone in the English or Journalism Department of a local college or university to edit the business plan for punctuation and grammar. It may be necessary to offer the individual editing the plan some compensation, but the expense will generally be worth it.

Print the business plan with a high-quality printer, preferably a laser printer. Do not use a dot matrix printer. When more than one copy of the business plan is needed, photocopies are acceptable, but these should be on quality paper, at least 20 pound bond. Photocopies should be scanned for smudges and smears, and those that are not completely clean should be discarded.

It may be helpful to bind the business plan. Alternatively, a two-pocket folder can be used in which the cover letter and business plan appear on the right side (so they are seen first when the folder is opened) and the appendices appear on the left side. This format is best used when the appendices are not all a standard size as, for example, when promotional materials of various sizes for a workshop are included.

The reasons to write a business plan are many and valid. Although a time-consuming and perhaps uncomfortable process for many, without such a guide most entrepreneurs may not be successful in translating an idea for a proposed venture into reality.

■ SUMMARY

This chapter discussed the development of ideas into new ventures within the notions of niche marketing. The process of developing an idea into a new venture through intrapreneurial or entrepreneurial approaches was discussed, along with characteristics of entrepreneurial individuals and organizations that support new ventures. Strategic planning, forecasting, and budgeting were discussed in relation to articulating the possibilities of an idea into the realities of a new venture. A discussion of business planning and guidelines for writing a business plan conclude the chapter, providing a practical application of these suggestions.

A business plan is an essential tool for nurses planning and implementing a new venture. The business plan provides information to the business owner and other publics about the venture. Preparing a business plan allows the potential entrepreneur to take an unemotional, objective look at the proposed venture. A business plan is an operating tool that will help the nurse entrepreneur manage the business and will provide the basis for obtaining financing for the venture.

ABBREVIATED SAMPLE BUSINESS PLAN

1. Cover Page

Business Plan
Continuing Education Consultation Services

Mary Jones, MSN, RN, C
Principal

Steven Grove, BSN, RN, C
Principal

1234 Any Street
Hometown, USA ZIP65-4321
(999) 987-6543
Fax (999) 123-4567

August 1, 1997

Plan number 1

2. Table of Contents:

Table of Contents

Executive summary. 1
Description of the company 4
The target market. 5
The product/service 8
Marketing strategies 10
Finances. 13
Appendices 17

3. Executive Summary (Abbreviated Version)

This business plan describes Continuing Education Consultation Services, a partnership of Mary Jones and Steven Grove. The company provides continuing education services including educational design of workshops, conferences, and in-service education classes. The company also provides workshops on topics such as stress management, case management, managed care, and clinical topics in pediatrics and rehabilitation. In addition, consultation on accreditation, approval, or evaluation of educational activities is available.

The principals hold a combined total of 34 years' experience in nursing education and practice. Both are certified in continuing education by the American Nurses Credentialing Center.

Current clients include University Hospital, Memorial Hospital, and the State Medical Center. Contracts are underway with Main University and the National Nursing Specialty Organization.

Marketing strategies include direct mail, advertising in national nursing publications, and word of mouth. Free consultation is provided to local chapters of national nursing organizations.

The company has shown a small profit (after direct expenses) after only 1 year. The principals also are employed part time in clinical settings in local hospitals.

4. Description of the Company

Continuing Education Consultation Services was started in 1995 by Mary Jones. Steven Grove joined the company early in 1996. The idea for the business began in the wake of restructuring and downsizing of staff development departments in hospitals. The need for consultation in educational design, approval of educational activities, and evaluation became apparent as fewer nurses were employed in staff development departments. Hospitals welcomed the cost savings of independent contractors providing educational services on an as-needed basis as opposed to having full-time employees provide these services.

The first contract with a hospital was signed in January of 1995. To date the company has signed contracts for educational services with 2 other hospitals and is negotiating contracts with a university and a national nursing specialty organization.

The company has as goals to provide continuing education consultation services to a majority of the hospitals in the tri-state area as well as to the 3 colleges/universities in the geographical area with continuing education departments in the schools of nursing. Two national nursing specialty organizations are headquartered in the tri-state area, and these are potential clients as well.

5. The Target Market

Continuing Education Consultation Services focuses on hospitals, primarily those which have or are contemplating reducing the number of staff development educator employees. The firm also offers services to local area colleges/universities with continuing education departments within the school of nursing.

A third market for the company's services is specialty nursing organizations with active programs for members.

6. The Product/Service

Continuing Education Consultation Services provides workshops on a variety of topics, including infection control, safety, and cardiopulmonary resuscitation (CPR). Sample workshop outlines appear in Appendix 1. The company also consults in educational design, using the adult learning model in Appendix 2. . . .

7. Marketing Strategies

Continuing Education Consultation Services uses a variety of marketing strategies. Among the most successful was an initial direct mailing announcing the formation of the company and the services provided. A response rate of 5% resulted in 2 contracts. . . . The principals of the company also conduct a direct sales campaign as described in a book by Robert O. Metzger entitled *Developing a Consulting Practice* (1993, Sage Publications, Inc.). . . .

8. Finances

Financial forms that may be included:

- Balance Sheet listing assets and liabilities
- Income Statement (quarterly; annual)
- Monthly Cash Flow Statement

9. Income Statement—1995

Income

Continuing Education Workshops	$2,225.00
Continuing Education Contracts	$3,000.00

Total Income	$5,225.00

Expenses

Clerical Services	$1,000.00
Printing/Copies	$ 100.00
Telephone	$ 150.00 (voice and facsimile lines; long distance)
Automotive	$ 250.00
Marketing	$1,035.00
Professional Development	$ 100.00 (dues; publications)
Supplies	$ 25.00
Accounting/Legal	$ 100.00
Taxes	$ 800.00
Equipment	$ 250.00
Postage	$ 100.00
Insurance	$ 175.00
Miscellaneous	$ 400.00

Total Expenses	$ 4,485.00
Income over Expenses	$ 740.00

■ BIOGRAPHICAL SKETCHES

Belinda E. Puetz is CEO and President of Puetz & Associates in Pensacola, Florida. The company offers association management services for national nursing specialty organizations. Current clients include the American Assembly for Men in Nursing, Home Healthcare Nurses Association, International Society for Psychiatric Consultation Liaison Nurses, National Nursing Staff Development Organization, Society for Vascular Nursing, Society for Education and Research in Psychiatric–Mental Health Nursing, and the Southern Nursing Research Society. She also serves as Editor for four nursing publications including *Gastroenterology Nursing,* the *Journal of Nursing Staff Development, Rehabilitation Nursing,* and *Rehabilitation Nursing Research.* She has been in business since 1983 and currently employs a staff of 12. Dr. Puetz has consulted with hospitals, colleges/universities, nursing organizations, and funded projects. She has written or co-authored five books, and has published numerous articles in the nursing literature. She is a diploma graduate of Henry Ford Hospital School of Nursing in Detroit, and received a baccalaureate in nursing from Indiana University in Indianapolis. Her masters and doctorate in adult education were awarded by Indiana University in Bloomington, Indiana.

Karen J. Kelly Thomas is an experienced nurse administrator and staff development specialist. In her 26 years' experience in nursing, she has focused primarily on administering developmental programs and projects in multiple settings. She is a founding member of the National Nursing Staff Development Organization and served as the 1992–94 president. Dr. Thomas owns and operates a private consultation practice called Kelly Thomas Associates. She recently served as Administrative Director at Suburban Hospital in Bethesda, Maryland. Presently, she is the Director of Practice and Research, Association of Women's Health, Obstetrics, and Neonatal Nurses in Washington, D.C.

Dr. Thomas also presents regularly to national and international groups, primarily on competence assessment systems, organization development, quality management, and strategic thinking. She has published more than a dozen articles and chapters in books. Her book, *Nursing Staff Development: Current Competence, Future Focus,* received a 1992 book of the year award from the *American Journal of Nursing.* (A second edition is in development now.)

Dr. Thomas received her diploma in nursing from Holy Name Hospital in Teaneck, New Jersey, a BSN from Regents College in Albany, New York, and an MS in Adult Education from Virginia Tech. She recently completed her doctorate in nursing and health care administration at George Mason University in Fairfax, Virginia. Her research is focused on the nature of intuition among staff development experts and expert practice.

■ SUGGESTED READINGS

Flanagan, L. (1993). *Self-employment in nursing: Understanding the basics of starting a business.* Washington, DC: American Nurses Publishing.

Gumpert, D.E. (1990). *How to really create a successful business plan.* Boston: Inc. Publishing.

Puetz, B.E., & Shinn, L.J. (1997). *The nurse consultant's handbook.* New York: Springer.

■ REFERENCES

Bangs, D.H., Jr. (1982). Business planning guide. In B.R. Riccardi & E.C. Dayani (Eds.), *The nurse entrepreneur* (pp. 103–136). Reston, VA: Reston Publishing.

Brookfield, S.D. (1993). On impostership, cultural suicide, and other dangers: How nurses learn critical thinking. *The Journal of Continuing Education in Nursing, 24,* 197–205.

Brown, A.D. (1995). Managing understandings: Politics, symbolism, niche marketing and the quest for legitimacy in information technology implementation. *Organization Studies, 16,* 951–969.

Dalgic, T., & Leeuw, M. (1994). Niche marketing revisited: Concepts, applications and some European cases. *European Journal of Marketing, 28* (4), 39–55.

Drucker, P.F. (1985). *Innovation and entrepreneurship: Practice and principles.* New York: Harper & Row.

Flanagan, L. (1993). *Self-employment in nursing: Understanding the basics of starting a business.* Washington, DC: American Nurses Publishing.

Gumpert, D.E. (1990). *How to really create a successful business plan.* Boston: Inc. Publishing.

Henry, B., Arndt, C., Di Vincenti, M., & Marriner-Tomey, A. (1989). *Dimensions of nursing administration: Theory, research, education, practice.* Boston: Blackwell Scientific.

Kotler, P. (1991). From mass marketing to mass customization. *Planning Review,* Sept./Oct., 11–47.

Lasher, W. (1994). *The perfect business plan.* New York: Doubleday.

Metzger, R.O. (1993). *Developing a consulting practice.* Newbury Park, CA: Sage.

Mintzberg, H. (1994). Rethinking strategic planning, Part II: New roles for planners. *Long Range Planning, 27* (3), 22–30.

Ornstein, R., & Thompson, R.F. (1984). *The amazing brain.* Boston: Houghton Mifflin.

Pinchot, G. (1985). *Intrapreneuring.* New York: Harper & Row.

Puetz, B.E., & Shinn, L.J. (1997). *The nurse consultant's handbook.* New York: Springer.

Rubenfeld, M.G., & Scheffer, B.K. (1995). *Critical thinking in nursing: An interactive approach.* Philadelphia: Lippincott.

Shenson, H.L., & Wilson, J.R. (1993). *138 quick ideas to get more clients.* New York: Wiley.

Vogel, G., & Doleysh, N. (1994). *Entrepreneuring: A nurse's guide to starting a business* (2nd ed.). New York: National League for Nursing Press.

Weber, J.A. (1994). Using purchase influence niching for better focus in industrial marketing plans. *Industrial Marketing Management, 23,* 419–438.

Wheelen, T., & Hunger, J.D. (1986). *Strategic management and business policy* (2nd. ed.). Reading, MA: Addison-Wesley.

Zoghlin, G.G. (1991). *From executive to entrepreneur: Making the transition.* New York: American Management Association.

CASE 7–1 Establishing a Care Management Business

Ann E. O'Neil

This case describes my development of a care management business and offers some information and lessons learned along the way. New business opportunities are always present and for the nurse who has a desire to be an entrepreneur, it is a matter of developing an awareness of the needs and wants in the communities and in society.

During my tenure as director of a hospice in the mid-1980s, I became aware of an unfulfilled need in the community. Many older people and their families were faced with lifestyle changes resulting from the older person's diminished capacity in the realm of physical, cognitive, behavioral or psychological functioning. Other families were trying to manage the care of an older relative from a distance, which created a hardship for all concerned. Hence, the idea to start a care management business.

Care and case management have been part of the health care arena for many years. Yet, in the initial stages of this business, there was little competition. The profession of geriatric care management was in the early phase of its development. The National Association of Professional Geriatric Care Managers had just been formed. Care and case management did not become a major player until insurance companies and their reimbursement policies became heavily involved in deciding what services from what provider an individual would receive and began to develop their own case management capabilities. Since the formation of this business, the numbers of providers have grown immensely as more people recognize the size of the market out there. In 1988, the National Association of Professional Geriatric Care Managers had less than 50 members. Today the association has over 900 members.

In 1988 as today, for the majority of people requiring ongoing care services, there was and is no insurance reimbursement for the complexity of services and care they require to maintain themselves in their homes or to ensure that the quality of their lives is not significantly compromised. This is the niche in the marketplace that was found.

■ COMMITMENT TO ACTION

An interval of several months was spent thinking, searching, discussing, and researching. The only nurse entrepreneur I knew of was Lucille Kinlein, a nurse practitioner from Maryland, who had opened a private practice in the 1970s. She influenced my dreams, ambitions, and the direction my career had taken. The literature disclosed others who had followed this path. Research also revealed that geriatric care management was an untried field with no one to serve as a mentor. On the other hand, the field was wide open.

Local government reports were obtained and reviewed. Discussions were

CASE: 7–1 *Continued*

held with an attorney, two accountants, experts in the field of geriatrics, and entrepreneurs. The most valuable piece of advice other entrepreneurs offered was to engage the services of an attorney and an accountant at the start. This enabled me to avoid many pitfalls and many uncomfortable situations. I was gaining momentum.

The next step was a course taken at a local university on "How to Operate Your Own Small Business for Profit." A useful discovery was the Small Business Administration's answer desk, at 1–800–827–5722. The Small Business Administration (SBA) offers a one-day seminar in many areas on "Owning Your Own Business." The SBA's web site, at http://www. sbaonline. sba. gov, also offers useful information.

It was interesting to observe the reactions of friends, family, and colleagues during this period. Although most people overwhelmingly encouraged the pursuit of the new venture, a few colleagues reacted negatively to the plans. They did not understand the need to pursue one's dream nor the driving force behind the entrepreneurial spirit. One cannot be offput by these negative attitudes and lack of understanding.

Finally, the time came to resign from a position that provided the security of a regular paycheck and a status that society understood and valued. I was on my way.

■ BUSINESS ARRANGEMENTS

The attorney assisted in determining the business structure that the company would operate under and explained the choices and regulations of the Commonwealth of Virginia. The types of organizations explored with the attorney were a sole proprietorship, a partnership, and a corporation.

A sole proprietorship requires a business license and a home occupancy license if the business is to operate from one's home. The profit and loss of this structure are grouped and tied to one's personal affairs. One advantage offered by this type of organization is the ability to deduct medical insurance. There is also no need to share the management of the business with anyone else.

The second structure, a partnership, is an association of two or more people carrying on business for profit. The individuals involved are considered the agent and the principal of the company. There are fiduciary responsibilities associated with these titles which denote a position of trust and a responsibility for each other as well as the company. The primary disadvantage of a partnership is the possibility that disagreements will arise from unclear expectations or new, unanticipated situations. The primary advantage comes from the additional capital of combined assets and resources. Partners also add a sense of stability to a business, as customers are not dependent on a single person for service.

The third structure, a corporation, was chosen for the business based on the advice of the accountant, the attorney, and the insurance agent. The main reason they cited was its limited liability. The corporation is considered a separate entity from its owner; it has separate rights and fiduciary responsibilities. The

CASE: 7–1 *Continued*

stock of a corporation can be sold, disposed of, or given away; this provides a continuity that banks may regard favorably in granting loans. The down side is the complexity of taxes.

The role of the accountant was invaluable as I wended my way through the maze of multiple tax entities, worker's compensation, business licenses, eligibility issues involving company benefits, such as pension plans, and the regulations governing such plans. The accountant assisted in setting up the account journals from day one. A general ledger was set up, as well as accounts payable (a list of what is owed), and accounts receivable for services rendered or products sold to the consumer. The accounting system was set out on a cash basis, not an accrual system.

A payroll system was also included. Two years later, when it became necessary to engage others, the accountant advised outsourcing the payroll. This proved to be an inexpensive option that allowed an expert to do a specific task more efficiently than could have been done in-house.

The accounting system can be implemented by several means. A combination of arrangements has been utilized to meet our accounting needs. Many computerized accounting programs are available. For our particular needs, the accountant advised a software program be used for our billing system, and a bookkeeper for the general ledger. A contract securing the expertise of a certified public accountant still remains necessary for overall direction of the system.

The design of the accounts format provides information on expenses, developing charges, pricing of items, and billing. Regular meetings are held with the accountant to review where the business is heading financially. Comparing monthly average figures, the level of current expenses, and current income enables better business decisions to be made as opportunities arise.

Having come from the non-profit world, it was surprising to me to encounter the multitude of tax entities that required payments. A deliberate decision was made to have the accountant track the taxes owed. The accountant follows the tax regulations, requirements, and changes in the law as part of routine work.

The next meetings were with the insurance agent, who arranged for general liability, business, health and disability, and professional liability insurance. Since the original office was in my home, the homeowner's insurance policy was reviewed. The insurance agent strongly advised adding a $1 million umbrella general liability clause to the current policy as there would be increased numbers of people coming onto the home property. This was certainly worthwhile advice. Business insurance was purchased to cover the public liability on the business premises, as well as theft, fire, and loss.

The cost of purchasing an individual health insurance policy came as a rude awakening. Every institution, facility, and organization I had ever worked with provided health insurance. The organizations I belonged to did not offer the health insurance package required for my needs. Eventually, a small business insurance policy was found.

CASE: 7–1 *Continued*

Until 1994, there was no specific policy to cover professional liability insurance for the role of a geriatric care manager. The National Association of Professional Geriatric Care Managers has been instrumental in the development and implementation of such a product. It is reassuring to have insurance specific to this type of professional work.

Within 3 years, the corporation had three employees. Worker's compensation and employer's liability insurance were required by law to be purchased. Interestingly, the insurance company did not understand the nature of the business and needed to be convinced we were not operating a nursing home.

■ THE BUSINESS PLAN

The original business plan developed in 1987–1988 is still in the office. Dogged-eared and yellow, it is reviewed on occasion. Most of the original goals have been met, but a few still remain to be reached. Updates have been added to the plan as new opportunities have arisen.

A business plan spells out the purpose and gives direction to the business. Built into the business plan are the means to be prepared for success—when to invest more money, add more staff, or market a new service/product. The plan allows one to organize ideas in a concrete manner, to describe the business, to test activities, to view what has been accomplished, to describe how the business will function out in the public, and to define who will manage the business and how it will be managed. It describes the market and identifies existing providers and services in the community.

Developing the business plan was a consuming but enjoyable task. A major portion of the research had been accomplished and now it was time to pull it all together. It took approximately one week to put down my dreams and thoughts into some kind of concrete business plan. This was an exhilarating experience which further heightened my determination to go forward. In the beginning, the plan was reviewed every week and then every 4 months. The original plan is still useful, summarizing as it does the mission of our corporation: to provide a highly individualized care management service to older people and their families by assisting older people to remain as independent as possible, balancing their functional limitations with their quality of life.

■ GETTING STARTED

Once incorporated with a business plan, the appropriate licenses, insurance, and accounting systems in place, the next task was to shop for equipment. The initial capital expenditure included the purchase of a computer, word processing software, a printer, an answering machine, a desk, a chair, a telephone, and a separate telephone line. A fireproof cabinet was also purchased, which proved beneficial 3 years later when there was a fire. Everything around the cabinet was burned but the contents were saved.

CASE: 7–1 *Continued*

The fixed costs included heat, light, car mileage, insurance, and licenses. The variable costs included brochures, stationary, advertising, and professional and secretarial services.

The initial pricing of the service proved to be a dilemma. Pricing of a product must take into consideration a variety of concrete factors. However, the process is the same, regardless of the service or product offered. The usual way to price a service is to calculate overhead expenses, materials needed to accomplish the job, and labor costs. It is essential to compare what similar services in the area cost. Based on information gathered from the literature, the cost of services around the country was $45.00 to $150.00 an hour. Similar local services—such as fees for psychotherapy charged by social workers and nurses—were also reviewed. A question to ask is, "What will the market bear?"

New entrepreneurs must remember that they are professionals and need to charge proper fees to survive in business as well as to be able to add competent staff for a growing business. A significant piece of advice provided by several business owners was, "Do not underprice the service or you will soon be out of business."

It was time to get to know my bankers. Introductions were made and we discussed the business plan. This proved beneficial 3 years later, when the business had grown to such a point that new premises were required.

■ MARKETING PLAN

In the early stages of the business, there was a lack of knowledge of care management services by the consumer and professional colleagues. After all, the number of older people in our society had just began to expand extensively. The care management services in existence in 1988 were mainly in New York, Pennsylvania, Florida, and California where there were higher percentages of older people, and the care managers there were mainly social workers. A heavy investment in marketing was required for the service to create a customer base.

During the first year of practice, 80 percent of my time was spent on marketing. The first major financial mistake was a marketing one—purchasing advertising that aimed at the wrong population group. While in business, one learns to live with one's mistakes and move forward. It is not sensible to dwell on mistakes and allow the mistakes to hold back the operation.

Paid advertising is still utilized, but only to narrow targeted groups. Public relations is essential to bring good will to the company and to spread the company's name out into the community. This includes sending out press releases, speaking to community groups, networking with local aging groups, writing articles, and responding to the editor of a newspaper.

Brochures and business cards are tools of the trade and are to be given to all potential sources of referrals, including other nurses, psychiatrists, attorneys, bankers, accountants, discharge planners, financial planners, friends, family, and acquaintances. Modesty and shyness must be put aside.

CASE: 7–1 *Continued*

Another valuable lesson, learned early, was the importance of having a graphic artist or public relations expert design the business logo, business cards, and brochures. An enormous amount of time was wasted struggling to write and design brochures and business cards that ultimately proved unsatisfactory. Eventually, the services of a public relations expert were engaged. The end results were brochures, business cards, and a logo design that are still being used today.

Geriatric care management is easily confused with home care agencies and nurse registries. To further confuse matters, some geriatric care management businesses have a separate component of a companion service or a registry. One must be prepared to explain the differences between these services— what is provided that is similar to competitors' services and what makes one's services unique. Our uniqueness has not changed over the years, a highly individualized service for older people and their families.

Keeping abreast of current market conditions is imperative. This means reading about the health care industry in many sources, including the business section of the newspaper, business journals, government reports on long-term care, and traditional clinical and professional journals and reports.

New markets appear on the horizon as often as there are changes in the health care industry and demographics. Managed care offers both a challenge and an opportunity for the geriatric care manager entrepreneur. It is difficult for the frail older persons to maneuver themselves through a large bureaucratic system. As the enrollments increase within these systems, the number of clients requiring an advocacy service increases.

To demonstrate how a potential new market was explored by our company, the long-term care insurance industry experience will be utilized as an example. Stories in the local media were discussing the increase in demand for long-term care insurance. The implications of this trend appeared to offer a new opportunity for our care management business. The next step was a number of discussions with a financial wizard, a stock broker who understood how the market works, an accountant, insurance agents, and the staff. From this process, it was determined that we could immediately participate in providing health assessment for the insurance companies for underwriting purposes and assessments for people who wanted to start utilizing the benefits under their policy agreements.

A staff meeting was held to determine a plan of action, which included obtaining from the Virginia Insurance Commission the list of insurance companies operating in Virginia who sell long-term care policies. We then engaged a consultant to make initial contacts and solicit contracts.

■ SCOPE OF PRACTICE OF CARE MANAGEMENT

A major goal of care management is to assist in the preservation of the person's functional status, recovery from an illness when possible, and preventing or delay-

CASE: 7-1 *Continued*

ing the progression of functional, physical, cognitive, and psychological problems. This service allows the care manager to work closely with the client to assess needs in depth and tailor care plans. The care plan maximizes the assistance of family, community resources, volunteers, and friends. The appropriate services are matched with the client. Unnecessary and inappropriate services are avoided by closely monitoring the care plan.

At the initiation of the business, I could not have conceived of the enormity of issues and problems that older people and their families encounter. My career had been hinged on assisting people with their health care needs. This proved too narrow a focus. A few of the problems the families were confronted with included home maintenance, long-distance caregiving, being victims of scams, succumbing to sweepstakes, entitlements, a room full of consumer items from home shopping that were left unopened, lack of durable power of attorney, sick pets, significant cognitive impairment, and worn-out caregivers. Families requested assistance with these issues and many more as the older person faced diminishing functioning and increased frailties.

The National Association of Professional Geriatric Care Managers defines a care manager as a "professional who specializes in assisting older people and their families with long-term care arrangements. GMCs have a minimum of a bachelor's degree or a substantial equivalent training in gerontology, social work, nursing, or counseling" (p. 10, 1996 Directory).

The services provided to a family can range from the provision of a single consultation to an extensive set of services, depending on the needs and resources of the family and the older person. The population served in our business includes frail older people, disabled adults, and their families. The payor may be family, guardian, power of attorney, or insurance company.

The services we provide include education; consultation; comprehensive assessment of the older person's physical, psychological, behavioral, and cognitive functioning with involved family or parties; assistance with finding alternative living arrangements; identifying available home care services; determining eligibility for services; developing short- and long-term care plans; crisis intervention; referrals to appropriate services, such as day care or legal services; monitoring the quality of care provided to the older person in the home; nursing home and assisted living facility recommendations; locating and coordinating services; ongoing liaison with family and concerned parties; and counseling. Other geriatric care managers provide adjunct services such as psychotherapy, guardianship, power of attorney for finances, companion registries, and day care.

The geriatric care manager requires education, skills, and experience in the field of aging in order to assist families and the older persons to deal with any number of issues, such as Alzheimer's disease, cardiovascular accident, depression, malnutrition, generalized frailness of aging, and/or behavioral problems.

The goal of the geriatric care management process is to assist older persons to remain as independent and in as

CASE: 7–1 *Continued*

much control of their lives as possible. Most of the clients presenting themselves to the care manager are over the age of 80 years. The following cases illustrate the range of situations that may lead to a call to our offices.

Case 1

Mrs. X., who is 89 years of age, lives independently in an apartment near her daughter. She moved here 10 years ago to be closer to her daughter, her only living child. In the last 6 weeks, Mrs. X. has called the police three times because the people in the apartment are sending "bad messages" to her. The woman upstairs "talks through the floor to her." She has forgotten to pay her electric bill. She is refusing all help from her concerned daughter and neighbors. The apartment manager has called the daughter "to do something."

Case 2

A more complex situation involves long-distance caregiving, such as that being provided by the son and daughter of Mr. and Mrs. Y. The daughter lives in New York; the son in North Carolina. Mr. and Mrs. Y. have lived in their home in Virginia for over 30 years. Mr. Y., who is 80 years of age, is experiencing increased symptoms of Alzheimer's disease, including memory loss, disturbed sleep patterns, agitation, and wandering. Mrs. Y. is losing weight and now weighs 90 pounds. At 83 years of age, she is the primary caregiver for Mr. Y. Both adult children have been alternating coming to Virginia every other month. They

acknowledge that their mother cannot manage the increased care needs of their father much longer, but they are at a loss as to how to help their parents. Their parents consider them their main support. The children are feeling overwhelmed by the responsibility and a sense of helplessness in providing the kind of care they feel their parents should be receiving. They both have growing families, and both are employed full time.

The services of a care manager are most likely to be utilized by the adult child of an older person. Others who commonly utilize or make referrals to the care manager are social service providers, trust officers of banks, hospital discharge planners, financial planners and managers, attorneys, health care professionals, senior housing agencies, and former clients.

The National Association of Professional Geriatric Care Managers has developed standards of practice to ensure that a high-quality of professional service is provided to a vulnerable and frail population. These standards, as well as the standards developed for each discipline in our service, provide the foundation for the provision of services as well as serving to judge the quality of the service by the professional care manager.

■ CARE AND MAINTENANCE OF A BUSINESS

Businesses are living organisms that need continual attention. The market-

CASE: 7–1 *Continued*

place is also in constant flux. Attention to both is necessary to maintain a competitive edge. This means being out in the marketplace, talking with the referral sources, continual networking, and looking for new challenges and directions to keep the business viable. These actions ensure that the marketplace is being served and the business can continue to compete with similar services. We continue to have a strong sense of our mission and a willingness to compete on a value basis.

The needs of older people require a diversity of skills. One business strategy was to deliberately expand the business by engaging staff from different disciplines. The first person engaged was skilled in administrative support; this released me to spend more time marketing and networking. Because this service is available 7 days a week, a relief care manager was engaged in the second year. Currently, the seven staff members are from disciplines that encompass nursing, social work, psychology, economics, and administration.

Over the years, nurses have been strong supporters of our care management business. In the initial stages of the business, the greatest number of referrals were from nurses.

Nurses who go into business for themselves do so for a number of reasons—to develop an idea, have more flexible hours, provide a unique service, be independent, be creative, do a better job. It is possible to succeed as a nurse entrepreneur. Society does value our services. The door is open. The choice of the business venture should include "how much happiness it gives," as the number of hours spent developing the business requires much energy. Believe and trust in yourself. For those with the willing spirit of an entrepreneur, good luck.

■ BIOGRAPHICAL SKETCH

Ann E. O'Neil is owner and president of Ann E. O'Neil, RN, MSN, Inc., a geriatric care management business located in Falls Church, Virginia. She is a graduate of St. Anselm's College and Catholic University of America. During her career, she has held positions in teaching, community, and international health, as well as clinical and administrative positions. She has held offices at the local level of the Virginia Nurses Association. She is currently on the Board of Directors of the National Association of Professional Geriatric Care Managers.

■ REFERENCES

1996 Directory of Members National Association of Professional Geriatric Care Managers. (1996). Tucson, AZ: Author.

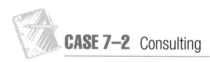

CASE 7–2 Consulting

Barbara A. Happ

When Phyllis Forrestor, RN, became Vice President of Operations for St. Elizabeth's Health System (SEHS), three facilities owned by SEHS were providing similar inpatient and ambulatory care services. Phyllis had limited in-house resources to deal quickly with merging and redesigning clinical operations, or to include the development of information systems that would be needed in the redesigned organization. Without these changes, SEHS was incapable of responding to the competitive health care environment in the community. "I needed a plan and assistance with changes to care for the contracted population under managed care and capitation," she recalled. Phyllis's goal included building an organization that was responsive to the current and future health care needs in her community and meeting the strategic objectives and financial objectives of SEHS.

Phyllis turned to consultants to provide these services, and 3 years later her goals are close to attainment. She successfully realigned the staff at SEHS, assimilated redundant services, and installed new information systems. SEHS is now winning contracts with major employers in the community. "I couldn't have done it without the help of good consultants," Phyllis said.

In a case study format, this chapter will describe the role and the selection process for health care consultants. Health care consulting will be defined and services will be described. Finally,

the critical success factors and management elements for nursing administrators will be outlined.

■ WHAT IS CONSULTING?

A *consultant* is a person with specialized expertise. Consultants have influence over an organization, a group, or an individual and provide strategic and operational insight and advice to these *clients*. They specialize in translating findings into specific recommendations. Consulting is an advisory service contracted for and provided to organizations by specially trained and qualified persons who assist the client organization to identify problems in an objective and independent manner. They recommend solutions to these problems, and may assist in the solution implementation. Consultants may be internal or external to the organization.

Clients purchase services for four key reasons:

1. Need for an objective, informed opinion from an outsider.
2. Lack of internal expertise to achieve goals or objectives.
3. Lack of necessary time to complete projects with internal resources.
4. Risk avoidance—projects so challenging or politically sensitive that an unbiased, expert opinion is warranted.

Phyllis identified the need for highly specialized skills for organizational re-

CASE: 7-2 *Continued*

design and information systems planning and development. These skills were unrelated to SEHS's core business of providing high-quality, cost-effective health care to the community.

■ CONSULTANT ROLES

Consultants perform as *experts,* and/or *collaborators* when working with clients (Block, 1981; Cordeiro & Bartik, 1996). Decision making, communication, fee structure, and control and performance of work differ for each of these modes of consulting. In addition, the *pair of hands* or "contractor" mode may be used when the organization simply does not have the people to get a job done.

Expert advice is sought by organizations with little or no experience in an area in which services are needed. Experts provide an unbiased, objective, second opinion. The collaborator mode is used when the organization would like to involve an outside expert in the decision-making process to assist internal personnel. The pair-of-hands mode is used for staffing projects in place of hiring new people for the job. Organizations may use one or all of these consultant modes to solve problems.

Consultant billing varies by the mode of service. Hourly fees are generally negotiated when the task and performance criteria are not well defined (expert and pair of hands), whereas a fixed fee is established for a well-defined product and period of performance. Consulting expenses (travel, meals, lodging, communication) are normally charged in addition to hourly or fixed fees.

Phyllis used the expert and collaborative modes for the SEHS project. She needed a shared decision-making process and joint control; she developed a partnership with the selected consultants. While she worked closely with the consultants on the merger and redesign, Phyllis needed expert advice for the information technology planning. Phyllis found this cooperative and expert style the best way for SEHS to engage consultants.

■ CHARACTERISTICS OF CONSULTING SERVICES

Consulting engagements are contracts between clients and consultants. Engagements or projects vary in size and duration. A small contract to develop an acquisition strategy for a respiratory therapy information system may employ one person for 6 weeks; a strategic information systems plan with implementation may engage six consultants for 2 years. A consulting engagement is characterized by:

- Provision of a skill or expertise that is not currently available within the organization.
- Unbiased evaluation and problem solving.
- Structured and formal business relationship.
- Well-defined scope of work.
- Services provided under a contract.
- Clearly defined schedule with performance objectives.
- Specific deliverables.

CASE: 7–2 *Continued*

The outputs of consulting services include new information, knowledge, skills, and changes in client organization, policy, procedure, or practice. Consultants provide products or perform services for clients under contract. *Services* are skills and experience applied to specific needs often related to solution implementation. *Products* are the results of consulting engagements and are the *deliverables;* i.e., reports, white papers, workshops, conferences, meetings, and training sessions.

Deliverables and Work Papers

Deliverables can be tactical recommendations or total business solutions. They are contracted in advance in partnership with the client and delivered according to a specific schedule. The first deliverable is often the *project work plan*. This plan provides the framework for the schedule and resource allocation. The work plan lays out the tasks and specific activities with start dates, duration, and the number and names of the people required. Typically, the second deliverable documents the results of the assessment of the problem with an analysis of findings. *Milestones* are significant events in the work plan, such as the date of completion of training. Consultants maintain *work papers* over the life of the contract. This is a complete record of all client interactions, plans, and deliverables.

■ TYPES OF CONSULTANTS

Phyllis had several decisions to make in the consultant selection. Could she use internal staff to do the job? Did she need an independent contractor who worked alone, or the services of a consulting firm?

The decision to use internal staff or external consultants is a critical issue for most organizations. The project costs, impact on staff morale, urgency, available skills and experience, and need for an unbiased, objective opinion require careful evaluation. Phyllis needed insight and impartial recommendations from consultants because she did not have the expertise within SEHS, and many politically sensitive merger issues had to be resolved. The decision needed objectivity, which could not be provided from within the organization. "With the rapid changes in the health care environment, it was difficult, costly, and inefficient to train and maintain in-house staff for strategic planning and change management. Hiring a consultant was the most cost-effective way to get the job done. "I did not want to increase permanent staff for this project," she said.

Consultants may operate independently or work for consulting firms. Consulting firms range in size from small (2 to 20) to large (100 plus) consultants and administrative staff. Consulting firms perform services for government-related health care organizations (federal, state, local), or private (for-profit or not-for-profit organizations). Consultants usually have a specific area of expertise, such as clinical information systems implementation or strategic planning, and they generally focus their products and services for a particular market (rural health care organizations, physician practices, military health care). Phyllis needed several

CASE: 7–2 *Continued*

related services and ruled out hiring an independent contractor.

Categories of Consultants

There are generally three types of consulting services:

1. Operations/Design.
2. Management.
3. Information technology.

Operations and design consulting services for health care include department or product line assessment, planning, development or redesign, and implementation. Design may span business process improvement of functional service areas (pharmacy, for example) or architectural and functional analysis and planning for services or product lines.

Management consulting covers a broad range of strategic and tactical planning services for the administration of health care. This may include organizational reengineering and merger and acquisition services. Information technology consulting involves assessing, planning, and deploying computer technology to meet current and future client needs.

■ PHASES OF THE CONSULTING PROCESS

From the consultant's point of view, there are generally three steps in the consulting process:

1. Understanding the client needs through interaction with the client; knowledge of the industry, client, and organization; researching the issue; and interviewing the client.

2. Developing effective solutions through creative problem analysis, solution design, pretesting, pricing, and presentation.
3. Implementing the solutions, and managing (scoping and controlling) and evaluating the engagement.

■ EFFECTIVE CONSULTANTS

Consultants must gain an understanding of the client's needs, organizational culture, and constraints. This will enable them to build rapport with the client and the organization, and to be effective in providing successful solutions. By questioning, listening, and articulating ideas effectively, consultants seek to gain a full understanding of the problems and develop effective solutions. They establish client confidence and buy-in working across organizational levels and by soliciting input from managers and employees who will be the target of resultant changes.

Consultants stay current in their field through industry publications, professional associations, peers, original research, and by working with clients. They need to have excellent technical, communication, interpersonal, and writing skills. They bring value to clients through their knowledge, analytical abilities, and specific expertise.

What Are the Critical Success Factors for Client Satisfaction?

From the consultant and client point of view, client satisfaction is the ultimate outcome of a consulting engagement.

CASE: 7–2 *Continued*

There are two essential elements for client satisfaction:

1. *Understanding client expectations.* The consultant must know the elements of the services that are most important to the client and what is needed to meet or exceed client expectations. This knowledge comes from clearly defined problems, understanding of the objectives, and negotiated completion criteria, fee schedule, personnel commitment, deliverables, and milestones. Consequently, setting and managing client expectations is critical. This is done through work plan validation, regular meetings, design reviews, briefings, and good written communication (meeting minutes, memorandums of understanding, standard operating procedures, etc.). Promises made to clients create a legal responsibility and should be considered carefully. Initial clarification of roles and responsibilities and the scope of the project are essential. The consultant for SEHS clearly defined the problem, identified objectives, set expectations, and outlined constraints. SEHS and the consultant negotiated completion criteria, fee schedule, milestones, and onsite work.
2. *Consultant reliability.* The consultant must deliver products and services on time and within budget. This includes not only work specified in the contract, and

contract modifications, but often other services as needed. In addition, when a consultant claims expertise in an area and presents information or recommendations as facts on which the client relies, consultants can be held liable for the representation. Credibility, integrity, and trust are critical elements of all business/consulting relationships.

■ SELECTING A CONSULTANT

Although the use of a consultant was the most cost-effective solution, Phyllis found that locating the right consultant and preparing and negotiating a well-defined contract were not trivial tasks. Consultants had to have the right technical expertise and experience to meet SEHS's needs. The consultants had to be internally justified, and their communication style had to match SEHS's organizational culture. In addition, the consultant cost had to be within the SEHS budget.

Consultant selection is a function of the type of work needed to be performed, and the size of the engagement. Here are six steps SEHS took to find the consultant for their project.

1. Write Requirements

Detailed project requirements were written as clearly as possible to outline needs, outcomes (deliverables), level of effort, period of performance, and technical requirements. SEHS wanted the selection to be a competitive process. A selection committee was formed and a

CASE: 7-2 *Continued*

request for information (RFI) was sent to selected consultants for initial capabilities exploration. Initial screening criteria included corporate qualifications such as financial stability, number of years in business, capabilities, and references for comparable work.

After peer, legal, and financial reviews, a formal request for proposal (RFP) was drafted and weighted selection criteria were designed. To ensure consultant credibility, responses to the RFP (proposals from the consulting firm selected) were included in the contract. "Through the RFP process, we were able to select the top candidates," Phyllis said. Follow-up work would be sought through a negotiated statement of work, assuming that the initial work was satisfactory.

2. Develop a List of Candidates

Where do you get a list of potential bidders? SEHS had used a consultant when acquiring physician practices and expanding ambulatory services. This referral, based on reputation, was a natural place to start. In addition, Phyllis contacted the American Organization of Nurse Executives, the American Association of Health Care Consultants, and the World Wide Web for a current list of health care consultants. Other consultants sources include: successful conference speakers, university teachers, book and journal authors, and advertisements.

3. Determine Evaluation Criteria

SEHS established four areas for consultant selection:

1. *Experience in the areas of need.* Phyllis needed change management experts with a track record of successfully integrating disparate health care organizations, and an in-depth knowledge of health care information technology and information system development strategy. She needed consultants who were successful in similar organizations. She focused on finding a firm with a reputation for quality products and services. She considered dividing the project among contractors if she could not find one firm with all the expertise. The initial capabilities statement from the candidate firms helped with the initial screening.

2. *Knowledge of the industry.* SEHS looked for consultant firms with core competencies in health care. "The firm that we selected understood the dynamics and economics of health care delivery and had a reputation for intellectual horsepower. They were critical, but independent thinkers with high regard in the health care industry. The firm had the integrity and industry knowledge to disagree with us," said Phyllis.

3. *Size of the firm.* The size and scope of the project directed the selection of a firm with sufficient depth and experience in business process change, mergers, and information systems. However, this need had to match the SEHS budget, so a smaller, local firm with

CASE: 7–2 *Continued*

the right skill set was considered. Consequently, the selection must go beyond size, requirements, and resumes. Can the firm do the job?

4. *Organizational culture match.* There must be a good rapport between staff and the consulting firm for the ongoing partnership to be nurtured. The chemistry between consultant, client, and organization must be a close cultural fit. Can they communicate well? Will the staff and managers be comfortable working closely with the consultants?

4. Send Out the Request for Proposals

Ten candidate firms were selected, and the RFP was mailed. Responses were requested within 6 weeks, and a bidders conference was scheduled. At the bidders conference, the selection committee described the work and answered questions from the candidates. During this time, consulting firms clarified expectations and obtained missing information. Consultant firms looked for new information that would have an impact on the project, such as changes in administration or other reorganizations.

Proposals are the written response to the client, outlining the consultant services necessary to complete the engagement. Proposals include the *technical solution* and a *cost proposal*. Proposals normally begin with a statement of the understanding of the needs of the client, the current situation, and the type of assistance needed. The technical solution must satisfy all organizational requirements. The second part of the proposal addresses the approach to the problem and answers the questions concerning the benefits of hiring the firm. A great deal of time is spent on the problem-solving methods to be used. A high-level work plan and management plan are included to describe the major tasks and responsibilities. A schedule and list of deliverables states the period of time and outputs the client can expect. Examples of similar engagements, similar problems solved, and the outcomes are included. Finally, the proposal identifies applicable firm experience.

The cost proposal outlines of the level of effort (hours) by job category (analyst, senior analyst) and other expenses, such as travel and communication or proposed subcontractors. For government proposals, the cost proposal must be very detailed.

5. Conduct Oral Evaluations for Best and Final Proposals

Based on the responses and evaluation criteria, three firms were selected for oral evaluation. In a 1-hour briefing, the firms described their understanding of the problem and the methodology for the solution. The SEHS selection committee then discussed and rated each firm using the selection criteria established for this acquisition.

6. Select Winner, Sign Contract, and Kick Off the Engagement

Within 3 months, SEHS had selected the partner they needed for the work and

CASE: 7–2 *Continued*

signed an agreement. The selected firm had excellent experience and references for business process improvements, including mergers and reengineering services. They proposed teaming with a subcontractor for the information systems work. As a result, Phyllis had one point of contact for the entire project. SEHS selected a consultant firm who understood the problems and the culture of the organization and had articulated an excellent methodology and tight plan. The consultants had exceptional educational and experiential credibility. Their communication style was professional, yet comfortable. Finally, the change management strategy was acceptable to SEHS personnel. A *kick-off* meeting officially began the engagement. The work was divided into several phases, and the complete contract spanned 18 months.

■ MANAGING THE CONSULTING CONTRACT

Phyllis had the responsibility for managing the contract with the SEHS consultants. However, she appointed a senior SEHS liaison to work on a day-to-day basis with the consultant project manager. The SEHS liaison arranged for administrative support and identified the points of contact. Weekly meetings were held and monthly formal in-process reviews were scheduled. These reviews focused on the planned verses actual budget, and work progress. At the reviews, potential risks to the project (delayed deliverables, unplanned scope changes) were discussed and risk mitigation strategies were identified.

■ CONCLUSION

This actual case, with the names and identification of the agency changed, illustrates and informs the reader about consultation. Phyllis Forrestor and the selection team led SEHS through problem identification, consultant service acquisition, and project administration. The project was highly successful because Phyllis had a clear understanding of her needs, focused on a structured consultant selection process, used a collaborative management approach and integrated quality management throughout the life of the project. Communication was open and project objectives were clear.

The project was not without challenges; risks were identified early and plans for joint resolution were developed. For instance, the information technology subcontractor firm merged with a larger firm during the engagement. This delayed part of the technology planning phase, but the project was subsequently completed on time and on budget. Another challenge was an unplanned visit by state health regulators. This removed Phyllis from the project for 1 week, slowing critical decision making and communication. A modification to the contract was made, and the project schedule was adjusted.

Engaging and managing competent consultants takes extensive planning and intensive communication. Nurse administrators must know when consultants are needed, how to hire and manage them, and when to terminate them. The model for engaging consultants that

CASE: 7–2 *Continued*

Phyllis Forrestor used was practical, flexible, acceptable, and most important, successful. The consultant firm assisted SEHS to become the provider of choice in the community while SEHS remained financially solvent.

■ BIOGRAPHICAL SKETCH

Barbara A. Happ is a Consulting Health Care Principal at Birch & Davis, Associates, Inc., Falls Church, Virginia. As part of the Federal Information Services Division, she provides leadership for client services to the Department of Defense. Projects include studies and analysis for the Computer-based Patient Record, the Clinical Integrated Workstation, and Clinical Information System. Dr. Happ's professional career has focused on commercial and government clinical systems consulting, research, teaching, health care administration, marketing, and technical writing. She resides in Reston, Virginia, with her family and can be found most weekends on the back of a tandem bicycle. Her email address is bhapp@birchdavis.com.

■ REFERENCES

Block, P. (1981). *Flawless Consulting.* San Diego: Pfeiffer & Company.

Cordeiro, W.P., & Bartik, S.A. (1996). How to consult to government. *Journal of Management Consulting,* 7 (4), 20–24.

■ ADDITIONAL READING

McCune, J.C. (1996). Bringing consultants onboard. *Beyond Computing,* March, 38–41.

Sherriton, J.C., & Stern, J.L. (1997). *Corporate culture, team culture.* New York: American Management Association.

■ RESOURCES

American Organization of Nurse Executives (AONE)
One North Franklin Street, 34th floor, Chicago, IL 60606
Tel: (312) 422-2800
American Association of Health Care Consultants
11208 Waples Mill Road, Suite 109, Fairfax, VA 22030
Tel: (703) 691-2242

THREE

Structuring Health Care Organizations

8

Assessing Organizations

Jacqueline A. Dienemann

Sensemaking itself is ongoing and the sense it makes, transient.

—Karl E. Weick, 1995

Organizations differ in their purpose, environments, internal structures, participants, and cultures. Patient care administrators are reeling under the pace of change. Like flood waters rising, new payment mechanisms, government regulations, business alliances, and emphases on cost containment are changing the world of patient care. Yet, patient care is still being delivered within an organizational context and nurses in administration continue to need tools and savvy to make sense of the context in which care is delivered. Viewing organizations from several theoretical perspectives can provide valuable insights into problems and their underlying issues. Many organizational problems arise from changes in the balance between ongoing tensions such as stability and change. Theories afford a moment of reflection to see a problem in a new light, providing insights beyond the present dilemma.

Administrators and consultants using organizational theory commonly use open systems models to guide organizational assessment, diagnosis, and planned change. Open systems models provide a comprehensive, holistic perspective of an organization. The applications vary widely; some identify types of organizational structures, others identify critical elements and processes within various structural types, and still others identify relationships among elements using diagrams of interactive processes (Burke, 1987). This chapter describes the concepts of general systems theory underlying all open systems models, presents the congruence model as a basic prototype of open systems theory, and then identifies three other theoretical perspectives: organizational life cycle stages, organizational environments, and organizational participants. Other chapters offer tools to gain alternative insights on specific aspects of organizational life, such as strategy or culture. Keep in mind that each theory is a simplification of the complexity inherent in organizations, and that by highlighting one aspect, it fails to examine others. Thus, no theory is sufficient alone to provide a full comprehension of organizational life.

■ OPEN SYSTEMS MODELS

Open systems models derive from the concepts of general systems theory, and thus share a holistic view of internal processes and basic analytical elements. However, labels for elements may vary due to independent development of general systems models in different disciplines. Moreover, each model offers a different emphasis.

The major concepts of general systems theory applied to organizations are summarized in Figure 8–1. The basic elements include: *inputs* from the environment that cross organizational boundaries; a *transformation process*

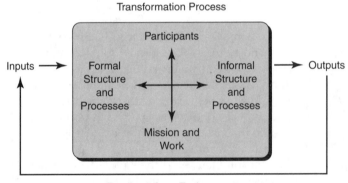

- *Open systems.* Permeable boundaries exist between the system and its environment.
- *Holism/synergism/organicism/Gestalt.* The *whole* is greater than the sum of its parts and is the focus of study.
- The four major analytical components of the transformation process are: *participants, formal sociotechnical structure and processes, mission and technology or work, and informal structure and processes.*
- Components/subunits/subsystems are interconnected and *interdependent.*
- *Input—transformation/throughout—output* process is goal oriented.
- *Feedback,* inputs, and feedforward provide information for self-regulation/dynamic equilibrium/cybernetic system.
- Systems are *resource dependent* on their environment.
- *Change/adaptation/homeostasis/steady state* processes are dynamic and ongoing.
- *Equifinality* of varying strategies to reach the same goals.
- Over time, systems *division of labor/internal elaboration* is reorganized and increasingly complex.

FIGURE 8–1. Major concepts in general systems theory.

that changes the inputs and transfers them to the environment as *outputs;* and *feedback,* which is information on outputs the organization receives through multiple channels. Desired inputs, transformation processes, and outputs (often called outcomes) are defined by the organizational mission, philosophy, and vision and are often stated as goals.

General systems theory has been described as cybernetic because of the way in which interpretation of feedback may lead to internal adjustments in recruiting types of inputs or the transformational processes to achieve more desirable outputs. General systems theory emphasizes the importance of the *structure of work and people,* and the formal and informal *interaction processes among work and people* as the critical analytical elements for understanding organizational life. Early writers in general systems theory had a "closed" perspective, emphasizing how internal processes resisted change and promoted internal stability. Recent general systems theorists have an "open" perspective, emphasizing the dependence of the system on the environment and the importance of rapid adaptation for survival (Scott & Christensen, 1995).

The concepts of general systems theory that apply to all open systems models are listed at the bottom of Figure 8–1. They include holistic view, interdependence of internal elements, constancy of change, multiple ways to accomplish the same output or equifinality, and periodic restructuring and increasing complexity as systems grow.

Open systems models use the metaphor of the living organism to depict a simplification of reality that captures the dynamic nature of organizations. Like all theories, they enable a person to critically analyze what would otherwise be too complex to comprehend. The organic metaphor allows us to understand our world by extending to new situations what we already know (Morgan, 1997). Open systems models can be used to direct administrators to look at how problems exist from the perspective of the entire organization, to recognize interconnectiveness of internal components, to value feedback and equifinality, to devise strategies to proactively shape their environment, to seek multiple channels of information, and to plan system change. Open systems models do not highlight the role the organization plays in creating its environment, the impact of culture on work patterns and outcomes, the interplay of power relationships, or tools for strategy formation.

Open systems models were developed within the human relations school of management theory, which began in the late 1920s with the Western Electric studies. These studies were the first to identify the presence of work group norms and the importance of worker motivation in determining productivity levels. Management research within this perspective focuses on motivation, values, traits, and other psychological and social characteristics of workers and managers. Consultants using this perspective promote humanistic, participative management. Open systems models became well established in the late 1960s and 1970s as academic behavioral scientists began to work more and more with management in large firms to develop and implement interventions based on research findings with the goal of increasing job satisfaction and productivity among workers. The applied field of organizational assessment, diagnosis, intervention, and evaluation uses open systems models as its theoretical base. Interventions continue to focus primarily on job design, team building, participative management, communication, cultural diversity, leadership, system redesign, and design of reward and compensations systems. The joint involvement of scientists and managers in the entire process is emphasized.

■ CONGRUENCE MODEL

Nadler and Tushman (Nadler, Gerstein, & Shaw, 1992) refer to their open systems model as a congruence model because it focuses on the fit between an organization and its environment at the levels of system functioning, work group behavior, and individual behavior (see Fig. 8–2). They also suggest using more specific middle range theories to examine the fit between pairs of transformation components. For instance, designing jobs that tightly fit work tasks with motivational needs of workers using the core job dimensions analysis of Hackman and Oldham (1975).

The four key inputs to the congruence model are (1) *environment,* (2) *resources,* (3) *history,* and (4) *strategy.*

The *environment* includes all stakeholders with an interest in this organization and the multitude of ways they relate to and influence the organization. *Resources* include the tangible resources such as the pool of potential organizational participants available, financial credit, organizational alliances and affiliations, physical plant, machinery and other capital assets, and consumable supplies. They also include the intangible resources such as govern-

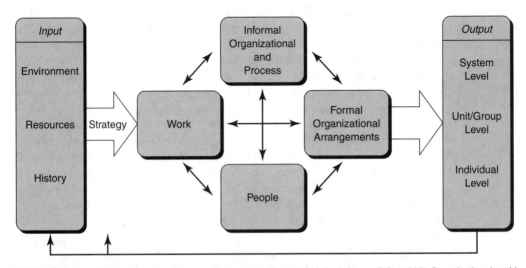

FIGURE 8–2. Organizational model. *(Source: Nadler, D.A., Gerstein, M.C., & Shaw, R.B. (1992). Organizational architecture: Designs for changing organization. San Francisco: Jossey-Bass, p. 54.)*

ment regulations, accreditation standards, standards of practice, credit rating, image, reputation, market composition and size, characteristics of competitors, public accountability, public expectations, locale, satisfaction of employees, and quality of client relations.

History describes the contextual fabric, which is a major contributor to organizational philosophy and culture. It includes age, patterns of key past decisions, patterns of leadership style, size, complexity, and sacred cows. Each factor is a unique characteristic of this organization. For example, sacred cows are those aspects of the organization that are taboo subjects for discussion with outsiders or in formal meetings, and that limit consideration of options for action. Sacred cows may refer to people who are heroes or "lepers." They may also refer to historical acts or situations that have become glorified or vilified over time. They are transmitted as "musts" or "nevers" in this organization. A newcomer often encounters sacred cows as illogical informal rules or incongruent actions of others that "old timers" may know the history of but most co-workers merely accept as an idiosyncrasy of that organization.

Strategy includes identification of the core mission, marketing plans, objectives for performance, and supporting systems for performance. Organizations vary widely in the degree to which strategy is a formal process, but a historical pattern may be discerned through retrospective analysis.

These four inputs shape the interactions of the four major components within the organizational boundaries: *tasks, individuals, formal organizational arrangements,* and *informal organization*. The outcomes of the transformational process are *outputs* and *feedback.*

Keep in mind that information being fed back as an input does not infer that reception will result in adaptive action. Due to distortion, time lapse, filtering, and mistargeting, much feedback is received but never used in decision making.

■ ORGANIZATIONAL LIFE CYCLE STAGES

An organization's life cycle stage shapes the managerial challenges facing administrators and affects the selection and application of an open systems model for analysis and planned change. Structures, policies, and practices need to reflect not only characteristics of the work being performed and the workers, but also the life cycle stage of the organization. Organizations spend most of their history in forms that are stable and enduring, but these forms change as an organization undergoes brief periods of reconfiguration. One compelling reason for reconfiguration is life cycle change. Others include: environmental changes, technology changes, organizational growth, changes in political climate, and leadership changes (Bolman & Deal, 1991). Life cycle models capture and describe patterns of change that are common, but not imperative. Mintzberg (1989) describes four stages in an organizational life cycle: formation, development, maturity, and decline.

Formation

Organizations usually begin their life cycle as small entrepreneurial ventures with a simple structure. The founding leader has great informal power and independence to "do his or her own thing" and often a driving vision of the venture. All employees and the owner interact face to face more or less as equals performing the daily work. Financial rewards are low, but intangible rewards of participation in creating a new enterprise are high. Some organizations also offer the potential for high financial rewards through stock or profit sharing. This informal structure tends to remain in place as long as the original leader remains in office, even in the face of pressures for division and specialization of work or more technocratic control. Increasing size often demands greater formalization and division of management from work, which the founding leader often resists. If the organization survives its own success and changeover in leadership, it will move to the next developmental stage and reconfigure itself into one of several forms. This movement will act as a source of renewal and energy.

Development

Organizations in this life cycle stage create a hierarchy and formal control systems. The reward system becomes formalized, job descriptions are developed, standards or organizational expectations are written, and departments for finance, human resources, and facilities management are created. The organization increases in complexity, sophistication, and division of labor.

Mintzberg (1989) points out that internal politics, work technology of the organization, and current environmental contingencies will influence the choice of configuration chosen. In the development life cycle stage, the organization reconfigures into one of four forms: the missionary, the machine, the innovative, or the professional. A small organization after the departure of a charismatic founding leader will have a tendency to assume the missionary form. It typically remains in a simple configuration and attempts to institutionalize his or her charisma. For instance, a nursing center founded by a charismatic leader with a strong network in one community will attempt to "continue in her spirit" after this leader leaves. This is a very precarious time, as the organization is held together by the shared values and beliefs of its members. It must institute indoctrination processes to pass on its ideology and internalized norms to others in order to survive over time. These norms are also what provides direction for growth and mediates conflicts among workers.

Long-term care facilities, larger ambulatory care centers, and small hospitals with 50 to 500 employees often become organized into a machine form due to the routine, repetitive, highly regulated nature of their work. They are typically internally organized as simple functional structures with centralized departments. As they grow beyond any one person knowing all about the operations, more departmental autonomy is delegated. As long-term care facilities are expanding to include subacute care, skilled nursing care, home care, assisted living, and continuing care, they often reconfigure to the professional form. In the current health care environment, fewer and fewer of these facilities are remaining independent; there is a definite trend toward being bought or merging with horizontally integrated chains or vertically integrated health care systems that allow for varying levels of local autonomy. The exceptions are small facilities with a specific market niche and direct payment, such as care management companies.

Organizations dependent on expertise will reconfigure into either the innovative or professional form. The innovative form is loosely coupled and supports creative work by project teams. Some home care agencies reflect this form with rapid growth of new project teams for pediatric care, oncology infusion services, adult hospice, pediatric hospice, and elder care. Each team is relatively autonomous and dependent on the expertise of its members. The employees are enthusiastic and entrepreneurial as they attempt to develop a corporate identity and survive in a competitive market. The central agency provides human resources and payroll support, access to documentation forms and billing, a logo, and office space. Leaders come together as directors of each project team. Over time these organizations usually evolve into the machine or professional form as they become more established.

The professional form provides bureaucratic supports for its mission of professional service delivery. The professional work maintains a hallmark of autonomy standardized through professional education, codes of ethics, mutual peer review, and standards of practice. Bureaucratic work emphasizes rationality through (1) a fixed division of labor, (2) a hierarchy of offices, (3) a set of rules governing performance, (4) separation of personal and organizational property, (5) technical qualifications for selecting personnel, and (6) employment as a long-term career (Weber, 1947). Historically hospitals have been prime examples of this hybrid structure. Currently, in health care, the configuration is evolving to expand technocratic control over professionals through the development of clinical pathways, performance improvement systems, standards of practice, and other mechanisms that reduce individual autonomy and expand multidisciplinary coordination and accountability for outcomes. This is shifting power from individual professionals to the administrative bureaucracy. The other trend is for hospitals to become members of integrated health systems and, thus, less autonomous.

Maturity

This life cycle stage is where the "iron law of oligarchy," as described by Michels (1958), moves an organization toward administration becoming the center of power. The organization becomes more of a closed system machine as it grows beyond 500 employees and gains a financial base that is less dependent on fluctuations in the external market and individual customers. Those at the top become more removed from the day-to-day reality of the service provided; they become focused on retaining their earnings and using them to enhance their size and influence. In this lies both the organization's power and seeds of later decline and destruction (Mintzberg, 1989). As organizations grow and become more complex, many political confrontations occur between the administrators, expert professionals, and external constituencies. These confrontations often result in shaky alliances between administration and other stakeholders in which neither side concedes, but all parties agree to tolerate the other's behavior.

As the organization grows beyond 500 employees it diversifies its products, services, and/or sites. Administrative control becomes more distant from service delivery. At this point, new managerial practices are needed. Local administrators assert that they lack the authority commensurate with their responsibilities. They are more aware of changing needs of their local market and need autonomy to respond rapidly to opportunities and constraints that often change as they await information and decisions from top management to filter down to them. Often the health care organization responds to this crisis and becomes revitalized by delineating levels of management and divisions by patient population. There is an elaboration of staff support roles and increasing decentralization of authority and responsibility. Control is more and more by system reporting of technical quality indicators, such as falls and nosocomial infections; financial indicators; and administrative indicators, such as turnover. First-line operational managers move away from direct service delivery and must now be trained to assume new functions, such as budgeting and then monitoring and explaining variances; tracking clinical pathway variances; marketing their services; and monitoring quality and administrative indicators.

The next stage of growth in size is external growth through merger or acquisition of other organizations or internal growth through horizontal or vertical integration. The other alternative is being bought and becoming part of an existing larger holding company or multidivisional organization. Certain regions of the country are presently in a period of rapid consolidation of health care financing and delivery. Regional integrated systems and national chains are forming with mergers and buyouts, collapsing the number of competitors in a local market. The reward system for managers in regional and national organizations changes to focus on financial performance of their subunit, using measures such as return on investment (ROI) and contributions to organizational profit.

As these corporations continue to grow, decisions to expand, terminate, or initiate sites and services are made impersonally using financial data and business plans with less emphasis on local concerns. Again, the complexity of the organization outgrows existing practices to direct multiple diverse operations, maintain control over entry and exit of services and sites, and allocate scarce resources such as capital funds between units. Lack of control leads to a major crisis, producing a metamorphosis into a multiple division structure to allow revitalization through simultaneous autonomy and control. This type of organization in health care is often found in national and multinational corporations. Growth is coordinated by corporate headquarters, which is usually separate from the operating divisions. Different types of management practices are now in place at differing levels within the organization. Participants may experience an entire career within one unit or organizational level. Most are neither familiar with nor know participants from other units of the organization, nor even all the sites or services of the organization. Units vary widely in size, technology, age, complexity, and autonomy from the corporate headquarters.

As the organization grows, it eventually becomes so complex it has a crisis of red tape (Griener, 1972). The organization is suffering from being top heavy and unable to coordinate its diverse, geographically dispersed enterprises with acumen. This crisis is resolved and renewal occurs if the organization can begin to free itself of centralized responsibility at the corporate level for all major allocations and new venture decisions through collaboration of major divisions acting in parallel with, rather than subservient to, a central hierarchy. The reward system shifts its focus from individual to team rewards. This collaborative structure often exists in successful multinational corporations with diverse holdings and service lines. Some health care organizations are beginning to approach this level of complexity.

Keep in mind that all organizations do not follow this stepwise pattern of growth, crisis, and renewal. Many do not survive at each level. Also, some organizations decide to stabilize at a particular size and complexity level and maintain vitality through environmental scanning and adaptation to their changing markets. Successful health care organizations today seem to be dividing into small, market niche, specialized organizations or complex regional or national corporations.

Decline

The absence of external control in large organizations tends to have a corrupting influence. As mature organizations become more and more self-sufficient, they become more like closed systems. The visible social responsibility of closed system executives acts as a smokescreen to ensure external influencers cannot penetrate their power base. As power produces corruption, then corruption produces conflict. Without the constraint of being responsive to their customers, these insiders are drawn into conflicts with one another. The professionals and administrators develop both arrogance and a desire for more and more power. This conflict becomes increasingly evident to customers and other outsiders who begin to challenge the insiders and the legitimacy of their power. With this long-term moderate conflict, the organization becomes politicized (Mintzberg, 1989).

Of course, this need not happen quickly or inevitably. Market competition, professional standards, ideology, or renewal can prevent decline into politicized configurations. Renewal and revitalization occur with resolution of each crisis described above.

Organizations that have become closed to their environment can be renewed through turnarounds. One means is economic turnaround through downsizing and restructuring in a way that is more responsive to environmental pressures. Another is strategic turnaround by changing direction through a coup d'etat with new leadership or through infusion of imperatives from the environment for survival and change because the organization is so large, and important to the nation's economy (e.g., the Chrysler turnaround by Lee Iacocca). Turnaround of extremely large organizations is very difficult as they are machines that are designed for stability, not dramatic change.

ORGANIZATIONAL ENVIRONMENTS

As we have seen, open systems models emphasize the separateness of the organization from its environment and the importance of influences from the environment for organizational growth, development, and vitality. The greatest danger of growth is insulation from environmental influences, leading to becoming closed systems that eventually decline and die. Another perspective on organizations and their environments is provided by theories of flux and transformation. Here, the environment and organization are perceived as never separate, and each is continuously participating in defining the other. In this model, the universe is a flowing and unbroken wholeness (Morgan, 1997): change is fundamental; and organizations are like a whirlpool having relatively constant form, with no existence other than the movement of the river. Four different bodies of literature offer four different insights into change using a wholeness approach. They are autopoiesis, chaos theory, cybernetic theory, and dialectical change.

Autopoesis

The term *autopoesis* was coined by two Chilean scientists, Humberto Maturana and Francisco Varela (1980). They observed that all living systems are actually closed systems that include their immediate environment. As we trace the nature of a system, it is necessary to trace the circular pattern of interaction through which it is defined. In doing so, the boundaries become less well defined.

Open systems theorists use the term *hierarchy of systems* to describe the nested relationships from individuals to their workgroup to their department to their organization. Maturana and Varela (1980) point out that this is a set of self-referring, autonomous, closed systems. Understanding the autopoetic nature of the total system requires acknowledgment that each element simultaneously combines the maintenance of itself with the maintenance of the others. Change does not come from the external environment, such as the department to the workgroup, but is coproduced through circular interactions. One cannot exist without the other. This theory does not question whether external environments exist; it questions causation of change. This view encourages organizations to view themselves and their environments much like a figure and the ground within the same picture. Survival can only be with, never against, the environment or context in which one is operating.

Chaos Theory

Chaos theory also focuses on the unity of change. If a system has a sufficient degree of internal complexity, randomness and diversity and instability become resources for change (Wheatley, 1992). This theory illustrates how an organization can experience catalyzing effects that ultimately shift a system from one configuration to another. Once an organization has moved away from one organizing "attractor," it may encounter another "attractor" and self-organize into a new form. The emphasis is on emergent properties rather than cause and effect, because each situation is so complex that linear relationships are impossible to predict change. Order always will emerge, but cannot be imposed. Those assessing organizations should look for patterns of change and emergent patterns indicating shifts to new configurations, rather than strategic plans. Excellence in management is demonstrated not by ability to control, but by (1) ability to assess what is locking the organization into an existing pattern, (2) ability to create instability when indicated, and (3) ability to manage through the edge of chaos and facilitate emergent self-organization.

Cybernetics

Cyberneticists encourage thinking of organizational causality as mutual loops rather than linear cause and effect. This theoretical perspective encourages analysts to look for patterns of organizational relationships rather than factors causing change. Processes of negative feedback, in which a change in one variable initiates counteracting forces leading to changes in the opposite direction, is useful in explaining organizational stability. Processes of positive feedback create conditions in which more leads to more and less leads to less, thereby offering explanation of escalating patterns of system change (Maruyama, 1982). Loops give a richer picture of processes than sequential linear charting. To avoid being overwhelmed by the implications, Senge (1990) recommends identifying archtypes of responses by a particular system. Does this organization tend to delay feedback, have positive escalating feedback loops, ignore feedback, or demonstrate another repeated behavior related to feedback? Those assessing organizations can map nests of loops that hang together, and identify key connections of loops and key patterns of loops. They may also recommend where to add or delete loops (Morgan, 1997).

Dialectical Change

The tension between opposites often leads to change. Whenever a situation develops extreme tendencies, it invariably turns around and assumes opposite qualities. This view that everything is in the process of becoming something else has been purported by Taoist philosophy for thousands of years.

The person assessing an organization using this approach (1) searches for the underlying contradictory tensions shaping the organization, (2) recognizes that all changes retain some of the old, and (3) recognizes that changes in quantity eventually lead to changes in quality (Morgan, 1997). Whenever planning a change in one direction, be aware of the latent arousal of the opposite. For instance, externally imposed change leads to resistance. It is by being aware of and capturing the power of the paradox that a manager becomes more effective. Continuous improvement may lead to a runaway system demanding ever higher productivity, thereby lowering morale and productivity. This can be checked by monitoring the costs and benefits of smaller increments of change as a work process improves. In other words, every solution leads to a new problem and the best solutions integrate some aspects of both opposites. There are no easy answers. Some of the paradoxes Morgan (1997) alerts the reader to are: (1) innovation—avoidance of mistakes; (2) thinking long term—delivering results now; (3) cutting costs—increasing morale; (4) reducing staff—improving teamwork; (5) being flexible—respecting the rules; (6) collaborating—competing; (7) decentralizing—retaining control; (8) specializing—being opportunistic; and (9) low costs—high quality.

■ ORGANIZATIONAL PARTICIPANTS

Open systems theory points out the importance of both individuals and the ways they interact within the formal and informal organizational structure and processes as vital to understanding organizational functioning. Keidel (1995) posits that it is the balance of three key types of human relationships in an organization that determine its "health." The types of relationships are autonomy (promotes separation), control (promotes subordination), and cooperation (promotes integration). Figure 8–3 provides a graphic representation of these relationships. These elements are useful concepts for assessing organizational strategies, structures, and systems in relationship to organizational participants.

Organizational strategies define what business an organization is in, what its identity is, and how it plans to compete with other similar businesses. Using autonomy, control, and cooperation to assess the impact of strategies on participants, the first question is, who is the point of reference? The three primary categories of participants are customers, shareholders, and employees. If an organization is customer oriented, it emphasizes autonomy, rewards individual players, and uses a strategy of differentiation of specific, novel, and/or stylish products for specific customers. An organization that is shareholder oriented utilizes control to reward compliance and uniformity and a strategy of low purchase price, low operating cost, and low transaction costs for competition. Finally, the employee-oriented organization highlights cooperation by rewarding teamwork and collaboration and using a strategy of flexibility to be responsive to customer initiatives, quick in development, and malleable to change. Obviously few organizations exist in these three pure

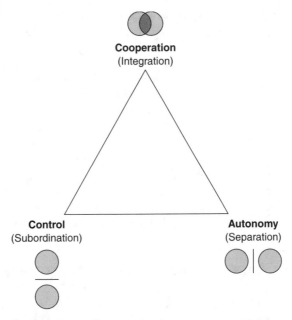

FIGURE 8–3. Types of human relationship. *(Source: Keidel, R.W. (1995). Seeing organizational patterns. San Francisco: Berrett-Koehler; Exhibit 1–1, p. 6.)*

forms, but they do illustrate a way to analyze organizational characteristics that result in a specific purpose, vision, mission, and culture.

In assessing organizational structure, one should focus on the relationships formed by structural arrangements. Is autonomy, control, or cooperation reinforced by work processes? What type of interdependence shapes work and information flow? The flat pyramidal structure shows a dominance of autonomy, which supports independent action and pooled interdependence. A steep pyramidal structure shows a dominance of control, which supports programmed interaction and sequential interdependence. An alternative measure is to calculate the ratio of managers to workers; the higher the ratio, the more control dominated the organization (Rosecrance, 1990). Finally, a flat, amorphous structure demonstrates a dominance of cooperation with spontaneous interaction and reciprocal interaction.

Again autonomy, control, and cooperation are useful concepts for assessing organizational systems. The reward system overlaps organizational character and plays a central role in influencing participants' behavior. In an organization that emphasizes autonomy, rewards are individualistic, meetings are held as forums for different ideas, and decisions tend to be decentralized to a specific issue. By contrast, in a control-oriented system, rewards are strictly by place on the organizational hierarchy, and meetings are held to build consensus, to solve tactical problems, or to mandate decisions on strategic problems. The cooperative system distributes rewards relatively equally through caps on executive salaries and collective rewards, such as profit sharing or gainsharing. Meetings are held primarily for teambuilding, sharing of feelings, and exploration. Decisions are primarily by consensus.

The strength of this perspective is to make the person studying an organization aware of trade-offs to look for. Any organization attempting to be cooperative, autonomous, and controlling simultaneously is without direction or clear priorities. Overemphasis on any one element to the detriment of the other two leads to organizational disaster. To only consider tensions between one dyad and ignore tensions with the third element is to court it rising up and biting you. Each organization must look at the *balance of all three dyads*—consistency from control and innovation from cooperation; local sensitivity from autonomy and a global perspective from control; synergy from cooperation and individual accountability from autonomy.

■ ORGANIZATIONAL DIAGNOSIS AND INTERVENTION

Newcomers to an organization seek to understand organizational norms of expectation and their own place, fit, and options for growth. Before joining an organization, people should spend time on the premises, read promotional materials, and interview others to garner information about the organization's mission, values, history, and any other information that will assist them to envision themselves in this organization. Creating profiles of different attributes of organizations and comparing them to your preferred profile can be helpful in assessing the desirability of your becoming employed there.

Managers are often faced with problems that they must resolve or make recommendations about. Organizational theories are tools to help them root out underlying issues that may not be self-evident at first. Often the problem itself will direct the manager to a specific theory for guidance. For instance, if a manager suspects an existing conflict is an artifact of organizational structure, he or she will look at theories describing implications of differing structures. Theory will direct the manager to examine whether positions are designed to include key responsibilities, to avoid gaps and overlaps, to balance overload and under use, to balance creativity and clear expectations, to allow autonomy without excluding interdependence, to provide structure without excessive control, to delegate authority appropriately, to provide goals but not mindless obedience, and to support responsiveness to customer and productivity (Bolman & Deal, 1991).

In other instances, the nurse patient care administrator may suspect an organization-wide issue to be the seat of several problems. Often referring to a book, such as those listed under suggested readings, with a description of several theoretical viewpoints will stimulate ideas and assist in identifying connections between problems. If an issue is especially knotty or complex, many administrators choose to hire a consultant instead of forming a task force, referring it to a standing committee or the management team. A consultant offers a fresh perspective that many executives find enhances communication concerning sensitive problems.

Theories can offer clues as to how problems are connected to critical elements throughout the organization and its environment. It is also useful to build scenarios that consider alternative strategies for problem resolution. Writings about organizational theory for practicing managers usually include suggested actions frequently used in resolution of common organizational problems.

In practice, the evaluation of organizational changes is complex and often problematic. It is important to target desired outcomes that are local and realistic before introducing change. Organizations are infamous for appearing to absorb attempts at change. For instance, the effect of a worthwhile change to reduce waiting time in one area may be offset by a resultant backup later in a work process, with the result of the same overall time to completion.

Cameron (1982), synthesizing research on organizational change, has identified the four most frequently used outcome criteria. They are goal achievement, ability to acquire needed resources, optimization of internal processes, and extent of satisfaction of all stakeholders involved in the organization. Managers often use a combination of these criteria.

Measurement of change is also complicated by the fact that outcome criteria may have conflicting dimensions. Goals are multiple and often conflictive; priorities of different stakeholders result in varying definitions of needed resources; and internal processes also conflict as managers attempt to satisfy different goals and/or stakeholders. Actions effective to achieve one goal such as client satisfaction block another such as lowest cost. Data comparing changes to organizational goals, benchmarks, local competitors, or ideal models will yield different results. Cameron (1982) suggests the evaluator take into account goals, constituencies, temporal frame, bias of data sources, and referent comparisons when designing an evaluation plan. Evaluation is for the support of decision making; therefore, desired outcomes should be stated in relation to specific problems to be addressed. Results need to be presented in a timely, useful, and understandable manner and need to include both intended and unintended consequences.

Health care organizations are increasingly employing consultants to support a culture shift to rapid and continuous change. No longer can work be designed primarily with efficient use of technology or the convenience of the provider in mind. Work design must include consumer and payer expectations. Health care has become a service industry in a competitive and uncertain market. Organizational development interventions have been used for over 30 years to develop and support participative management practices in traditional businesses. They are now a popular choice to assist health care employees in change transitions and reengineering. Nurse patient care administrators may find consultants a valuable adjunct to change management.

▪ BIOGRAPHICAL SKETCH

Jacqueline A. Dienemann is currently Associate Professor and Coordinator of Nursing Systems and Management at The Johns Hopkins University School of Nursing, where she has worked since 1992. She is responsible for all students and programs that focus on nursing management and business. These include: BS to MSN option, MSN, MSN/MS dual degree program in Nursing Administration and Business, and MSN to PhD option. She also teaches in the MSN/MPH joint degree program. She also holds a joint appointment as a Nursing Systems Expert at Johns Hopkins Hospital where she assists on program evaluation and management development. Previously, she was at George Mason University where she also coordinated the masters program in Nursing Administration. Her consultation, publications, and research have focused on development and evaluation of organizational power, research programs, domestic violence interventions; cultural competence, continuous quality improvement; collaboration between service and educational institutions; and nurse performance.

Dr. Dienemann is active in the Academy of Nursing and the American Nurses Association. She is currently chair of the Council on Nursing Service and Informatics of the American Nurses Association and a commissioner for the Magnet Recognition Program for the American Nurses Credentialing Center. She also belongs to Sigma Theta Tau, Maryland Organization for Nurse Executives, the Council for Graduate Education for Administration in Nursing, the Academy of Management, and the American College of Health Care Executives.

Her background includes a BS in Nursing from Mount St. Mary's College in Los Angeles; practice as a public health nurse and home health nurse; an MSN in Psychiatric Mental Health Nursing from Catholic University of America; teaching nursing at Columbia Union College; and a PhD in Sociology from Catholic University of America.

▪ SUGGESTED READINGS

Bolman, L.G., & Deal, T.E. (1991). *Reframing Organizations*. San Francisco: Jossey-Bass.

Morgan, G. (1997). *Images of Organization* (2nd ed.). Thousand Oaks, CA: Sage.

Nadler, D.A., & Tushman, M. (1997). *Competing by Design*. New York: Oxford University Press.

▪ REFERENCES

Bolman, L.G., & Deal, T.E. (1991). *Reframing organizations*. San Francisco: Jossey-Bass.

Burke, W.W. (1987). *Organizational development*. Reading, MA: Addison-Wesley.

Cameron, K. (1982). *Organizational effectiveness: A comparison of multiple models.* New York: Academic Press.

Griener, L. (1972). Evolution and revolution as organizations grow. *Harvard Business Review, 51* (4), 37–46.

Hackman, J.R., & Oldham, G.R. (1975). Development of the job diagnostic survey. *Journal of Applied Psychology, 60* (1), 159–170.

Keidel, R.W. (1995). *Seeing organizational patterns.* San Francisco: Berrett-Koehler.

Maruyama, M. (1982). Mindscapes, management, business policy and public policy. *Academy of Management Review, 7,* 612–619.

Maturana, H., & Varela, F. (1980). *Autopoesis and cognition: The realization of the living.* London: Reidl.

Michels, R. (1958). *Political parties: A sociological study of the oligarchical tendencies of modern democracy.* New York: Free Press.

Mintzberg, H. (1989). *Mintzberg on management.* San Francisco: Jossey-Bass.

Morgan, G. (1997). *Images of organization* (2nd ed.). Thousand Oaks, CA: Sage.

Nadler, D.A., Gerstein, M.S., & Shaw, R.B. (1992). *Organizational architecture.* San Francisco: Jossey-Bass.

Rosencrance, R. (1990). Too many bosses, too few workers. *New York Times,* July 15, F11.

Scott, W.R., & Christensen, S. (1995). *The institutional construction of organizations.* Thousand Oaks, CA: Sage.

Senge, P. (1990). *The fifth discipline.* New York: Doubleday.

Weber, M. (1947). *The theory of social and economic organization* (T. Parsons translation). New York: Free Press.

Wheatley, M. (1992). *Leadership and the new science.* San Francisco: Berrett-Koehler.

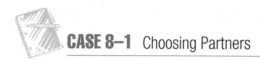

CASE 8–1 Choosing Partners

Emilie M. Deady

This case study describes the process one visiting nurse association went through to assess its own strengths and weaknesses and the environment's opportunities and weaknesses. The outcome was to join into an alliance and become part of an integrated health system while preserving the organization's strengths.

The Visiting Nurse Association system of home care is an integral part of the healthcare delivery system in northern Virginia. Services are provided through the parent Visiting Nurses Home Care (VNHC), and the two subsidiary corporations, the Visiting Nurse Association (VNA) and VNA Community Hospice. The VNA is the flagship corporation within the system that was founded in 1937; it provides traditional skilled intermittent home care services. VNA Community Hospice provides the full range of hospice Medicare services; VNHC provides management services, development, and prevention service. The structure of the VNA system is more a product of the current reimbursement environment established by the federal government than a conscious business strategy for delivery service.

The VNA system operates within a 120-square-mile area of northern Virginia. Since its inception in 1937, the main purpose of the system has been to provide quality in-home health services to the sick and disabled in our service area. The Board has a commitment to providing care to all in need within the

financial constraint of the agency's resources. In fiscal year 1997, the combined budget is over $20 million, with approximately 85 percent of revenues from the Medicare system. Additional revenues come from fee for service from other third party payors and patient paid fees.

Approximately 5 percent is funded through the application of community resources. These resources include United Way allocations, grants, and contributions given for the purpose of providing care. The VNA system is the largest nonofficial home health care provider in the state; is Medicare/Medicaid certified; and is accredited by the Community Health Accreditation Program (CHAP) of the National League of Nursing.

The VNA system is governed by a voluntary Board of Directors, which hires a Chief Executive Officer/President to carry out the day-to-day operations. The President is the same individual for all three corporations. The system employs over 500 multidisciplinary direct care providers and support staff. It is known and recognized as a leader in the provision of specialty services, especially in enterostomal therapy, maternal–child health, psychiatric–mental health, oncology, and infusion therapy. The Extended Hours team (services provided after 6 P.M. throughout the night) has received commendation for outstanding quality service to clients from CHAP in 1994 and 1995.

CASE: 8–1 *Continued*

The VNA system has changed and expanded services in response to the needs of the community and the changes in the environment in which it interacts. The VNA system is seen as a system that responds to other systems and the supersystems in which it functions. Many internal changes have occurred in response to our environment and to our commitment to customer service through self-directed work teams. We have increased efficiency as we have moved to reduce costs and maintain quality.

In the past several years, the health care industry has been undergoing a revolution and a major transformation. External forces and systems are dramatically changing the face of home care. This major transformation in all of health care is occurring very fast and independent of any health care reform legislation. It has been market driven, with the need to reduce the cost of health care and control the expenditure within the Medicare/Medicaid systems. A recent article in *Modern Health Care* (August 5, 1996) reported that in 1996, merger and acquisitions for all types of providers were 2.4 per day. All of this activity is based on the current strategy that integration of services is the future. The assumptions are that vertical and horizontal service integration will achieve access for all, quality services, and cost containment. The patient will receive the right treatment in the right place and at the lowest price. Vertical integration includes linking facility-based services such as acute care hospitals, subacute units, and long-term care facilities with community-based services such as home care, hospice, pharmacy/infusion services, private duty, and home medical equipment. Horizontal integration is having a number of the same type of facility- or community-based services in one integrated system. Our belief is that home care is the bridge that unites the facility- and community-based care together and aides the smooth transition of services for patients within the system.

To be financially successful, an integrated system needs to focus on keeping a defined population well through prevention and risk reduction, early detection and intervention, and restorative care for the disabled. All services should be given at the less expensive level of appropriate care. In order to be efficient, an integrated delivery system must have a large number of clients, a large number of primary care physicians with access to specialty services, and strong community-based services with home care. This usually requires a large geographical area of service.

Home care within an integrated system must include all products (equipment, supplies, intravenous solutions) and services (nursing, physical and other therapies, counseling, hospice, etc.) for all ages of people that work in close collaboration and integration. The home care component often is critical to providing a seamless system to the client or patient. This is how the VNA system envisions the direction for the future of health care and its role within this future. The VNA system staff hope that this future will again make the patient central to the delivery of health services.

CASE: 8–1 *Continued*

These changes in the health care system have put pressure on all providers, especially hospitals, as they look to diversify and remain profitable. Home care and its products have appealed to many hospitals as a way to shift patients and services. In the 1980s, the VNA survived a threat from two local hospitals to develop their own Medicare-certified agency by joining with the VNA in the formation of the parent company, Visiting Nurse Home Care. The VNA became, for these two hospitals, their home care program while at the same time remaining a community-based corporation. This relationship proved beneficial for the community, the hospitals, and the VNA. In January 1996, these hospitals moved to join different integrated health care systems that would have placed them in direct competition with each other. These decisions placed the VNA system in the position of having to redefine itself and its affiliations. It was decided that an alliance was strategically necessary for VNA's future health.

The VNA Boards and staff anticipated the hospitals' decisions and established a VNA Future Task Force in September 1995. The purpose of the Task Force Committee was to establish clear direction for the VNA system in selecting an integrated health care system with which to partner or join. The Board members selected to serve gave unselfishly of their time, expertise, and desire to "save the VNA." They were truly the support that staff needed. The process and recommendations were of extreme importance to the staff because of our values and commitment to each other, our community,

and patients. We also enlisted the services of a consultant with whom we had worked on various projects over the past 10 years. In addition to the consultant, staff sought the advice of our outside accounting firm and our legal attorneys. These specialists were current not only with the local marketplace, but also with national changes. The charter for the Task Force was:

- To develop a plan to address the changing market conditions and relationships.
- To identify and develop a framework for future relationships.
- To solicit, review, and negotiate the best alternative for the VNA system.
- To present a recommendation to the full Boards of the system.

The first task that the committee tackled was the development of principles to guide the committee in its recommendations. The principles were:

1. Preserve the VNA institutional presence as the voice of the community for home care.
2. Continue the VNA name, mission, and philosophy in the delivery of home care in Northern Virginia.
3. Continue to manage a vertically and horizontally integrated home care system. Our alliance would be part of development of a vertically and horizontally integrated system with a regional delivery capacity.
4. Establish a patient care coordinator system within a large system.

CASE: 8–1 *Continued*

5. Provide staff with the opportunity to reinvent home care in the field.
6. Affiliate with a system aggressively growing home care.
7. Implement an ownership structure that yields high growth and access to capital in order to improve technology and fund indigent care.
8. Provide VNA personnel with opportunities to continue employment.
9. Position the executive team to deliver on all agreements.

These principles were sorted into three categories: governance, operations, and participation.

In order for us to achieve these objectives as defined through the principles, staff identified seven possible scenarios for the committee to consider (see Fig. 8–4). They also drew a conceptual model reflecting the impact of the reimbursement system and an integrated delivery system on VNA (see Fig. 8–5). A traditional strategic planning process was used by the committee in considering the options. First, an internal assessment of the VNA was done to clarify the strengths we had to offer and the weaknesses we would like to augment in the affiliation. Then each scenario was considered in relation to the strengths and weaknesses of the VNA and the opportunities and threats of possible affiliations. Models of organization options were developed as working tools for the committee. The committee then recom-

mended three system options to the Boards.

The three systems approached were each interested in merging with VNA. The committee then asked for proposals from each system in relation to the established principles. The committee work also included reviewing proposals and meetings with the three final systems representatives.

The staff was anxious about which systems would be chosen. They were hearing rumors in the community and among themselves that were either not valid or misleading. We utilized the "town meetings" that our executive team routinely holds at our different offices throughout our service area as a forum to control rumors. The town meetings discussed the issues of the change in health care environment, our current market, and the progress of the Task Force. The staff were informed of who the final three systems were and the principles for evaluation through announcements on our voice mail system and our internal newsletter. I asked for staff input and did receive several phone calls and suggestions both at the office and my home. It has always been my management philosophy that staff involvement in change and decisions will influence the outcome positively.

Prior to the Task Force committee's final selection phase, we had a mini-Board retreat, including all three corporate Boards within our system as well as our senior and middle management staff. The purpose of the meeting was to discuss the following questions:

VNA Organizational Models

	I. VNA of the United Way	II. VNA of the County	III. VNA of the City	IV. VNA of Multi-Hospital Holding Co.	V. VNA of ABC Hospital	VI. VNA of XYZ System	VII. VNA of QRS Health Plan
Ownership	Freestanding	Freestanding	Freestanding	Hospital partnership	Hospital owned	System owned	Payor owned
Mission	Community based	Community based	Community based	Community based	Community oriented	System oriented	Reimbursement oriented
Market Share	Not dominant in the market	Dominant in the market (little hospital-based competition)	Special relationships with certain hospitals	Hospital-based referrals; some community referrals	Hospital-based referrals	Single system referrals	Single payor source
Patients	Dominant in Medicaid and indigent care	Makes money to deliver indigent care	May manage some home health programs	Takes some Medicaid and indigent care	Takes some Medicaid and indigent care	Limited indigent care	No indigent care
Payors	Dependent on United Way and charity funding	Good payor mix	Good payor mix	Good payor mix	Good payor mix	Good payor mix	Plan participants must use

VNA autonomy

High ———————————————————→ Low

Community based

High ———————————————————→ Low

Referral risk (covered patients)

High ———————————————————→ Low

FIGURE 8–4. VNA organizational models.

CASE: 8–1 *Continued*

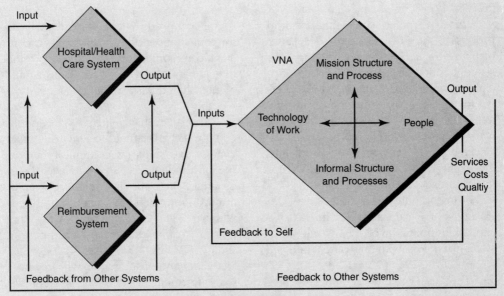

INTERACTION

FIGURE 8–5. Impact of reimbursement system and integrated delivery system on VNA.

1. What is going on in the health care system nationwide and in our region that makes it imperative for the VNA to seek out new relationships?
2. Is there anything special about the VNA that must be preserved in any new relationship?
3. What primary mechanisms can or should we use in preserving these special things as we begin developing our new relationship(s)?
4. What elements need to be considered in order to ensure that the VNA plans a leadership role in developing a horizontally and vertically integrated delivery system?

Each participant was given information before the meeting on the agency's mission and values statement. We were fortunate that the Boards had recently reaffirmed the mission statement.

The information from that meeting was synthesized and analyzed to clarify the consensus on expectations of the Boards and management staff for the Task Force. This information was then utilized in the final selection process. A final written and oral presentation by the three systems under consideration was made within the same week.

CASE: 8–1 *Continued*

Based on these presentations and proposals, the President drafted a Letter of Intent for each system clarifying their stated positions in regard to VNA's principles. The letters of intent were different for all three systems. One of the systems was for-profit; its letter of intent was one of a sale of the corporation, advisory capacity only for the Board, and the exclusion of the VNA name except in a foundation. The two nonprofits' letters of intent indicated a merger with the existing home care agencies in the system, high Board involvement with one system and less with the other, and retention of the VNA name.

The Task Force presented their recommendation for a final selection to the Boards and asked for permission to sign the Letter of Agreement with one of the nonprofit systems. The decision was based on agency mission, compatibility, economies of scale, the capability to expand the market, and perceived opportunity to achieve synergy. The VNA would bring to the merger a well-functioning home care system with a strong management. The other corporation would bring a home care company that had undergone constant turnover and needed the stability and quality focus of the VNA. It also brought with it a vertically integrated system with a strong financial base that the VNA needed. All three Boards agreed with the recommendation and the letter was signed.

The next phase will involve due diligence and implementation of the letter of intent. These implementation plans will need to be well-developed with clear time tables and benchmarks to be achieved. We anticipate that the implementation phase will involve constant communication within and outside the agency. Above all, the phase must assure that quality patient care is provided.

The VNA has, since its inception, continuously adapted to environmental change and shifts on community needs. In our adaptations, we have been grounded in a mission to serve a community and defined health problems within that community. We have evolved from a charity organization, to a sliding scale fee-for-service, to a Medicare and insurance payor revenue reimbursement system. The current demand that organizations have an increased level of interaction and larger, more integrated systems requires another structural change to be achieved through this merger. The response must be creative, looking beyond the traditional boundaries that each subsystem has established. The system, to be successful, must be open to the flow of ideas between the subsystems in order to adapt and prosper in the future. Regardless of changes in services, revenue systems, and structure, the VNA remains grounded in the same mission to provide patient- and family-centered, quality, cost-effective care.

■ BIOGRAPHICAL SKETCH

Emilie M. Deady has been President/ CEO of the Visiting Nurse Association of Northern Virginia since 1979. In addition, she is President/CEO of the Visiting

CASE: 8–1   *Continued*

Nurse Home Care, Inc., and VNA Community Hospice. She currently serves on the Board of Directors of the Visiting Nurse Association of America and the Community Health Accreditation Program. Ms. Deady has been involved at national, state, and local levels in areas relating to home care. She was one of the Washington Women in 1985 and is in Who's Who in Nursing.

9

Financial Skills
for Department Managers

Michelle Robnett and Alissa Schaub-Rimel

Financial skills, particularly budgeting proficiencies, are vital for department managers. Navigating the budgeting process and understanding the many pieces involved is crucial to effective and responsible managing. Additionally, it is important to comprehend how budgets can impact other aspects of business and how budgets can be impacted. Although the scope of financial responsibilities for nurse managers will vary among institutions, the necessity of financial skills for nurse managers will remain a constant.

Budgeting empowers managers, creating greater opportunities for decision making but also for greater responsibility. More than a statement of figures, a budget acts as a formal, but not binding, guide and framework for many other activities. These activities include: prioritizing efforts, implementing goals, planning, developing rational contingency plans, establishing the scope and breadth of initiatives, creating proactive action plans, and evaluating performance (Finkler & Kovner, 1993). In addition, a budget can and should act as a communication tool. Such an important activity becomes a work in progress, coordinating with the overarching development of corporate strategies, operational planning, and ultimately resource allocation.

It is easy to understand why budgeting and other financial skills are so important for nurse leaders to learn and develop. Such skills are especially important in nursing today, since an ever-growing focus is being placed on financial performance and viability in health care institutions. Well-developed financial skills can enhance managerial performance because managers with such skills are better able to prioritize efforts and communicate to staff and administrators. Financial skills also allow nurse managers to adjust their expectations. More importantly, financial skills permit managers to fulfill responsibilities more completely with ever-limited resources. Most people already possess these skills but are not familiar with the business-oriented language used to define them (Decker & Sullivan, 1992).

This chapter is divided into three sections covering the budget preparation process, cost concepts and controls, and the context of departmental financial management. Throughout this chapter, the term *unit* refers to any of three types of departments: a clinical service unit, such as an operating room or rehabilitation laboratory; an inpatient unit, such as a critical unit or medical cardiac unit; or an ambulatory care unit, such as an emergency department, opthamology clinic, or home care unit. The last example may or may not be physically contiguous to the agency itself.

■ BUDGET PREPARATION PROCESS

The budget preparation process is a continuous one. Organizations are constantly preparing projections for future budgets, implementing current budgets, and analyzing performance in relation to the budget. A budget is the financial definition of an organization's vision and strategies to implement that vision through allocation of monetary resources (Hoffman, 1984). A budget establishes the financial expectations of the organization for each unit and is the standard against which they are measured. Control is accomplished at the start of each fiscal period when management determines whether achievement of the financial expectations set in the budget will enable the organization to accomplish the goals and objectives established by its planning processes. In other words, will the expected revenues cover all the expenses implied by these goals and objectives? Control is again accomplished at each reporting period and annually when actual performance is compared to the standard of expectations set forth in the budget.

Corporate Strategy Development

Prior to the allocation of resources, it is necessary and important to develop long-range plans. A strategic plan establishes the goals and objectives for an institution, department, or other defined unit. Assumptions about external and internal forces are factored into the strategic plan and updated at least annually. Consideration is given to the institution's environmental position, as well. In short, this is a qualitative process that describes an organization's vision and strategies to achieve that vision. The parallel financial process is budget forecasting of expenses and revenues for specified periods of time based on alternative proposed strategies. This is often done for worst, typical, and best case scenarios. Also included in financial planning is analysis of financial performance in previous years. These forecasts are considered in choosing options, setting priorities, and goal setting. Priorities for the organization must be established and strategies chosen in order to determine what goals and objectives will require resource allocation.

Making Projections

A unit manager is often asked to predict the number of service units he or she will provide for a period of time. Average number of patient days is the common service unit for inpatient services, although some agencies are now moving to patient hours for some short-term units. Average number of visits or visits by category (short, intermediate, long) are used as service units for ambulatory care clinics, home care, and other discrete services. Clinical units define service units in differing ways depending on service provided—operating rooms are often by minute, radiography is often by type of x-ray, and dietary by type of meal delivered.

Projections for any of these units are by defined unit of service and often are based on past records of delivery through trend analysis. This technique is the process of examining patterns in the level of phenomenon (service unit) over time. In long-term forecasting, this is usually by year; intermediate is by month, and short term is by day or hour. Regardless of time period, the method involves two important assumptions: (1) there has been a recognizable trend in the past; and (2) the trend will continue into the future.

Trend analysis is a powerful tool to verify the first assumption. The second may only be verified by expert opinion, common sense, and time (Finkler, 1993). As a first step, the unit manager creates a line graph with units of time across the bottom (x axis) and units of service along the perpendicular edge (y axis). Each number of units delivered for each time period is then plotted. The manager then looks at the chart to see whether the dots form, or cluster around, a line. If a linear trend can be detected, a line can then be drawn and possible future projections derived from the position at future time points. This approach is forecasting trend analysis in its simplest form. Several pitfalls must be examined before accepting such a projection. One pitfall to avoid is failing to test the numbers using statistics to verify the fit with the line. A manager may wish to consult a resource person in the performance management (or quality assurance or continuous quality improvement, etc.) office who can test for fit and determine whether the fit is actually linear or curved by using inferential statistics such as regression. Another pitfall to avoid is not seeking another expert opinion about assumption two, the continuation of the trend. Often, the marketing department may be helpful in offering environmental information and commonsense guidance. Sources of referrals and publications in the specialty may also be helpful in offering observations based on trends in practice.

Operational Planning

This phase of the budgeting process should include specific and measurable operating goals and objectives that will guide the resource allocation process. These goals and objectives should be communicated to all involved in the budget process before resource allocation begins. Not only will there be greater time to build consensus on organizational goals, but considerable thought and planning can be done to devise the most effective departmental plans for attaining goals.

The other basic decision is to make *incremental* adjustments to this year's budgets or to prepare *zero-based budgets* as if each service unit were new to the organization. There is no preferred basic approach, but significant participation by persons at all levels of the organization utilizes the expertise they have and increases their commitment to the final budget. Everyone in the decision-making process will be using actual performance in this year's budget as one guideline as to the "reality" of projections. It is, therefore, desirable to establish the expectation that all budget items will be examined with the attitude espoused in the zero-based budgeting approach: Is this item needed and, if yes, at what level of expenditure (Meigs & Meigs, 1990)?

The preparation of budgets requires managers to solicit the participation of many individuals and spend many hours in an iterative process of submission, review, and adjustments. The first step in the resource allocation process is often senior management's review and revision of the budget manual outlining the steps to follow and the forms to standardize information. Such a review and revision will enable the remainder of the organization involved in the budgeting process to take appropriate and timely action in the budget's development. Timeliness is guided by the timetable that sets forth the sequence of activities to be followed and the due dates for each step in the budget preparation process. This timetable varies for each organization, but usually requires at least 4 to 6 months of activity before the budgets are submitted to the Board of Trustees for its approval.

Operating guidelines to be included in all manuals should address:

1. Operating decisions made, such as salary increases; projected change in total employment; adjustments in rates charged; and addition, deletion, or modification of services or products offered.
2. Assumptions about the external environment stated in terms of their anticipated financial impact from the effect of (a) the projected level of reimbursement by third-party payors, including Medicare and contractual allowances being given to preferred providers and managed care companies and any global pricing or capitated payment contracts; (b) the impact of changes in activities by competitors, such as new ambulatory care services, birthing centers, primary care centers, or mergers; or (c) the anticipated modification of the Certificate of Need (CON) laws or other governmental laws or regulations on gross revenues.
3. Assumptions about operations, such as average length of stay, numbers of patient visits, units of service for new integrated services such as inpatient–outpatient hospice, and expected changes in level of demand for particular services or products.

Once the manual is finalized, it is distributed to all unit managers. When there is any major change, this should be presented to the Board of Trustees or an appropriate group within the Board, for its review and acceptance. This forms consensus about the parameters within which the final budgets will be prepared and facilitates final Board approval.

In some institutions, the financial department still prepares budgets that are given to unit managers for review and comment. This approach lacks the benefits of financial savvy and commitment that come with involvement of unit managers in budget preparation. The preferred approach is for unit managers to develop projections and subsequent revisions for operating budgets, capital budgets, and cash budgets.

The operating budget includes projections for the statistics budget and service estimates. The statistics budget will forecast the volume or amount of activity for the budgeting period. Service estimates will forecast dollars in revenue that can be expected as a result of the volume, as well as the resources necessary to provide that volume of services. Resource allocations are typically presented as full-time equivalents (FTEs) for each category of personnel. The resource allocation forecasts are not financial budgets because of the range of costs that may exist for each category of personnel. For instance, staffing for six FTEs of registered nurses in staff nurse positions may cost more for a unit with experienced staff at the higher end of the salary scale or when temporary nurses are used (Ward, 1994).

The capital budget establishes what expenditures will be made for plant and equipment. Each organization has definitions that define capital versus supply expenses. The organizational capital budget covers a period of several years so that the organization will know what total funds it will need to finance these large expenditures. When doing a unit capital budget, the appropriate elements of the organizational long-term capital budget should be used.

The cash budget forecasts cash receipts and payments for the fiscal period. This usually encompasses supplies and miscellaneous expenses for units.

After completing the first unit projections for each type of budget, a series of meetings of managers by division is then held to continue work on the budget. These are usually referred to as technical budget meetings for unit managers and administrative meetings for executive managers. At the administrative meetings, budgetary priorities are ranked in order of importance and then communicated to the unit managers.

Senior management then develops the operating, capital, and cash budgets for the organization, organized into revenues and expenses. These budgets may also be broken down into several smaller pieces, such as supplies, labor, administrative and general expenses, and nonoperating expenses.

Unit managers then review and revise their budgets and resource specifications in line with priorities and new projections of volume. This iterative process may involve several rounds before goal and objective priorities, available resources, and projected volumes are aligned. Budget integration is completed and executive management makes its final administrative review. At this point, the budget is complete, pending the Board of Trustees' approval. In some instances, outside agencies also must give budget approval due to local laws, or lease or loan agreements. Once the Board and all other required bodies give their approval, the budget becomes the standard for implementation and review for that fiscal year. It should be stressed that preparation of next year's budget begins with submission and approval of the current year's budget.

■ COST CONCEPTS AND CONTROLS

Cost control has become a more salient concept as health care organizations are being asked to share risks with payors and to enter into prospective payment agreements such as global prices and capitation. In response to this new monetary constraint, administrators must develop policies and procedures that do indeed keep costs in line with operating revenues. There are two parts to a cost control program. One is to understand and properly use the concepts that describe different types of cost behavior. The second is to use the budget process and the budget itself as standards for monitoring costs and variances. Table 9–1 groups cost concepts into four categories: asset val-

TABLE 9–1. Categories of Cost Concepts

Asset Valuation
Historical/replacement
Cash/accrual
Managerial Control
Controllable/noncontrollable
Direct/indirect
Committed/noncommitted
Budgeted/actual
Decision Making
Sunk costs
Incremental costs
Opportunity costs
Avoidable or escapable costs
Volume
Fixed costs
Variable costs
Semifixed or semivariable costs
Step costs

Adapted from Neumann, Suver, & Zelman (1984).

uation, managerial control, decision making, and volume. The concepts in each category focus on a particular set of problems with which management must deal.

Asset Valuation

Management needs an accurate valuation of the organization's assets to know whether the results of operations are increasing the value of the assets and to have a basis for persuading investors to provide additional capital when needed.

Historical/Replacement

These concepts are concerned with the valuation of the fixed assets on the balance sheet. Use of a historical basis means the fixed assets are valued at their purchase price and this value is used when computing the depreciation expense incurred from operations. Through the process of charging depreciation expense against operations and accumulating a depreciation reserve, an organization retains asset values in the business that can be used for future replacement of the fixed asset. When the cost of a new fixed asset is increasing due to inflation, depreciation will not offset replacement cost. When this occurs, the additional funds needed for the actual replacement of the fixed asset must be obtained from the excess of revenues over expenses kept as a retained earnings and/or an infusion of additional capital (Horngren & Sundem, 1993).

Cash/Accrual

These concepts affect when the cost of using a fixed asset is recognized on the statement of revenues and expenses. With cash accounting, the cost is recorded when the expenditure is made. With accrual accounting, the cost is recognized as the asset is used up in producing goods or services. The latter basis is used more often, because it records on the balance sheets within the same fiscal period both the cost of producing revenues and revenues earned.

Managerial Control

These cost concepts are used by patient care administrators in their management of costs associated with operations.

Controllable/Noncontrollable

When evaluating the financial performance of a unit manager for a fiscal time period, one should consider which costs the manager can control and which are outside his or her control. For example, if the unit manager determines the scheduling of nursing personnel, and chooses to use overtime, agency personnel, float personnel, or no replacement when someone calls in sick, then this is controllable. On the other hand, the unit manager does not control the timing or range of raises in nursing salaries, this then is a noncontrollable cost.

Direct/Indirect

Direct costs are those that can be traced to a specific unit or activity that incurred the cost, whereas indirect costs are shared by or common to two or more units or activities. Indirect costs are usually distributed using a formula such as square footage for costs of heat, light, and electricity. These concepts are used when administrators are determining whether the revenues generated by a given unit or activity are sufficient to cover its costs.

A particular cost may be a direct cost for one analysis and an indirect cost for another. For example, the operating cost of the magnetic resonance imaging (MRI) machine is a direct cost to the radiology department, but an indirect cost to each of the departments whose patients use the MRI scanner. For these latter departments, the administrators must use a standard accepted as providing a good estimate of "fair shares" as a basis for allocating the MRI costs.

Committed/Noncommitted Costs

These concepts are used in the budgeting process to define which costs have been committed to a particular activity (e.g., nurses' salaries) or to the acquisition of certain assets (e.g., supplies, pieces of equipment). Normally, certain funds will be left uncommitted to be available to cover fluctuations in operations, or an unanticipated acquisition or repair of fixed assets. These may also be referred to as discretionary funds.

Budgeted/Actual

These concepts are used as an integral part of the budgeting process. Budgeted costs are the operating costs planned for the next fiscal period given the assumptions of levels of activity, whereas actual costs are those actually incurred from the operations. A comparison of the actual costs to the budgeted costs is frequently used by administrators to determine the quality of performance at each level of the organization. Large variances from the budget are a signal that the organization may be in serious trouble.

Decision Making

The cost concepts in decision making are used by administrators in making decisions about adding, deleting, or modifying a service. This involves a comparison of alternative uses of resources. A subgroup of these decisions are called make-or-buy decisions.

Sunk Costs

This recognizes that a cost incurred cannot be undone and should not be considered when deciding whether to delete a service. Frequently, these are costs associated with the replacement of a fixed asset. For example, a health care organization should not decide to continue to use its present computerized billing system solely because it owns it. Its purchase is a sunk cost that should not be "charged" in a replacement decision.

Incremental Costs

These are added costs that occur when a complementary service is added or represent the additional cost for one alternative as compared to another. The use of the incremental costs concept in decisions recognizes only the additional costs the new service or alternative will incur and does not consider other costs that are already present in the organization, such as building costs or top management salaries, that will not increase with the addition of a new service. It is expected that the projected revenues for any new service minus the incremental costs will provide a contribution to the general overhead of the organization and to its excess of revenues over expenses.

Opportunity Costs

These costs are the value of the benefits foregone because the organization invested a set of resources in one new service and not in another. Thus, when one is evaluating what the new service will contribute to the organization both the operating costs and the opportunity costs will be deducted from the projected revenues to arrive at the contribution this use of resources will make to the organization. Then management can focus on the question, is this contribution sufficiently large enough to support the risk associated with this investment of resources? Once the resources are invested, they are not available for another use.

Avoidable or Escapable Costs

This cost concept is used in decisions to delete a service. It recognizes that not all costs will be reduced or saved if a given service is discontinued. If an organization needs to reduce its total costs, it needs to identify those services that will, in fact, result in a reduction of costs when deleted. In such decisions, management must also recognize that the contribution from that service to the general overhead and the excess of revenues over expenses for the organization will also be lost.

Volume

Volume concepts deal with the behavior of costs as the volume of operations changes. In examining cost behavior with respect to changes in volume, the patient care administrator must keep in mind that these observed behaviors only hold true for a relevant range of volumes and a specific period of time.

Fixed Costs

These are costs that do not change with a change in volume of operations; for instance, rent for the building.

Variable Costs

These are costs that do change in a definite relationship with a change in volume of operations.

Semifixed or Semivariable Costs

These are costs that are mixed as to how they react to changes in volume; they are partially fixed and partially variable. The labeling of these costs reflects which cost element is dominant.

Step Costs

This term describes costs that are fixed to a certain volume level and then increase by a fixed amount when this volume level is exceeded. An example of a step cost is the increase in salary costs from the addition of one nurse to a staff when patient volume increases above a threshold level.

These costs concepts for the category of volume are used in doing break-even analysis to answer the question, what volume in units or revenues is needed to equal the total cost of producing that volume? The break-even volume is the number of units at which total revenues equal total costs (total fixed costs plus total variable costs). If the organization has established some level of expected dollar or rate of return for any new venture, this amount is also included as part of the total costs. An example is provided in Table 9–2.

The real value of break-even analysis is that it forces the patient care administrator to understand what costs are involved in providing the new service, their relationship to changes in volume, and what volume is needed to achieve a break-even volume. After doing the break-even analysis the management question then becomes, will the organization achieve this volume? If management has done the break-even analysis carefully, it can have confidence that the answer to this question is accurate as to what would happen if the new service were indeed begun.

An adaptation to break-even analysis can be used by nurse managers to see what volume changes are needed, that is, what new volume level, to maintain the same amount of excess of revenues over expenses if a contractual allowance is provided to a health maintenance organization (HMO) or managed care organization in exchange for becoming a preferred provider to their members. Also, if an organization is not achieving a positive excess of revenues over expenses, it may wish to do a break-even analysis to see what volume is needed to achieve break-even, or the specific dollar amount of excess revenues over expenses above break-even desired.

Monitoring

Budget monitoring is an ongoing process intended to keep managers abreast of the effectiveness of the tools and measures established to control costs, as well as a department's ability to meet budgetary goals. Within the monitoring process, managers will compare budget goals against actual performance to ensure that goals are met and to devise corrective action when indicated. When disparities exist, these differences between budgeted amounts and actual reported amounts are known as variances.

TABLE 9–2. Break-Even Analysis at the Goodhealth Clinic

The Goodhealth clinic plans to provide clinical services in its clinic as well as an in-home vis-itation service. Staff for the clinic includes two physicians and two RNs. The one LPN does the in-home visitation service.

These are the operating assumptions management made to have a basis to determine the volume needed for a break-even operation and to earn an excess of revenues over ex-penses equal to 4% of gross revenues.

1. The expected revenue per visit is $45 for a clinic visit and $20 for an in-home visit.
2. The annual salaries are $30,000 for each RN, $65,000 for each employed physician, and $21,000, for the LPN.
3. The telephone charge is $23.50 per line per month. There are two lines for the clinic and one line for the in-home service.
4. The LPN is paid $0.21 per mile traveled and it is assumed each patient visit re-quires 8 miles of travel.
5. The rent is $2,000 per month.
6. The cost for supplies is $200 per month plus $3.50 per patient visit for the clinic, and $1.00 per in-home visit.
7. The laundry cost for the clinic is $3.00 per patient visit.
8. The custodian works 20 hours per week to clean the clinic and is paid $7.50 per hour.
9. Depreciation expense for medical and office equipment used in the clinic is computed by use of the straight-line method.

The steps for completing the break-even analysis demonstrated below are:

1. Determine the total costs for the time period for which you wish to determine volume needed to achieve break-even or a volume that results in an estab-lished dollar amount of excess of revenues over expenses;
2. Identify each cost as fixed, variable, or semifixed or semivariable;
3. Determine the total fixed costs, the unit variable cost, and the revenue per unit;
4. Determine the break-even volume and/or the volume needed to achieve a given level of excess of revenues over expenses.

	IN-HOME		CLINIC	
	Fixed costs	Unit variable costs	Fixed costs	Unit variable costs
Employed physicians			$130,000	
RN salaries			60,000	
LPN salary	$ 21,000			
Telephone	282		564	
Rent			24,000	
Supplies		$ 1.00	2,400	$ 3.50
Laundry				3.00
Custodial services			7,800	
Mileage		1.68		
Depreciation			10,000	
Totals	$ 21,282	$ 2.68	$234,764	$ 6.50

(continued)

TABLE 9–2. (continued)

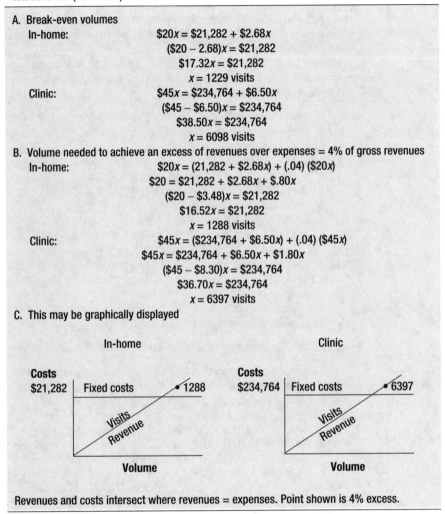

A. Break-even volumes
  In-home:
$$\$20x = \$21,282 + \$2.68x$$
$$(\$20 - 2.68)x = \$21,282$$
$$\$17.32x = \$21,282$$
$$x = 1229 \text{ visits}$$
  Clinic:
$$\$45x = \$234,764 + \$6.50x$$
$$(\$45 - \$6.50)x = \$234,764$$
$$\$38.50x = \$234,764$$
$$x = 6098 \text{ visits}$$

B. Volume needed to achieve an excess of revenues over expenses = 4% of gross revenues
  In-home:
$$\$20x = (21,282 + \$2.68x) + (.04)(\$20x)$$
$$\$20 = \$21,282 + \$2.68x + \$.80x$$
$$(\$20 - \$3.48)x = \$21,282$$
$$\$16.52x = \$21,282$$
$$x = 1288 \text{ visits}$$
  Clinic:
$$\$45x = (\$234,764 + \$6.50x) + (.04)(\$45x)$$
$$\$45x = \$234,764 + \$6.50x + \$1.80x$$
$$(\$45 - \$8.30)x = \$234,764$$
$$\$36.70x = \$234,764$$
$$x = 6397 \text{ visits}$$

C. This may be graphically displayed

In-home

Costs
$21,282 | Fixed costs   • 1288
                Visits
                Revenue
Volume

Clinic

Costs
$234,764 | Fixed costs   • 6397
                Visits
                Revenue
Volume

Revenues and costs intersect where revenues = expenses. Point shown is 4% excess.

Generally, managers receive monthly reports from which they can monitor budget progress and track budget variances. The basic information contained in these reports is actual revenue and expenses, as reported in the institution's general ledger. Reports will likely contain even more detailed and specific information, including labor distribution for each payroll period, supply utilization, purchasing, and departmental service volume and revenue. The primary report used for budget implementation and monitoring is the revenue and expense statement or income statement (see Table 9–3).

TABLE 9–3. Goodhealth Hospital Statement of Revenues and Expenses for the Period Ending December 31, 19XX (amounts in thousands)

Revenues		Totals
Inpatient revenues		$135,040
Outpatient revenues		19,422
Emergency room revenues		8,176
Total gross patient revenues		$162,638
Less: Deductibles (uncollectible accounts, contractual		
allowances, Medicare, Medicaid, indigent care)		34,154
Net patient revenues		$128,484
Other operating revenues		4,673
Total operating revenues		$133,157
Operating Expenses		
Salaries	$ 61,450	
Wages	18,940	
Employee benefits	10,762	
Employed physicians	10,684	
Interest expense	3,186	
Utilities	9,168	
Supplies	5,632	
Depreciation	8,944	
Total operating expenses		$128,766
Net operating income		4,391
Nonoperating revenues		2,277
Excess of Revenues Over Expenses		$ 6,668

Looking at the Table 9–3, note how it is arranged by revenues, operating expenses, net operating income, nonoperating revenues, and excess of revenues over expenses. This particular format is used in a nonprofit organization.

Let's start with revenues. Under revenues, you have reports of outpatient revenues and inpatient revenues. Outpatient revenues can consist of independent billing for procedures done by staff physicians, nurse practitioners, or other health care providers and clinic or facilities fees. The same applies to emergency room revenues. Inpatient revenues consist of basic room and board charges as well as any additional fees for care provided in an inpatient setting. For example, many hospitals charge for variable intensity of nursing care with fees in addition to the basic room and board charge. Pharmaceutical fees, supply fees, and others also are included here. Notice how discounts to HMOs, uncollectable patient charges, and differences in fees received and billed as for Medicare are deducted here under "Less."

Operating expenses include direct expenses that relate to salaries, wages, and employee benefits; employed physicians; supplies; and usually other broad categories such as purchased services, photocopying, and leases.

Interest expense on loans, utility costs, and depreciation on capital equipment is also included here for the entire hospital, but would not appear on the monthly income statement for a department, since this would be an indirect expense for that department. No upper management, medical records, housekeeping, or other support department expenses are reported on department monthly revenue and expense statements; they are included on a hospital's organizational income statement once a year. It is unfair to compare relative amounts in categories by departments, as much variance is directly related to the services provided. For instance, supply expenses are often the largest category for the operating room, but salaries are the largest category for intensive care units.

Next is the category of operating income. Revenues minus expenses equal operating income. From a unit perspective, managers always need revenues to be greater than expenses because their operating budget does not include the indirect expenses or expected rate of return on investment that are charged to the unit in calculating its break-even point. In a cost-based pricing environment, the quotient for expenses required to break-even divided by the number of service units needed to break-even would be the service unit charge (daily room rate for inpatient units, visit charge for an ambulatory visit).

Revenue

Let's go back now to look in more detail at the category identified as revenue. As shown in Table 9–4, an analysis of budget variances is based on comparison of budgeted and actual revenues. Budgeted revenues come from volume projections that are made for the unit and aggregated across units for divisions, and then totaled for an institution. Volume projections are made at the beginning of the budget cycle. Projected or budgeted revenues are determined by multiplying the volumes by the rates (rate × volume = revenue). Actual refers to the gross revenue the unit was able to generate. The variance is the difference between what was budgeted and actual. If actual figures are greater than budgeted figures, this is called a positive variance. There are many reasons for changes in volumes, but they usually relate to market conditions, as well as the quality of service.

Expenses

Let's move down to expenses on Table 9–4. For expenses, there are the same kinds of categories as revenues: budgeted, actual, total, variance, and volume. Budgeted expenses in a financially solvent department should always be less than budgeted expenses because revenues minus expenses equal operating income and this does not include costs of indirect expenses. The exception is the department that is losing monies, but is kept because it (1) meets a community need, (2) provides business to another department that generates enough money to cover the loss, (3) provides another function

TABLE 9–4. Analysis of Budget Variances at Goodhealth Clinic

	BUDGET	ACTUAL	TOTAL	VARIANCES PRICE	VOLUME
Revenue					
Patient visits	$278,280	$262,773	($15,507)	($12,222)	($3,285)
Expenses					
Employed physicians	$130,000	$130,000			
RN salaries	60,000	65,000	$ 5,000	$ 5,000	
Telephone	564	591	27	27	
Rent	24,000	24,000			
Supplies	24,044	25,316	1,272	1,528	$ (256)
Laundry	18,552	18,700	148	367	(219)
Custodian services	7,800	7,800			
Depreciation	10,000	10,000			
Totals	$274,960	$281,407	$ 6,447	$ 6,922	$ (475)
Excess of revenues over expenses	$ 3,320	$(18,634)	($21,954)	($19,144)	($2,810)

These facts were used by management in completing the variance analysis for the patient visits to the Goodhealth Clinic for the past year.

1. In determining the budgeted revenues it was estimated there would be 6,184 visits at an average charge of $45 per visit. Analysis of the records show that there were 6,111 actual visits at an average charge of $43.
2. Each of the two RNs was given an annual salary increase of $2,500, on July 1.
3. As of April 1 this year, the monthly charge for each telephone line increased from $23.50 to $25.00 per line. The clinic uses two lines.
4. The cost of supplies was budgeted at the rate of $200 per month plus $3.50 per patient visit to the clinic. Analysis of the records shows that the variable cost of supplies per patient visit last year was $3.75.
5. Laundry was budgeted at the rate of $3.00 per clinic patient visit. Analysis of the records for the past year shows that the average cost for laundry per patient visit was $3.06.

such as prestige or image to the organization and all the other services can cover the loss, or (4) a mix of the three. For instance, pediatric service may attract obstetric and gynecologic business to an institution. Such expenses must be balanced by other profitable units, because overall the business cannot survive without financial health.

Now that we have budgeted expenses, we can look at actual expenses. Actual expenses consist of the same list of expenses. One area of contention between staff and management is often the level of staffing. The clinicians would like to provide all the care that they possibly can to a patient, and this maximum may exceed what was budgeted or needed to give quality care. Working with clinicians to assist them to include in their care planning value to the patient for the cost of nursing services is an important fiscal function for the department manager. Realistic budget projections are essential for the appropriate quality and cost management of clinical units.

Variances

Variance analysis compares the budgeted dollars to actual dollars. Negative variances are negative amounts and positive variances are positive amounts. A manager is expected to explain all variances. A common budget item with variances in a patient care department is salary and benefits. Variances in salary and benefits budgets tend to occur for four reasons:

1. Patient volumes are either higher or lower than projected.
2. Intensity of care is higher or lower than projected.
3. Efficiency of staff in providing care is higher or lower than projected.
4. Cost of personnel is higher or lower than projected.

These are typically labeled as: price variance, volume variance, and usage variance (sometimes called intensity/efficiency variance). The formula and steps for calculating each of these variances are listed below with examples from Table 9–4. Interestingly, variance analysis uses the same process for all categories of expenses and revenues.

Price Variance

First calculate budgeted rate: RN salary for the 2 RNs

$$\frac{\text{Budgeted amount}}{\text{Budgeted volume}} = \text{Budgeted rate} \qquad \frac{\$60,000}{2} = \$30,000$$

Second, calculate actual rate:

$$\frac{\text{Actual expense}}{\text{Actual volume}} = \text{Actual rate} \qquad \frac{\$65,000}{2} = \$32,500$$

Budgeted rate − Actual rate = Variance $30,000 − $32,500 = −$2,500

Variance explanation: The negative RN salary variance was due to the uncontrollable cost to the manager of the RNs getting a $2,500 raise per year on July 1.

Volume Variance

Number of budgeted visits − Number of actual visits = Variance

Visits budgeted were 6,184
Visits actual were 6,111
The volume variance was 6,184 − 6,111 = 73
Expressed in dollars at $45 each ($45 × 73) is $3,285

Volume variance explanation: In examining the monthly and weekly reports, the lower than expected volumes primarily occurred in January. This January had an unusually high amount of snow; perhaps patients were unable to come due to weather. This will be monitored more closely in the future. Clinic closure on snowy days would reduce costs.

Usage Variance

$$\frac{\text{Amount category budgeted}}{\text{Number of budgeted units}} = \text{Budgeted category per unit}$$

$24,000 budgeted for supplies at 6,184 visits budgeted

$$\frac{\$24,000}{6,184} = \$3.88 \text{ per visit}$$

$$\frac{\text{Amount of actual}}{\text{Number of actual delivered}} = \text{Actual category per unit}$$

25,316 actually spent for supplies
6,111 visits actually delivered

$$\frac{\$25,316}{\$6,111} = \$4.14 \text{ per visit}$$

Budgeted category per unit − Actual category per unit = Usage variance

$$\$3.88 - \$4.14 = -\$.26$$

Variance explanation: This extra .26 per visit spent on supplies was analyzed by examining categories of supplies for variances. A volume discount was offered by a supplier if we bought a volume actually higher than we needed monthly in the twelfth month of the fiscal year. This supply lasted 3 months and we anticipate supplies to have a positive variance for next year.

Supplies

Although agencies may define supplies differently, generally, supplies are defined as consumable goods used directly in patient care. Ambiguity can exist where equipment purchases are concerned, as in some instances these purchases are not consumables, but do not qualify as capital equipment purchases. To rectify this potential discrepancy, many agencies establish a dollar figure threshold under which equipment purchases are included in the supply budget.

Unit supplies can originate from many sources, including central storage and/or sterilization departments within the institution or from direct vendor purchases. It is important for nurse managers to know which sources of supplies result in direct costs to their budgets and which are included in indirect costs.

Another important issue for nurse managers to consider when budgeting for and purchasing supplies is how to make projections. Generally, supply needs can be anticipated and budgeted for fairly accurately by using historical data, reviewing care trends, and considering new factors that may increase or decrease supply needs, such as new treatments or changes in procedures. Often, reports generated within institutions can be helpful in predicting future supply needs and evaluating past supply budgeting efforts. These reports include an analysis of supply expense and variance from budget, a listing of supplies used by unit, statement of supply expenses charged against units, as well as daily and monthly unit average census reports. If needed, the finance department may be a resource to use more advanced formulas to provide budget projections for specified time periods.

However, there are some unpredictable instances in which supplies must be purchased that may create a budget deficit situation. Such instances include start-up costs for an unbudgeted, new, or expanded service; one-time purchases of replacement parts or small equipment; and items purchased infrequently but directly from supply vendors.

Operating Income

The business goal of a nurse manager is to achieve a positive operating income. Managers are also evaluated by their operating margin, which is a profitability ratio computed by dividing operating income by revenues to render the profit per dollar of sales. This margin should be monitored by managers to help determine capability and need for growth in clinical services (i.e., more exam rooms to increase the number of clinic visits). When an operating margin is growing as a function of volume increases, managers can be fairly certain that an increase in salary and supplies will be approved by administration. Further, when the operating margin is small or negative, the manager may need to initiate actions to control expenses to regain a certain budgeted operating margin.

■ FINANCIAL CONTEXT

The nurse who is a patient care manager is operating a department that is part of a larger organization. In order to actively participate in financial management of the department, she or he needs to become knowledgeable about basic accounting concepts and language used by accountants. This will be of assistance in discussing problems with the accounting department, such as when tracing a major transaction from journal entry to the ledger account, the statement of revenues and expenses, and finally to the organizational balance sheet. This chapter does not include this material; it is available in basic accounting textbooks, which are readily available.

The patient care administrator also needs to be able to assess the financial health of the organization and understand how that is affecting her or his area of responsibility. For instance, when asked to delay a purchase due to "cash flow" problems, the administrator should ask, is this due to longer lag from time of transaction to payment? To lower numbers of transactions? Or to unusual expenses occurring during this period? What percentage of monies are kept aside for discretionary expenses and what is designated to certain budget categories?

Familiarity with common indicators used in financial analysis will hold the manager in good stead when seeking to understand the finance context their unit operates within. One set of indicators are financial ratios. None of these alone determines the financial status of an organization, but together they draw a picture of financial status. The four most commonly reported indicators are: *liquidity ratios,* indicating the extent to which short-term obligations can be met; *profitability ratios,* indicating the extent of net revenue and its comparison to a given level of equity; *activity* measures of efficiency; and *leverage* ratios, showing the amount of financing from debt compared to that from equity. Formulas for these ratios are available in any health care financial management text. The Health Care Management Association annually publishes a set of industry data that organizations often use as a benchmark to assess their financial health compared to other health care organizations.

■ BIOGRAPHICAL SKETCHES

Michelle Robnett is currently the President of the Medical Group Management Company, a firm specializing in practice management, strategic management, and billing. She is the former Director of Special Program Development at The Johns Hopkins Bayview Medical Center in Baltimore, Maryland. In this role, she worked to develop a Nurse Practitioner Group Practice for the Johns Hopkins Bayview Medical Center. Dr. Robnett was formerly the Vice President, Patient Care Services at the same institution. She received her doctorate in Hospital and Health Administration from the College of Medicine, her MBA from the College of Business, her MA from the School of Nursing at the University of Iowa, and her BSN from Marycrest College, Davenport, Iowa.

After completing her Masters of Health Administration degree at the Pennsylvania State University in 1991, **Alissa Schaub-Rimel** served as a Health Insurance Specialist at the Health Care Financing Administration (HCFA) in the Social Security Administration specializing in Medicaid issues. In 1993, she became a Management Analyst for the Chief Operating Officer and Vice President of Patient Care at Johns Hopkins Bayview Medical Center in Baltimore, Maryland. She returned to HCFA in 1997 to work in the area of Medicare Medical Review.

■ SUGGESTED READINGS

Finkler, S., & Kovner, C. (1993). *Financial management for nurse managers and executives.* Philadelphia: Saunders. This book is aimed at the more proficient financial manager and covers more advanced topics.

Neumann, B., Suver, J., & Zelman, W. (1988). *Financial management: Concepts and applications for health care providers* (2nd ed.). Owings Mills, MD: National Health Publishing.

Ward, W. (1994). *Health care budgeting and financial management for non-financial managers*. Westport, CT: Auburn House. This book is excellent for beginning readers seeking to familiarize themselves with financial terms and applications, and offers pragmatic methodologies for the monitoring of operational issues.

■ REFERENCES

Decker, P., & Sullivan, E. (Eds.) (1992). *Nursing administration: A micro/macro approach for effective nurse executives*. Norwalk, CT: Appleton & Lange.

Finkler, S. (1993). Issues in cost accounting for health care organization. Gaithersburg, MD: Aspen Publisher.

Finkler, S., & Kovner, C. (1993). *Financial management for nurse managers and executives*. Philadelphia: Saunders.

Hoffman, F. (1984). *Financial management for nurse managers*. Norwalk, CT: Appleton-Century-Crofts.

Horngren, C., & Sundem, G. (1993). *Introduction to management accounting*, (9th ed.). Englewood Cliffs, NJ: Prentice Hall.

Meigs, R., & Meigs, W. (1990). *Accounting: The basis for business decisions* (8th ed.). New York: McGraw-Hill.

Ward, W. (1994). *Health care budgeting and financial management for non-financial managers*. Westport, CT: Auburn House.

CASE 9–1 Financial Issues in Opening a New Patient Care Program

Alejandra M. Dreisbach

The only way to predict the future is to have power to shape the future.
—Eric Hoffer, *The Passionate State of Mind* (1954)

This case centers on Karen, a nurse manager, on a hospital team given the task of defining and evaluating the feasibility of a new hospital venture—a cosmetic surgery center. The hospital where Karen works faces increased competitive pressures from rival institutions and has seen its revenues decrease because of the managed care environment. Sensitive to the media's prognostications about increased consumer demand for ways to diminish the effects of the aging process, the administrators decided to evaluate setting up an organized program for cosmetic surgery and skin laser treatments. A team with members from operations, marketing, and finance departments was formed to determine the feasibility of the venture.

Karen found that the members of her team approached their tasks with very different perspectives. Joan, the representative from marketing, was primarily concerned about competitive issues and how the program would be received by the public and physicians. Darlene, Manager of Finance and Budgets, made sure that the program was analyzed rigorously and that the group presented both the upside and negatives to the undertaking. The Director of Reimbursement, Don, helped the group understand the methods for setting charges and projecting net revenue generated by the program. Karen, representing operations, often pointed out the clinical implications of various options. George, the plastic surgeon, offered information on new developments in laser technology and the demand for various procedures based on his practice.

The team members were aware that their program proposal would be competing with other programs for funding. They would have to prove that their program would produce the best results for the hospital and put the finite resources of the organization, such as capital, labor, and physical space, to their best use.

The team had its work cut out for it. Team members needed to decide the feasibility of the program with accurate and realistic projections for the revenue and expense budgets. To begin, the team defined program objectives in detail. Cosmetic surgical cases had been done sporadically, but this new program was designed to provide a well-organized and comprehensive service for cosmetic and laser skin procedures. The goals for the new program were to position the hospital for longer term success by providing additional sources of revenue, additional patient traffic, visibility in the community, and the opportunity for physicians to use state-of-the-art technology. As an added benefit, it would help to maintain high utilization of the same-day surgery suites.

CASE: 9–1 *Continued*

■ REIMBURSEMENT ISSUES AND PAYMENT METHODOLOGIES

Karen's team recognized that its efforts had to begin with the revenue budget. To get their hands around the revenue budget, team members needed to understand the complex issues regarding reimbursement and the net revenue projected to be generated by the new program. Hospital administration would not authorize the program if the financial projections could not show a reasonable timeline for the program to cover its initial costs and generate a positive contribution to the bottom line.

Identification of net revenue in the current health care environment has become more difficult as the complexity of payment venues and the number of payors have increased. In most instances, patients do not assume full responsibility for their health care costs. They have insurance, the third-party payor. Third party is any agent other than the patient who contracts to pay all or part of the patient's hospital bill. The hospital and patient are the first two parties. Most third-party payors do not pay full price. Consequently, the identification of the payor mix and revenue stream is very important. Income for today's hospital is much like an airline—for the same service there is a mix of fares. Business travelers on a flight often pay three or four times more than the lowest price tickets "through special offers or advance booking with Saturday overnight stays." So, too, full-price patients receive the same services as those from insurance companies or Medicare patients with discounted fees.

In today's hospital, few patients pay the full rate. The provider's full rate covers all expenses incurred to deliver the service and provides a net contribution to the hospital's bottom line. Care is rendered with charges per episode, and inflationary or other increases in the costs of care are passed through to the payors of the health care services. Most payors now have negotiated a predetermined, or discounted, rate or fee for a particular package of services. The traditional form of indemnity insurance that paid 80 percent of full-rate reimbursement and required the patient to co-pay 20 percent of the hospital's full charges, as determined by the hospital, seems to have practically disappeared.

Public payors, which cover about 42 percent of the total cost of health care, consist of the federal, state, local governments, and CHAMPUS, the Civilian Health and Medical Program of Uniform Services. The other 58 percent of payments are made by private payors: Blue Cross, Blue Shield, commercial insurance companies, health maintenance organizations (HMOs), self-insured corporate entities, and individuals.

Medicare, the Biggest Payor of All

Medicare was enacted in 1965. It was the intention of Congress that Medicare would provide health insurance to protect the elderly or disabled from the substantial costs of acute health care services. The Medicare program was designed to cover services ordinarily furnished by hospitals, skilled nursing facilities (SNFs), and physicians. The

CASE: 9–1 *Continued*

Medicare Act prohibits payment for any expenses incurred for items or services "which are not reasonable or necessary for the diagnosis or treatment of illness, or injury, or to improve the functioning of a malformed body member" (Section 1862(a)(1)(A)). This statutory provision has been interpreted to exclude from Medicare coverage of those medical and health care services that have not been clinically shown to be safe and effective. Medicare approval of coverage for new procedures is followed carefully, as it often prompts third-party payors and state Medicaid plans to also cover a newly developed procedure.

The Medicare program today uses the prospective payment system (PPS), in which hospitals are paid using a rate designated in advance for treatment of a specific diagnosis. Hospitals are paid these fixed amounts or rates irrespective of the costs that they might have incurred. If the hospital can provide care at a lower cost than the amount paid by the Medicare program, the hospital has a positive contribution to the bottom line.

The basis for the PPS is the Diagnostic Related Groups (DRGs) system. The DRG refers to a classification system in which the disease codes are identified by the *International Classification of Diseases, 9th Revision, Clinical Modification* (ICD-9-CM) system. Codes are assigned to groups, within organ-related diagnostics categories. Patients are classified under a DRG based on their principal diagnosis. The principal diagnosis is determined based on the real reason for admission as known after treatment. The DRG is further subdivided according to the presence or absence of a surgical procedure, age of the patient, and presence or absence of complications. A complication is a condition that arises during the clinical stay and often increases the length of stay.

Any hospital that provides services at a cost below the standardized national payment rate makes a profit on that case. Any discharges provided at costs above the national rate results in a loss for the hospital.

The Medicare program is now developing and testing a prospective payment system for outpatient care called ambulatory patient groups (APGs). Medicare is looking at APGs as a means to control costs. Because of the way ambulatory care is now priced, Medicare now pays for certain outpatient services at a cost that exceeds a hospital inpatient day. With APGs, all charges for outpatient services, such as emergency room visits, will be lumped together (except the physician's fees).

Medicaid

The Medicaid program is administered by states and funded jointly by the federal government and states. Medicaid pays for the medical services of low-income pregnant women and children, and low-income elderly, blind, and disabled people. Each state sets its own level of income to qualify for Medicaid. There is no age limit for Medicaid; the only test is need. After elementary and secondary education, Medicaid is the largest component of state benefits. Because Medicaid spending has skyrock-

CASE: 9–1 *Continued*

eted, states have turned to managed care as a way to hold expenditures down. Although there are variations of the managed care program, typically the Medicaid program pays a capitation amount to an HMO to provide a set of services to Medicaid enrollees.

Other Third-Party Payors

Managed care is a convenient shorthand description for the range of alternatives to traditional health insurance programs. The largest managed care organizations are HMOs. An HMO is commonly defined as an organized system providing inpatient and outpatient health services to a voluntary enrolled population. The HMOs get an annual fee from the enrollees themselves or their employers as full payment for health care. The HMO is both a health insurer and a health care provider when it runs its own outpatient sites for primary and specialized care and, in some cases, its own hospitals. HMOs contract directly with outpatient providers and hospitals for services they do not provide in their own facilities.

Managed care organizations (MCOs) typically pay hospitals based on negotiated, discounted fee schedules. The hospital submits its claim in full and the MCO pays only their rate. The hospital, in turn, accepts this reimbursement as payment in full. Listed below are some payment modes associated with managed care:

- *Per diem.* Single payment for a day in the hospital irrespective of actual charges or costs incurred delivering services to a patient (flat per diem). In a staged per diem, the payment depends on the length of stay.
- *Sliding scales for discounts.* A percentage discount is applied to the total volume of admissions and outpatient procedures. An example of a sliding scale is a 10 percent reduction in charges for the level from zero to 500 bed days per year and a 15 percent reduction from 501 to 999 bed days per year.
- *Case rates.* Also called global contracts, the most common type is for obstetrics, with negotiated flat rates for a normal vaginal delivery and for a cesarean section. Specialty procedures at tertiary hospitals, such as coronary artery bypass surgery or heart transplants, are also more commonly being paid as flat rates.
- *Capitation.* This refers to the reimbursement that hospitals receive for providing care to a defined population. The payment is usually set at a rate per member per month (PMPM) basis to cover all institutional costs and may vary depending on the age and sex of the insured.

For the cosmetic surgery and skin laser program under evaluation, there would be limited potential for third-party reimbursement. Payors consider most cosmetic procedures as not medically necessary and would not cover them. Karen's team identified which procedures might be covered and the actual

CASE: 9–1 *Continued*

payment to be received after applying per-case rates or negotiated discounts from the total fee. For most procedures, the patient would be responsible for the entire bill. Therefore, the team recommended that charges be set to compete with other local programs, noting that volume would be highly dependent on meeting patient's financial expectations.

■ CHARGES

Karen was familiar with hospital charges. She knew that her hospital included the cost of inpatient nursing services as part of the room and board charges. A different amount was charged depending on the intensity of nursing care given to the patient, ancillary and special services commonly provided, and the average amount and types of supplies consumed. This was calculated for each of the different patient care areas of the hospital, such as intensive care, step down, or a medical/surgical unit.

In establishing the charge rate for the cosmetic and skin laser program, Karen's team was not constrained by regulatory agencies or rate-setting commissions that, in certain states, set specific rates for clinical procedures. Instead, they could recommend to hospital administration rates that would make the program successful while covering the program's costs.

Hospitals use many methodologies to set up charges or "list prices" of their services. One technique is to calculate the charge by first determining the actual payment to be made by the third-party payor and adding to that amount the out-of-pocket cost to the patient, and a certain markup factor set by the hospital. In other situations, the charge may be established after making a decision on what the market will bear. While working on this new program, Karen became involved in cost-based pricing, a more sophisticated method for establishing the charge rate. The team sought to identify the total cost of each procedure including the direct labor, supplies, and indirect costs such as an allocation for administrative expenses. Team members wanted to make sure that the charges reflected the real costs of the program. Simultaneously, they were aware of the aggressive and competitive environment in which the hospital operated. As a result, the hospital might have to discount its charges, for example, by not including all indirect costs, to be competitive. This would give the program a fair chance to get off the ground and capture volume from competing institutions. Because of the current reimbursement environment of heavily discounted charges negotiated by payors, the hospital administration regarded charges as more nearly a measure of actual costs rather than as costs plus desired return on investment.

The team went on to project the annual revenue budget, taking into account the number and type of procedures, gross charges, and potential net revenue. The team members struggled to reach a compromise about the number of procedures to be done. Some members were optimistic the program would take off quickly and fill in the available surgical time in the ambulatory care center. Others argued that because of the

CASE: 9–1 *Continued*

competition and the entrenched habits of physicians it would take a long time to get the program up to its full capacity. Eventually they compromised by reducing the utilization rates in the first 3 years of the 5-year plan. Accurate projections of the utilization rate may be the single most difficult and critical input into a program analysis. It has a major impact not only on the projected revenues, but also on the cost associated with hiring staff or spending capital for changes required for the new endeavor.

■ IDENTIFYING THE COSTS OF THE PROGRAM

Once the team projected the revenue budget, members worked on various models to decide the projected costs of the program. Karen helped identify the clinical resources needed to carry out the program. Initial investment or start-up costs of a program may include marketing, advertising, and capital equipment required to build and equip the program. Joan from marketing had conducted a survey of the competition and potential market. All the organizations that offer or might offer this service in the future had been assessed. Joan had information on their prices, service packages, facility setups, and the perceived level of client satisfaction.

Darlene led the team in the preparation of an analysis of capital costs for equipment, and the renovation and enhancement of the physical plant for the cosmetic surgery and skin laser setup. For their analysis, classical financial evaluation techniques such as net present value and internal rate of return were effectively used. The team was aware that because the hospital had several projects competing for finite capital resources, administration might apply a profitability index (PI) methodology to rank the alternatives. The PI is calculated by dividing the present value of cash inflows of each program by the present value of cash outflows. Using this index, the project with the highest ranking, rather than the highest net present value, is selected for investment.

One specific concern of the team considering the program was the high expense of the laser skin equipment. The equipment would have to be depreciated quickly (3 years or less) to cover the equipment's high cost and potential for rapid obsolescence. The depreciation expense would have to be added as part of the total cost. If the same-day surgery center were not used, examination tables, supply carts and some renovation would be needed. However, if all the procedures were to be done in the center, the physical setup would require only minor modification and very little additional equipment.

Karen provided the clinical information required to estimate the operating costs for each year of the project. She based her assumptions on the volume of procedures projected for the program. The team then evaluated costs based on the type and length of the procedures and the length of stay of the patient in the facility.

For any intervention, there are direct expenses such as staff salaries. In

CASE: 9–1 *Continued*

this case, direct expenses included salaries for nurses and technicians with laser and intravenous certification, salary benefits, and supplies. Some expenses would be variable; they would fluctuate with the volume of procedures done. Others would be fixed expenses, which are incurred regardless of the quantity of patients seen. The lease cost of equipment is an example of a fixed expense. Karen identified needed patient supplies and other related expenses, such as maintenance of equipment. The team decided which expenses would be part of the base charge and which would be charged separately, only when needed. Drugs and anesthetics, for example, were chosen to be separate charges because use of these items varied by specific procedure and patient.

Besides direct charges, indirect expenses needed to be charged to the program to get an accurate picture of the total cost to the hospital. At Karen's hospital, indirect costs charged to all programs include an allocation of general expenses, such as hospital administration; nonpatient care departments, such as billing, dietary, housekeeping, and security; utility fees; and routine building maintenance and repairs. Overhead costs specific to the program, such as program management and computer equipment, are also included.

Any revenues left after all direct, indirect, and overhead costs are charged to the program or deducted from the payment, become the positive (or contribution) margin. Ideally, all hospital endeavors should have a positive margin. Health care institutions, like other organizations, need to generate enough net income to be able to fund future activities and continue to carry on their mission through the purchase of new equipment and other capital assets.

■ STAKEHOLDERS

With this new program, there are many interested parties or stakeholders. One interested party is the admitting physician. Increasingly, physicians are interested in services that are not paid by insurers due to the limits on fees set by managed care. Plastic surgery, dermatology, and podiatry are some specialties best positioned to have the patient be a self-payor. Physicians provide the essential link between the patient and the hospital. To a large extent, physicians will decide where a procedure is to be performed based on their association with institutions, their normal practices, and the perceived quality and experience of the hospital staff.

Another significant stakeholder is the patient. Patients' interest in value for their dollar is increased when they are paying out-of-pocket. Potential patients have an array of choices and decisions to make. They need to choose a physician, a location for a procedure—in a physician's office, freestanding surgical center, or a hospital's same-day surgery area—and much more. Patients will also decide how much of an intervention to have—one or several procedures at one time. These decisions will have a significant impact on cost.

Karen's group considered the total cost to the patient for a procedure. The

CASE: 9—1 *Continued*

total cost includes different fees: the physician's, the facility's (hospital, surgical center, or physician's office), and the anesthesia fee. The total cost of the procedure will also vary according to the complexity and time involved. Patients need to be keenly aware of what will be considered reimbursable, if anything, by their insurance company.

Third-party payors represent a third leg of interested parties. With surgical cosmetic procedures, payors often consider medical necessity on a case-by-case basis.

While Karen's team sought to analyze the cosmetic surgery and laser skin programs from a strict financial perspective, the team recognized that patients and physicians as well as third-party payors, are really looking for value. All the participants will inevitably consider the quality received in relation to the price paid. Value has been defined by Nauert (1996) as the beneficial relationship of quality divided by cost: Value = quality/cost. From the patient's standpoint, quality consists of variety of choice; the provider's image, service experiences, and convenience of access. The cost most considered in determining value is the amount out-of-pocket as a deductible or co-payment or the total amount paid all at once or by installments by cash or credit. Value to patients is generally understood to mean getting the desired outcome—the fundamental criteria, with a minimum of suffering, at a minimum out-of-pocket cost.

For the payor, reliable information on cost and quality, improved health status for beneficiaries, providers' image,

lines of services, and outcomes are important. Providers must raise the perceived worth or quality of their services and/or reduce the cost of their services to secure insurance contracts. Both costs and quality are examined by the payor.

The admitting physician is probably in the best position to compare quality of service and care. Nurses can have a powerful impact on the perception of all these stakeholders because of their skills and capabilities and their willingness to make the extra effort.

Tabbush (1994) described a technique of value analysis based on estimating which components of a provider's costs are out of line with the benefits they deliver to the customer. The patient identifies a series of outcomes as desired, ranking them by importance. The health care provider identifies alternate modalities of care that may be acceptable to a patient and approximates how each approach relates to the patient's desired outcomes. Then, the cost factor is added and the intervention with the highest value index is identified. A major implication of value analysis is that individuals may (1) value the same outcomes differently, and (2) place different values on alternative modalities of care. Because of these individual differences, the appropriate clinical modality of treatment that maximizes value must be individually determined. Value analysis increases a hospital's awareness of customer differences in both desired outcomes and commensurate costs that will be competitive in today's marketplace.

CASE: 9–1 *Continued*

■ TEAM RECOMMENDATION

Karen's team concluded that the new program made sense for the institution. The team's report showed the cosmetic surgery program would be financially beneficial and positive for the hospital's image. However, the financial analysis for the skin laser component argued against its implementation. The cost of the equipment was very high, the predicted volume only moderate, and there was every indication that new technologies in skin lasers would force the hospital to replace equipment on an accelerated schedule. The team decided not to recommend proceeding with the skin laser program.

As it happened, hospital management accepted the team's recommendation and the cosmetic surgery program was initiated. The hospital found that it had to adjust pricing as it implemented the program. Admitting physicians complained about some charges for procedures when compared to those previously performed in the freestanding surgery centers. The hospital began promoting the cosmetic surgery center in its advertising and organized a series of open houses for patients considering cosmetic surgery. These marketing activities began to pay off in increased volumes. A year and half later, the cosmetic surgery center was considered a success.

■ BIOGRAPHICAL SKETCH

Alejandra M. Dreisbach is the Director of Value Management, Budget and Reimbursement for Robert Wood Johnson University Hospital in New Brunswick, New Jersey. Her initial assignment at Robert Wood was as Finance Manager of the Nursing Division. Previously, Ms. Dreisbach held financial positions at the Bendix Corporation and the American Cancer Society. She holds an MBA with a concentration in finance from the Wharton School, University of Pennsylvania, and an undergraduate degree in psychology. Ms. Dreisbach is the author of several articles and chapters for health care publications and has given presentations to national audiences. She is an Advanced Member of the Healthcare Financial Management Association and a Diplomate of the American College of Healthcare Executives.

■ REFERENCES

Nauert, R.C. (1996). The quest for value in health care. *Journal of Health Care Finance, 22* (3), 52–61.

Tabbush, V. (1994). Improving health care through an economic approach to health care management. *Clinical Obstetrics and Gynecology, 37* (1), 216–234.

10

Information Systems for Managing Patient Care

Susan K. Newbold

Nurses in all settings need data for decision making about patient care and organizational management. Data are the raw facts—the building blocks of information. The key task is to filter through the vast amount of data collected in the course of patient care activities and to organize that data into information needed to guide patient care, run the organization, and manage human resources.

Although much effort is taking place in automating information processes, the use of technology in health care is 5 to 10 years behind other industries (Crowe & Eckstein, 1995). The expenditures for information technology in health care have averaged 2.6 percent of the total budget compared to the manufacturing industry, which averages 5 percent, and 7 percent for banking. Considering the low investment coupled with the dynamic nature of the health care environment, it is no wonder that information technology in health care lags behind other industries.

The purpose of this chapter is to describe the development of management information systems (MISs) and identify the trends and issues that affect health care MISs today. The environment in which these systems are implemented has an important influence on the success of any project. The nurse in patient care administration has an important role in understanding MISs—how they impact patient care and how they facilitate or frustrate the providers of that care. This chapter will not provide basic information on computer applications in nursing. See the suggested readings for resources describing computer functions, types of hardware and software, and nursing roles.

■ MANAGEMENT INFORMATION SYSTEMS

An automated MIS is a combination of hardware, software, and people for the purpose of accomplishing a specific task. The hardware, which is the physical equipment, such as the computer, monitor, modem, printer, and cables, has changed rapidly within the 40 years computers have been used in health care. Hardware is now more powerful, smaller, and less expensive than in previous years. In the past, large mainframe computers were needed to handle the workload of the health care environment; today, many functions can be undertaken by notebook computers.

Cost Effectiveness

Although computer-based MISs have been part of most organization's activities for more than 40 years, there are many fundamental issues of MISs that are still as important today as they were at the onset of the computer revolution. The essential concept of MISs has always been to harness technology for the reduction of unit costs and improvement of productivity. The verb *harness* is particularly appropriate, as it brings to mind the problems encountered by a farmer in the preindustrial era to bring an earlier technology— horses and mules—to productive use. Early uses were primitive and limited to a few jobs. Effective use of horses and mules involved farmers having a detailed knowledge of both the animal's capabilities and the commands and training processes to improve productivity.

The harnessing of MISs requires similar knowledge. It has always been associated with the productive use of computer hardware, software, and computing experts along with the careful nurturing of the users and computer system. Nurses today typically receive some instruction in use of computers and health care applications in their basic education. Agencies are also aware of the need for both those with expertise in computers and clinical issues to work together to improve the health information systems (HISs) in all types of provider agencies from an isolated physician's office or nursing center to a national or international corporation.

The fundamental importance of the concept of unit costs per service in an MIS is shown in Figure 10–1. The vertical scale shows unit costs of delivery of a service, and the horizontal scale reflects the total volume of services delivered. The horizontal line labeled manual system shows that the unit cost of a completely hand-operated process changes little over different ranges of volume. For example, a patient order entry system that involved writing down each entry with a pen and paper would have a unit cost that varies lit-

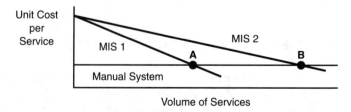

FIGURE 10–1. Effect of increased volume on unit cost per service.

tle with volume of orders. Each order would take about the same amount of time to transcribe. But if automated systems are introduced, such as the two downward sloping lines in the diagram, there is an opportunity to seize major cost advantages—as long as there is sufficient volume to overcome the investment cost and to take advantage of the computer's relative speed in performing the task. These are the fundamental questions in purchasing systems—Will it be capable of reducing unit costs, and how many ways may it increase unit productivity? Without this framework of decision making, the computer resource may be left unharnessed and many potential benefits never realized. In fact, it may be a poor investment.

It can also be seen from Figure 10–1 that points A and B represent the minimum volumes of services in which automation will save money, using reduced unit cost of service delivery as the criterion. Notice also, that automated systems 1 and 2 are not the same. One is more expensive to operate than the other. The decision whether to purchase system 1 or system 2 would be based on cost and other criteria, such as the number of ways each might increase unit productivity. These criteria are discussed later in the chapter.

Who Benefits from MIS?

The "M" in MIS was included originally because the benefits were thought to accrue primarily to top management. In fact, it is now generally agreed that all levels of management and patient care providers benefit from an MIS. The patient care provider benefits from the MIS with knowledge of the patient's status, services received, scheduling, and resources available for care. The first-line manager, often called the operational manager, is the individual responsible for day-to-day decisions. These decisions have a time horizon of days or weeks. In the nursing context, this person is the equivalent of a unit or ambulatory center manager. An MIS would be used by that person for scheduling personnel, budgeting, quality improvement, patient classification, and appointment or admission scheduling (if decentralized).

The second-line or tactical manager has broader responsibilities and a longer time horizon for decision impact. The director of a patient care service or division whose responsibilities focus on the implementation of organizational change and strategic initiatives is an example of a tactical manager. These individuals have to make plans for months or even years ahead. They need aggregate data related to the performance of units, equipment, and facilities. They have input in major financial decisions affecting their functional area. They use MISs for reports on exceptions, projected budgets and variances, comparisons of costs and performance, and so forth.

The early MISs were directed toward meeting the needs of these two types of managers. These systems are capable of furnishing reports, inventory balances, shift data, and patient population comparisons quickly and accurately. In fact, nearly all the popular success stories of MISs were framed in the context of greater availability of timely summary data and the great improvements in productivity that have resulted.

The most information-starved manager of all is at the third level. These managers—called top management, executive management, or strategic management—had historically been little served by MISs. Nurses who are executive directors of home care companies, in corporate positions of health systems or managed care organizations, or part of the top executive team of large hospitals are in this type of position. Their decision span is several years, with ongoing adjustments to fit the dynamic environment. They need information to support decision making, monitor environmental trends, and benchmark their competitors. Recently, more decision support systems have been developed to meet their needs.

The MIS Growth Cycle

Nolan (1979), in his classic article, elaborated the six stages in the growth of MIS development. He also points out that different divisions in the same organization may be experiencing different stages of growth. This model has been widely applied to many disciplines, including nursing information systems (NISs) (Suding, 1984). Table 10–1 describes this cycle. It consists of six stages of computer system (CS) development, each characterized by behaviors in CS applications, CS planning and control, and user versus CS personnel involvement. Applications slowly expand from automation (stages I, II) to include management decision making (stages III through V) and then strategic planning (stage VI). Nolan argues that many organizations never even approach stage IV, where major benefits can be attained due to issues of user acceptance, control of information, and poor communication between CS personnel and users. Development of MIS growth needs to be assessed periodically by administrators for pervasiveness of functional applications and adequacy of technology. Growth should be systematically planned using a CS steering committee in the early stages and placement of CS experts in executive management positions in later stages.

Fortunately, a cadre of nurses specializing in nursing informatics has developed. There are now two masters degree programs in Nursing Informatics, and many graduate courses available in schools of nursing. There are also many nurses who have developed expertise in information systems and telecommunications on the job. Nursing informatics was officially recognized as a specialty by the American Nurses Association in 1992 (Milholland, 1992), and certification became available at the generalist level in 1995. Nurses with this expertise work both for health care providers to assist in the selection, implementation, and ongoing monitoring of the adequacy of MISs and for vendors, assisting in the development of new health care applications and the sales of products.

TABLE 10–1. Stages of MIS Growth

	I INITIATION	II CONTAGION	III CONTROL	IV INTEGRATION	V DATA ADMINISTRATION	VI MATURITY
CS applications	Financial automation	Widespread automation	Upgrade and restructure systems for databases	Apply database technology	Integration of internal information	Integration of internal and external information
CS plan and control	Financial application demonstrates savings	Facilitate and expand applications	Formalize planning and control over applications	Refine to match supply and demand	Network sharing databases	Balance supply and demand
User vs CS personnel involvement	User: "hands off"; CS: accountable	Limited number of users receive data CS: controls and designs	User: "more" active role but still CS: dependent and few trained	User: defines needs CS: designs solutions	User: designs solutions CS: support	Joint user and CS accountability

CS, computer systems.
Adapted from Nolan (1979), pp. 115–126.

Health Care Management Information Systems

Computers are used to support nursing management in all settings—hospitals, long-term care, home health agencies, and nurse-managed centers. A nursing management information system typically consists of the components in Table 10–2.

A classification and acuity system categorizes clients individually or in a group, based on nursing care needs. The results are transferred to systems that manage and schedule nurse resources. Cost accounting systems identify the cost of providing nursing services and running the organization. Software to prepare department budgets, prepare the payroll, and manage finances are used by nursing administrators. Quality management systems gather data from other automated sources to provide a "report card" of department activities. Many of the word processing and communication activities of the nursing department can be provided by various office automation functions. Integrated packages that include word processing, databases, spreadsheets, presentation packages and scheduling are useful for sharing data between the applications.

■ SELECTION

Key Variables

In designing an optimal MIS, managers need to consider both people and computer variables. These have been summarized by Emery (1987) as:

People Variables

- Availability of relevant inputs.
- Timeliness of the database, including response time between an event and its recording in the database.
- Accuracy; agreement between stored and actual data.
- Backup; redundancy; frequency with which copies are made to provide protection against loss.
- Adequacy of training programs.
- Performance standards that include computer-based reports and presentations.

TABLE 10–2. Nursing Administration Applications of MISs

Client classification and acuity
Cost accounting
Budgeting and financial management
Resource scheduling
Resource utilization
Quality management
Office automation

Hardware Variables

- Variety of transactions that can be handled.
- Flexibility; relative ease with which the system can be modified.
- Reliability; probability that the system will operate satisfactorily without breakdowns.
- Availability of support and maintenance personnel, including that supplied by contract from the vendor.
- Space and special environmental requirements, such as air conditioning and electricity demands.
- Peripherals available; input and output devices.
- Capability of network server for internal communications.
- Cost to purchase and to maintain.

Software Variables

- Robustness; the extent that the system safeguards against user errors.
- User friendliness; the degree of familiarity with computer language that the user needs in learning the system.
- Security; protection against unauthorized access or loss of system resources.
- Generality; the range of functions provided.
- Degree of "intelligence," or the complexity of logical steps the programs can perform.
- Availability of packaged programs versus programmer-created programs.
- Transportability of programs between computers and of information between programs.
- Lack of errors in the source code (program itself).
- Maintainability or ease of updating and correcting.

The nurse manager must actively participate in the selection, installation, and evaluation of any system that affects patient care. Several documents written by nurses are available to assist the nurse manager in learning specifically about selecting and installing an information system (Abbott, 1996; McAlindon, 1995; Mills, 1995; Mills, 1996). Nurses must be involved to make certain that the systems selected meet the patient care needs and those of the nursing workforce.

■ TRENDS AND ISSUES IN PROFESSIONAL PRACTICE

The demand in health care organizations today is for meeting enterprise-wide needs for data while continuing to manage financial, human resource, and clinical data systems. Organizations need to integrate existing information systems and add new information systems. The move to prospective and capitated financing is forcing organizations to change from charge-based accounting systems to cost accounting. This requires integration of clinical and financial data. The other new environmental demand is for the collection and analysis of significant amounts of data to measure clinical outcomes. This is moving efforts to standardize nomenclature ahead as an essential precursor to comparing quality and outcomes data between delivery organizations.

A multitude of activities focusing on computing in the health care environment are taking place today. The principal activities of interest to nurses in patient care administration are: the computerized patient record, managed care, advances in information technology, and changes in regulation and accreditation requirements.

Computerized Patient Record

In April 1991, the Institute of Medicine of the National Academy of Sciences completed an 18-month study on improving patient records in response to the need for better information management and increasing technological advances. The study committee examined the current state of medical record systems, identified impediments to the development and use of improved record systems, identified ways to overcome impediments to improved medical records, and developed a research agenda to advance medical record systems. Finally, the multidisciplinary committee recommended policies and other strategies to achieve these improvements. The conclusions and recommendations of the study were described in *The Computer-based Patient Record: An Essential Technology for Health Care* (Dick & Steen, 1991).

The Institute of Medicine advisors cited the advantages of a computized patient record as including: the ability to maintain longitudinal records, the instantaneous availability of information, the increased possibilities for health care research, the improvement in legibility, the provision of data to support decision making, and the capability to use triggers and reminders to reduce liability. The limitations of implementing the computerized patient record were judged to be: the varying levels of provider readiness, the varying levels of security and confidentiality capabilities, the complexity and amount of data, the nonexistence of a standardized method to assign each person a unique identifier, and the knowledge that reengineering and change are painful. One outcome of this study was the incorporation of an organization in Chicago, Illinois, in 1992, the Computer-Based Patient Record Institute, to facilitate the creation and implementation of a computerized patient record. Much work by the participating organizations has been accomplished, but work is ongoing. The computerized patient record is not yet a reality in the majority of health care organizations today. Achievement of a computerized patient record will take many years. Meanwhile, many sections of this record, such as nursing progress notes, physician order entry, and laboratory reporting, are being developed and used.

Managed Care Trends

Managed care, case management, and consolidation of providers over the continuum of care are trends taking place in today's health care environment that are having an impact on the way nursing conducts business. New information infrastructures are being developed to integrate information between agencies in the same system over a continuum of care.

Managed care is a clinical system that organizes and sequences the caregiving process to better achieve cost and quality outcomes. The goals of managed care include the achievement of expected and standardized patient outcomes, appropriate use of health services, a continuity of care, collaborative practice, and client discharge within the appropriate length of stay. With a case management approach, clinicians become accountable for patient outcomes and continuing contact beyond one episode of care. Case management facilitates the consumer's lifelong access to health care–related services. To achieve a managed care approach, organizations are being reshaped to reduce costs, become more comprehensive, and provide better health outcomes. Enterprises that a few years ago consisted of one hospital and possibly a physician office building now include complex networks of physicians' offices, clinics and ambulatory centers, hospitals, home health agencies, long-term and specialized care facilities, health maintenance organizations, insurance policy options, and medical device and pharmaceutical companies. The information technology demands are enormous to support this complex business infrastructure.

Advances in Information Technology

In the past, health care software applications provided the health care professional with limited flexibility. This has led to poorly installed systems with limited benefits that are difficult for individual organizations or departments to use and modify. Newer health care applications are incorporating technologies that enable the users to modify information processes to fit unique needs or to change as business processes change. For example, the graphical user interface (GUI) is a personal computer-based application that allows the user to easily open and navigate through applications. The GUI has been adopted by most health care information system vendors and enhances the ability of the organization to train users to do multiple applications and to install new applications as needed.

Natural language processing (voice recognition) and handwriting recognition are emerging technologies not yet widely integrated into MISs. Voice-recognition software can be trained to recognize and understand an individual voice and can be used to input and process data. A few applications of voice technology have been used by radiologists and emergency room physicians with limited success. Difficulties in computers recognizing the wide variety of ways individuals form letters has slowed the development of hand-writing recognition technology for admissions, patient records, and other health care applications.

The use of advanced telecommunications in the health care arena is called telehealth or, more popularly, telemedicine. Telecommunications (Skiba, 1995) is the use of wire, radio, optical, or other electromagnetic channels to transmit or receive signals for voice, data, and video communications. Nurses use telecommunications in its simplest form when providing advice over the telephone system. For more advanced use of telecommunications, nurses in pilot projects use sound, video, and text to send and receive data in home care. There is much unexplored potential for this technology within the nursing field.

The Internet and the World Wide Web are technologies that are beginning to be exploited by nurses. Online resources for nurses fall into categories of communications with other people, reference materials, and continuing education. Communication between health care professionals within and between organizations is increasingly occurring through the use of electronic mail. Nurses are also using Internet interactive options to pose questions about clinical care dilemmas and quickly receive comments and suggestions from nurses anywhere in the world with an Internet connection. Communication links from the office or nursing station can promote efficient retrieval of reference materials with clinical, administrative, research, and educational information. Literature searches for reference materials can be conducted locally using a variety of databases at the National Library of Medicine in Maryland from worldwide sites. Some services provide for the delivery of the actual text of a requested article. Continuing education and credit course work can now be delivered using distance technologies. Nurses who are geographically distant from universities offering desired programs or those in isolated, rural areas can now have access to electronic classrooms. Online resources can also be accessed by the public seeking either scientific knowledge about a health problem or support and coping ideas from others experiencing similar health problems. Nurses can begin to evaluate the implications of Internet technologies for health care processes and outcomes.

Regulatory and Accreditation Requirements

Federal laws and accreditation requirements affect the development and use of information systems for managing patient care. The Safe Medical Devices Act and Joint Commission on Accreditation of Healthcare Organizations (JCAHO) guidelines are highlighted as examples of this impact on health care.

The Food and Drug Administration (FDA) published final rules for the Safe Medical Devices Act of 1990, which took effect in April of 1996 (Pub. L. No. 101-629, 1990). The Act and the regulations establish a uniform system for all medical device user facilities and manufacturers to use in reporting adverse events related to medical devices. The breadth of the Act and the regulations, both with respect to the variety of providers covered and the definition of what constitutes a medical device, will have implications for a large number of health care providers. An FDA software policy is under development at this time. For example, the emerging use of computer-aided diagnostic equipment is subject to this rule. Implications for nurse practitioners using such equipment or participating in the development of computer-aided diagnostic equipment have yet to be explored.

The JCAHO (1996) published guidelines for information management across all disciplines. There are no requirements specific to nursing, although examples of practical applications of managing technology are indicated that can directly affect the nursing workforce. Nurses may be called upon to conduct an internal needs assessment, to include such information as: the time needed to document patient care activities; a definition of hospital information-management needs; an evaluation of existing systems; criteria for selecting software and hardware; and the value of documenting on bedside terminals. As agencies incorporate more computer technology, nursing work may include receiving laboratory and radiology reports electronically; aggregating patient-specific data; querying health care literature databases; comparing the performance of the organization to other organizations using external databases; and compiling performance improvement statistics to report rates and trends. Nurse executives need to be aware of opportunities to harness technology and prepare clinicians to confidently make full use of technology's potential contribution to information management.

■ BENEFITS OF TECHNOLOGY

In this age of process reengineering, nurse managers can use technology to promote better use of staff resources. Documentation of patient progress notes, word processing for correspondence, electronic mail, personnel databases, and budget spreadsheets can be used to improve documentation, communication, and planning in the nursing office and at the patient care site. Nursing practice can be assisted by using standardized assessment and documentation forms online to promote a uniformly high level of patient care. Services to clients, including nursing interventions, can be tracked and outcomes of care can be documented and measured. Costs can be tracked more readily using automated systems. All these benefits of technology lead toward the goal of providing improved patient care at an affordable cost. These benefits are summarized in Table 10–3 and discussed in more detail in the monograph by Saba, Johnson, and Simpson (1994).

TABLE 10–3. Benefits of Information Technology for Nursing

Better utilization of nursing staff resources

Improved documentation, communication, and planning

Standardized nursing practice

Tracking of nursing services

Measurement of outcomes

Improved cost accountability

Improved patient care

Summarized from: Saba, Johnson, & Simpson (1994), p. 1.

■ INFORMATION SYSTEMS FOR MANAGING PATIENT CARE

Nurses first used automated systems in hospitals to manage patient care orders and results. Later, the planning for and documentation of that care was added in many information systems. Many health care information systems now have modules that admit, discharge, and transfer clients; order tests and receive results; document patient progress; access patient status; manage patient appointments and bills; and provide for trending and graphics. Some organizations are installing the second and third generation of information systems, while others have not yet provided applications that directly assist nurses in providing and managing patient care.

Nurse managers need to be familiar with the use of administrative decision support systems for budgeting, managing, planning, and evaluating care delivery and to consider further developing the MIS infrastructure surrounding these processes. Development includes the assessment of information needs, system selection and implementation, and ongoing interest in current and future applications in nursing administration. The nurse administrator must be able to utilize information management skills for the purpose of managing the delivery of health care. The primary intent of using a nursing MIS is the provision of information to make decisions about the effective and efficient allocation of resources for the highest quality of patient care (Hannah & Shamian, 1992).

Information Technology Affects Nursing Practice

All nurses have a role in managing information whether or not it is part of an automated health care information system. A task force of the American Nurses Association created *The Scope of Practice for Nursing Informatics* (1994), which clearly indicated minimum informatics competencies for all graduates of basic nursing programs. It is the work of *all* nurses to:

identify, collect, and record data relevant to the nursing care of patients; analyze and interpret patient and nursing information as part of the planning for and provision of nursing services; employ health-care informatics applications designed for the clinical practice of nursing; and, implement public and institutional policies related to privacy, confidentiality, and security of information. These include patient care information, confidential employer information, and other information gained in the nurse's professional capacity. (p. 12)

Nursing informatics as defined by Graves and Corcoran (1989, p. 227) is a combination of nursing science, information science, and computer science to manage and process nursing data, information, and knowledge to facilitate delivery of health care. The definition highlights the goal of nursing informatics as supporting the delivery of nursing care.

Issues and Strategies

Shamian and Hannah (1995) reviewed issues and challenges regarding data for health information systems and proposed strategies for managing data. They indicate reliability and validity; real-time data versus retrospective data, and availability of data across the episode of care as current issues. One suggested strategy for promoting the collection of data that are reliable and valid is conducting regular checks for accuracy and completeness of data. Many individuals have the erroneous belief that data found in a computer system are correct. This will only be true if compliance with procedures for data input are monitored and corrected as needed. Regarding timeliness of data needed, one needs to document a time component when specifying data needs. Systems that provide real-time data may generally suit the need of the nurse executives.

Integration of data available across the continuum of care is a new need that nurses in patient care administration must make a high priority to support case management and capitated payment. Another need for integration is the linking of clinical data with financial and administrative data for clients in all settings. These links are needed to define cost, quality, and outcome components. Partnerships with nursing, other care providers, finance, human resources, and information services will facilitate integration. Other strategies suggested by Shamian and Hannah (1995) include: establishing a solid nursing informatics expertise in the department to remain current with health care information system innovations, educating nonclinical administrators about clinical care, and learning the language and detail of data requirements.

To improve both tactical and operational management within nursing, nurse administrators need to actively promote automation of their work areas and the corresponding training necessary to promote the health care organization's information technology. One option to support management decision making is to implement use of a nursing management minimum data set (Huber et al., 1992). This core data will assist in decisions comparing units/ division productivity and quality.

Due to the rapid changes in information technology, patient care administrators need to monitor the need to upgrade hardware and software. To remain competitive, they should recruit or internally train a member of their management team to be an expert in information technology in order to spearhead the design, implementation, and ongoing maintenance of the relevant components of the information system.

As nurse administrators are involved in strategic management for the total organization, they also need to be involved in the strategic vision for the technology that supports patient care and the work of nurses. The challenge of using information systems in patient care will always be one of integrating people systems and computer systems to increase productivity and quality while decreasing cost. Only by keeping this challenge as a top organizational priority will the information systems of the future become a reality.

■ BIOGRAPHICAL SKETCH

Susan K. Newbold is Manager, Database Administration for University Physicians in Baltimore, Maryland. She is also a doctoral candidate at the University of Maryland at Baltimore School of Nursing, where her emphasis area is Nursing Informatics. She received her BSN from Ball State University in Muncie, Indiana, and her MS in Nursing from the University of Maryland at Baltimore. She was previously employed by a hospital, hardware and software vendors, and a consulting firm in various roles relating to health care informatics in over 15 years of practice. She is a leader in nursing informatics, having co-founded the first regional nursing informatics group, and conducts intensive workshops for informatics nurses. She has published extensively in this field and has spoken at national and international conferences in the United States, Singapore, and Australia. In 1996, she received a Certificate of Appreciation from the National League for Nursing Council for Nursing Informatics to honor her contribution in nursing informatics, and she is certified in Nursing Informatics by the American Nurses Credentialing Center. She is President of the second largest chapter of the Sigma Theta Tau International Honor Society of Nursing.

■ SUGGESTED READINGS

Basic Information on Computers in Nursing

Joos, I., Whitman, N.I., Smith, M.J., & Nelson, R. (1996). *Computers in small bytes: The computer workbook* (2nd ed.). New York: NLN Press.

Saba, V.K., & McCormick, K.A. (1996). *Essentials of computers for nurses* (2nd ed.). New York: McGraw-Hill.

Simpson, R.L. (1993). *The nurse executive's guide to directing and managing nursing information systems.* Ann Arbor, MI: The Center for Healthcare Information Management.

Information on New Developments in Information Technology and Nursing

American Nurses Association. (1995). *Nursing data systems: The emerging framework.* Washington, DC: American Nurses Publishing.

Computers in nursing. Philadelphia: Lippincott-Raven.

Field, M.J. (Ed.). (1996). *Telemedicine: A guide to assessing telecommunications in health care.* Washington, DC: National Academy Press.

Kissinger, K., & Borchardt, S. (Eds.). (1996). *Information technology for integrated health systems: Positioning for the future.* New York: Wiley.

Newbold, S.K. & Jaffe, M. (1995). Electronic resources for nursing. In M.J. Ball, K.J. Hannah, S.K. Newbold, & J.V. Douglas (Eds.), *Nursing informatics: Where caring and technology meet* (2nd ed.). New York: Springer-Verlag.

Zielstorff, R.D., Hudgings, C.I., & Grobe, S.J. (1993). *Next-generation nursing information systems.* Washington, DC: American Nurses Publishing.

■ REFERENCES

Abbott, P.A. (1996). The nursing manager's role in successful system implementation. In M.E. Mills, C.A. Romano, & B.R. Heller (Eds.), *Information management in nursing and health care.* Springhouse, PA: Springhouse Corporation.

American Nurses Association. (1994). *The scope of practice for nursing informatics.* Washington, DC: American Nurses Publishing.

American Nurses Association. (1995). *Standards of practice for nursing informatics.* Washington, DC: American Nurses Publishing.

Crowe, G.D., & Eckstein, M.G. (1995). Health information networks. In M.J. Ball, D.W. Simborg, J.W. Albright, & J.V. Douglas (Eds.), *Healthcare information management systems: A practical guide* (2nd ed.). New York: Springer-Verlag.

Dick, R.S., & Steen, E.B. (1991). *The computer-based patient record: An essential technology for health care.* Washington, DC: National Academy Press.

Emery, J.C. (1987). *Management information systems: The critical strategic force.* Oxford, England: Oxford University Press.

Graves, J.R., & Corcoran, S. (1989). The Study of Nursing Informatics. *Image, 21* (4), 227–231.

Hannah, K.J., & Shamian, J. (1992). Integrating a nursing professional practice model and nursing informatics in a collective bargaining environment. *Nursing Clinics of North America, 27,* 31–45.

Huber, D.G., Delaney, C., Crossley, J., Mehmert, M., & Ellerby, S. (1992). A nursing management minimum data set. *Journal of Nursing Administration, 22* (7/8), 35–40.

Joint Commission on Accreditation of Health Care Organizations. (1996). *1996 Comprehensive accreditation manual for hospitals.* Oakbrook Terrace, IL: JCAHO.

McAlindon, M.N. (1995). Choosing and installing an information system. In M.J. Ball, D.W. Simborg, J.W. Albright, & J.V Douglas (Eds.), *Healthcare information management systems: A practical guide* (2nd ed.). New York: Springer-Verlag.

Milholland, D.K. (1992). Congress says informatics is nursing specialty. *The American Nurse, 24* (4), 1.

Mills, M. (1995). Computerization: Priorities for nursing administration. In M.J. Ball, D.W. Simborg, J.W. Albright, & J.V. Douglas (Eds.), *Healthcare information management systems: A practical guide* (2nd ed.). New York: Springer-Verlag.

Mills, M. (1996). Nursing participation in the selection of healthcare information systems. In M.J. Ball, K.J. Hannah, S.K. Newbold, & J.V. Douglas (Eds.). *Nursing informatics: Where caring and technology meet* (2nd ed.). New York: Springer-Verlag.

Public Law 101–629 (H.R. 3095), November 28, 1990.

Nolan, R. (1979). Managing the crisis in data processing. *Harvard Business Review, 57* (2), 115–126.

Saba, V.K., Johnson, J.E., & Simpson, R.L. (1994). *Computers in nursing management.* Washington, DC: American Nurses Publishing.

Shamian, J., & Hannah, K.J. (1995). Management information systems for the nurse executive. In M.J. Ball, K.J. Hannah, S.K. Newbold, & J.V. Douglas (Eds.), *Nursing informatics: Where caring and technology meet* (2nd ed.). New York: Springer-Verlag.

Skiba, D.J. (1995). Health-oriented telecommunications. In M.J. Ball, K.J. Hannah, S.K. Newbold, & J.V. Douglas (Eds.), *Nursing informatics: Where caring and technology meet* (2nd ed.). New York: Springer-Verlag.

Suding M.J. (1984). Decision making: Controlling the computer input. *Nursing Management 15* (7) 44–52.

CASE 10–1 Cutting the Gordian Knot: Implementing OrderNet in an Academic Health Center

Cynthia A. Dolan and Linda Kisamore

The Johns Hopkins Hospital (JHH) is a private, nonprofit academic health center that is part of a larger system of medical institutions. With more than 1,000 licensed beds, and 1,300 active physicians, JHH offers an extensive range of primary, secondary, tertiary, and quaternary inpatient and outpatient care. During fiscal year 1996 alone, there were 39,298 discharges and more than 400,000 outpatient visits.

The Johns Hopkins Medicine Center for Information Services (JHMCIS) provides systems development, operations and network services, technical support, desktop support, and training to all affiliates of Johns Hopkins Medicine. JHMCIS has more than 180 employees and manages a complex computing environment of multiple hardware platforms and software packages.

■ THE PROJECT INITIATIVE

A Total Quality Management (TQM) initiative at JHH in 1991 identified the need for a computerized physician order entry (POE) system. Because of this recommendation, a decision was made to purchase the necessary hardware and software for a computerized POE system.

A multidisciplinary group was convened to draft a Request for Proposal (RFP). Group members were responsible for identifying requirements the system must have to be acceptable to their disciplines. Identified requirements included the ability to (1) handle a large volume of orders; (2) handle complex orders, e.g., sliding scale insulin and taper doses; (3) interface with existing laboratory, radiology, and pharmacy systems; and (4) support online documentation of medications.

In the spring of 1992, the committee chose Invision, a product of Shared Medical Systems (SMS), after evaluating all responses to the RFP.* The Invision product met all specifications and had the additional capability of allowing physicians to enter all patient orders online. Because the hospital had several SMS systems already installed, and to prevent confusion for the Help Desk staff, the SMS Invision order management system at JHH was named OrderNet.

The original scope of the project was a two-part implementation. Phase I would include the following functions for inpatient areas only: order entry, physicians' view, nurses' view, nursing unit clerk view, clinical observations and results (COR), and medication charting. Phase II would include outpatient areas, and additional charting applications.

---

*SMS and INVISION are registered trademarks of Shared Medical Systems Corporation.

CASE: 10–1 *Continued*

■ COMMITTEE STRUCTURE

The committee structure for the POE system includes a steering committee and a hospital review team. Memberships of the steering committee and hospital review team are interdisciplinary, consisting of representatives from various departments including nursing, lab, pharmacy, radiology, and information systems.

The steering committee, composed primarily of physicians, department directors, assistant directors, supervisors, and managers, is the governing body that determined the pilot site and the roll-out plan for implementation throughout the hospital. The steering committee is responsible for periodically reviewing the status of the project and making high-level decisions.

The hospital review team consisted of managers, staff nurses, representatives from pharmacy, radiology and lab, and the POE project team. The hospital review team was responsible for (1) assuring that the system could be used hospital-wide, (2) assuring that the system upheld hospital policies and procedures, and (3) providing ideas regarding the design of the system and hardware requirements.

HRT meetings occurred during the design and pilot phases. Members saw the system developed from the prototype to a fully functional system.

■ PILOT PHASE

The steering committee and JHMCIS agreed that the OrderNet system should be piloted on one nursing unit before rolling-out to the rest of the hospital. The main requirement in choosing the pilot unit was that the unit provide a good cross-section of orders to test the functionality of the system. Likewise, a geographically stable patient population, experienced nurse manager, and physician practice group were wanted.

The decision was made to pilot the system on a 21-bed medical unit covered by a medical director, attending physicians, and rotating residents. The pilot unit had a stable nursing staff with a low turnover rate.

Getting Ready for Pilot

A JHMCIS project team worked for 2½ years customizing the system to prepare for the pilot. The project team started workflow analysis in the fall of 1992 and had a prototype system for physician review in early 1993. Major areas of customization included ordersets or standing orders; nursing orders; complex pharmacy orders, such as taper doses, hyperalimentation, and sliding scale insulin; limiting access for the various physician levels, such as medical students; and countersigning functions. Extensive unit, system, and integration testing was completed before the system was piloted. Samples of inpatient orders were used to develop realistic testing scenarios. The goal of the final integration test was to mimic typical nursing unit ordering activity over several days.

JHMCIS hired several physicians from various specialties to work 4 to 10 hours

CASE: 10–1 *Continued*

each week to help customize the system. Physician consultants helped with system design issues, evaluation of order screens, training plans for physicians, and advocacy for the OrderNet system. The consultants also attended committee meetings and helped develop procedures.

An implementation team consisting of representatives from the project team, lab, pharmacy, radiology, and the pilot unit met regularly to prepare for implementation. Pilot unit representatives included the nurse manager, a physician assistant, a senior clinical nurse, and a nursing unit clerk. These individuals provided (1) information regarding what would work, (2) thoughts about how to make the system easier to use, (3) information about hardware requirements for the unit, and (4) suggestions to make the electronic system more closely resemble the manual one.

The implementation team was effective in identifying ways to streamline the ordering process. Pilot unit representatives developed ordersets for the core group of diagnoses seen on the unit, and for frequently ordered tests and procedures. Ordersets were submitted to JHMCIS implementation specialists for building into the system.

After 14 months of planning and development, a 4-week pilot on the medicine unit was conducted. Delays in getting approval for electronic signature for order entry from the state and specific pathway issues in the system extended the pilot from 1 to 11 months. Thus, the pilot unit remained the only unit on OrderNet for nearly a year.

Emerging Committees

During the OrderNet pilot, several issues emerged that resulted in new task forces being created to deal with computer downtime and the special needs of intensive care unit (ICU) staff, and to support wider implementation throughout the medical division.

The Clinical Downtime Committee, consisting of interdisciplinary representatives, was convened to develop a procedure for handling orders during scheduled and unscheduled downtime. The goal was to develop a procedure that would reduce the number of manual orders written during downtime without compromising patient care and provide a simple, effective method for sending orders without OrderNet.

The Medicine Implementation Team and the ICU Subgroup emerged to plan the implementation schedule and process for the entire medical division. The Medicine Implementation Team consisted of nurse managers, nurse educators, clinical nurse specialists, JHMCIS implementation specialists, and representatives from the ancillary services. The group focused on developing the roll-out schedule and preparing the individual units. The ICU Subgroup was formed to address the need for ordersets specific to critical care and other ICU issues. The subgroup consisted of physician and nursing representatives from the intensive care and pilot areas and JHMCIS representatives. The group addressed a variety of issues including how to handle documents and labels

CASE: 10–1 *Continued*

produced by OrderNet and the development of ordersets to streamline time spent by clinicians entering orders.

■ POSITIONS ON THE PROJECT TEAM FILLED BY NURSES

When JHMCIS management formed the project team for the POE system, they recognized the need to include clinicians. Nurses continue to serve in several roles, including that of project manager.

Project Manager

The project manager is responsible for the project as a whole and reports to the Director of Clinical Systems. The manager provides the overall plan of work for the team, and ensures that deadlines are met and that important issues are addressed and resolved appropriately. The manager chairs project meetings and is involved in other interdisciplinary committees and projects that relate to clinical systems. The manager is responsible for personnel activities, including hiring and evaluating team members. A nurse with a masters degree in Nursing Informatics was chosen for this position.

Project Leader

The two project leaders, one of whom is a registered nurse, are responsible for assigning tasks to the team members and ensuring that these tasks are completed appropriately. They meet with each team member weekly to discuss assigned tasks and responsibilities. The

project leaders chair some committee meetings and the weekly project team meeting. The project leaders are responsible for updating the project plan and keeping the project manager informed of the day-to-day progress of the team, and any issues that need to be addressed.

Implementation Specialist

The JHMCIS OrderNet project team has five implementation specialists. Registered nurses fill four of the positions, while a pharmacist fills the other. The implementation specialists are responsible for workflow analysis, system design, screen and pathway building using the SMS Online Architecture System (OAS), system testing, and support for maintenance and implementation. The implementation specialist serves as a liaison between the end users and the technical information systems staff.

Nurses work well as implementation specialists because they have an intimate understanding of order processing for patient care. Nurses are quick to point out to other clinicians the inefficiencies of the manual process and can easily communicate the benefits of the automated process for patient care.

Support Analyst

Support analysts are responsible for providing 24-hour on-site support during roll-out. Support analysts are trained to be expert users of the system and can provide one-on-one user training as needed. They are trained to triage problems and accept requests for system en-

CASE: 10–1 *Continued*

hancements. They help with system analysis, design, and documentation. Clinical experience is a requirement for the support analyst. Two of the four JHMCIS support analysts are registered nurses.

Roll-out Coordinator

The roll-out coordinator position was created to facilitate the dissemination of OrderNet to the clinical areas. Each clinical area or product-line department is responsible for identifying a clinically experienced individual to function in the role.

The roll-out coordinator is responsible for helping the JHMCIS staff to understand the needs of the department during the implementation period. The coordinator consults with JHMCIS to help solve problems with OrderNet during implementation and roll-out. The coordinator also helps the department solve problems related to existing practice patterns or policies that need revision. The roll-out coordinator works closely with the training team to address educational issues, including customizing learning materials to suit the needs of staff and faculty and helping to ensure that the appropriate individuals receive training. Most of the roll-out coordinators are registered nurses.

■ PLANNING FOR ROLL-OUT

The Department of Medicine Implementation Team was formed in the fall of 1995 and met biweekly. This group reviewed the pilot system, listened to users about lessons learned on the pilot unit, and determined the changes and additions needed before the system could roll-out to other units. For example, nurses thought that online documentation of medications and intravenous fluids was critical for roll-out. Automating this process would eliminate the need for transcription of medication orders to a paper medication administration record.

During the pilot, several system problems were identified. The pharmacy pathways were confusing and had too many screens. The lab terminology was not familiar to physicians and ordering morning labs was taking too long. The team spent several months modifying these pathways with the help of the clinicians and the ancillary staff.

Ordersets developed before the roll-out were too cumbersome and complex. Physicians worked on revising the existing ordersets and developing new ones for the roll-out. Nurses provided detailed analysis about documents generated by the system and helped to design a nursing worklist that could be generated automatically at specified times of the day.

Training

A key aspect in planning for roll-out was training. End users must have sufficient training to become knowledgeable about how the system works. The time allotted for training varied by position. Nurses and unit clerks were scheduled for 3½ hours of training. Physicians, who assisted in developing the physician training class, recommended limiting physician training to 2 hours.

CASE: 10–1 *Continued*

Each unit identified at least one "super user" to receive additional training. The content of the super user training mirrored that of the regular nurse training, but was delivered in two, 2-hour sessions. Additional practice sessions, including supervised practice, were required. Super users were also encouraged to meet with individuals responsible for building various screens in the system (e.g., pharmacy and lab) to gain a better understanding of the work behind the screens and the limitations of the system.

JHMCIS' training coordinator worked closely with the roll-out coordinators and nurse managers to schedule nurse and house staff training. Scheduling nurses and unit clerks was difficult because nurse managers were asked to schedule staff for 4 hours off the unit. Likewise, physician 2-hour training needed to occur around the house staff's schedule. Additional training was provided on the unit during the roll-out.

Trainers were nonclinical staff well versed in OrderNet but not clinically knowledgeable. Trainees became frustrated when clinically pertinent questions were asked but could not be answered. The addition of clinically experienced individuals to help trainers was welcomed by both trainees and trainers.

Because it was thought that the attending physicians could not clear their schedules for formal classes, an initial decision was made to train them on-the-spot or just-in-time. For some physicians, this approach was adequate. Others requested full training sessions. Now, the JHMCIS training coordinator contacts attending physicians and schedules full training sessions.

Coordinating Support

Adequate user support is critical during and immediately after implementation of a new system. The goal was to satisfy the user support needs identified by the department. Minimum support for the first several days consisted of three people on the day and evening shifts, and two people on nights to support an average 27-bed unit.

JHMCIS hired four full-time support analysts to support users, and pilot unit nurses were recruited as well. In addition, nursing students from Johns Hopkins University and the University of Maryland's Nursing Informatics program were recruited and trained to help with roll-out support. These clinically experienced support persons were more often sought by the users than those who had no clinical backgrounds.

Hardware

Each nurse manager determined the hardware needed to support electronic order entry on her or his unit. Input devices included both dumb terminals and public workstations. The public workstations operated under Windows NT and ran HIP, a host interface program, and Rumba.* Pointing devices included light pens for the dumb terminals, and a

---

*Windows NT is a registered trademark of Microsoft Corporation. Rumba is a registered trademark of Wall Data Incorporated.

CASE: 10–1 *Continued*

mouse or trackball for each workstation. Laser printers that could print 12 pages per minute were used for OrderNet-generated documents. A thermal label printer printed barcoded labels that replaced the laboratory requisitions and specimen labels used in the manual system.

Ideally, hardware should be in place at least 2 weeks before implementation to provide trained users the opportunity to practice in their own environment. Sometimes hardware was not available and fully functional until the evening before, or morning of, implementation. The problems that prevented the hardware from being fully functional included failure to load the software on the workstation, incorrect cards in printers, and absence of necessary cabling. Lessons learned were the importance of facilities work and that requisitioning of hardware needs to start early in the process to avoid delays.

■ IMPLEMENTATION

The OrderNet project team developed a task list of all of the change requests and enhancements that would be necessary before the system could be rolled-out to the rest of the medicine units. This list added up to approximately 1,700 hours of work to be done. This list was then reviewed by the Medicine Implementation Team and the steering committee. A subgroup was formed to help with refining the list and determining the priorities. From this list, a project plan was developed that included time to build the

changes and enhancements, test integration, train people, and roll-out.

The Medicine Implementation Team was charged with determining the order in which the patient care areas would roll out. This turned out to be a difficult task. At first, the goal was to order implementation so that patients would have all electronic or all manual orders on their charts. The procedure units, such as cardiac catheterization lab and dialysis, protested that it would be too cumbersome to switch between electronic and manual orders just to keep the charts consistent. The decision was made to schedule roll-out for procedure units at a point when the majority of patients seen in these areas would be on electronic orders (and to change over all at once).

The Medicine Implementation Team developed guidelines for handling orders for the procedure areas. The guidelines included the development of ordersets from pre- and post-procedure standard orders. This ensured that all orders for the inpatient unit would be electronic and only the intraprocedure orders would be on paper.

The order of roll-out was decided to flow from most acute to least. Thus, the ICUs were selected to be the first units to implement OrderNet post pilot. This approach was not successful because of the combination of high patient acuity, type and location of input devices, amount and type of support necessary, and the extreme differences in workflow between the pilot unit and the ICUs.

The ICU subgroup was formed to work on these issues, and implementa-

CASE: 10–1 *Continued*

tion was switched to the general nursing units. One nursing unit was brought onto the system each week. A roll-out team, consisting of pilot unit staff, JHM-CIS staff, and a pharmacist, assisted with conversion of existing patient orders from paper to electronic form. Nurses from the unit summarized patients' active orders. Nurses on the roll-out team entered them as verbal orders. The pharmacist verified pharmacy orders. The active orders (see Fig. 10–2) were printed and reviewed for accuracy. Once assured of the accuracy, worklists were printed (see Fig. 10–3) and distributed to the nursing staff. Several units requested a separate worklist (see Fig. 10–4) for the nursing support technicians (NSTs). Once this process was completed for all patients, physicians were notified that they could begin entering orders.

Problem Solving: Online Documentation Problems

Before online documentation of medications (ODM), nurses gathered, prepared, administered, and documented the administration of medications using the Medication Administration Record (MAR). With OrderNet, the MAR was replaced by the nursing worklist. Unlike the MAR, the worklist is not a permanent part of the medical record; thus, nurses would have to record the administration of drugs again, online, for the permanent record. Nurses use the worklist to prepare, administer, and keep track of medications given. Within 4 hours of administering any medication or before leaving the unit, the nurse is required to document electronically the medication administration. This duplication of work on the worklist and the online record was deemed inefficient.

A management engineering team was consulted and agreed to examine the medication documentation process. The team reported three ways to document medication administration: handwritten on the MAR, by electronic data entry at a terminal or workstation, or through barcoding and scanning devices. Reverting to handwritten documentation on the MAR was not acceptable given the institution's move toward a paperless medical record. Barcoding and scanning were appealing but expensive and not well tested for medication administration using this software. The option of electronically documenting medications at the bedside had the most possibility.

Electronic documentation of medication administration at the bedside requires either point of care workstations or portable devices. We decided to test wireless portable devices. Representatives from the Johns Hopkins University Applied Physics Lab conducted studies to determine if radio frequency interfered with other medical hardware. The results of the studies were satisfactory and three wireless laptops were mounted on carts and placed in operation.

Several observations have been made since the wireless laptops have been used: (1) there has been no problem with loss of signal; (2) the few times the laptops have lost power were results of staff failing to plug the units in for

```
ACTIVE ORDERS FOR: PHSUEONE ,TEST                     PAGE: 1
DATE: 08/28/96    TIME: 12:35


OSL8 816SB         PT NO:   200032746   MED REC NO: 36565656
                   AGE:   63 SEX:  F   ATN DR: CHAISSON, RICHARD E
DIAGNOSIS: CHF
WEIGHT: 75.0  KG  BSA: 1.9093 M2  HEIGHT: 5 FT 8.75 IN


ALLERGIES:
CODEINE          AMINOGLYCOSIDES      HEPARIN          CHLORAMPHENICOL
CALCIUM BLOCKER     ETOPOSID, TENIPO
------------------------------------------------------------------------

DEPT          ORDER INFORMATION           START DT/TM  STOP DT/TM  ORD #

ADM  ALLERGIES: CODEINE,AMINOGLYCOSIDES, *MORE*  08/28 0915     /        1
        CODEINE:COCOS                      AMINOGLYCOSIDES:AAA
        HEPARIN:HEP                        CHLORAMPHENICOL:CHCH
        CALCIUM BLOCKER:CCC                ETOPOSID,TENIPO:ETO

ADM  ADMIT TO: OSL8 INFECTIOUS DISEASES    08/28 0916     /        2

ADM  DIAGNOSIS: CHF                        08//28 0916    /        3
        COPD

ADM  CONDITION: FAIR                       08/28 0916     /        4

DTY  REGULAR DIET                          08/28 1200     /       13
        ENTER DIET IN NUTRITION SYSTEM

LAB  URINALYSIS DIPSTICK URINE OTHER       08/28 0936  08/28 0936  25

LAB  URINALYSIS MICROSCOPIC URINE OTHER    08/28 0936  08/28 0936  26

LAB  CULTURE BACT URINE CC URINE CC        08/28 0936  08/28 0936  27

LAB  APTT # A                              08/29 0600  08/29 0600  19

LAB  CHEMISTRY PANEL,SERUM (M12) # A       08/29 0600  08/29 0600  20

LAB  ELECTROLYTE PANEL,SERUM (M6) # A      08/29 0600  08/29 0600  21

LAB  HEME-8 # A                            08/29 0600  08/29 0600  22

LAB  MAGNESIUM, SERUM # A                  08/29 0600  08/29 0600  23

LAB  PROTHROMBIN TIME # A                  08/29 0600  08/29 0600  24

NUR  LATEX PORT                            08/28 0916  08/28 0916  17

NUR  DAILY WEIGHT                          08/28 1000     /        7
        AND ON ADMISSION

NUR  VITAL SIGNS QSHIFT                    08/28 1400     /        5

                                              CONTINUED
   PT. NAME: PHSUEONE ,TEST        MED REC NUMBER: 36565656
```

FIGURE 10–2. Page 1 of the active orders list. (Printed from SMS Invision.)

```
ACTIVE ORDERS FOR: PHSUEONE ,TEST                    PAGE: 2
DATE: 08/28/96    TIME: 12:35


OSL8 816SB        PT NO:    200032746   MED REC NO: 36565656
                  AGE:    63  SEX:  F   ATN DR: CHAISSON, RICHARD E
DIAGNOSIS: CHF
WEIGHT: 75.0  KG  BSA: 1.9093 M2  HEIGHT: 5 FT 8.75 IN


ALLERGIES:
CODEINE           AMINOGLYCOSIDES    HEPARIN         CHLORAMPHENICOL
CALCIUM BLOCKER   ETOPOSID, TENIPO
-----------------------------------------------------------------------


DEPT              ORDER INFORMATION              START DT/TM  STOP DT/TM  ORD #
                                                             CONTINUED


NUR  UP AD LIB QSHIFT                            08/28 1400    /            6

NUR  I & O QSHIFT                                08/28 1400    /            8

NUR  NHO TEMP >38.4                              08/28 1400    /            9

NUR  NHO PULSE >100 <60                          08/28 1400    /           10

NUR  NHO SB/P >180 <90                           08/28 1400    /           11

NUR  NHO DB/P >95 <60                            08/28 1400    /           12

PHM  FUROSEMIDE 20. MG PO QD                     08/28 0936    /           28

PHM  VITAMIN MULTIPLE 1. EA PO QD                08/28 1000    /           14

PHM  ACETAMINOPHEN 650. MG PO Q4HPRN             08/28 1000    /           15

        FOR TEMP > 38.5 AFTER INITIAL CULTURE

PHM  CHLORAL HYDRATE 500. MG PO QHSPRN           08/28 1000    /           16

        SLEEP

PHM  D5 1/2NS 1000. ML CONT 24 ML/HR            08/28 1000    /           30

        D5 1/2NS                   1000.  ML

        Q24HRS

PHM  *RTY ALBUTEROL - MDI 17. GM INHL Q4H        08/28 1000    /           32

        2 PUFFS

PHM  INSULIN SSI REGULAR SUBQ QACHS              08/28 1200    .           29
        IF B.S. < 60, NHO       AND GIVE ORANGE JUICE
        IF B.S. > 400, NHO
        INSULIN SSI REG HUMAN          8.    UNT
        B.S. 61 TO 200 GIVE 0 UNITS
        B.S. 201 TO 250 GIVE 2 UNITS
        B.S. 251 TO 300 GIVE 4 UNITS
        B.S. 301 TO 350 GIVE 6 UNITS
        B.S. 351 TO 400 GIVE 8 UNITS


  PT. NAME: PHSUEONE ,TEST            MED REC NUMBER: 36565656
```

FIGURE 10–2. Page 2 of the active orders list. (Printed from SMS Invision.)

CASE: 10–1 *Continued*

```
Name: PHSUEONE ,TEST              Worklist Report
Date: 082896   Time: 0944            For: 0701 thru 1900              1

# HOURS ONE TIME ORDERS APPEAR: PHM=2, LAB=120, DTY=24, NUR=24, Others=2

OSL8  816SB  Pt. No:   200032746  Med Rec No: 36565656
 75 KG            Age: 63 Sex: F  Attending DR: CHAISSON, RICHARD E

ALLERGIES:
CODEINE           AMINOGLYCOSIDES    HEPARIN          CHLORAMPHENICOL
CALCIUM BLOCKER   ETOPOSID,TENIPO
-----------------------------------------------------------------------

DEPT      ORDER INFORMATION                STOP DT/TM FREQ    DUR  ORD #

PHM VITAMIN MULTIPLE 1. EA PO QD            08/28 1000 QD     999D   14
 08/28 10:00 ____


PHM D5 1/2NS 1000. ML CONT 24 ML/HR         08/28 1000        999D   30
     D5 1/2NS                                1000.     ML
 08/28 10:00 ____
   Q24HRS


PHM *RTY ALBUTEROL - MDI 17. GM INHL Q4H    08/28 1000 Q4H    999D   32
 08/28 10:00 ____
 08/28 14:00 ____
 08/28 18:00 ____
   2 PUFFS


PHM INSULIN SSI REGULAR SUBQ QACHS          08/28 1200 QACHS  999D   29
                  SUBQ QACHS   DAILY
    IF B.S. < 60, NHO          AND GIVE ORANGE JUICE
    IF B.S. > 400, NHO
    INSULIN SSI REG HUMAN                  8.     UNT
    B.S. 61 TO 200 GIVE 0 UNITS
    B.S. 201 TO 250 GIVE 2 UNITS
    B.S. 251 TO 300 GIVE 4 UNITS
    B.S. 301 TO 350 GIVE 6 UNITS
    B.S. 351 TO 400 GIVE 8 UNITS
 08/28 12:00 ____
 08/28 16:00 ____


PHM SOD CHLORIDE 0.9% LOCK 1. ML IV FLUSH Q8  08/28 1400 Q8H  999D   18
 08/28 14:00 ____
    IV PUSH
    IV PUSH                         LATEX PORT FLUSH


PHM FUROSEMIDE 20. MG PO QD                 08/28 0936 QD     999D   28
 08/28 09:36 ____
*** END OF RX NON-PRN ORDERS -- (08/28/96 07:01 TO 08/28/96 19:00)   *****
-----------------------------------------------------------------------

PHM ACETAMINOPHEN 650. MG PO Q4HPRN         08/28 1000 Q4HPRN 999D   15
                                                     CONTINUED
```

FIGURE 10–3. Nursing worklist. (Printed from SMS Invision.)

```
--------------------------------------------------------------------------------
```

                                                                    CONTINUED
          FOR TEMP > 38.5 AFTER INITIAL CULTURE

PHM   CHLORAL HYDRATE 500. MG PO QHSPRN   08/28 1000 QHSPRN   999D   16
          SLEEP
*** END OF RX PRN ORDERS ---- (08/28/96 07:01 TO 08/28/96 19:00)   *****

```
--------------------------------------------------------------------------------
```

DEPT	ORDER INFORMATION	STOP DT/TM	FREQ	DUR	ORD #
LAB	URINALYSIS DIPSTICK URINE OTHER 08/28 09:36 ___	08/28 0936	ONCE	0H	25
LAB	URINALYSIS MICROSCOPIC URINE OTHER 08/28 09:36 ___	08/28 0936	ONCE	0H	26
LAB	CULTURE BACT URINE CC URINE CC 08/28 09:36 ___	08/28 0936	ONCE	0H	27
LAB	APTT # A	08/29 0600	ONCE	0H	19
LAB	CHEMISTRY PANEL,SERUM (M12) # A	08/29 0600	ONCE	0H	20
LAB	ELECTROLYTE PANEL,SERUM (M6) # A	08/29 0600	ONCE	0H	21
LAB	HEME-8 # A	08/29 0600	ONCE	0H	22
LAB	MAGNESIUM, SERUM # A	08/29 0600	ONCE	0H	23
LAB	PROTHROMBIN TIME # A	08/29 0600	ONCE	0H	24

```
*****   END OF LAB ORDERS ----- (08/28/96 07:01 TO 08/28/96 19:00)   *****
--------------------------------------------------------------------------------
```

DEPT	ORDER INFORMATION	STOP DT/TM	FREQ	DUR	ORD #
DTY	REGULAR DIET ENTER DIET IN NUTRITION SYSTEM	08/28 1200	TID	999H	13

```
*****   END OF DTY ORDERS ----- (08/28/96 07:01 TO 08/28/96 19:00)   *****
--------------------------------------------------------------------------------
```

DEPT	ORDER INFORMATION	STOP DT/TM	FREQ	DUR	ORD #
NUR	LATEX PORT	08/28 0916	ONCE	0H	17

                                                                    CONTINUED

FIGURE 10–3. Nursing worklist, continued. (Printed from SMS Invision.)

```
Name: PHSUEONE ,TEST          Worklist Report
Date: 082896   Time: 0944        For: 0701 thru 1900              3

# HOURS ONE TIME ORDERS APPEAR: PHM=2, LAB=120, DTY=24, NUR=24, Others=2

OSL8  816SB  Pt. No:   200032746  Med Rec No: 36565656
  75 KG           Age: 63 Sex: F  Attending DR: CHAISSON, RICHARD E


----------------------------------------------------------------------------

DEPT              ORDER INFORMATION           STOP DT/TM FREQ      DUR   ORD #
                                                                 CONTINUED


NUR  DAILY WEIGHT                             08/28 1000 QD       999H    7
         AND ON ADMISSION
NUR  VITAL SIGNS QSHIFT                       08/28 1400 QSHIFT   999H    5
NUR  UP AD LIB QSHIFT                         08/28 1400 QSHIFT   999H    6
NUR  I & O QSHIFT                             08/29 1400 QSHIFT   999H    8
NUR  NHO TEMP >38.4                           08/29 1400 QSHIFT   999H    9
NUR  NHO PULSE >100 <60                       08/29 1400 QSHIFT   999H   10
NUR  NHO SB/P >180 <90                        08/29 1400 QSHIFT   999H   11
NUR  NHO DB/P >95 <60                         08/29 1400 QSHIFT   999H   12
*****    END OF NUR ORDERS ----- (08/28/96 07:01 TO 08/28/96 19:00)    *****
----------------------------------------------------------------------------

DEPT              ORDER INFORMATION           STOP DT/TM FREQ      DUR   ORD #
ADM  ALLERGIES: CODEINE,AMINOGLYSOSIDES,*MORE 08/28 0915 QD       999H    1
         08/28   09:15 ____
         CODEINE:COCOS            AMINOGLYCOSIDES:AAA
         HEPARIN:HEP              CHLORAMPHENICOL:CHCH
         CALCIUM BLOCKER:CCC      ETOPOSID,TENIPO:ETO
ADM  ADMIT TO: OSL8 INFECTIOUS DISEASES       08/28 0916 QD       999H    2
         08/28   09:16 ____
ADM  DIAGNOSIS: CHF                           08/28 0916 QD       999H    3
         08/28   09:16 ____
         COPD
ADM  CONDITION: FAIR                          08/28 0916 QD       999H    4
         08/28   09:16 ____
RAD  CHEST AP                                 08/28 0938 ONCE      0H    31
         08/28   09:38 ____
*****    END OF ORDERS ----- (08/28/96 07:01 TO 08/28/96 19:00)        *****
```

FIGURE 10–3. Nursing worklist, continued. (Printed from SMS Invision.)

CASE: 10–1 *Continued*

```
Name: PHSUEONE ,TEST              NST Worklist Report
Date: 082896   Time: 0944          For: 0701 thru 1900                1

# HOURS ONE TIME ORDERS APPEAR: DTY=24, NUR=24, Others=2

OSL8  816SB  Pt. No:   200032746  Med Rec No: 36565656
 75 KG           Age: 63 Sex: F   Attending DR: CHAISSON, RICHARD E


-------------------------------------------------------------------------------

DEPT            ORDER INFORMATION            STOP DT/TM FREQ    DUR    ORD #
DTY  REGULAR DIET                            08/28 1200 TID     999H    13
        ENTER DIET IN NUTRITION SYSTEM
*****    END OF DTY ORDERS ----- (08/28/96 07:01 TO 08/28/96 19:00)    *****
-------------------------------------------------------------------------------

DEPT            ORDER INFORMATION            STOP DT/TM FREQ    DUR    ORD #

NUR  LATEX PORT                              08/28 0916 ONCE     0H     17
NUR  DAILY WEIGHT                            08/28 1000 QD      999H     7
        AND ON ADMISSION
NUR  VITAL SIGNS QSHIFT                      08/28 1400 QSHIFT  999H     5
NUR  UP AD LIB QSHIFT                        08/28 1400 QSHIFT  999H     6
NUR  I & O QSHIFT                            08/29 1400 QSHIFT  999H     8
NUR  NHO TEMP >38.4                          08/29 1400 QSHIFT  999H     9
NUR  NHO PULSE >100 <60                      08/29 1400 QSHIFT  999H    10
NUR  NHO SB/P >180 <90                       08/29 1400 QSHIFT  999H    11
NUR  NHO DB/P >95 <60                        08/29 1400 QSHIFT  999H    12
*****    END OF NUR ORDERS ----- (08/28/96 07:01 TO 08/28/96 19:00)    *****
-------------------------------------------------------------------------------

DEPT            ORDER INFORMATION            STOP DT/TM FREQ    DUR    ORD #

ADM  ALLERGIES: CODEINE,AMINOGLYSOSIDES,*MORE  08/28 0915 QD    999H     1
        08/28   09:15 ____
        CODEINE:COCOS              AMINOGLYCOSIDES:AAA
        HEPARIN:HEP               CHLORAMPHENICOL:CHCH
        CALCIUM BLOCKER:CCC        ETOPOSID,TENIPO:ETO
ADM  ADMIT TO: OSL8 INFECTIOUS DISEASES       08/28 0916 QD     999H     2
        08/28   09:16 ____
ADM  DIAGNOSIS: CHF                           08/28 0916 QD     999H     3
        08/28   09:16 ____
        COPD
ADM  CONDITION: FAIR                          08/28 0916 QD     999H     4
        08/28   09:16 ____
RAD  CHEST AP                                 08/28 0938 ONCE    0H     31
        08/28   09:38 ____
*****    END OF ORDERS ----- (08/28/96 07:01 TO 08/28/96 19:00)    *****
```

FIGURE 10–4. Nursing support technician (NST) worklist. (Printed from SMS Invision.)

CASE: 10–1 *Continued*

recharging; (3) in a survey of all nurses, 12 percent reported that eliminating double documentation saved an estimated 1 hour per 12-hour shift; 59 percent reported that having wireless devices available has added convenience but indicated a reluctance to change their method for documenting medication administration; and 29 percent reported rarely using the wireless devices. The group of nurses reporting rare use of the laptops are the evening and night shift nurses who have larger patient assignments. They report that the carts on which the wireless devices are mounted are too small to accommodate the laptop and medications for their assigned patients.

The Medical Implementation Team is now working with the nurses to increase utilization of the laptops and searching for larger carts to allow for the larger patient assignments on off-shifts.

■ LESSONS LEARNED

The OrderNet roll-out to the Department of Medicine took longer than anticipated. The roll-out was complicated by system and network problems. Some of the problems could not have been anticipated, and delays were unavoidable. Despite the problems, overall implementation has been successful. Many lessons have been learned during the OrderNet roll-out which can be used to make future roll-outs go more smoothly.

- *Secure support from senior clinical and administrative leaders.* Because of the complexity of POE and the cultural changes that need to occur, having senior management available at a moment's notice to address major issues and make decisions is critical. Even with the best planning, some part of the implementation will not go as smoothly as predicted and senior management must be available to make decisions quickly.

- *Plan early.* Scheduling meetings and getting added to committee agendas takes time and energy, especially when physician schedules are involved.

- *Involve all Information Systems (IS) areas from the start.* Each area plays an important part in the roll-out and everyone needs to understand that a POE system must be available 24 hours a day, 7 days a week. The IS group needs coding, documentation, and change control standards in place and enforced throughout the process. Delays in one area of IS can mean greater delays in another area. For example, hardware has to be installed and tested a few weeks before going live. The Help Desk should be involved so those who staff it can prepare for the increase in the number and complexity of queries.

- *Hold productive, well-attended meetings.* Meeting attendance needs to be a priority to avoid delays and to assure the appropriate people are making the decisions. Each department needs to be represented by both a physician and

CASE: 10–1 *Continued*

nurse who have decision-making authority for the department. In fact, physicians and nurses need to be involved at every level of planning. Actual system users are important to have as committee members.

- *Change existing policies and procedures to be consistent with the move to an electronic system.* Moving to an electronic system cannot occur with policies and procedures written for a paper system. Policies and procedures will need to be revised. For example, user procedures must be documented, well-communicated, and readily available for reference.

- *Diagram the medication process using flowcharts.* Nursing needs to be aware of the impact a POE system will have on all levels of unit staff and on workflow. Flow diagrams of unit processes, with and without the POE system, are helpful in determining potential impacts. It was difficult to anticipate all of the changes before implementation, which is why a small controlled pilot was essential. As unanticipated issues arose, JHMCIS staff were readily available to assist nursing staff in resolving them.

- *Select both a physician and nurse as roll-out coordinators.* The roll-out coordinator plays an important part in the roll-out process. Each understands the issues others in their professions will face with respect to POE.

- *Provide 24-hour support during the roll-out.* Staff are more tolerant of change when sufficient support is available to assist in adapting to the change. When possible, use people with clinical experience for support. For example, nurses from the pilot unit were knowledgeable about both OrderNet and workflow on the units.

- *Plan the roll-out for the quietest day of the week and at the time of day when most patients being discharged have been identified.* Enter existing orders before the start of the nurses' shift. Schedule additional clinical staff for the first few days to allow the extra time staff need to become accustomed to the change. Having extra staff available during the first 3 to 5 days helps in getting through the sometimes steep learning curve without compromising patient care.

- *Plan downtime and have procedures established.* Staff handle downtime effectively when familiar with the downtime procedures and when assured that patient care will not be compromised. Well-documented procedures also reduce the number of phone calls to the Help Desk during system outages, which can delay the communication of important information to oncall IS staff.

- *Keep users informed of changes in the system.* An effective means for communicating information to all users needs to be working before roll-out begins.

CASE: 10–1 *Continued*

- *Meet with the emergency response team daily to identify problems that have occurred and plan how to resolve them*. User input is valuable in identifying the problems and offering suggestions for enhancements.
- *Develop online help screens for users*. It is distracting to flip through manuals looking for help in maneuvering through a particular screen when online help could be available. Users from the pilot unit were helpful in identifying key areas where help screens could prevent mistakes and save time during order entry.

■ BENEFITS TO NURSING

Computer-based POE offers several benefits to nursing. Improvements in the medication administration cycle, availability of medical information, efficiencies in work flow, and compliance with regulatory agencies are a few of the benefits.

The timeliness of the medication administration cycle depends on transmitting orders to the pharmacy for processing. Lost orders can be eliminated with POE. Direct communication of the order by the physician to pharmacy virtually eliminates medication errors that occur when handwriting is misinterpreted (Sittig & Stead, 1994). Elimination of the transport of handwritten orders to the pharmacy improves the response time for getting medications to the unit.

Orders can be entered at any terminal or public workstation in the hospital, eliminating the need for a physician to be physically present on the nursing unit. Availability of terminals and workstations throughout the hospital will decrease the number of verbal or telephone orders.

The worklist offers a view of the patient's orders by department. Worklists can be printed with or without medications for the nurse or nursing technician. Organizing work is simplified. The amount of time needed to take report is decreased with the presence of the active orders on the worklist. Checking charts is no longer a hassle. Orders are readily available online for review and verification even when the patient is off the unit.

Nurses document their review of the chart online. All information entered is stamped with the date and time of entry, eliminating any confusion concerning when orders were entered by an authorized prescriber, verified by a pharmacist, or checked by the nurse.

Verbal orders requiring countersignature are often the focus of regulatory agencies. Nurses have frequently accepted the responsibility for assuring that orders requiring countersignature are signed by the appropriate physician. OrderNet has been set up to alert physicians that there are orders to be countersigned. Reports are generated at specified intervals showing those orders that have not been countersigned.

Documenting medication administration, reasons why medications were not given, and response to as-needed medications are areas reviewed by both regulatory agencies and third-party

CASE: 10–1 *Continued*

payors. OrderNet requires the nurse to document the reasons medications are omitted and the reasons as-needed medications are given. Nurses are also required to document the site in which injections are administered. The nurse cannot move from the screen until these essential data are entered.

Managers also benefit from Order-Net features. Reports can be generated providing necessary information for follow-up. For instance, the medicine units receive a daily report specifying orders that require countersignature. The report is used to follow up with physicians who need to countersign their orders. The charge nurse receives a report at the end of each shift that lists medications uncharted for that shift. The charge nurse follows up with the appropriate nurse to assure documentation is complete before leaving the unit. The nurse manager receives a similar report covering the previous 24-hour period that indicates uncharted medications. This report can be used for performance improvement and performance management.

Performance improvement activities can be automated through OrderNet. For example, random audits of documentation of medication administration can be replaced by a report comparing all medications prescribed and all medications documented as administered over a specific period of time. The report is thorough and eliminates the manpower required for data collection.

Implementing POE can be likened to cutting the Gordian knot. With proper planning, support, and creativity, an implementation team can cut through the complexities of POE just as Alexander cut through the mythical Gordian knot to be crowned king of Phrygia.

■ BIOGRAPHICAL SKETCHES

Cynthia A. Dolan has been a Registered Nurse for 14 years. Her experiences in clinical nursing include: ophthalmology, pulmonary medicine, cardiovascular and thoracic surgery, gastrointestinal surgery, telemetry, burn care, and liver and renal transplantation. She was a staff nurse and assistant nurse manager before returning for her Masters Degree. She received her MS in Nursing Informatics from the University of Maryland in Baltimore in 1992. Since then she has worked on the design, implementation, and management of the physician order entry system at Johns Hopkins Hospital. She is presently a manager at the Johns Hopkins Medicine Center for Information Services.

Ms. Dolan is a member of Pi Chapter of Sigma Theta Tau. She is also active in the Capital Area Roundtable on Informatics in Nursing (CARING) and the American Medical Informatics Association (AMIA).

Linda Kisamore has worked at Johns Hopkins Hospital since 1976. She began her career in nursing as a Licensed Practical Nurse in 1970. Her experience includes medical nursing, emergency nursing, and specialty practice in poly substance abuse and now HIV/AIDS. While working, she obtained her Associ-

CASE: 10–1 *Continued*

ate Degree in Nursing from the Community College of Baltimore in 1980 and her BSN from the College of Notre Dame in Baltimore, Maryland, in 1986. She is now a graduate student in nursing at Johns Hopkins University. During this time, her positions have included staff nurse, shift coordinator, and nurse manager.

She is currently the nurse manager on a dedicated AIDS unit that is scheduled to begin providing inpatient services for an AIDS Health Maintenance Organization later this year. During the pilot program for the OrderNet, a computer-based physician order entry sys-

tem, she served in the dual role of nurse manager and roll-out coordinator.

Ms. Kisamore is a member of Sigma Theta Tau, Mu Eta Chapter and Alpha Sigma Lambda. She is also active in the American Association of Nurse Executives (AONE).

■ REFERENCE

Sittig, D.F., & Stead, W.W. (1994). Computer-based physician order entry: The state of the art. *Journal of American Medical Informatics Association. 1* (2), 108–123.

Job Design and Work Processes in Patient Care

Theodore L. Gessner

A central function of any organization is to take complex tasks and to divide those tasks so that they can be completed by the individuals who are members of that organization. The division of labor for these tasks is an important component of organizational architecture, and the way in which the components of the work are divided and coordinated is a major determinant of the efficiency of the organization. Once the division of tasks has been identified, the organization is responsible for selecting, training, rewarding, and motivating individuals to complete the tasks. In the delivery of health services, the job and the identity of the nurse has been associated with the provision of day-to-day care of sick individuals in a human and personal manner. The question is, How much of this task and what other tasks are the responsibility of nursing? In attempting to answer this question at different times and in different settings, many methods have been employed to define the nature of the work and to coordinate the different work components.

Two general approaches to the design of work are job design and system redesign. Job design has been the more traditional approach to structuring the nature of work. The focus of this approach is on changing a job or a cluster of jobs within the organization without altering the total structure of the organization. The system redesign approach is relatively new and is seen as a necessary step to make modern organizations more flexible and competitive in an uncertain and complex business environment. This chapter will look at these two general approaches to designing the process of work.

■ JOB DESIGN

The history of systematic job design can be divided into three major periods. In the first period, between the early 1900s and the 1950s, most of the job design effort was directed toward the use of job simplification for unskilled work. This was the heyday of the assembly line, and the task of job design was to break the job into its simplest parts. Skilled or professional work was standardized through the use of extensive education, codes of ethics, supervised training, peer review, and licensing. The second period, which lasted until the early 1960s, was an era of job enlargement for unskilled work. This change was in reaction to the morale problems that had resulted from job simplification. The third period, which extends from the 1960s until the present, involves the redesigning of jobs to allow for personal and professional growth of workers. Interestingly, the current trends in outcomes measurement, clinical pathways, and clinical guidelines are to add greater standardization to skilled and professional work and reduce individual variation.

Job Simplification

The concept of *scientific management* has been attributed to Taylor (1910). This approach focused on the simplification of jobs through standardization of unskilled work to increase efficiency. The major method is to observe the efficient worker and analyze the component parts of each task in a job. This process was called management engineering. The concepts supporting this approach are very simple. The workers are more efficient if their work is standardized and broken into simple discrete components. The smaller, standardized units of work may then be easily learned, supervised, and rewarded. Using this approach, work can be more precisely planned by managers. The parts of the job can be prescribed and the timing of the task can be calculated, controlled, and coordinated. This is the approach from which efficient production lines were made. Scientific management represents an important movement in modern organizational thought and, in terms of job design, was the preeminent model for over 50 years. The primary value of this approach was that it provided managers with tools for controlling the quantity and speed of production. Deviations from expectations could be identified and corrected with direct action. The planning and scheduling of work became a rational enterprise. The negative effects of this approach were workers' perceptions that they were being treated as cogs in a machine. Jobs were designed to be simple and routine (mechanical), low in skill requirements, and involving little interaction. Workers often felt that their jobs were boring, unchallenging, and meaningless. They had little control over their work. Many people reacted with a lack of pride about the quality of their work.

Job Enlargement

After World War II, there was increased recognition that many jobs had become so routine and boring that they were causing serious worker morale problems. Low productivity and high turnover became serious management problems. New job design techniques were developed to deal with these problems by introducing variety in unskilled jobs through horizontal enlargement.

The first new technique was job rotation where the tasks performed by the workers were considered to be simple and interchangeable. Unskilled workers could be rotated from one simple task to another without extensive retraining or a detrimental slowing of production. There was no major change in job functions but the worker gained a variety of skills. It was expected that job rotation would reduce fatigue and boredom and increase job meaning and involvement as workers participated in an entire task through rotation. Usually, the process of job rotation resulted in only short-term gains. The jobs in the rotation were usually very similar and very routine. It took a little longer for the worker to become bored. The most important impact of this method was that it considered the worker's morale in job design.

The next step in the evolution of job design was the focus on job enlargement. Proponents of job enlargement recognized that the small, simplified parts of a job could be connected into larger, more complex jobs to be carried out by a single worker. The worker's job then increased in task variety and complexity. This approach was designed to increase job satisfaction but, like job rotation, it proved to be only a short-term solution. It did little to increase the meaning of work or the personal involvement of workers. The enlargement and job rotation approaches enjoyed relative success, and they opened the way for more complex and theoretically based approaches to job design.

Job Enrichment

The phase of job design referred to as job enrichment involved three major theoretical contributions. They were: Herzberg's theory (Herzberg, Mausner, & Snyderman, 1959) of job motivation, expansion of this theory by Hackman and Oldham (1975), and the sociotechnical design approach (Trist, 1981) to job design. The concept of job enrichment is grounded on the theoretical framework developed by Herzberg (1966). This theory identified two sets of motivational factors: hygiene factors and motivators. Hygiene factors are the external characteristics of the job (e.g., pay, job content, security, benefits). The job rotation and enlargement approaches dealt with hygiene factors. These factors are important because they reduce job dissatisfaction, but according to Herzberg's theory, they do not result in an increase in satisfaction. Job dissatisfaction and satisfaction are viewed as two separate dimensions related to the motivational factors. It is the motivators (e.g., job challenge, autonomy, responsibility) that are the basis for the feelings of job satisfaction. The motivators are important for all jobs, but they take on greater importance in professional jobs where job challenge, autonomy, and responsibility are expectations of both the employee and the employer.

Job enrichment approaches are concerned with changing the motivators. An increased sense of achievement and involvement is the goal. Worker accountability and responsibility is increased, and feedback is provided. The job is not just increased in terms of horizontal complexity, but there is the opportunity for the worker to vertically shape the job's contribution to organizational tasks and experience personal growth. The thrust of this approach is that enlarging the job vertically as well as horizontally will increase job satisfaction and there will be a concomitant increase in quality of production.

The cost of this approach from the managerial viewpoint is that there is greater investment in each employee and less control as each employee participates in decision making. More skill is required to carry out the enriched job, and there is greater investment of time, training, and pay in each worker. Success of a job enrichment program was measured by reduction in absenteeism and turnover and by improved outcomes. Savings resulted from reducing the cost of recruiting and training replacements. The idea of job enrichment is to deal with both the hygiene factors and motivators to reduce sources of dissatisfaction and increase sources of satisfaction. Basically, it considers the skills and needs of the employee in the design of the job.

Herzberg's approach was modified by Hackman and Oldham (1975). Their expansion of this theory is based on the idea of altering core job dimensions to fit the specific needs of the employee (Fig. 11–1). In this approach, the core job dimensions are linked to specific psychological states. The psychological states are linked to specific production and work behavior

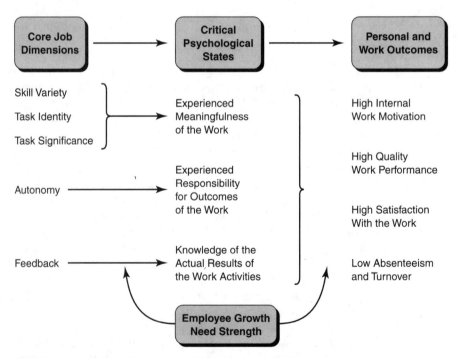

FIGURE 11–1. Relationships among core job dimensions, critical psychological states, and on-the-job outcomes. *(Copyright © by the Regents of the University of California. Reprinted/condensed from the* California Management Review, *17 (4), by permission of the Regents.)*

outcomes. The total linkage between job dimensions and productivity is moderated by the employee's needs.

The five core job dimensions are skill variety, task identity, task significance, autonomy, and feedback. Skill variety refers to the degree to which the job requires different skills and talents. Task identity is the extent to which the job requires the completion of a visible, identifiable product. Task significance is the extent to which the product impacts on others or is valued within and outside the organization. Autonomy is the extent to which the employee can exercise discretion in how and when the job will be done. Feedback is the extent to which the job and the organization provide clear information about the employee's performance.

When the core job dimensions of skill variety, task identity, and task significance are maximized, the employee experiences the critical psychological state of meaningful work. When autonomy is maximized, the individual experiences a sense of responsibility for the work outcome. When feedback is increased, the person has knowledge of work activities. The theory predicts that the combination of these three critical psychological states results in high productivity and job satisfaction.

The caveat in this theory is the assumption of a direct linkage between core job dimensions, personal and work outcomes, and the needs of the employee. If the employee is concerned primarily with having work meet lower order needs (*hygiene factors*) the attempts at job design are likely to be resisted. If the employee places a high value on meeting higher order needs through his or her work, then the attempts at job design are more likely to increase job satisfaction, reduce absenteeism and turnover, and improve work outcomes. There is some evidence that over time employees can be trained to change their expectations of their work to include meeting higher needs.

The sociotechnical approach (Trist, 1981) focuses on the work group as the appropriate place for job redesign. The task of the group is defined, but the methods used to accomplish the task are determined by the members of the work group. With this type of approach, the work group becomes the unit that controls the planning and assignment of work. The performance of the work group becomes the criteria for the distribution of pay and other rewards. Within this approach, there is change in both the work of individuals and the structure of the organization. One of the most successful and best known examples of this approach is the design of the Volvo plant in Kalmar, Sweden. In this situation, the replacement of assembly lines with autonomous work groups increased morale, reduced turnover, and improved quality and volume of productivity.

The major lesson that can be garnered from the theories of job design is that there is no single best approach or clear set of guidelines. The literature on the effectiveness of job design is basically case history research without rigorous studies comparing the relative effectiveness of one job design strategy over another. These case studies have been done in different industries, and few of the studies have been concerned with service organizations.

■ JOB DESIGN IN NURSING

Historically, nursing had been under the administrative control of physicians and, more recently, the professional hospital administrator. The nurse was a key care provider, but there was little acceptance of the nurse as a professional. The nurse carried out the orders of physicians as well as other tasks; the services of nurses were paid for out of daily operating budgets. The responsibility of the staff nurse was seen by many administrators as using skills only within the constraints of the prescribed medical regimen. The nurse was perceived as providing the routine medical care that was too time consuming for the physician to perform. The nurse was viewed as a physician extender, with little recognition given to the nurse's independent functions. The physician's job was simplified through delegation of certain tasks to nurses. The physician was seen as having the professional part of the job (e.g., diagnosis, treatment planning, prescription) and the nurse as having the semiprofessional part (e.g., monitoring the patient, delivering medications). Decisions about the patient's care were seen as the primary responsibility of physicians. This job distinction was clearly codified in the structure of many health care organizations and in licensing laws.

The question that faced the nurse executive in this type of structure was, how could the professional status of the nurse be either established or enhanced? Within the nursing profession a number of models of nursing practice were developed that provided the basis for executing a program of job design within an organization. Some of the models were nurse extenders, service-line managers, primary care nursing, case management, clinical ladders, and nurse-administered units. Each of these models provided the structure upon which a comprehensive program of job design could be built. Each of these models has strengths and weaknesses in bringing about limited change within a nursing environment.

Work sampling to describe the components of nurse's work was one of the earliest forms of nursing job redesign. The usual categories sampled were direct care, indirect care (including documentation), and nonpatient activities (including unit management, errands, and housekeeping). Innovations were often targeted to increase direct care time. Examples of efforts to reduce documentation time include: standardization of documentation, use of flow sheets, use of bar codes, physician order entry, and documentation by exception (Sittig, 1990). Prescott and associates (1991) reviewed work sampling studies of nursing, noted the substantial time nurses spent in unit management, and offered suggestions to increase efficiency of information flow and reassigning work, such as ordering supplies to unit clerks and other personnel. The primary limitation of this approach is the focus on actions, which does not include the timing and processes involved in clinical decision making.

The *nurse extender* model was one of the easiest models to implement. This model may best be employed to deal with situations in which there is a shortage of nurses, patient care includes a great deal of routine work, or the organization has to economize to survive. Nurse extender programs can be implemented relatively quickly and efficiently. The strategy is one of job simplification. The job of the registered nurse (RN) on a unit is analyzed into component parts and more routine tasks are assigned to licensed practical nurses (LPNs), nursing assistants, or other unlicensed assistive personnel (UAPs).

The job design task becomes a matter of deciding (1) what tasks can be most easily and legally carried out by the paraprofessional, and (2) what kinds of training the paraprofessionals need to do these jobs and the RNs need to delegate and supervise these employees. These kinds of programs have an immediate impact on the professional status of the nurse because they free the nurse to perform the more challenging parts of the job and they increase the responsibility of the nurse to include more direct supervision and training of the paraprofessionals. These kinds of changes are usually not met by much resistance within the organization as they are a response to immediate crisis and they do little to alter the structure of the organization other than to increase the supervisory responsibility of the staff nurse.

The major problem with this type of job design is that it has very little impact on the structure of the organization and does very little to change the autonomy and responsibility of the nurse in the process of determining the care of the patient. It may, in some cases, remove the nurse from direct involvement in patient care, resulting in both a reduction in stress and a reduction in job satisfaction. It may also increase stress if the nurse does not receive training and/or legitimate authority commensurate with the responsibility of supervising the paraprofessionals.

Another model of job design is *primary care nursing* (Grau, 1984; Zander, 1985). Within this model, there is a central concern with the progress of the client through an episode of care within a nursing unit. The primary care nursing model is tied to a specific patient care unit, the traditional setting of nursing care. This model of nursing care is an extension of accountability from one shift to the entire patient stay on the unit. The primary care nurse becomes an administrator who has the autonomy and the responsibility to provide patient care without losing the rewards that come from being directly involved in the provision of care. The job is enriched in terms of task, responsibility, and autonomy. The staff nurse has to exercise professional judgment and is accountable for that judgment. This model of nursing care increases the meaningful nature of the work because the primary care nurse must oversee and evaluate the total treatment process for an episode of care on her geographical unit. Difficulties in implementation have centered on 24-hour accountability, scheduling of nurses, training, and lack of authority to enforce other RN's and paraprofessional nursing personnel's implementation of the primary nurse's plan of care.

The implementation of primary nursing involves some organizational change. The nurse manager no longer is responsible for coordinating care for the unit stay of patients and is thus further removed from direct involvement in the provision of patient services. The staff nurse must learn new responsibilities for evaluation, advocacy, and delegation as a primary nurse and adherence to other nurses' care plans with patients for whom she or he is not a primary nurse. In addition to changes in nursing roles, this model affects the roles of other professionals (e.g., social workers, physicians) and paraprofessionals (e.g., UAPs, rehabilitation therapists). These changes may present an impediment to the implementation of this program of job design. The *case manager* or *service-line manager* model (Bruhn & Howes, 1986) is a job design strategy that was designed to increase the responsibility of the nurse within the organization. Case management is sometimes referred to as second-generation primary nursing. Here, the nurse is assigned a patient upon admission and becomes a case manager for the entire course of treatment for that episode of care. The nurse may be unit based and follow patients from admission to that unit or be service-line based and follow all patients within one diagnostic group. An example is the case manager on an orthopedic patient unit or a diabetic nurse case manager for all diabetic patients. The responsibilities of the case manager at the individual patient level are to oversee the process of providing treatment within the health care setting and to provide for continued treatment outside the setting. The nurse plays an active role in planning, providing treatment, negotiating with insurers for payment, cost monitoring the evaluation of treatment effectiveness, and providing aftercare. At the system level, the case manager often has responsibilities for monitoring quality of care (quality assurance); initiating and implementing activities to improve the system of care (performance improvement); and developing, implementing, and improving clinical pathways, protocols, or guidelines. This strategy increases the job variety and responsibility of the nurse and the duties of coordinating services and negotiating with insurance payors may represent an increase in autonomy within some systems. Issues of requisite authority in both patient progress through the system and quality responsibilities often occur.

This type of change does involve a change in some areas of the institution's chain of command and from a status perspective can be seen as enhancing the professional status of nurses. One drawback of this approach, however, is that if the services provided for a particular type of patient are fairly routine or if any change in routine requires the permission of a physician, then there may be no reason for this type of function to be carried out by a nurse. If no clinical judgment is needed, there is no reason that the job needs to be done by a nurse.

Another model of nursing care that can provide the foundation for increasing the professional status of nurses is the *clinical ladder* (American Nurses Association Cabinet on Nursing Service, 1984). Two problems noted in the nursing turnover literature are that the nurse quickly reaches the salary ceiling and that advancement within many organizations involves becoming an executive. The clinical ladder in its prototypic form differentiates the lines of advancement into a clinical track and an administrative track using delineation of competencies for different levels of clinical nurses. Benner's work on nursing expertise is often used as a guide in leveling competencies (Benner, 1984). In some systems, case manager or acute care nurse practitioner positions are the top level on the clinical ladder (Knaus et al., 1997). To implement this type of system, criteria for advancement that include both skill and education must be developed, and within the organization the pay scale of the nurse must be modified to accommodate the differentiation of skills within the nurses' work.

This model affects the organization by modifying the pay ceiling primarily for the clinical nurse; it may also lower the pay for new graduates. It also contributes to the professional status of nursing because it codifies the competencies, responsibilities, and duties that are performed by the nurse. The problem with the model is that there is a great deal of work and soul searching involved in developing the criteria and, except for the pay schedule changes and some organizational recognition of the status of nurses, there is often little concomitant change in the organizational structure.

The final model that is considered is the *nurse-administered unit* (Dear, Weisman, & O'Keefe, 1985; Gordon et al., 1993). In this model, there is increased self-governance for the nurses. In this particular example of the model, a group of nurses who are hospital employees develop an informal contract with the hospital for the total management of the unit. This can also be applied by nurses in an ambulatory nursing clinic. The contract involves a budget, agreements about amounts of institutional support, and specification of criteria for quality of care. In effect, a team of nurses negotiates a contract with the organization, and within that contract the team of nurses is free to develop a system for providing a program of health care. The nursing team experiences increased responsibility, autonomy, control, and accountability. The redesigning of the nurses' job is not a sweeping change and can be implemented quickly because it is localized within the contracting unit. Its success is dependent on both the acceptance of accountability by the nurses and cooperative working relationships with physicians and other professionals working on the unit.

■ IMPLEMENTING JOB DESIGN

Job design can be as simple as changing the duties of a single nurse or as complex as redesigning the role of nurses within the unit or organization. Under ideal conditions, the decision about job design can be incorporated within the long-term planning processes of the organization. Ideal conditions, however, rarely exist in complex organizations, and the nurse who is a patient care administrator has to make decisions that are at best only partial solutions to complex problems. This should not stop the process of job design. Many of the activities that have been included under the title of job design are not exotic activities for an administrator. They are frequently routine responses to problems that arise within the day-to-day commerce of an organization. Job design should not be looked at as a single discrete event, but rather as an ongoing process. Understanding this process involves awareness of what is happening within the organization, the profession, and the health care industry. At the organizational level, there is a need to know how the organization is structured and what plans are being made for continued and innovative services. At the professional level, there is the need to know the major trends in the provision of nursing care. There are a number of models of nursing practice that can provide the skeleton upon which nursing and patient care jobs can be shaped.

The process of job design that involves changing the model of delivering patient care services can be conceived as an organizational developmental process. To carry out a program of *organizational change,* it is necessary for the patient care administrator to engage in a systematic program that can be conceptualized as involving three stages: planning, implementation, and evaluation. Each of these stages involves a great deal of effort, and the success of any program of organizational change requires attention to detail at every stage.

Planning Stage

The planning stage can be seen as having four steps. The first step is to perceive a need for change. The second step is to identify the existing problems within the organization. The third step is to select and modify a specific model for change. The final step is to systematically plan for the implementation of the change. The careful execution of the steps in this first stage can reduce, although not eliminate, problems in the later implementation and evaluation stages.

The first step in planning for job redesign is to be aware that the redesigning of the nursing job is possible. *Perceiving the need for change* is not as simple as it appears. Within organizations the daily demands on an administrator of a large service are frequently both exhilarating and exacerbating. The demands on time and resources can limit one's ability to look at the organization objectively. There are constant problems to be dealt with and often there is neither the time nor resources available to plan for the long term. Without consideration of long-term objectives, the process of job redesign turns out to be a crisis intervention and not a thoughtful enhancement of the jobs of the people within the organization. Many administrators hire consultants to assist in diagnosing problems and planning job redesign. The ability to perceive the need for change involves an acute awareness of both the organization and the total environment within which that organization is embedded. Periodic retreats and self-studies often support an administrator's ability to perceive a need for change.

The second step in the planning stage is the identification of problems. *Diagnosis of problems* within a nursing staff requires knowledge of the nurses' professional concerns and their views of their job duties and responsibilities. This information is sometimes available through the normal interaction with the staff nurses and others delivering care, but as an organization gets larger, informal methods of obtaining information are often inadequate. Other methods are needed to obtain information. Structured group techniques can be used to clarify the concerns of staff nurses and paraprofessionals. These might include routine procedures, such as unit meetings, or more directed interactions, such as quality circles or focus groups. These techniques provide a way to learn about concerns, and they encourage those delivering care to participate in the planning, which can prove invaluable in diagnosing underlying problems. In addition to group interaction approaches, there is often the need to collect more precise empirical data about the entire staff and their views of patient care and the work that nurses and others do.

At the level of measuring attitudes toward the work, there are measures already developed to look at the attitudes of nurses (Prestholdt, Lane, & Mathews, 1987). In addition to these nurse-specific attitudinal measures, structured measures of staff member self-reports of their work have been developed, including the job diagnostic survey (Hackman & Oldham, 1975) and the multimethod job design questionnaire (Campion & Thayer, 1985). These questionnaires provide a relatively cheap and effective method to assess the staff's evaluations of their work. Another source of information is the behavioral assessment of patient care staff productivity (e.g., Rantz & Hauer, 1987). This method involves taking a time sample of the staff at work, and it gives a complete picture of how staff actually spend their working time. The diagnoses that are made by the patient care administrator are only as good as the information on which they are based, and the administrator has to make conscious choices about the amount and quality of information that is necessary to identify problems of the patient care staff. In most cases, it is prudent to collect information using more than one method, and if job design is an ongoing process, routine collection of this type of data should be considered.

The next step after problems have been identified is to develop *methods to remedy or reduce the problems*. The information collected about the staff and the organization become important data for the planning of change. The choice of an alternative design of patient care duties and responsibilities should be based on a realistic assessment of the attitudes and needs of the nursing and paraprofessional staff, with full awareness of organizational constraints. The models of job design developed within the nursing profession can provide both structure and justification for organizational change, but any model of patient care delivery must be molded to fit the needs of that particular nursing and paraprofessional staff and organization. At this step in the planning stage, it is important to involve professional staff in the decision-making process.

The final step in the planning stage is to *plan for the implementation* of the job redesign. At this point, the plan begins to move from an abstraction to a concrete reality, and it becomes necessary to deal with resistance to change. This resistance comes not only from management but also from the nursing and paraprofessional staff. Change represents a threat to established patterns of relationships, and if there is animosity between management and staff, the threat posed by change is magnified by the lack of trust and communication. One strategy that can be helpful in overcoming this resistance is to include organizational staff in this choice process. Treating staff in a professional manner by involving them in the choice process can increase both their involvement and investment in the change process. The short-term cost of this approach is that it often broadens the scope of the changes, but in the long term it reduces some of the resistance. It keeps the new program from being perceived as being imposed by the administrators, and, in many cases, the people included in this planning stage become the core group of the implementation stage.

Implementation Stage

The implementation stage is the major action component in organizational change. In most cases, the success of this stage is dependent on the thoroughness of the planning and the involvement of middle management. It also depends on the ability of the administrators and staff to translate plans into action. Often, insufficient resources are allocated to this stage, resulting in fragmented implementation. For example, deadlines have to be established, staff members must be trained, responsibilities of staff and management must be defined, mechanisms must be established to deal with the problems that inevitably arise, and methods for obtaining feedback from the staff and communicating information to the staff must be established. The implementation is not a one-time occurrence, but an ongoing process.

Evaluation Stage

The final stage is evaluation of the effectiveness of the job redesign. This evaluation involves measuring the impact of the changes on staff, clients, and the organization. The measures should be chosen to reflect the stated goals of the job redesign effort. These measures should include measures of clients (e.g., desired outcomes, quality of care processes, client satisfaction), staff (e.g., absenteeism, turnover, job satisfaction), and organizational effectiveness (e.g., competitive advantage, cost–benefit analysis). The job redesign program has been designed and implemented to improve the organization, and it has involved a great deal of effort. Thought and effort alone, however, do not insure that the job redesign will work. The evaluation component of organizational change is designed to provide objective standards for justifying continued implementation and for identifying components of the effort that require modification. The administrator must realize that the job redesign usually will not fulfill all of the stated goals, and there will be the need for modification over time.

Job design has played an important part in changing the manner in which work gets done. In nursing, a series of job design approaches have attempted to deal with specific problems (i.e., nursing shortages, failure to recognize clinical expertise, power differentials, coordination of care across a continuum of services). An overall evaluation of these approaches suggested that no method has been dramatically successful, but each of these approaches has been successful in dealing with important problems. The focus of the job design approaches, however, has been limited to subsystems (i.e., units, services, departments) within the larger organization. This focus has led primarily to local change within the organization. Local change is manageable, and there is no doubt that attempts to deal with local change will benefit from a review of the available models of patient care delivery and from an understanding of how the changes were implemented. These job design methods are a valuable source of ideas for dealing with subsystem-based problems. However, job design is not simply a matter of selecting and implementing a model. Job design is a change process and is subject to all of the challenges and pitfalls of any change process.

■ SYSTEM REDESIGN

The reality of organizations today and at the start of the 21st century is that traditional, multilayered, bureaucratic organizations could become an endangered species. Business environments have become more competitive and less predictable. We are in the midst of a technological and information revolution. The new business organization is being visualized as lean and flexible. Organizational survival will depend on the ability to improve internal and external communications, to constantly monitor the environment, to make effective use of personnel and resources, and to negotiate and form alliances with other organizations. Organizations will become parts of an interconnected network.

In light of these realizations, organizational scientists have proposed a number of prescriptions for managing organizational change. The proposals have included ideas such as quality circles, total quality management (TQM), matrix organizations, learning organizations, and reengineering the organization. All of these methods share the view that technology has changed both the nature and speed of information exchange and expectations of customers, and that these changes will continue. Organizations have to adapt, and adaptation requires more accountability and efficient use of information. The employees are central to both generating and making proper use of the information for efficiency and accountability. Decisions have to be made quickly; to implement this rapid response, each individual becomes a part of the process and takes on new responsibilities and authority.

These changes have engulfed production and service-based industries, and they certainly apply to health care delivery systems. Health care still has as its primary goal the provision of quality care to its customers, but the importance of providing care in an affordable and accountable manner has increased. The health care industry has become competitive, and the need for redesign of health care systems is clear. The freestanding community hospital that offers only inpatient and emergency care is no longer economically viable. The new health care system has to become comprehensive and seamless. The product is not just treatment for illness, but also wellness, education, and information sharing among service providers and clients. Health care is increasingly being provided by multidisciplinary teams operating across different organizational boundaries, rather than by an independent physician.

The work of health care has become more complex, and the system redesign approaches hold that organizational structures and functions must be redesigned to accommodate these changes and to prepare for changes that are on the horizon (Dienemann & Gessner, 1992). The problem is how best to accomplish these changes and plan for the future. In nursing, four broad and interrelated frameworks have been proposed to accomplish the redesign of health care systems. The first is the creation of structures to involve more nurses in decision making. The second is an extension of the primary care and case management approaches to job design. The third is the use of TQM and other group-based performance improvement methods to modify organizations. The fourth is to reengineer the work environment. Despite their different methods, all of these approaches are designed to make organizations more responsive to customers, more accountable, and more cost efficient.

One of the first attempts to enrich nursing jobs through system redesign was the introduction of *shared governance*. This approach creates an infrastructure for decentralization of decisions about nursing work. Council or committee structures are initiated to involve staff nurses in organizational issues of patient care delivery. Often they include informational meetings, practice committees or councils, unit-based and system-wide quality improvement, and nursing standards committees or councils (Peterson & Allen, 1986; Porter-O'Grady, 1994).

The second of these approaches to system redesign has its origins within the nursing profession and is an extension of case management. Examples of these approaches include *ProACT* and *ProACTII* (Brett & Tonges, 1990; Brett et al., 1977; Tonges, 1989), and *CareMap* (Zander, 1995). These methods for systems redesign view the care of the customer as the basic job of the health care system. They seek to redirect the organizing center of care from the individual hospital unit to the person and his or her family. Health care is seen as being provided by a multidisciplinary team and involves planning and coordinating entire sequences of interventions. The person is seen as requiring a continuity of care across a number of different services or settings, and the job of providing care involves a coordination of these diverse activities. Service can no longer be perceived as happening in one unit or even one organization, and the nurse's responsibility is to coordinate the total care process. The nurse, as coordinator of care, assumes a central role. Nursing has the primary responsibility for planning and implementing the redesign of the system, parallel to and in conjunction with the organizational evolution of health care delivery.

The third model for the redesign of the work systems is *TQM*. This approach has as its focus the removal of waste and non-value added work (Carefoote, 1995). TQM depends on input from employees, and views employees' input as essential for the development of proposals for streamlining work processes. The approach strives to shift management styles from directive to facilitative and the culture of the organization from top down decision making to top stimulation of decision making. The impetus and prescription for change is seen as coming from within the organization at the direct care level. There may be a champion or facilitator of change, but the TQM groups are the source of innovation. The process must be management supported, but not management controlled. This process involves extensive employee involvement to insure that an accurate analysis of the work process occurs and that employees are committed to creating and implementing innovations. The process of change is seen as evolutionary in nature. Many organizations that adopted this approach in the 1980s are reporting disillusionment because the underlying issues remain unresolved. Proponents point out that TQM is a continuous process and requires ongoing commitment to evolutionary change to resolve problems; processes of work will never be perfected and can only be improved.

A fourth approach to system redesign has been labeled *reengineering*. This approach, like the others, focuses on changing old techniques and structures and moving toward a flexible organization (Hammer & Champy, 1993). It differs however in its focus and in its call for rapid, revolutionary change. The goal of reengineering is to improve performance while reducing costs. The simplest approach to cost reduction is restructuring (combine, disaggregate, or spin off) to reduce the workforce. This may create an economically viable future and less bureaucracy. It may also demoralize the survivors or be ineffective (Cameron, 1993).

Reengineering is a more complex approach than those previously mentioned as it involves the changing of work processes. The job of change agents is to dramatically change the way in which work gets done. The reshaping of work is revolution, not evolution. The method of revolution is to focus on the solution and not the problem. The assumption is that insufficient gains can be made by incremental change to redesign existing jobs; total redesign is the only effective solution. The task in reengineering is to look at desired outcomes and the entire work process, and to identify the existing steps in the process. Once the steps have been identified, reengineering attempts to reconfigure the process to reduce the steps, assign the lowest appropriate level of worker, and reduce costs of coordination and control. The reengineering team is to begin "with a clean slate." For instance, if the work is presently being done by five different specialists in five different departments but the same outcome could be done by two generalists in one department, then the reengineering will involve getting rid of the specialists. Two generalists are then trained to become the work team within one department. The work is the focus, and the people have to be selected and/or trained to fit the work. If the work changes, then the individuals and teams have to adjust to the new role demands. This is a top down approach to innovation, and change is based on the rational qualities of the work, not on the politics of functional units or professional identity. It has proven to be most effective in bureaucratic organizations that need to become more responsive to customers.

Keidel (1994) suggests another approach to reengineering, which he labels rethinking. The target for change in this instance is individual and collective mindsets. It is the most expensive type of reengineering and involves changes in the balance of technical control, personal autonomy, and organizational cooperation. This approach is limited to firms that are not under current threat to survival and that value change through development of employees to maintain strategic advantage.

■ IMPLEMENTING SYSTEM REDESIGN

System redesign has been perceived as being necessary for organizational survival in a turbulent environment. The problem is that large scale organizational change is a challenging, even daunting, task. There are different perspectives on what needs to be changed and how that change should be accomplished. There are calls for radical change, but change within an existing organization is often a slow process that can evoke fierce resistance. The process of system redesign involves altering, replacing, or eliminating existing structures and changing the coordination and interrelationships among many stakeholders both within and outside the organization. The role of the nurse patient care administrator is to be an advocate for quality of care, and to provide a sense of direction during the planning, implementation, and evaluation phases.

The questions are those of how to manage the change and what the roles of different stakeholders in the redesign process are to be. The systems redesign approaches views change as a radical necessity. Continual monitoring and assessment is needed to evaluate the success of the process and to improve outcomes.

Planning

The planning stages for job design and system redesign can be seen as having similar steps: a perceived need for change, diagnosis of problem, identification of method, and planning for implementation. In the present era, there is consensus that change is necessary and beneficial. The problems arise at the level of diagnosis of problem. The diagnosis often seems to be determined by the orientation of the practitioner, whose method prescribes steps for implementation.

Successful planning to redesign an organization might depend more on the quality of administrator than on the particular strategy selected. Some of the qualities desired are system awareness, a vision or sense of direction, and a flexible leadership style (Smeltzer, Formella, & Beebe, 1993). Of these characteristics, system awareness of the interactive consequences of the internal dynamics of the organization and its external environment is most critical. Systems change, whether revolutionary or evolutionary, requires an awareness of the total environmental context of the organization. Edwards and Roomer (1996) suggest that nurse managers are frequently focused on the operations of individual units and are less aware of the relationship among units and among health care organizations. It is vital for the future of nursing that their awareness is expanded to the entire health care industry. Closely tied to systems awareness is developing a sense of vision or direction. In an uncertain environment, there is no clearly defined path to the goal of affordable quality care, but the goal itself provides guidance in choosing among alternatives. The planning for system redesign requires being able to tap the knowledge and experiences of a large number of stakeholders, because they have valuable expertise and their involvement and energy are essential to the implementation of change. The leader must persuade, influence, facilitate, and actively listen to the groups involved in the planning process. Too many innovations have been stifled by leaders who try to impose their solutions to problems.

Implementation and Evaluation

The process of implementing a systems redesign plan in an existing organization requires an extremely high level of effort and involvement. This is a job that requires partnership, teamwork, and organizational support. Change reverberates throughout the system. The evaluation and monitoring processes have to involve the entire system. Sovie (1995) has enumerated some of the implications of redesign efforts. Management will have to change assumptions about control and move toward sharing both responsibility and authority with employees. People will have to expand and create new role relationships and relinquish others. Some functions will be centralized and others decentralized; some jobs will disappear and others will be created. Traditional mixes of staff will be altered. New technology will be introduced and the need for effective communication will be heightened.

Implementation of system redesign must be a collaborative effort that involves people both inside and outside of the organization. People are not accustomed to the rapid pace or extensiveness of change in reengineering. Multiple, unanticipated and undesirable short-term consequences are inevitable. The implementation of the plan and the evaluation of its impact must be a continuing and recursive process that includes quick responses.

Implementation of the initial reengineering design is not an end in itself. Everyone from top management to maintenance workers needs to "keep their eye on the prize" and be empowered to redesign their work in response to unanticipated outcomes. Personnel, at all levels, will also need ongoing support for long-term growth through massive transitions.

■ BIOGRAPHICAL SKETCH

Dr. Theodore L. Gessner is an Associate Professor of Psychology at George Mason University in Fairfax, Virginia. Dr. Gessner received his PhD in Social Psychology from the University of Maryland. Before joining the faculty at George Mason University, he was employed as a research psychologist in both private and public mental hospitals. His research interests include adaptation to organizations, destructiveness in organizations, and sense of humor. Dr. Gessner teaches undergraduate and graduate courses in social psychology and psychological research methods.

■ SUGGESTED READINGS

Blancett, S.S., & Flarey, D.L. (1995). *Reengineering: Nursing and health care.* Gaithersburg, MD: Aspen.

Porter-O'Grady, T., & Krueger, C. (1995). *The leadership revolution in health care: Altering systems, changing behaviors.* Gaithersburg, MD: Aspen.

Rousseau, D.M. (1995). *Psychological contracts in organizations.* Thousand Oaks, CA: Sage.

For a review of basic theories of motivation and job design, see any textbook on organizational behavior or organizational development.

■ REFERENCES

American Nurses Association Cabinet on Nursing Service. (1984). *Career ladders: An approach to professional productivity and job satisfaction.* Kansas City, MO: American Nurses Association.

Benner, P. (1984). *From novice to expert: Excellence and power in clinical nursing practice.* Redwood City, CA: Addison-Wesley.

Brett, J.L., Bueno, M., Royal, N., & Kendall-Sengin, K. (1997). ProACTII: Integrating utilization management, discharge planning, and nursing case management into the outcome manager's role. *Journal of Nursing Administration, 27* (2), 37–45.

Brett, J.L.L., & Tonges, M.C. (1990). Restructuring patient care delivery: Evaluation of ProAct model. *Nursing Economics, 8* (1), 36–44.

Bruhn, P.S., & Howes, D.H. (1986). Service line management: New opportunities for nursing executives. *Journal of Nursing Administration, 16* (6), 13–18.

Cameron, K.S. (1993), cited in Richard A. Melcher, How Goliaths can act like Davids. *Business Week, 193.*

Campion, M.A., & Thayer, P.W. (1985). Development and field evaluation of an inter-disciplinary measure of job design. *Journal of Applied Psychology, 70* (1), 29–43.

Carefoote, R. (1995). The TQM-reengineering link. In S.S. Blancett & D.L. Flarey (Eds.), *Reengineering Nursing and Health Care* (pp. 50–59). Gaithersburg, MD: Aspen.

Dear, M.R., Weisman, C.S., & O'Keefe, S. (1985). Evaluation of a contract model for professional nursing practice. *Health Care Management Review, 10* (2), 65–77.

Dienemann, J., & Gessner, T. (1992). Restructuring nursing care delivery systems. *Nursing Economics, 10* (4), 253–259.

Edwards, P.A., & Roemer, L. (1996). Are nurse managers ready for the current challenges of health care? *Journal of Nursing Administration, 26* (9), 11–17.

Gordon, D.L., Wiesman, C.S., Cassard, S.D., Bergner, M., & Wong, R. (1993). The effects of unit self-management on hospital nurses' work process, work satisfaction and retention. *Medical Care, 31* (5), 381–393.

Grau, L. (1984). Case management and the nurse. *Geriatric Nursing, 5* (8), 372–375.

Hackman, J.R., & Oldham, G.R. (1975). Development of the job diagnostic survey. *Journal of Applied Psychology, 60* (1), 159–170.

Hammer, M., & Champy, J. (1993). *Reengineering the corporation: A manifesto for business revolution.* New York: Harper.

Herzberg, F. (1966). *Work and the nature of man.* New York: World.

Herzberg, F., Mausner, B., & Snyderman, B. (1959). *The motivation to work.* New York: Wiley.

Keidel, R.W. (1994). Rethinking organizational design. *The Academy of Management Executives, 8* (4), 12–30.

Knaus, V.L., Felten, S., Burton, S., Fobes, P., & Davis, K. (1997). The use of nurse practitioners in the acute care setting. *Journal of Nursing Administration, 27* (2), 20–27.

Peterson, M.E., & Allen, D.G. (1986). Shared governance: A strategy for transforming organizations, Part 1. *Journal of Nursing Administration, 16* (1), 11–16.

Porter-O'Grady, T. (1994). Whole system shared governance: Creating the seamless organization. *Nursing Economics, 12* (4), 187–195.

Prescott, P.A., Phillips, C.Y., Ryan, J.W., & Thompson, K.O. (1991). Changing how nurses spend their time. *Image, 23* (1), 23–28.

Prestholdt, P.H., Lane, I.M., & Mathews, R.C. (1987). Nurse turnover as reasoned action: Development of a process model. *Journal of Applied Psychology, 72* (2), 121–127.

Rantz, M., & Hauer, J.D. (1987). Analyzing acute care nursing staff productivity. *Nursing Management, 18* (4), 33–44.

Sittig, D.F. (1990). Work sampling: A statistical approach to evaluation of the effect of computers on work patterns in healthcare. *Methods of Information Medicine, 71* (7), 58–63.

Smeltzer, C.H., Formella, N.M., & Beebe, H. (1993). Work restructuring: The process of decision making. *Nursing Economics, 11* (4), 215–222.

Sovie, M.D. (1995). Tailoring hospitals for managed care and integrated health systems. *Nursing Economics, 13* (2), 72–83.

Taylor, F.W. (1910). *The principles of scientific management.* New York: Harper & Row.

Tonges, M.C. (1989). Redesigning hospital nursing practice: The professionally advanced care team (ProAct) model, Part 1. *Journal of Nursing Administration, 19* (7), 31–38.

Trist, E. (1981). The evaluation of sociotechnical systems as a conceptual framework and as an action research program. In A.H. Vandiven & W.F. Joyce (Eds.), *Perspectives in organizational design and behavior* (pp. 19–75). New York: Wiley.

Zander, K. (1985). Second generation primary nursing: A new agenda. *Journal of Nursing Administration, 15* (3), 18–21.

Zander, K. (1995). CareMap systems and case management: Creating waves of restructured care. In S.S. Blancett & D.L. Flarey (Eds.), *Reengineering nursing and health care* (pp. 50–59). Gaithersburg, MD: Aspen.

CASE 11-1 Challenges in Evaluating Redesign

Marcelline Harris, Alice P. Weydt, Holly Frohling, and Annette McBeth

Immanuel-St. Joseph's-Mayo Health System (ISJ) is a 272-bed hospital located in south-central Minnesota. In the mid-1980s, the nursing department was experiencing difficulties with recruitment, retention, and difficult contract bargaining sessions with the contract bargaining unit. Concerns were voiced about the lack of staff input into decision making. The nursing department was characterized by other departments as having a sense of "entitlement" regarding hospital support for nursing work. Throughout the hospital, there was a pronounced internal department focus. It was not unusual for one department to make changes in procedures or processes that affected multiple departments without any notification, let alone collaborative planning, about changes. Meanwhile, in the broader health care arena, there was a dawning realization that hospital work had to change in very fundamental ways to fit the federal prospective reimbursement system associated with Diagnostic Related Groups (DRGs). Cost containment was a theme. Consequently, at the time a new nurse executive was hired as vice president in 1988, there was serious interest and broad support from within nursing, as well as the broader hospital organization, in redesigning the way work was done.

This case study is about the challenges we faced in evaluating the redesign project, and recommendations based on our experience. Details of the redesign are described elsewhere (Mc-Beth, Schweer, & Aadalen, 1995; McBeth & Weydt, 1996). A brief summary is presented here only to give readers a sense of the broad scope of the redesign effort and the most significant process changes.

■ BASIC BELIEFS ABOUT REDESIGN

The overall goal of the redesign was to focus responsibility and accountability for decision making at the point of care with awareness of the ramifications for the patient across a continuum of service settings. Expectations were that this would be the best way to manage the use, quality, and cost of services throughout the course of a person's illness. At the time redesign was planned, the basic beliefs of the nursing management team were that:

- Nurses involved in direct care should be given responsibility and accountability for the care delivery system.
- Nursing services delivered beyond the hospital walls would require a "seamless continuum of care" approach.
- Collaboration within nursing and across disciplines is necessary for work redesign to succeed.
- New processes needed to support the changes in nursing care delivery should complement broader changes within the hospital.

CASE: 11-1 *Continued*

Primary nursing was selected as the model for redesign of inpatient nursing care delivery, and case management was selected as the model for external, or "beyond the hospital walls" care delivery. The other new nursing role was use of clinical nurse specialists (CNSs) to provide clinical support to both primary nurses and case managers. Implementation of this redesign required a more highly educated nursing staff. The hospital supported the educational preparation of the nursing staff at all levels: licensed practical nurse (LPN) to registered nurse (RN), RN to baccalaureate of science in nursing (BSN), and graduate preparation, through service/education partnerships and tuition reimbursement. Consultants were used extensively. Job descriptions and evaluations were rewritten to reflect performance in new job roles.

Predictions were that emerging health care systems would demand that the patient and family move between episodes and settings of care without fragmentation or duplication. Nurse case manager positions, expanded home care, parish nursing, occupational health, and a nurse-run health center were created to support nursing care delivery beyond the walls of the hospital.

Improved collaboration within nursing (between nursing management and the contract bargaining group), and without nursing (between nurses and those in other disciplines) was sought through several channels. Labor–management forums were initiated and convened monthly between nursing management and the nursing contract bargaining unit. A primary objective was to facilitate communication about work redesign. Staff nurse representation was achieved on a broad array of hospital committees. A physician was hired by the hospital to focus on quality improvement, and serious work was put into relationship management issues between nursing and medicine. Clinical paths were developed and implemented by nurse and physician partnerships to enhance standardization of care within specific clinical populations.

Changes in the hospital to support the redesign also supported wider needs of the hospital. The physical plant was remodeled, and structural changes on patient care centers supported decentralized patient care delivery. A new information system was installed, including handheld computers for nursing staff. The budgeting process was restructured across hospital departments, and a patient acuity system designed to distribute nursing resources according to patient needs was implemented. As part of a regional consortium known as "Health Bond," ISJ received consultation and financial support for redesign through participation in the Robert Wood Johnson Foundation/Pew Charitable Trusts (RWJF/Pew) initiative "Strengthening Hospital Nursing, Improving Patient Care." ISJ's administrator and board members were participants along with nursing in patient-focused, interdisciplinary activities supported by the grant.

■ CHALLENGES IN USING EXISTING DATA TO EVALUATE REDESIGN

The end of funding from the RWJF/Pew grant in 1995 required submission of an evaluation of changes within the consor-

CASE: 11–1 *Continued*

tium as a whole, and also stimulated an internal evaluation of redesign within ISJ, specifically. Several interconnected issues that emerged as we tried to identify, retrieve, analyze, and interpret "hard data," have been carried forward into future plans for ongoing evaluation of nursing services. These include: evaluation model issues, ratio issues, numerator issues, denominator issues, and interpretation issues.

Model Issues

A shift from measuring change based upon a goal-driven, management by objectives (MBO) model to a resource-driven model occurred nationally between the 1980s and the mid-1990s (Barnum & Kerfoot, 1995). ISJ's redesign effort was planned using a goal-driven MBO model to measure quality of the nursing redesign product. Goals were set, objectives articulated related to nursing care delivery, plans designed to meet the objectives, resources obtained to meet the objectives, and plans made for evaluation and data collection; the plan was then carried out. Several years later, when the final evaluation was due, the value of the original model was questioned. The need for answers to different questions was evident.

In the resource-driven model the concern is whether, given the available resources, goals have been prioritized, the most feasible methods determined, the plan put into effect, and outcomes analyzed within the context of resources used. Subsequently, analytical ratios such as cost–benefit and cost–effective-

ness became the focus of the evaluation effort. Retrospective data analysis was necessary, as data elements to answer questions posed in this new model were not identified at the start of the project and collected concurrently. An evaluation focused on demonstrating whether the objectives designed in the MBO model were met was of limited interest within or outside the hospital.

Ratio Issues: Cost–Benefit and Cost–Effectiveness

Ratios are the desired data to analyze outcomes in the context of resources used in the resource-driven model. Ratios represent the magnitude of one occurrence in relation to another. Issues related to constructing cost–benefit and cost–effectiveness ratios included obtaining data from comparable time periods in the numerators and denominators, and defining data elements in the numerators and denominators. Our hospital is typical of all health care organizations; many data elements are collected in different time periods by different databases for different purposes. Each database had been developed independently without provision for standardization or integration. Therefore, data such as births are reported as total annual or average annual, patient satisfaction is reported quarterly, and patient days are reported monthly. Data about salaries are most accurately available for 2-week time periods. It is time-consuming to extrapolate different data to comparable time periods, and concerns arise about the accuracy of the extrapolated values.

CASE: 11–1 *Continued*

The greater concern, however, was defining and identifying data elements for the ratios. We referenced Rossi and Freeman (1993), who defined cost–benefit as an "analytical procedure for determining the economic efficiency of a program, expressed as the relationship between costs and outcomes, usually measured in monetary terms" (p. 362). Cost–effectiveness was defined as "the efficacy of a program in achieving given intervention outcomes in relation to the program costs" (Rossi & Freeman, 1993, p. 362). Overall, we have found that "true" hospital costs are extremely difficult to obtain with accuracy, and that neither costs, nor benefits, nor outcomes are easily identified or retrieved.

Numerator Issues: Cost Data

Charge data is readily available; cost data is not. The problem of detecting costs by using hospital charge data is an issue widely discussed in the current literature. Charges in most hospitals have been skewed to fit reimbursement systems, with little attention to whether those charges are consistent with resource inputs (costs). Additionally, the data capturing systems in our hospital, like most hospitals, was not designed to look at nursing costs. At present, the controller uses a percentage of the cost–charge ratio as an estimate of "true" cost. Other challenges we faced in obtaining data to report the costs are whether nursing cost data was *available, useful,* and *comparable* over time.

In searching for *available* data, the nursing department at ISJ tapped two in-formation sources to try to abstract nursing cost data. First, we looked to the hospital's internal accounting system. Complicated formulas and adjustments are applied before hospital-generated financial data is available in budget packets. Interpretation of this data is subsequently neither simple nor straightforward, and requires close consultation with the hospital's financial officer. Additionally, although our acuity system is used within nursing for resource allocation, it is not yet a formal part of the hospital's budgeting process. The second source we used to obtain cost data was a large, national consulting company that provides ongoing productivity reports to the hospital. ISJ's productivity is reported by department and nursing center, and we receive data about comparable organizations in the region and the nation that also contract with this consulting company. (See Examples 1 and 2, later in this case study.)

In some situations, cost data was available but not *useful* because data elements did not measure value for a resource-based paradigm. An example was the effort to analyze the cost–benefit of tuition reimbursement for the formal education of nursing department employees. Although the Human Resources (HR) department processed tuition reimbursement checks, and required evidence that the class was passed, HR did not track information on actual completion of degrees. Remember, the original objective of providing tuition reimbursement was to support continued formal education, not necessarily achievement of higher degrees. Thus, we could say

CASE: 11–1 *Continued*

that the objective of nurses achieving additional formal education was met, but we could not measure benefits in value added to the organization or improved patient outcomes. Also, the impact of a single course was believed to be too small to show any value or outcome change.

Some elements of cost data were not *comparable* because similarly labeled categories changed composition over time. For example, interpreting nursing full-time equivalent (FTE) changes by unit over time was not comparable. Unit nursing FTEs had been reported differently in different years—for some years, unit reports included just direct care staff; for other years, nursing middle management and administrative positions were included. In addition, in some instances unit definition changed because of the physical remodeling of the hospital. Reconstructing this data would have been very labor intensive and it was not clear that it was possible to do so accurately.

Denominator Issues (Benefits and Effectiveness)

Identifying and retrieving relevant data for the denominator when analyzing cost–benefit and cost–effectiveness ratios is challenging because of the range of factors that may be of interest. For us these included: defining beneficiaries of costs, identifying the outcome measure that would endure over time, and calculating unit productivity for the system.

In cost–benefit analyses, when outcomes in the denominator are expressed in monetary terms, one must first determine *to whom the benefits will be ascribed*. Many potential beneficiaries of redesigned nursing care delivery systems are suggested in the literature: the hospital, the as-yet-unrealized-but-expected-to-emerge "system," patients, providers, and society. Decisions about benefits to whom, ways to put dollar values on those benefits, and then collection of relevant data must be made before cost–benefit ratios can be computed. Cost–effectiveness ratios present similar challenges. Many varied clinical and satisfaction outcomes are of interest in the denominator; some are "generic" across clinical populations, and some are specific to clinical populations. The complex, unresolved issues associated with inferring effectiveness of specific activities by reporting clinical outcomes and perceptual outcomes, such as satisfaction, are well described.

A second issue was finding an *enduring outcome measure*. Patient days are presently the most easily retrieved denominator because of the tracking systems in place within the organization. Medical records, fiscal services, and information services departments all track this data. We regularly retrieved this data for annual retrospective trending as part of our budgeting process. Interpretation of this data in the context of nursing care is less straightforward than it first appears. For example, the category of patient days reflects inpatients on nursing care units at midnight but does not capture any patients on an inpatient unit classified as outpatients. (Depending on the service, a substantial number of

CASE: 11–1 *Continued*

patients may be classified as outpatients because their planned length of stay [LOS] is less than 24 hours.) Another invisible user of nursing services not captured by this measure is the midday overlap experienced with discharges and admissions to the same bed. Consequently, it can be difficult to reconcile the costs of nursing care with the "official" counts of patient days.

Recently, statistical adjustments have been made to address this issue, and we are fine-tuning the concept of "adjusted patient days." One source of data to assist this endeavor has been the detailed, 4-hour records of census counts, acuity, and staffing kept by the nurse manager of the intensive care unit (ICU) for several years. Unfortunately, this data was recorded on paper and requires a great deal of time to enter into a database and analyze. We also fear our new "adjusted patient day" measure may not be useful for long as it may not capture costs for capitated payment. Capitated systems are less likely to be as interested in tracking admissions and patient days, and more likely to be interested in other means of tracking resources used to achieve specific patient outcomes. This is another issue in evaluating anything in a natural environment that is rapidly changing; no measure seems to endure long enough to have great value over time.

Demonstrating unit productivity for the system with available data has been especially problematic within our organization. There is a need to present data that administrators and controllers accept as "true." Anecdotal stories about

what "might" have happened without case managers or primary nurses are not acceptable. For example, what didn't happen as a result of primary nursing and case management being in place? Our efforts to examine avoidance of rehospitalization and physicians' visits in behavioral health and medical/surgical populations are presented later in this case study (see Example 3).

Separating productivity measures by department when costs span more than one department leads to misleading productivity outcomes. This is especially problematic when rewards are based on department productivity reports. For example, although the pharmacy department report shows high productivity from generating revenues in the form of charges and low wage costs, the costs of nursing time are not included in calculations. ISJ has a centralized pharmacy that sends out 3-day supplies of patient medications to the unit. Nursing time (cost) is needed to submit medication orders, monitor timeliness and accuracy of delivery, break down supplies into daily dosages, and return unused medications for patient credit, but is not reflected in the pharmacy productivity report. All nursing time is charged to the nursing department's productivity reports.

We are also concerned about interpreting productivity as the switch to capitation is made. For example, services presently viewed as high revenue generators (e.g., cardiac catheterization lab) are likely to be viewed as high-cost liabilities. Identifying ways to quantify productivity to the system represent significant challenges.

CASE: 11–1 *Continued*

Interpretation Issues

No data is interpretable without some point of comparison, or benchmark. Within most organizations, historically trended data is of interest (assuming issues presented above are adequately reconciled). We were very pleased that the internal, trended data suggested we accomplished not just cost containment, but also true cost reduction within the nursing department. This interpretation was supported by the controller and administrator. However comparisons with hospitals in the region and nation, available through ISJ's productivity reporting service, somewhat tempered our eagerness to attribute cost reduction to redesign, as most of our comparison hospitals have also experienced progress in cost reduction. (See Example 2, later in this study.) Reports in the literature are available to use for benchmarking purposes, but at this point we are hesitant to compare our results to published reports on the benefits of redesign because there is rarely enough supporting documentation about how data elements were defined and measured. Additionally, important contextual variables such as details of redesign, severity of illness, and physician practice patterns are rarely available.

■ CHANGED BELIEFS ABOUT REDESIGN

Several beliefs that guided the planning of the redesign have been modified in response to our evaluation efforts and results.

- Giving nurses involved in direct care responsibility and accountability is not enough.
- The "seamless" continuum of care is not the correct analogy for a redesigned system of nursing care delivery.
- Collaboration is more than desirable; it is absolutely essential.
- Changes in processes to support nursing care delivery and the organization's mission will never be complete.

At ISJ, accepting responsibility and accountability requires access to information to support decision making, as well as on a shared perception of responsibility and accountability. Demonstrating accountability with "hard data" has become a focus within the total organization, and many inconsistencies have been uncovered. Our case management executive committee and intensive care concurrent review activities act as a crucible for struggling with these issues.

An executive case management committee was formed to review cases and attempt to develop cost–benefit and cost–effectiveness measures to demonstrate value. Membership includes the case managers, physicians, and the heads of utilization review, fiscal services, quality improvement, home care, information services, the vice president, and two clinical directors. This committee meets quarterly to review cases the nurses believe may highlight that the redesign effort has made a difference in clinical, satisfaction, or financial outcomes. We use these cases to try to

CASE: 11–1 *Continued*

construct cost–benefit and cost–effectiveness ratios. The availability, retrievability, and interpretability of data within ISJ across the continuum of care is examined and debated at these meetings.

A concurrent review is conducted twice a week in ICU and includes primary nurses, utilization review, medical records coders, and other clinical services such as physical therapy and speech. The availability, retrievability, and interpretability of data within ISJ as it relates to patients currently in the hospital is discussed. The focus of this meeting is identification, delivery, and timely use of resources to support care throughout the anticipated length of stay. This has been very effective in limiting resource consumption in ICU, but has not been expanded to other patient centers because of the limited availability of the medical record coders.

Issues associated with shared responsibility and accountability emerged during our evaluation of redesign. Consultants were used extensively to work with the entire staff on articulating the primary nursing model within ISJ, and on individual leadership and empowerment skills that could make the redesign happen. Nonetheless, our evaluation showed many patients did not have a primary nurse assigned or the assigned primary nurse was not consistently available to the patient. We believe that the learning curve was more extended than we anticipated, that several barriers impeded implementation, and that multiple new nursing roles were initially not well understood, nor fully embraced.

Noting that even the best-tailored garments have seams, we have shifted our goal from seamless care to ensuring that the plaids match and the seams are not obvious. Two issues in this area were the barriers of contract agreements about floating and scheduling with low census and part-time nurses being primary nurses. We had firm guidelines in our bargaining contract, using seniority as the criteria for floating a nurse off a unit or sending a nurse home on low census days. It became difficult to stay true to the philosophy of primary nursing for a patient's tenure on a unit when primary nurses were floated to other units or canceled as low census days occurred. At present, the behavioral health unit staff has developed an alternate plan to address this issue with seniority being only one of the factors considered.

The use of part-time RNs as primary nurses was unexpectedly problematic. We had not sufficiently considered that the effectiveness of nursing work is often influenced through relationships established over time with patients, families, and others in the system who interact around the patient's care. There were too many opportunities for important information and activities to be omitted when part-time RNs functioned as primary nurses. One director uses the analogy of running a relay with too many runners and too many opportunities to drop the baton. We have changed our qualifications for the primary nurse position to include being full time. We are also scheduling primary nurses to support their role. In addition to full-time primary nurses, two full-time nurse case managers have been put in place within the past 2 years. Presently, primary

CASE: 11–1   *Continued*

nurses refer to case managers for coordination of services outside the hospital.

This redesign, separating coordination of care inside and outside of the hospital walls, influenced the evaluation effort in two ways. First, we were unwilling to launch an extensive evaluation before the full redesign was in place. Second, we are still searching for the points in time where the "benefits" or "productivity" of primary nursing and case management are best captured. Delineating the scope of influence and effect of redesign in the midst of so many other changes is a continuing difficulty.

We mentioned the importance of and attempts to improve collaboration earlier. Despite all our efforts, physicians and other departments within the hospital did not initially act collaboratively; the redesign was seen as belonging to nursing and not the hospital. Outsiders were initially critical of the redesign. Frequent comments were heard about not understanding "who to go to" and "who to make rounds with." Looking back, we believe insufficient attention was paid to the losses experienced during the transition. The loss of relationships with previous head nurses was genuinely grieved. Under the old model, head nurses were reliable and easily identifiable sources of information. It takes time to establish and trust new relationships, especially when substituting one for several. The reality is that without "hard data" to demonstrate the benefits of redesign, it was often very difficult to defend the changes.

Multiple data sources must constantly be analyzed to inform process changes related to practice. One-shot evaluations do stimulate a useful intense and focused look at the effects of total redesign. However constant, concurrent use of data such as LOS, recidivism, relevant clinical data, and patient and staff satisfaction may better support the continuous quality improvement processes that are needed to best respond to a rapidly changing environment.

■ EXAMPLES OF EVALUATING FINANCIAL OUTCOMES

Although this case study has focused on the challenges in evaluating the redesign of nursing care delivery systems using existing data, we believe opportunities exist. Three examples of using financial data to demonstrate effects of redesign within this organization are presented here.

Example 1: Evaluating the Financial Impact of Redesign Using Internal Benchmarks

Dollar expenses attributed to nursing did not decrease over the 5 years from the start of the redesign effort to the point of evaluation, even when the numbers were adjusted for inflation. As we sought to understand this, we examined different ratios and found nursing expenses as a percentage of total hospital expenses demonstrated a consistent decrease. Had nursing expenses remained at 18.79 percent of total hospital expenses over this 5-year period, we estimate that nursing costs would have been over $5.6 million higher than they were (see Table 11–1).

CASE: 11–1 *Continued*

TABLE 11–1. Decreasing Nursing Expenses After Redesign*

	NURSING EXPENSES	HOSPITAL EXPENSES	NURSING HOSPITAL (%)	EXPECTED NURSING EXPENSES AT 89/90 RATE (18.79%)	VARIANCE (ACTUAL – EXPECTED AT 18.79%)
1989–1990	5.829	31.018	18.79	5.829	—
1990–1991	5.851	34.273	17.07	6.44	0.589
1991–1992	6.073	36.639	16.58	6.885	0.812
1992–1993	6.739	42.105	16.01	7.912	1.173
1993–1994	7.009	44.332	15.81	8.33	1.321
1994–1995	6.737	45.441	14.83	8.458	1.721
Total	—	—	—	—	5.616

*In millions of dollars.

We believe this is because the nursing care delivery system prevented losses from extended LOSs that would have occurred under prospective payment. This was the result of primary nurses initiating very early referrals to CNSs and case managers for patients requiring complex care. Because nursing costs are closely tied to LOS, well-coordinated and timely discharges reduced nursing costs per patient admission.

Example 2: Evaluating the Financial Impact of Redesign Using External Benchmarks

Our productivity consulting service provides comparative regional and national LOS data. (LOS has traditionally been used as a proxy for cost, although this assumption is now challenged.) We compared the interquartile range of LOS in the first 3 months of the year regionally and nationally for five patient care centers in 1991 and 1995 to actual average LOS for those months in our facility (see Fig. 11–2). Although LOS changes at ISJ "improved" in all patient care centers, we maintained or improved in only two centers *relative to reported changes in the region and the nation:* medical/surgical services and women's and children's services. This must be interpreted cautiously, because while we know about the factors in our environment that make interpretation over time difficult (physical remodeling with rearranging of clinical populations, increased volume, increased patient complexity), we do not know about changes within the environments of the comparison organizations that may have influenced their data. Evaluating the financial impact of redesign without comparable information is not meaningful.

Example 3: Evaluating Cost Avoidance Benefits of Nurse Case Management

Full-time nurse case managers were employed to coordinate services for patients discharged from the behavioral

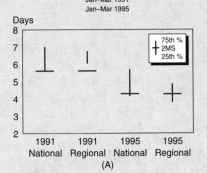

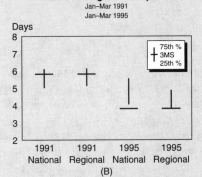

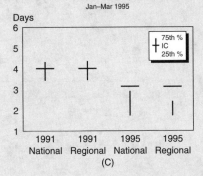

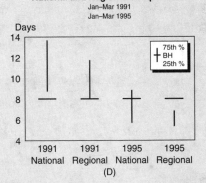

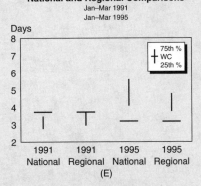

FIGURE 11–2. Data from five patient care centers. (A) Two month average LOS: national and regional comparisons, January–March 1991, January–March 1995. (B) Three month average LOS: national and regional comparisons, January–March 1991, January–March 1995. (C) Intensive care unit (ICU) average LOS: national and regional comparisons, January–March 1991, January–March 1995. (D) Behavioral health average LOS: national and regional comparisons, January–March 1991, January–March 1995. (E) Women's and children's average LOS: national and regional comparisons, January–March 1991, January–March 1995.

CASE: 11-1 *Continued*

health unit and medical/surgical units. Although the potential cost savings of this role are widely recognized within the organization, there is not sufficient definition of the role within the cost-accounting system so that the controller and top administrators are confident they were actually saving money. Utilization data from 28 behavioral health and 36 medical/surgical case-managed patients were reviewed for 6-months prior to the patients being case managed and 6-months after case management (see Table 11-2). It is important to note that

the controller and director of information services participated in the review, and it took many hours to retrieve the data. (Despite the multiple electronic databases in our organization, we are not yet able to get the information in the formats that reflect nursing costs.)

Patients in both groups were admitted less often after case managers began working with them, and patients in both groups had fewer inpatient days and costs when admitted. Reviewing emergency room costs and physician office fees (for the behavioral health group

TABLE 11-2. Cost–Benefits of Case Management

	BEHAVIOR HEALTH CASE MANAGEMENT (n=28)			MEDICAL/SURGICAL CASE MANAGEMENT (n=36)		
	6-mos. pre	6-mos. post	% change	6-mos. pre	6-mos. post	% change
Number of admissions	37	11	−70.27	32	16	−50.00
Total inpatient days	357	89	−75.07	313	51	−83.71
Average LOS	9.65	8.09	−16.17	9.78	3.19	−67.38
Average admission acuity	6.25	6.3	—	6.88	6.88	—
Total inpatient costs ($)	213,673	59,150	−75.32	321,758	130,602	−59.41
Total ER costs ($)	11,312	3,585	−68.31	11,081	5,774	−47.89
Total hospital costs ($)	224,985	62,735	−72.12	332,839	136,376	−59.03
Total physician/clinic fees ($)	38,225	41,335	+ 8.14	N/A	N/A	N/A

ER, emergency room; LOS, length of stay; N/A, not available.

CASE: 11–1 *Continued*

only) does not suggest a shifting of care to other settings. (Note: Clinic data was not made available for the medical/surgical patients.) Limitations in interpreting this information include the lack of comparison with similar patients who were not case managed, and the lack of control for insurance changes that may have influenced findings (although we believe these were minimal during the time of this study).

■ RECOMMENDATIONS

The following recommendations are based on our experiences:

1. *Use an evaluation model that supports a formative evaluation rather than summative evaluation.* Continuous feedback is needed not only to respond quickly and appropriately in rapidly changing environments, but also to provide the foundation for continuous modifications and improvement.

2. *Define, both conceptually and operationally, system indicators that will be used for cost–benefit and cost–effectiveness evaluation early in the redesign effort.* The definitions must be supported by the controller, information services, and quality improvement people. Ideally, these definitions can be referenced in the literature so there is some assurance that comparisons with other organizations and reports in the literature will be possible.

3. *Learn the details about existing data within your organization.* Consider what is presently being collected, how it is used, who has access to the data, how much people within the organization trust the validity of the data specific to your intended use, how much people within the organization trust the accuracy of the data, whether the data is available in an electronic format, and whether it can be linked to other databases. Foster relationships that help identify ways to obtain data to support your information needs. It is especially important to include the financial officer and information systems manager.

4. *When using consultants, require that they provide evaluation plans directly applicable to any changes based on their recommendations.* Have the consultants help identify sources for the data within your organization. Do not ever assume that data to support evaluation within a specific organization is available, accessible, and in the form the consultant recommends and you desire.

5. *Allocate resources to train nursing staff on data management skills.* Some of these resources will go to obtaining access to the data, because it is costly to retrieve data if it is not stored electronically or if it needs to be broken down in new ways. Other money needs to be allocated to

CASE: 11–1 *Continued*

training and supporting staff to construct, maintain, and analyze spreadsheets and databases.

6. *Use a process in staff and management meetings that incorporates data-based evidence rather than anecdotal evidence of success.* This has many benefits: it forces an analysis of data requirements for meaningful information, it encourages interpreting and critiquing data before it is used for evaluative purposes, and it suggests gaps in obtaining the data.

7. *Finally, and most importantly, retain a sense of humor and perspective.*

■ BIOGRAPHICAL SKETCHES

Marcelline Harris was a research associate at Health Bond, the consortium that received the Robert Wood Johnson Foundation and Pew Charitable Trusts grant in the Strengthening Hospital Nursing Program, at the time this work redesign was completed. Immanuel–St. Joseph's Hospital, a 272-bed community hospital, was one member of the Health Bond consortium. Presently, Ms. Harris is a PhD candidate in Nursing at the University of Nebraska School of Nursing in Omaha, completing her dissertation related to measuring outcomes of care. Her BS in Nursing is from the College of St. Catherine in St. Paul, Minnesota, and her MS in Nursing is from South Dakota State University.

Alice P. Weydt began her nursing management career in 1976 as the Director of Nursing at a 32-bed hospital in rural Minnesota. Presently, she is Director of Patient Care Services at Immanuel–St. Joseph's–Mayo Health System in Mankato, Minnesota, and responsible for the clinical management of patient care across multiple clinical and continuum of care service areas. Ms. Weydt received her BS in Nursing from Montana State University, her MS in Health Services Administration from Cardinal Stritch College in Milwaukee, Wisconsin, and has obtained ANA certification in Nursing Administration.

Holly Frohling has over 30 years experience in hospital-based nursing. Starting her career as an LPN in 1965, she received a BSN in Nursing at Mankato State University in Mankato, Minnesota, and an MBA with a concentration in health care management from the University of St. Thomas in St. Paul, Minnesota. She also has obtained ANA certification in nursing administration. As a Director of Patient Care Services at Immanuel–St. Joseph's–Mayo Health System, Ms. Frohling's primary responsibility is financial data management and budgeting for the Nursing Department.

Annette McBeth is Vice President, Immanuel–St. Joseph's–Mayo Health System in Mankato, Minnesota. She has a BSN and an MS in Nursing from the University of Minnesota in Minneapolis. She is presently a doctoral student at the Fielding Institute in Santa Barbara, California. Ms. McBeth is active in many

CASE: 11–1 *Continued*

professional nursing administration groups and is a frequent speaker on strategies to promote innovations in patient care delivery and systems redesign. In 1996, she became a Fellow in the American Academy of Nursing.

■ REFERENCES

Barnum, B.S., & Kerfoot, K.M. (1995). Nursing resources: Pricing and productivity. *The nurse as executive* (pp. 173–184). Gaithersburg, MD: Aspen.

McBeth, A., Schweer, K., & Aadalen, S. (1995). In M.K. Kohles, W.G. Baker, & B.A. Donaho (Eds.), *Transformational leadership: Renewing fundamental values and achieving new relationships in health care* (pp. 209–219). Chicago: American Hospital Publishing.

McBeth, A., & Weydt, A. (1996). Innovative delivery systems: Freedom, trust, caring. In E. Cohen (Ed.), *Nurse case management in the 21st century* (pp. 105–116). St. Louis: Mosby

Rossi, P.H., & Freeman, H.E. (1993). Measuring efficiency. In P.H. Rossi & H.E. Freeman (Eds.), *Evaluation: A systematic approach* (pp. 362–401). Newbury Park, CA: Sage.

CASE 11–2 Integrating the Work of Nurse Practitioners in an Acute Care Setting

Marie Collins Donahue

Since the 1980s, health care has been undergoing rapid change. One such change has been reductions in medical residencies in many specialties resulting from fewer approved residency programs, as well as voluntary and legislative constraints on resident work hours (Asch & Parker, 1988; Karnell, 1991). In response to these reductions, in September 1989, the Department of General Surgery at the Children's Hospital in Boston introduced a program to utilize pediatric nurse practitioners (PNPs) to supplement the decreasing numbers of available house staff to care for an increasing number of inpatients on the general surgery service.

■ **THE INPATIENT PEDIATRIC NURSE PRACTITIONER PROGRAM**

A pilot program began with two pediatric nurse practitioners on a 21-bed infant–toddler surgical unit. With the exception of performing operations, and handling ICU and on-call responsibilities, the PNP role paralleled that of the surgical residents with some additional advanced practice nursing responsibilities. Responsibilities included surgical admission histories and physical examinations, management of a selected caseload of inpatients, discharge planning, telephone triage, surgical clinic follow-up, family teaching and follow-up, consultation with nursing staff, and various other activities

in collaboration with the attending surgeons. The PNP's scope of practice was defined by Children's Hospital in accordance with Massachusetts law and the Board of Registered Nurses Advanced Practice Regulations. Guidelines for practice were collaboratively developed by the PNPs and members of the Departments of Nursing and General Surgery. The PNPs had direct reporting lines to the Associate Chief of Surgery and to the Director of Nursing Research and Quality Assurance (who also was a PNP).

The two PNPs initially hired for the pilot program were masters-prepared graduates of pediatric nurse practitioner programs, credentialed by a national nursing organization, and had 20 years of combined pediatric nursing experience, including physical assessment, growth and development, family counseling, critical care management, and surgical care. One PNP had prior experience on a pediatric surgical service at another institution.

■ **8 WEST: THE INFANT–TODDLER SURGICAL UNIT AT CHILDREN'S HOSPITAL**

Patients

8 West, the unit in which the pilot program was initiated, is a 21-bed infant–toddler surgical unit. Children cared for there are admitted to several surgical services,

CASE: 11–2 *Continued*

including general surgery, urology, plastic surgery, and otolaryngology and, therefore, had a multitude of surgical diagnoses. On the general surgery service, children experienced a wide variety of surgical conditions as well as a large variation in acuity. Patients had conditions ranging from inguinal hernia to intussusception, tracheoesophageal fistula, and benign and malignant tumors; still others had complex congenital anomalies, such as cloacal malformations, gastroschisis, and omphalocele. Although some infants experienced relatively short and uncomplicated hospital stays, many infants had very prolonged inpatient courses with subsequent readmissions for complications that developed after discharge; still others had anomalies that required staged surgical corrections. Most children on the unit required care from a variety of specialties while inpatients and had complicated discharge and home care needs.

The Nursing Staff

The nursing staff on 8 West consisted of 37 registered nurses (RNs) who reported directly to the Nurse Manager of the unit. The primary nursing model was utilized on the unit, with every patient assigned to a primary nurse who coordinated that patient's nursing care throughout the entire hospital stay as well as during any subsequent readmissions.

Surgical Attendings and Resident House Staff

Because Children's Hospital is a teaching institution, the surgical house staff rotated from neighboring adult surgical programs for periods of 1 to 3 months to obtain the necessary pediatric experience to qualify them for board certification. Under the supervision of 12 attending surgeons and a Chief Surgical Resident, first-year residents or interns were assigned to 8 West for 1 month. None had any prior pediatric experience or education, and most did not intend to pursue pediatric surgery as a specialty upon completion of their residency programs.

Other Staff

Because of the complicated nature of the unit's inpatient population, nearly every other specialty and discipline in the hospital had interaction or consultation with the staff on 8 West. These included physicians from nonsurgical subspecialties, most frequently radiology, gastroenterology, nutrition support, neurology, cardiology, and infectious disease. The more complicated patients also often required the services of physical therapists, developmental therapists, pharmacists, and social workers.

■ DESCRIPTION OF THE DAY-TO-DAY ACTIVITIES OF THE PNP

The PNPs cared for a particular caseload of patients mutually agreed upon with the surgical resident assigned to the unit. One PNP would arrive before morning surgical rounds, "pre-round" on all her patients to review the progress from the previous night with the staff nurses, collect and analyze all clinical and laboratory data from the previous 24 hours,

CASE: 11–2 *Continued*

and formulate a plan for the day. She would then join the surgical team for morning rounds led by the Chief Resident and present her patients and the daily plan to the team. After morning rounds, the PNP would write the daily progress note, and, because nurse practitioners have prescriptive authority in the Commonwealth of Massachusetts, write any necessary orders for medications, intravenous solutions, hyperalimentation, diagnostic studies, and so on. She would also consult with the patient's attending physician, primary nurse, and any other specialties involved with the patient's care to help formulate the care plan. At midday, the second PNP would arrive, and receive "sign-out" from the morning PNP in order to continue the care plan formulated during the morning. This would include following up on any diagnostic studies arranged for or laboratory data obtained, and presenting the PNPs' caseload of patients during evening rounds. After evening rounds, the junior resident on-call for the night would assume responsibility for the PNPs' caseload. For the sake of continuity, a written or verbal sign-out would be left by the afternoon PNP for the morning PNP. In addition, the PNPs were responsible for preoperative evaluation of patients scheduled for elective procedures, writing admission histories for unscheduled admissions, and serving as consultants to staff nurses on other units about surgical issues such as central line management, gastrostomy tube complications, and so on. Often the PNPs would facilitate transfer of patients from other units such as the intensive care

unit (ICU) or neonatal intensive care unit (NICU) to 8 West. If a patient's condition deteriorated the PNP would, after consulting with the Chief Resident or Attending Surgeon, coordinate stabilization of the patient and arrange for transfer from 8 West to the appropriate ICU. The PNPs also consulted by telephone with parents of patients known to the surgical service when they became ill at home. They would facilitate emergency room evaluation or direct admission to 8 West for these patients.

■ EVALUATION OF THE PILOT PROGRAM

One year after the initiation of the pilot program, several surveys were developed to evaluate the impact of the program. Participants in the surveys included the nurses on 8 West, the surgical house staff, attending surgeons, and parents of patients. The results of these surveys as well as additional comments and analysis follow.

Nurses

A survey of the nurses on 8 West prior to implementation was conducted to examine the RNs' perception of the PNP program. Eighty-eight percent of the nurses had never worked with PNPs and consequently, upon initiation of the program, the surgical nurses openly expressed fears about having their roles as primary nurses usurped or diluted (Nemes & Barnaby, 1992). Others feared that the PNPs might interfere with their access to the attending physicians or

CASE: 11-2 *Continued*

other subspecialists, while yet others worried that the PNPs would interfere with the relationship the RNs had with families. Some nurses expressed the belief that the PNPs did not have sufficient education or experience in pediatric surgical issues.

Results of the evaluation survey indicated that these fears were generally unfounded. Seventy-two percent of the nurses felt that the PNP had not interfered with the primary nurse role, while 92 percent of the nurses felt that the PNPs had enhanced patient care and felt positively about the PNPs' knowledge base (Nemes & Barnaby, 1992). Ninety six percent of the nurses felt that the PNP was much more accessible to the staff nurse than the resident for consultation and problem solving, and 86 percent felt that this availability decreased the number of telephone calls to the attending physicians and residents (Nemes & Barnaby, 1992). This is probably largely due to the fact that PNPs did not perform operations, whereas the residents and attending physicians did. When the nurses were asked about PNP involvement if their own child were hospitalized, 96 percent responded that they would welcome this involvement (Nemes & Barnaby, 1992).

Perhaps one of the best indicators of the positive impact of the PNP role on staff nurses was that, over time, the RNs often requested that the PNPs rather than the surgical residents care for the more complicated patients.

Probably the biggest barrier to overcome in implementing the PNP program was to achieve acceptance by the 8 West staff nurses. As stated earlier, most had no experience with PNPs and many of the nurses had extensive years of experience working on the surgical unit. Many of these staff nurses had more experience caring for surgical patients than the PNPs did. In order to achieve acceptance by the staff nurses, the PNPs had to show that they did not view their role as superior to that of the primary nurse, and that they had no intention of becoming the primary nurse for the patient. One of the biggest obstacles to acceptance of the role was the implicit hierarchy that exists among nurses; the perception that those nurses practicing in advanced roles had really "moved up," "left" nursing, and were actually "physician wannabes." Unfortunately, this implicit hierarchy is reinforced by nurses themselves as well as by members of other disciplines. The PNPs overcame this barrier in several ways. First, they acknowledged that the primary nurses had a unique role in patient care: they still spent more time with the patient and family than anyone else on the patient's team. Therefore, rather than impose the patient plan of care onto the primary nurse, the PNPs strove to collaborate with the nurses in developing this plan. This point may seem obvious, but in the few circumstances where this was not done, much conflict arose.

Second, and of profound importance to the success of the new role, the PNPs did not function merely as a resident would, but brought the experience and education gained as nurses to their advanced clinical practice. This involved spending time doing patient teaching

CASE: 11-2 *Continued*

with families, assisting with discharge planning, and at times, whenever possible, assisting the nurses to perform nursing tasks. On one occasion, after conducting a physical examination on an infant, a PNP changed the diaper and the bedding of the infant to the amazement of the nurse who exclaimed, "I thought those tasks were beneath you now that you are a PNP."

Finally, the PNPs were able to bring their advanced practice education and experience to the unit in formal and informal ways. Although many of the nurses were experienced in the management of surgical issues, they had knowledge gaps in primary care issues and in the management of nonsurgical problems. Because many children remained hospitalized for months at a time, current immunization practices, nutrition management, growth and development issues, and the management of common pediatric illnesses were an important part of patient management. Before the arrival of the PNPs, resources to recognize and address these issues did not exist on the unit. The PNPs provided formal inservice education for the nursing staff about these issues, and shared this knowledge informally as well during patient care conferences and during formulation of the patient care plans. It was also important that the PNPs acknowledged that they had much to learn from the experience of seasoned surgical nurses.

Attending Surgeons

Of the 12 attending physicians surveyed, only 2 had prior experience working with a nurse practitioner. All surgeons were positive about the PNPs involvement in managing their patients, and 92 percent felt that PNPs had actually enhanced communication with their patients' families (Nemes, Barnaby, & Shamberger, 1992). All attending surgeons felt the PNPs had decreased the resident workload, and 83 percent felt that the PNPs had not interfered with resident learning (Nemes, Barnaby, & Shamberger, 1992). Fifty-eight percent felt that implementation of their plan of care was more expeditious with a nurse practitioner than with a resident (Nemes, Barnaby, & Shamberger, 1992).

Surgical House Staff

Only 8 percent of the residents had prior experience with nurse practitioners (Nemes, Barnaby, & Shamberger, 1992). All of the junior residents and 91 percent of the senior residents felt that PNPs were a valuable resource in the daily management of patients (Nemes, Barnaby, & Shamberger, 1992). Although 87 percent of the junior residents felt that the PNPs decreased their workload, none of the residents felt that the PNPs interfered with their learning. Seventy-three percent of the junior residents and 55 percent of the senior residents felt that the PNPs actually enhanced their learning (Nemes, Barnaby, & Shamberger, 1992).

These survey results indicated that there was great benefit to the PNP role on the general surgery service. The resident house staff was accustomed to caring for adults and their rotations to Children's Hospital were of fairly short

CASE: 11–2 *Continued*

duration. In addition, upon their arrival at Children's Hospital, they had no formal orientation or instruction on how to care for children, much less manage the complicated issues of acutely ill infants. Recognizing this educational gap, the PNPs began conducting an orientation session with each new resident, which included reviewing all patients on the unit as well as common pediatric management issues. The PNPs also served as a resource on pediatric issues and illnesses both to the resident during the rotation as well as to the surgical team on morning and evening rounds. One PNP developed a formal lecture, entitled "Pediatric Pearls," that used case studies to illustrate important aspects of pediatric management issues commonly found on 8 West such as sepsis workups, common pediatric infections, and the appropriate use of specialty infant formulas. This lecture became part of the Surgical Resident Teaching Series. Conversely, the residents served as a resource to the PNPs regarding the technical aspects of surgery.

Parents

Of all the groups surveyed, parents had more prior experience with nurse practitioners as 40 percent of the parents had worked with PNPs before their hospital admission. Ninety-six percent were comfortable with involvement of the PNPs in their child's care, while 84 percent felt that the PNP facilitated communication between them and their attending surgeon (Nemes, Barnaby, & Shamberger, 1992). Although some parents expressed

frustration at not having more communication with their attending surgeons, parents of chronically ill children who had prolonged or repeated hospitalizations felt that the PNPs provided continuity in a system they viewed as fragmented because of the frequent change in residents.

Quality of Patient Care

No formal methods of evaluation of the impact of the PNP role on quality of care were conducted; however, many observations can be made. First, as discussed in some detail above, the PNPs brought much knowledge and expertise regarding pediatric issues to the patients on the unit. Quite often in specialty units, the main focus is on the management of the specialty problem, sometimes to the exclusion of other pediatric issues. The neglect of these issues can be particularly detrimental to the infants who often spend several weeks or even months hospitalized. Recognizing the importance of growth and developmental issues, for example, the PNP would consult with an appropriate specialist who would then evaluate the infant for potential problems and collaborate on a plan of care that sought to prevent delays resulting from prolonged hospitalization.

Through education and experience, the PNPs were also able to recognize or anticipate conditions specifically found in pediatric populations that differed from the adult populations with which surgical residents commonly dealt. Often, even the attending surgeons had

CASE: 11–2 *Continued*

little knowledge of these considerations. For example, the work-up for a postoperative fever in an adult is very different from that of a neonate whose immature immune system makes meningitis a dangerous possibility. Although at times, the surgical residents were resistant to recommendations made by the PNPs, in almost all cases, the attending physicians did defer to the PNPs' unique pediatric knowledge base.

The PNPs also worked very closely with the variety of other subspecialties that were consulted during the patients' prolonged hospitalization. Because the PNPs did not perform surgery, as the residents and attending surgeons did, they were able to bridge communication gaps that previously had existed because of the long hours that the surgeons spent in the operating room. The attending surgeon's plan of care could be explained to members of other consulting teams, and recommendations of the consultants and their rationales could be explained to the surgeons. Changes in care could be implemented much more quickly because of this. For example, changes recommended by the nutritional support service regarding the proper concentration of electrolytes, minerals, and other nutrients in patients who received hyperalimentation, could be made without delay since the PNP was present on the unit at the time the team made rounds.

Finally, the PNPs, by virtue of their education, brought research skills to their clinical practice. The survey conducted after the first year of the program was one example of applying these skills (Nemes, Barnaby, & Shamberger, 1992). The PNPs also conducted a clinical research project that resulted in changes in clinical practice for infants undergoing preoperative bowel preparation (Donahue, Evangelista, & Shamberger, 1994). Patients and staff were not the only beneficiaries of these projects; both were accepted for publication and presented at the American Academy of Pediatrics Annual Surgical Section meeting.

After 1 year, the pilot program was determined to be so successful that two additional positions were created and the role was expanded to include an additional inpatient unit, the school age and adolescent surgical unit.

■ IMPLICATIONS

Pioneered by Henry Silver, MD, and Loretta Ford, RN, PhD, the nurse practitioner role began in the 1960s in response to the shortage of physicians willing to serve in certain geographical and practice areas. Since then, nurse practitioners have been the specific focus of hundreds of effectiveness studies. The most comprehensive of these studies was a case study released in 1986 by the Office of Technology Assessment that demonstrated the advantages of the nurse practitioner in improving access to care, and providing quality care in a cost-effective manner. Safriet (1992) points out that this is all the more remarkable given the significant constraints and barriers on advanced nursing practice. In addition, nurse practi-

CASE: 11–2 *Continued*

tioners bring additional skills to practice. They are more likely to talk to patients and adapt medical regimens to a patient's preferences, family situation, and environment (Brown & Grimes, 1993). They are also more likely to provide disease-prevention counseling, health education, and health promotion activities, to know about and use community resources, such as nutrition programs, parenting, and stress reduction programs (Avorn, Everitt, & Baker, 1991; Office of Technology Assessment, 1986). The training and perspective gained in nursing education account for the extra time nurses spend on these aspects of care.

Although this research is valuable in describing the benefits of advanced nursing practice roles, it has been limited to those nurse practitioners who practice in the ambulatory setting. Similar research is necessary that specifically evaluates the role of the inpatient nurse practitioner and its impact on patient outcomes, patient and family satisfaction, length of stay, readmission rates, and cost-effectiveness.

One additional challenge is to assure that nurse practitioners, traditionally educated in preventive and ambulatory care, are adequately prepared for roles that require specialized knowledge and expertise. The first two PNPs in the Children's Hospital pilot program had many years of prior nursing experience, including critical care and pediatric surgical experience, in addition to several years of experience in the advanced practice role. This previous experience was most relevant to their ability to provide excellent patient care and undoubtedly crucial to their success

in establishing a new role on 8 West. Later in the program, a recent graduate of a PNP program with few years of nursing experience was hired. In addition to having no experience practicing as a PNP, her prior nursing experience did not involve critical care or pediatric surgery. This inadequate preparation for the inpatient role caused significant problems with job performance and problems with her own transition into the advanced practice role.

Several pioneering graduate programs have been developed to address this challenge. The American Nurses Credentialing Center (ANCC) began certifying Acute Care Nurse Practitioners in 1996. Keane and Richmond (1993) describe the "tertiary nurse practitioner" (TNP) role and its curricular essentials; these curricular changes should reflect the strengths of both the nurse practitioner and the clinical nurse specialist roles. Aspects crucial to the delivery of care by a nurse practitioner in a highly specialized setting include: first, an in-depth knowledge of the specialty's health problems and the technology used; and second, retention of a "generalist" approach—the cornerstone of most nurse practitioner programs currently. This approach is valuable because it retains nursing's holistic view of the patient and family. If this approach in graduate programs is not retained, the inpatient nurse practitioner will lose the qualities and skills that make him or her a unique member of the hospital health care team and merely a "resident substitute."

Nurse practitioners are in a unique position to meet some of the most formidable challenges facing health care

CASE: 11–2 *Continued*

today. Since the 1960s, nurse practitioners have demonstrated that they can provide high quality, accessible, and cost-effective care to those in underserved communities. In this new advanced practice role, inpatient nurse practitioners are well on their way to demonstrating that they can do the same for yet another patient population.

■ BIOGRAPHICAL SKETCH

Marie Collins Donahue received her BSN from The Catholic University of America, an MS with a major in Pediatric Primary Care from Columbia University, and an MPH with a major in Public Management and Community Health from Harvard University. As a pediatric nurse practitioner, she has worked in both primary and tertiary care settings and has lectured on the evolving role of the nurse practitioner. She is a regular contributor to the National Certification Board of Pediatric Nurse Practitioners and Nurses National Qualifying Examination. She is a Fellow of the National Association of Pediatric Nurse Associates and Practitioners (NAPNAP). Currently, she is the Pediatric HIV Clinical Trials Study Coordinator and a pediatric nurse practitioner at the Women and Children's Care Center, Columbia Presbyterian Medical Center.

■ REFERENCES

Asch, D.A., & Parker, R.M. (1988). The Libby Zion case. *New England Journal of Medicine, 318* (12), 771–775.

Avorn, J, Everitt, D.E., & Baker, M.W. (1991). The neglected medical history and therapeutic choices for abdominal pain: A nationwide study of 799 physicians and nurses. *Archives of Internal Medicine, 131,* 694–698.

Brown, S.A., & Grimes, D.E. (1993). *A meta-analysis of process of care, clinical outcomes, and cost-effectiveness of nurses in primary care roles: Nurse practitioners and certified nurse-midwives.* Washington, DC: American Nurses Association.

Donahue, M.C., Evangelista, J.E., & Shamberger, R.C. (1994). The effects of golytely on hydration status and serum electrolytes in infants. *Journal of Pediatric Surgery, 29* (8), 1095–1096.

Karnell, L.H. (1991). *Longitudinal studies of surgical residents in 1989–90.* Washington, DC: American College of Surgeons, p. 33.

Keane, A., & Richmond, T. (1993). Tertiary nurse practitioners. *Image, 25* (4), 281–284.

Nemes, J., & Barnaby, K. (1992). The pediatric nurse practitioner in a surgical in-patient setting. *Nursing Management, 23* (1), 44–46.

Nemes, J., Barnaby, K., & Shamberger, R.C. (1992). Experience with a nurse practitioner program in the surgical department at Children's Hospital. *Journal of Pediatric Surgery, 27* (8), 1038–1042.

Office of Technology Assessment. (1986). *Nurse practitioners, physicians assistants, and certified nurse-midwives: A policy analysis.* Washington, DC: Government Printing Office.

Safriet, B.J. (1992). Health care dollars and regulatory sense: The role of advanced practice nursing. *Yale Journal on Regulation, 9* (417), 419–487.

FOUR

Nursing Administration

12

Leadership and Management in Patient Care Delivery Systems

Karen B. Haller

There may be no social commodity more in demand and less understood than leadership. It has been said that leaders are born, and it has also been said that leaders are made. Actually, both perspectives hold a portion of the truth. Regardless, leaders and leadership are chronically in short supply.

There are no clear-cut, universally accepted definitions of leadership. The only consensus seems to be that all leaders have followers, and it is the nature of the relationship between the two that defines leadership. To be a leader means that others must cooperate and collaborate to achieve a goal. When strong leaders look over their shoulders, they see strong followers. What else do we know? We know that leadership is an intentional process demonstrated only in action and that the outcome is accomplishment.

Complicating the definition of leadership is the need to distinguish it from management. For our purposes here, *leadership* implies effective use of influence that is independent of one's position in an organization. *Management* implies formal authority and power based on one's position in the organizational structure. The two functions and roles overlap: Many leaders become managers, and effective managers must also lead.

This chapter will begin by tracing the development of theories on leadership, then explore the proposition that leadership is adaptive work. Next, the particular demands and issues of leadership in health care delivery systems will be highlighted. Finally tools of leadership and the art of leadership will be described.

■ THEORIES OF LEADERSHIP

Theories of leadership rise and fall. Theories rise, in part, as a reflection of the prevailing social perspectives at a point in time; they fall because they fail the tests of both research and reality. Each emerging theoretical perspective builds on the new knowledge acquired by research done to test earlier perspectives. Over time, the complexity of leadership and the inadequacy of simple definitions have become evident.

The Great Man Theory

An early 20th century theory was the "great man" or trait theory of leadership. This theory—that leaders are born, not made—dominated into the 1950s; it held that some individuals have charisma, intelligence, and certain physical features or other heroic attributes that enable them to assume responsibilities that not everyone can execute (Bolman & Deal, 1991). Early research was primarily in the form of biographical studies of military and political leaders. Later, psychologists carried out studies to identify a list of traits found in leaders, but not followers. Stodgill (1974) examined 287 studies undertaken from 1904 to 1970 and identified intelligence, dominance, self-confidence, high energy level, and task relevant knowledge as the most commonly identified traits of leaders. The great man theory fell into disrepute when studies failed to demonstrate consensus or strong statistical relationships between traits and outcomes. In addition, there was mounting evidence that a leader could be effective in one setting but ineffective in another (Fiedler, 1969). It appeared that leadership depended less on "being born a leader" than on being in a situation in which leadership was needed or in a context in which one's traits fit the need for leadership at that time.

Contingency Theory

Contingency theory holds that it takes more than personal traits to be a leader; rather, leadership depends on the person's behavior, the setting, and the environment. There were several major studies of leadership undertaken immediately after World War II that focused on these three variables. Leadership theorists using this perspective investigated individual propensity for a leadership style, which was assumed to be relatively fixed and inflexible. They believed one is an effective leader when there is the right match of style with a historical time or a particular managerial situation. The style could vary from being task oriented to being relationship oriented (Fiedler, 1967). On one end of the continuum were authoritarian, task-oriented leaders who were leader centered in their actions. At the other end were democratic, relationship-oriented leaders who granted subordinates the freedom to function within limits. Another type of leader essentially abdicated influencing both task and relationships, and was labeled the laissez faire leader. The contingency variables that influenced leadership success were the quality of the leader–follower relationship, the degree to which the task was structured, and the level of positional power held by the leader. Fiedler (1967) predicted the authoritarian leadership style was the best for most favorable situations (where all three contingency variables were positive) or the least favorable situations (where all three contingency variables were negative). Democratic leadership was best in all mixed situations. The critical variable was not the person's traits or prevailing style, but the fit between style and what the situation needed. In this view, leaders do not make history; history makes leaders because a person happens to be at the right time and in the right place. Again, despite its intuitive attractiveness, the theory was found insufficient to explain leadership.

Situational Theory

In reality, many leaders vary their style with the situation. Situational theorists assert that effective leaders are those who can diagnose accurately the needs of the followers, select the most appropriate style and behaviors, and help people get their work done. Early studies expanded leadership to include instrumental behaviors to define and specify work, supportive behaviors, participative behaviors, and achievement-oriented behaviors that define leader expectations of performance (House & Mitchell, 1974). Hersey and Blanchard's (1993) tridimentional leader effectiveness model is widely known in both academic and practice arenas. The theory presents a two by two grid of *high and low task structure* and *high and low relationship* behavior. The third dimension adds characteristics of the followers, which they name *work group maturity*. This is defined as the mix of job ability and psychological willingness to do the job, with four levels from high to low. The leader is to diagnose both the task and the group, and choose one of four leadership styles that vary from most authoritarian to most participative. Along this continuum, the styles are telling, selling, participating, and delegating. Again, the theory pulls together the factors identified in earlier theories into a cohesive conceptual framework. There has been no research to confirm the framework; however, managers and students find the model simple to use, practical, and intuitively appealing.

Transactional Leadership

Transactional theory approaches leadership as a set of functions and roles that develop from the interaction—or *transaction*—between two or more people. The focus is on what happens between leaders and followers, and what factors directly or indirectly influence them. Transactional theorists go beyond situational and contingency theories by asserting that each failed to include all pertinent variables. Additional variables included by transactional theorists are organizational structure and size, market conditions, and the expert or technical knowledge required of the employees. Transactional theory is complex because of the large number of variables that are considered. As a result of this complexity, it has had more academic interest than practical application. One enduring concept used by practitioners is that authority consists of reciprocal interactions between leaders and followers. People in authority influence constituents, but constituents also influence authorities (Heifetz, 1994).

Transformational Leadership

By the 1970s, leadership theorists became interested in how to change organizational culture. The seminal work was done by Burns (1978) in his studies of politicians. He identified two types of politicians: transactional leaders, whose actions were focused on change *within* an existing organizational culture, and transformative leaders, whose actions led to a change of culture (Bass & Avolio, 1990). Transformational theorists contrast transactional leadership for incremental change with transformative leadership for radical change.

By the 1980s, transformational leadership was the dominant theory. Transformational leaders are characterized by a charismatic personality, visionary projections for the organization, and belief in empowering employees. Jack Welch of General Electric and Lee Iacocca of Chrysler are often cited as exemplary transformational leaders. In some sense, leadership theory had come full circle—back to the "great man" perspective.

Administrative Conservatorship

Currently competing for theoretical prominence with transformational leadership are theories of administrative conservatorship. Conservatorship theorists rely less on scientific rigor and quantitative testing than on qualitative case studies. These theories include concepts of systems thinking, visioning, facilitation of learning, stewardship, and empowering followers. Much more attention has been paid to the role of followers and how leaders are able to elicit collaboration and cooperation, especially in unpredictable and changing environments. Interest has turned from the leader's ability to combine intuitive thinking and rational problem solving—and to know the right answers—to the leader's ability to challenge and assist others in discovering and testing transient answers for changing situations.

Unlike transformational leadership, where the visionary leaders know the right choices and are the catalysts for organizational transformation, administrative conservatorship theories focus on preserving an institution's distinctive competence within an environment of flux and change.

Administrative conservatorship is grounded in sociology, and specifically in open systems thinking. An open systems orientation causes those in the organization to consider themselves in a constant interaction with a changing environment (new services, new competitors, new partners, changes in regulations) and with new technologies—both of which are major sources of uncertainty. This perspective also emphasizes organizational participants' adaptive ability to remain competitive in the marketplace. Leaders adopt strategies to effectively guide the organization during times of uncertainty.

■ LEADERSHIP AS ADAPTIVE WORK

Anyone can hold the helm when the sea is calm, but leadership is a foul weather job (Drucker, 1990). And there is a lot of foul weather, risk, and uncertainty in health care today. The changes that are listed below are but a reminder of the uncertainties in the environment and the need for adaptation:

- The societal shift from viewing health care as a public utility to treating it as a market commodity introduces dramatic change in health care finance and promotes competition.
- Competition, by definition, requires winners and losers. All organizations will not survive.
- The radical shift of hospitals from being revenue centers to being cost centers portends a change in where and how health care will be delivered.
- The continued rapid pace of technological advances is expensive and will need to be managed.
- The information explosion increases the rate of change, and puts information in the hands of consumers and competitors.
- An increasingly heterogeneous work force brings diverse views and skills to employing organizations.
- An aging population with high expectations for care will place demands on the current system.

Facing these conditions, Heifetz (cited in Flowers, 1995) believes that leadership is an activity: "It is what people do in mobilizing other people . . . to do adaptive work. When you have a problem or a challenge for which there is no technical remedy, a problem for which it won't help to look to an authority for answers—the answers aren't there—that problem calls for adaptive work" (p. 32). Adaptive work requires people to change their values, their behavior, their attitudes, their skills, or the way they work.

Heifetz (1994) contrasts two different views of leadership. In the first, leadership means influencing a community or organization to follow the leader's vision. If this approach solves problems (or fails to solve them), then the credit (or blame) lies with the leader. In the second view, leadership means influencing the community or organization to face its own problems. The leader needs the courage to turn down easy solutions and guide the group to struggle with dilemmas, realizing that many issues are not permanently solvable. The leader also needs to monitor the stress level of followers to keep it at a productive level by managing information flow, supporting transitions, and accepting limited solutions. Success or failure, credit or blame, accrue to both the leaders and the community. Heifetz argues that the second type of leadership is best suited to dealing with uncertainty and change. Influence and authority are tools in the leader's kit, but they are not ends. The end is robust adaptation—not adaptation to survive, but rather adaptation to thrive.

The biological concept of adaptation is comfortable to nurses, but it is not a perfect metaphor for the change facing us in health care. As Heifetz (1994) argues:

> Species change as the genetic program changes; cultures change by learning. Evolution is a matter of chance—a fortuitous fit between random variation and new environmental pressures; societies, by contrast, can respond to new pressures with deliberation and planning. (p. 30)

The concept of leadership as doing adaptive work is also appealing because it is simple and practical, unlike grander theories such as transformational leadership or administrative conservatorship. It is consistent with democratic principles, including respect for conflict, diversity, and negotiation (Heifetz, 1994). Furthermore, it fits with the "baby boomer" culture, which distrusts autocratic leadership and prizes community participation, freedom of choice, and social justice. Many "boomers" are now in positions of leadership and authority, and currently define the dominant organizational culture.

Finally, the concept of leadership as adaptive work is appealing because it allows a melding of viewpoints and disciplines. As health care moves away from functioning as a collection of guilds (medicine, nursing, social work, etc.) to working as teams in integrated delivery systems, then all views and all skills need to bear collectively on the problems we face. No one discipline has the answer or the vision. Leaders need to mobilize the multidisciplinary community to tackle health care's problems and meet patient needs.

■ LEADERSHIP WORK IN HEALTH CARE

The need is for broad-based leaders who can work effectively in complex situations, which by definition require expertise and competence that is greater than any single individual or discipline offers. As hospitals evolve into health care systems, there has been a shift toward organizing leadership by programs instead of by disciplines.

The Shift Toward Patient-Focused Care

Traditional functional departments are disappearing, and cross-functional departments with multidisciplinary teams are cropping up like grass in spring. The shift is reflected in the term *patient-focused care*. The chief nursing officers in many institutions no longer have titles with the word *nursing* in them.

Rather the chief nurse is likely to be the Vice President for Patient Care or Vice President for Women's Services (or other population of patients)—a term that implies a broader scope than nursing, often including other professions and paraprofessional workers.

Likewise, hospital nursing units are increasingly called patient care units and some are encompassing more than one geographical area and even outpatients or home care patients. The title of head nurse gave way in many hospitals in the 1980s to nurse manager, and now there seems to be a trend to patient care manager. The change in title is reflective of the increasing scope of work to include all activity within the unit—not just nursing care.

There are pros and cons to these broader scopes of responsibility given nurses at all levels of management. In a recent survey of 7,500 nurses, 45 percent of the participants reported a reduction in the number of nurse managers at their institutions and 38 percent claimed that they had lost their nurse executive without replacement (Joel, 1996). Joel, commenting on these results, fears that "for want of nurse managers and administrators who understand clinical nursing, the care environment has become destabilized" (p. 7). She emphasizes:

> Managers are the leaders at the direct care level who facilitate practice and access resources. . . . In contrast, nurse administrators represent the caregiver at the executive level. They are the chieftains of the macrosystem, supplying the kind of vision that is only possible when you're situated at the boundary between the internal and external environments, and serving your constituency best with direct access to the ultimate decision makers. (Joel, 1996, p. 7)

Fagin (1996) has asked whether we are seeing a denigration of the nursing ethics of advocacy and accountability as our chiefs of nursing services leave out the nursing word in their assumption of broader portfolios; she adds that "whether in hospital or community care, if we lose our accountability, we lose our discipline" (p. 35). Yet, these broader scopes of responsibility lend themselves to thinking of leadership as adaptive work; this adaptive work aims at melding constituencies in search of solutions to shared problems.

■ THE TOOLS OF LEADERSHIP

Leaders have two primary tools—authority and influence. Authority is the power given to a person because of the position he or she holds. Authority may be further broken down into formal authority and informal authority. When the President of the United States is sworn in during inaugural ceremonies, formal authority is being granted and the President promises to carry out the roles and responsibilities of the Oval Office. The President also has informal authority, which comes from perceptions that he is ethical, judicious, fair, and trustworthy; the extent of his informal authority is measured both in the share of votes he garners at elections and his ratings in the popularity polls. Formal authority is static, but informal authority rises and falls (Heifetz, 1994, p. 102). Each of us—in our professional positions—has both formal and informal authority.

Using Authority

From a position of authority, the leader has a tool kit of seven strategies that can be used to mobilize people (Heifetz, 1994, pp. 103–104). One of these is control over the amount of change, and therefore stress, placed on people. The leader wants to place enough challenge and urgency before people to motivate and move them, but not so much as to overwhelm and immobilize them. This is the strategy of *providing a holding environment.*

The leader in authority also has a public platform from which to diagnose systems problems, *direct attention* to them, identify the plan for addressing them, and focus collective effort on finding solutions. The authority has *access to information* and can *control the flow of information,* including *framing issues* in constructive ways. Leaders with authority can *orchestrate conflict,* and perhaps most importantly, *choose how decisions will be made.* Heifetz (1994) notes that these tools are limited, but are all that leaders have to work with.

Using Influence

Not all leaders have authority. One becomes a leader through doing the work of a leader (DePree, 1992). When this work is engaging people to make progress on changing—and that is the work needed in health care—then many can rise up and carry out the tasks of leadership. Influence is the main tool of the leader who has no positional authority.

In 1996, Pinchot described three approaches for empowering people and bringing forth many leaders within organizations. First, in a traditionally organized hierarchy, the leader delegates authority and allows leadership to emerge from subordinates. In a home care agency, for example, the executive director may delegate authority and accountability for a nursing office's operations to the nursing supervisor. The supervisor may demonstrate great leadership in mobilizing the resources available to deliver high-quality care at a low unit cost.

Second, in organizations that view themselves as communities, an environment is created that allows leaders to arise from many quarters. "Community is a phenomenon that occurs most easily when free people with some sense of equal worth join together voluntarily for a common enterprise," notes Pinchot (1996, p. 28). In the community model, local leaders strive to accomplish a common goal. This model may work best in smaller hospitals or agencies, which allow a great deal of face-to-face contact, or in larger institutions that are decentralized to maintain cohesiveness on the local level.

Third, and most radical in Pinchot's taxonomy, is empowering people and bringing forth leaders by establishing a free-market system within an organization. Applying the concept to hospitals, the core business—patient care—would be run by groups of nurse managers who buy services from competing teams inside the facility. For example, there would be several internal suppliers of meals from whom the manager could choose. Meal service would not be imposed from above and enforced by an internal monopoly.

Pinchot's (1996) taxonomy is ordered by degrees of freedom: From a traditional hierarchical model to a community model to free *intra*prise. The freer the system—that is, the more it mimics a free-market economy—the greater the chance for leaders to rise at local (departmental) levels. The role of the senior leadership is to create an environment where indirect leadership flourishes.

Max DePree, chairman of the board of directors at Herman Miller, Inc., a company known for innovation in the furniture business, describes his company as a community in which there are both hierarchical leaders and roving leaders. Hierarchical leaders have positional authority and can delegate, but roving leaders are those people who take charge on their own initiative because they believe they can solve the problem at hand. "In special situations, the hierarchical leader is obliged to identify the roving leader, then support and follow him or her, and also to exhibit the grace that enables the roving leader to lead" (DePree, 1989, p. 42).

■ THE SCIENCE AND ART OF LEADERSHIP

The science of leadership has evolved over time—from the great man theory to Pinchot's recent concepts of free *intra*prise—but each theory has flaws and none has yet stood the test of time. Each theory leads to techniques that are espoused as the recipe for leadership; however, techniques alone do not make leaders. Leadership, like nursing, is both a science and an art.

DePree believes that leadership is more about ideas than techniques. "The art of leadership," he says, is "liberating people to do what is required of them in the most effective and humane way possible" (1989, p. 1). His concept of liberating people is consistent with Heifetz's view that great leaders motivate people to solve their collective problems, as well as with Pinchot's value on freedom as a tool to promote leadership in our institutions.

Like all art, there is no formula to produce leadership. Great leaders—with or without formal authority—have influence. People trust them. This trust is earned. The following list itemizes how trust and influence are earned by leaders, whether global or local leaders, hierarchical or roving leaders.

Leading by Example

As medical missionary Albert Schweitzer said, "Example is not the main thing in influencing others, it is the only thing" (cited in Bridges, 1991, p. 61). De-Pree (1992) tells a story of arriving at a tennis club after a group of high school students had vacated the locker room: "Like chickens, they had not bothered to pick up after themselves. Without thinking too much about it, I gathered up all their towels and put them in a hamper" (pp. 218–219). Then he ponders whether he picks up the towels because he is the president of a company, or whether he is the president because he picks up towels. He does not answer the question, but the lesson is clear: Effective leaders are doers and lead by example.

Maintaining Integrity

Telling the truth gives leaders integrity. Boldt (1993), in his iconoclastic career guide, reminds us that truth-telling is more than a matter of not telling lies: "It includes the capacity to be precise in your statements and measured in your judgments" (p. 423). Leaders with integrity avoid exaggeration and distortion, and refuse to take credit for what others have done.

Living on Purpose

Leaders find a purpose in their work, and it provides them with focus. They love their work and become intimate with its craft. They care. Mintzberg (1996), in an article in which he promises to "insult almost everyone," ends by flattering the nursing profession's management of its craft. Because organizations need continuous care, not interventionist cures, Mintzberg finds nursing to be a good model of management. He followed a head nurse around as she practiced her "craft style" of managing: "It is about inspiring, not empowering, about leadership based on mutual respect rooted in common experience and deep understanding. Craft managers get involved deeply enough to know when not to get involved" (pp. 66–67).

Being Available

The head nurse who Mintzberg followed spent most of her day on the floor, not in her office—literally a roving leader! Effective leaders watch and listen more than they talk. Their antennae are up to test reality, perceive change, and gather information. They talk with employees, followers, peers, and customers (in our case, patients).

Thriving on Relationships

Leaders respect and enjoy people. They promote diversity. They eschew carbon copies of themselves, and seek out strong peers and subordinates. What matters is a person's performance, standards, and values. Leaders assist others to use their strengths and do not focus on weaknesses (Drucker, 1996).

Following Teaches Leadership

Effective following is a skill. Good followers make the leader effective by practicing self-discipline; holding themselves accountable for outcomes; delivering solutions, or at least options, rather than problems; and serving as the eyes and ears of the leader. Followers learn that the leader can only accomplish something by permission of the followers (DePree, 1989). Therefore, the follower who becomes a leader knows that he or she is vulnerable, and "vulnerable leaders trust in the abilities of other people" (DePree, 1992).

■ CONCLUSION

Leaders are neither born, nor made. Both nature and nurture influence leaders. The line between leaders and followers is fragile, as leaders are vulnerable to their followers' knowledge, skills, and abilities. The line between leaders with authority and leaders without authority is equally thin. Both must work with the tool of influence—a tool that is hard earned by integrity, purpose, availability, and positive human relationships. Although scientists have tried to reduce leadership to a set of traits, styles, or skills, the pursuit remains elusive. Leadership—like nursing—is as much an art as a science.

■ BIOGRAPHICAL SKETCH

Karen B. Haller is the Director of Nursing for the Department of Medicine at The John Hopkins Hospital in Baltimore, Maryland. She also serves as an Associate Professor in the Johns Hopkins University School of Nursing, where she has taught nursing administration. Dr. Haller earned her BSN, MPH, MSN, and PhD degrees from the University of Michigan in Ann Arbor. In her spare time, Dr. Haller provides editorial leadership for *JOGNN* (Journal of Obstetric, Gynecologic, and Neonatal Nursing). She has served as editor since 1991.

■ SUGGESTED READINGS

Keep reading and studying. Experience is perhaps the single best teacher of leadership. Reading and studying provide vicarious learning, new ideas, models to organize your thinking, and new energy to go out each day and continue developing. Leadership, being a process and not a thing, is never fully known.

Atchison, T.A. (1990). *Turning health care leadership around: Cultivating inspired, empowered and loyal followers.* San Francisco: Jossey-Bass.

DePree, M. (1992). *Leadership jazz.* New York: Bantam Doubleday Day.

Hesselbein, F., Goldsmith, M., & Beckhard, R. (Eds.). (1996). *The leader of the future* San Francisco: Jossey-Bass.

Kelly, R. (1992). *The power of followership: How to create leaders people want to follow: and followers who lead themselves.* New York: Doubleday.

Senge, P. (1990). *The fifth discipline: The art and practice of the learning organization.* New York: Doubleday/Currency.

■ REFERENCES

Bass, B., & Avolio, B. (1990). *Transformational leadership development: Manual for the multifactor leadership questionnaire.* Palo Alto, CA: Consulting Psychologists Press.

Boldt, L.G. (1993). *Zen and the art of making a living.* New York: Penguin.

Bolman, L.G., & Deal, T.E. (1991). *Reframing organizations.* San Francisco: Jossey-Bass.

Bridges, L. (1991). *Managing transitions: Making the most of change.* Reading, MA: Addison-Wesley.

Burns, J.M. (1978). *Leadership.* New York: Harper & Row.

DePree, M. (1989). *Leadership is an art.* New York: Bantam Doubleday Day.

DePree, M. (1992). *Leadership jazz.* New York: Bantam Doubleday Day.

Drucker, P.J. (1990). *Managing the nonprofit organization.* New York: HarperCollins.

Drucker, P. (1996). Not enough generals were killed. In F. Hesselbein, M. Goldsmith, & R. Beckhard (Eds.), *The leader of the future* (pp. 25–39). San Francisco: Jossey-Bass.

Fagin, C.M. (1996). Executive leadership: Improving nursing practice, education, and research. *Journal of Nursing Administration, 26* (3), 30–37.

Fiedler, F.E. (1967). *A theory of leadership effectiveness.* New York: McGraw-Hill.

Fiedler, F.E. (1969). Style or circumstance: The leadership enigma. *Psychology Today, 2* (10), 38–43.

Flowers, J. (1995). A conversation with Ronald Heifetz, MD: Leadership without easy answers. *Healthcare Forum Journal, 38* (4), 30–36.

Heifetz, R. (1994). *Leadership without easy answers.* Cambridge, MA: Harvard University Press.

Hersey, P., & Blanchard, K. (1993). *Management of organizational behavior: Utilizing human resources* (6th ed.). Englewood Cliffs, NJ: Prentice-Hall.

House, R.J., & Mitchell, T.R. (1974). Path-goal theory of leadership. *Journal of Contemporary Business, 3* (4), 81–98.

Joel, L. (1996). Decrying the loss of organizational leadership. *American Journal of Nursing, 10* (7), 7.

Mintzberg, H. (1996, July–August). Musings on management. *Harvard Business Review,* pp. 61–67.

Pinchot, G. (1996). Creating organizations with many leaders. In F. Hesselbein, M. Goldsmith, & R. Beckhard (Eds.), *The leader of the future* (pp. 25–39). San Francisco: Jossey-Bass.

Stodgill, R.M. (1974). *Handbook of leadership.* New York: Free Press.

CASE 12–1   Shared Governance in an Academic Health Center

Linda M. Herrick

The purpose of this case study is to look at the implementation of shared governance in an academic health center. During the 1980s, shared governance was promoted as a means by which to increase nurse job satisfaction (Pinkerton et al., 1989) and to give nurses more control over their work environment, thus enhancing professional practice (Kardos, 1990). Shared governance has been implemented since 1991 in the Department of Nursing, Mayo Medical Center, Rochester. This case study will describe key elements of success for implementing shared governance, implementation on one patient care unit, the nurse manager role, and evaluation.

Shared governance is a systems concept that promotes involvement in decision making and partnerships in the workplace (Porter-O'Grady, 1990). Most shared governance models provide a structure through which employees participate in decisions and are accountable for those decisions. Shared governance provides equity and horizontal relationships rather than vertical reporting relationships (Porter-O'Grady, 1995). Shidler and associates (1989) state that shared governance models provide for sharing of power and promote interdependence and cooperation. These principles underlie shared governance models, although structures and implementation may vary.

■ KEY ELEMENTS FOR SUCCESS WITH SHARED GOVERNANCE

In the Department of Nursing, shared governance was adopted to move decision making to the people closest to the patient, the staff on the patient care units. This type of shift from traditional management to staff provides equity and increases cooperation, accountability, and ownership of practice. We have found key elements for success in implementing shared governance to include a patient focus, decision making structures, consensus management, free expression, individual responsibility, timing issues, and a common language (Frusti, 1996).

At the department level and unit level, a *patient focus* is maintained by asking four questions in the following order: (1) What is best for the patient? (2) What is best for the institution? (3) What is best for the department? and (4) What is best for the individual nurse? One example that demonstrates this focus was related to changes in the floating model. The Staffing and Scheduling Committee reexamined issues related to floating between units. The goal was to revise the model to meet needs from all perspectives. Staff identified that patients should have adequate and competent staff to meet their needs; therefore, it would not be in the patient's best interest to have extra staff on one unit and

CASE 12–1 *Continued*

too few on another unit. From the institutional and departmental perspective, reallocation of staff to meet workload fluctuation was cost-effective. From the nurse's perspective, there were concerns related to specialty knowledge and not feeling a welcomed part of the unit. The revised model includes unit-to-unit floating, but a nurse from the unit is teamed with the nurse floating and both together are given an assignment. Work is divided according to the patients' needs and the expertise of the unit float nurse.

The shared governance structure includes the departmental committees and unit councils. The department has encouraged staff participation in *decision making* by requiring that at least 60 percent of the membership of departmental committees be nonmanagement staff. Four major or standing departmental committees exist, including the Nursing Council and the Practice, Education, and Research Committees. The Nursing Council is responsible for seeing that the tenets of shared governance are maintained in committees and unit councils. The Council mentors unit councils, educates, and showcases successes. The other committees support the work of the department and coordinate efforts between other committees, such as documentation or procedural guidelines. Communication between committees occurs through minimal joint membership and sharing of minutes.

Each committee is asked to establish ground rules or norms for working together. These may be used during the meeting to keep the meeting focused or to confront behavior. They are used at the end of the meeting for processing, which includes stating the positives of the meeting and those things that should be changed.

The organizational reporting structure serves as a communication system by which information flows between administrative levels and the units rapidly. Communication of decisions also occurs through a weekly announcement sheet, a monthly nursing newsletter, and a weekly institutional newsletter.

Consensus management was chosen over democratic forms of voting, including a simple majority. The voting mechanism is often detailed in the bylaws of shared governance. Our nursing department felt that if decisions were made by vote, there would be times when a large percentage of the staff would not agree with a decision and might impede the change. A division between staff could occur and separate people into those who "won" and those who "lost." When consensus is used, solutions are negotiated until one is reached that all can accept. Time may be needed to reach consensus, especially in committees where one person is representing a group and may need to go back to that group in order to decide priorities and items to be negotiated. Frusti (1996) notes that the timing of issues is a key element and shared governance is a process requiring sufficient time for planning, implementation, and evaluation. Rushing the process may jeopardize the result. The consensus-making model promotes the principles of partnership, equity, accountability, and ownership that Porter-O'Grady (1995) states are critical to shared governance.

CASE 12–1 *Continued*

Shared governance is based on open, honest communication and respect for different perspectives. Porter-O'Grady (1994) notes that shared governance builds relationships necessary to do the work while achieving mutually acceptable outcomes. At committee meetings, participants are encouraged or requested to express their ideas and opinions. *Free expression* and mutual respect concepts are included in the ground rules of most committees.

Porter-O'Grady (1994) states that shared governance obliges members to own decisions. This highlights another key element, *individual responsibility*. In the Department of Nursing, shared governance has increased individual involvement in committees, councils, and groups. Members involved are responsible for sharing information, getting input from their peers, and communicating decisions. Those not directly involved in the committees are responsible for staying informed and giving input to members in a timely manner. All are responsible for supporting decisions made by peers. The focus is on professional practice and involvement rather than on traditional hierarchy and managers.

A consultant was used to introduce the principles of shared governance, expectations, skills, and a *common language*. The strategy was to promote a sense of cohesion and unification through use of a common language (Frusti, 1996). As shared governance was implemented in the department, some of the language and meaning was unfamiliar to people in other areas. Explanations were required so others in the organization could share this language and comprehend the key elements, such as patient focus, which were driving decisions.

■ A CASE EXAMPLE OF UNIT IMPLEMENTATION

Prior to the adoption of the formal shared governance model, there was an emphasis on participative management on this unit. Staff had been involved in decision making and activities on the unit for over 5 years. The patient care unit for this case example was a 30-bed medical/surgical gastrointestinal (GI) and general surgery unit. The unit staff included registered nurses (RNs), licensed practical nurses (LPNs), nursing assistants (NAs), unit secretaries, and a nurse manager. Other personnel frequently present on the unit included the dietitian, dietary assistant, housekeeper, decentralized pharmacist, and physician teams.

Several philosophical themes have been identified that assisted staff in successfully transitioning to shared governance. One theme was that the *staff RNs were viewed as clinical experts* and professional nurses. This was important, as they were seen as credible and had the self-confidence to speak up, especially about practice and clinical issues. Another theme was that the *unit "belonged" to the team,* nurses and others, who worked there and the team was responsible for the success or failure of the unit. The role of the nurse manager was to facilitate the work, but not control it.

CASE 12–1 *Continued*

Mutual respect was a theme at the unit level as well. Mutual respect included acceptance of people from different cultures and backgrounds, but it also meant respecting each person for his or her knowledge and valuing the skills that person contributed to patient care and to the unit. All staff, including the nursing assistants and housekeepers, were recognized for the importance of their work, their knowledge, and the role they played on the unit. The importance of different perspectives was valued. When groups were formed, they were often multidisciplinary and people were chosen for the perspectives they brought.

Finally, a *learning environment was encouraged*. It was acceptable to say "I don't know ... " as long as it was followed by " ... but, I'll find out"—and people did. Staff were encouraged to use resources, including clinical nurse specialists, nursing education specialists, journals, books, and each other, to find answers or better ways to practice. Questions often focused on why and how things are done, and there was a sense of inquiry. One staff member asked why a surgical communication card for families was used at the desk. A brief explanation was provided including the fact that it had been developed as part of a master's thesis that was available in the library. The RN and unit secretary obtained the thesis and discovered that the unit could improve use of the form. They took action posting notices on the bulletin board and informing key people of the rationale and changes in practice.

Lastly, *change was embraced*, but not necessarily passively accepted. Members of the staff on various committees volunteered the unit for numerous product and practice trials. They felt it was an opportunity to give input and influence changes. They could then accept the change or outcome if the process for the decision could be understood.

■ STRATEGIES FOR SUCCESS

Before and after the implementation of shared governance, staff on the unit were involved in numerous unit and departmental activities. This process took time and did not occur simply with the initiation of shared governance and formation of a unit council. A discussion of strategies for implementation and staff development that contributed to success over time follows.

A consultant was hired to use a "train the trainer" approach to teach concepts and skills related to shared governance. A representative from each patient care unit agreed to attend classes and to serve as a facilitator and instructor on the unit. Related skills that were taught included consensus decision making and the plan, do, check, act (PDCA) model of problem solving. The unit facilitator taught the rest of the staff these concepts and skills. Although concepts were taught in a relatively short time, implementation of skills took more than 1 year.

Units were responsible for forming a unit council and identifying how to communicate decisions and information

CASE 12–1 *Continued*

to all staff, but membership and the process were left to the unit to decide. Since this was a relatively small unit, it was decided that all staff would be a part of the unit council; other units chose or elected representatives to make up the council. A steering group was identified to assist in setting agendas for meetings. Unit council meetings replaced traditional staff meetings. Methods for communicating information to those not at council meetings or new information that arose between meetings were identified. These methods included the communication book, posting notices, and individual mailings. Staff were accountable to read the information.

One issue that arose early in implementation was the scope of authority of the unit council in decision making. Staff were excited about making meaningful changes and chose first to work on changing the unit dress code. At the time, white uniforms were the standard for general care units and many staff wanted to wear scrub suits. An institutional work group was already in process to address multiple issues related to scrub suit use. Staff were disappointed to learn they could not make the change they wanted, but they quickly learned to examine their scope of authority on issues they wanted to address. Later, when institutional policies related to scrub suits were communicated, unit level decisions on dress code could proceed.

One area of deficiency for many staff was systems thinking. Staff were oriented to their unit and not all were clear about how it fit into the context of the broader institution. Although some staff had insight as to why decisions had to be integrated, others viewed the need for coordination as a road block. The constraints affecting decision making, such as wage and labor laws, accreditation requirements, and institutional policies, needed to be reviewed and discussed as topics and ideas were considered.

At times, the information and perceived constraints were overwhelming to staff and they would become discouraged. This was especially true at the beginning when the council chose to struggle with topics that were broad in scope and impact. The time and effort required to get the information and the constraints were perceived as excessive. The process of shared governance was blamed as being too burdensome. A successful strategy to support the shared governance process and reduce frustration was to teach staff how to break down each decision or project into manageable components early in the process. Having the council work on one manageable component at a time also provided a feeling of progress toward a goal.

New skills were needed by some staff. Basic presentation skills were helpful in presenting information or the concern at hand. More difficult were the negotiation skills needed for a work group to come to consensus. There were many times when everyone on the unit, including the nurse manager, thought voting might be much easier, but no one wanted to be on the side that lost and so negotiations continued. It took a great

CASE 12–1 *Continued*

deal of facilitation by the unit facilitator, the nurse manager, and, sometimes, an outside facilitator from the department. People needed to be reminded that the goal was a decision with which all could live and work.

One "small" decision that nearly threatened to split the work team was related to the placement of stock items on a newly remodeled unit. A group consisting of an RN, LPN, NA, and unit secretary volunteered at a council meeting, and the unit staff agreed this group would decide where items would go and work with central services. The group used blueprints, sought input from all staff members, and drew up plans well before the unit opened. A plan was agreed to, the unit was stocked, and the patients and staff returned. It was a major remodeling effort and everyone had a difficult time finding items for the first few days. By the second or third day, people were moving items to more "logical" places in different drawers and shelves. The work group members were frustrated at seeing their work disintegrate and angry that their co-workers who had given input were not following through with the plans. The work group asked for a halt to the moving of items for 1 week and posted a paper on which staff were to log their complaints/concerns. Staff were reminded of the shared governance process and their responsibility to give the decision a chance. All of us needed to remember that decisions by consensus meant a commitment to live with them, even though we might not like every component or, in this case, where

every item was placed. There was a new appreciation for the consensus decision and shared governance. At times, educational efforts and personal counseling were needed to separate the topic from the person. It took a while for some staff to learn how to debate an issue rather than taking all disagreement personally.

Ground rules were established by the unit council during the implementation of shared governance. One of the most difficult rules was to avoid doing business outside a meeting. Sometimes as information was being collected, and discussed, negative discussions ensued related to the people involved. A new ground rule was established stating that each person on the unit had a responsibility to refrain from such conversations and to assist others to discuss issues, rather than people. At first, it was difficult to confront others in a thoughtful, respectful way that maintained positive relationships. Receiving feedback and graciously accepting it was also hard.

■ NURSE MANAGER ROLE

The nurse manager role in shared governance becomes one of coach, mentor, and facilitator. For some managers, this entails a considerable shift in emphasis. Reflections and examples of changes in the role are shared here.

Nurse managers successful in the shared governance environment appear to believe in the staff and to believe they will try to do well given a chance with skills needed to succeed. The nurse manager needs to be comfortable with

CASE 12–1   *Continued*

unit personnel trying, failing, learning, becoming competent, and gaining recognition for activities. This can be difficult if the activity being given up is something the nurse manager has enjoyed and been praised for doing well. As a nurse manager known for scheduling expertise and fairness, it was difficult for this author to turn that function over to staff nurses, but the pride when one of the nurses became recognized as an expert by peers throughout the institution more than made up for it. The shift from gaining satisfaction from doing to gaining satisfaction from assisting others can be difficult.

The time commitment by the nurse manager to implement shared governance is considerable. Time is needed to share concepts and put the structures in place, but even more demanding is the time to mentor and coach staff. Change is slow and often painful.

Performance evaluations serve as a base for mentoring and coaching. Feedback is given by the nurse manager and peers through peer review; time is also set aside to discuss the employee's professional and personal goals related to work and opportunities related to unit activities. Discussion may include the time the employee is willing to commit to a project, skills the employee thought he or she had, skills to be developed, and interests. This may also be an opportunity to challenge the employee to develop new skills or take on a different project or set priorities Although formal evaluations occur once a year, the number of formal and informal meetings with employees and groups increases.

In our experience, peer delegation skills became especially important as staff continued to become more involved in unit activities. As a group began to work on a project, all members needed a clear picture of each person's role, their own responsibilities, the timeline, and where to obtain more information. The manager had to decide when to be a source of information and when to allow staff to find their own information. Issues that needed to be weighed included avoiding spoon feeding, respecting their resourcefulness, and not overwhelming staff with too much information at once. Often this balance was a fine line and hard to judge.

Periodic follow-up served to give work groups a chance to clarify expectations, ask for more information, and receive positive feedback. It also gave the nurse manager a chance to assess project progress against the timeline to be met and intervene as necessary.

Time and scheduling can be an issue if many staff are involved in committee work. Having a calendar of meetings and incorporating it in the schedule is helpful. Adequate coverage for the unit was critical. Staff became adept at covering for one another and setting priorities between patient care and other activities. Commitment to the process was required of those caring for the patients as much as of those attending meetings.

■ EVALUATION

Evaluation is important to the success of shared governance. Many research

CASE 12–1 *Continued*

studies have looked at the relationship between shared governance and staff satisfaction (Kreitzer, 1991; Wilson & Laschinger, 1994). In 1995, members of the Nursing Council asked the question, "Does shared governance make a difference in patient care and patient outcomes?" However, with additional discussion, they agreed that shared governance was only one change affecting outcomes. The question was revised to, "What are the perceptions of personnel in the Department of Nursing regarding the impact of shared governance?" It was felt these perceptions could be significant to the success of implementation and ongoing commitment to the process. A research team was formed of Council members. All staff in the Departments of Nursing and Surgical Services were surveyed. The study provided information regarding perceptions and an impetus for some changes. It also served as a baseline for periodic evaluation.

Shared governance promoted professional practice and development of staff. Patient care and the working environment were enhanced. The accountability and responsibility of staff bring about an environment in which it is a pleasure to work.

■ BIOGRAPHICAL SKETCH

Linda M. Herrick is Director of Nursing Research, Mayo Medical Center, Rochester, Minnesota. She was nurse manager for 12 years on the patient care unit described in the case study. She received her BSN from Winona State University, Minnesota, and her MS in Nursing from the University of Minnesota, and is currently a doctoral candidate at the University of Minnesota.

■ SUGGESTED READING LIST

Atwood, J.R., & Hinshaw, A.S. (1980). Job satisfaction instrument: A program of development and testing. *Communicating Nursing Research, 12,* 55.

Blegen, M.A., Goode, C., Johnson, M., Maas, M., Chen, L., & Moorhead, S. (1993). Preferences for decision-making autonomy. *Image, 25* (4), 339–344.

Brodbeck, K. (1992). Professional practice actualized through an integrated shared governance and quality assurance model. *Journal of Nursing Care Quality, 6* (2), 20–31.

Edwards, G.B., Farrough, M., Gardner, M., Harrison, D., Sherman, M., & Simpson, S. (1994). Unit-based shared governance can work! *Nursing Management, 25* (4), 74–77.

Jenkins, L.S. (1993). Impact of shared governance: Instrument development and testing. *Proceedings: Sigma Theta Tau International, 32nd Biennial Convention* (p. 77). Indianapolis, IN: Sigma Theta Tau International.

Jones, C.B., Stasiowski, S., Simons, B.J., Boyd, N. J., & Lucas, M.D. (1993). Shared governance and the nursing practice environment. *Nursing Economic$, 11* (4), 208–214.

Kanter, R.M. (1977). *Men and women of the corporation.* New York: Basic Books.

Kusserow, R.P. (1988). Nurse participation in hospital decision making: Potential impact on the nursing shortage. *Nursing Economic$, 6* (6), 312–316.

Ludemann, R.S., & Brown, C. (1989). Staff perceptions of shared governance. *Nursing Administration Quarterly, 13*(4), 49–56.

CASE 12–1 *Continued*

McDaniel, C., & Patrick, T. (1992). Leadership, nurses, and patient satisfaction: A pilot study. *Nursing Administration Quarterly, 16* (3), 72–74.

Neis, M.E., & Kingdon, R.T. (1990). *Leadership in transition: A practical guide to shared governance*. Schaumberg, IL: Nova I, Ltd.

Parkman, C.A., & Loveridge, C. (1994). From nursing service to professional practice. *Nursing Management, 25* (3), 63–68.

Thrasher, T., Bossman, V.M., Carroll, S., Cook, B., Cherry, K., Kopras, S.M., Daniels, L., & Schaffer, P. (1992). Empowering the clinical nurse through quality assurance in a shared governance setting. *Journal of Nursing Care Quality, 6* (2), 15–19.

Van Tassel, M. (1993). Reallocating power. *Canadian Nurse, 89* (8), 55.

Zelauskas, B., & Howes, D.G. (1992). The effects of implementing a professional practice model. *Journal of Nursing Administration, 22* (7/8), 18–23.

■ REFERENCES

Frusti, D.K. (1996). Perspectives of a chief nurse executive. *Journal of Shared Governance, 2* (1), 11–12.

Kardos, B.C. (1990). Governance? Who governs? *Journal of Post Anesthesia Nursing, 5* (1), 60–62.

Kreitzer, M.J. (1991). *Impact of staff nurse participation in decision-making on job satisfaction and organizational commitment*. Minneapolis, MN: University of Minnesota Press.

Pinkerton, S.E., Eckes, A., Marcouiller, M., McNichols, M.B., Krejci, J.W., & Malin, S. (1989). St. Michael Hospital: A shared governance model. *Nursing Administration Quarterly, 13* (4), 35–47.

Porter-O'Grady, T. (1990). *The reorganization of nursing practice: Creating the corporate venture*. Rockville, MD: Aspen.

Porter-O'Grady, T. (1994). Whole system shared governance: Creating the seamless organization. *Nursing Economics, 12* (4), 187–95.

Porter-O'Grady, T. (1995). From principle to practice: Whole systems shared governance. *Journal of Shared Governance, 1* (3), 21–26.

Shidler, H., Pencak, M., & McFolling, S.D. (1989). Professional nursing staff: A model of self-governance for nursing. *Nursing Administration Quarterly, 13* (4), 1–9.

Wilson, B., & Laschinger, H.K. (1994). Staff nurse perception of job empowerment and organizational commitment. *Journal of Nursing Administration, 24* (8), 39–47.

13

Professional Development

Brenda S. Cherry

In the past 5 years, professional development has become more critical to maintaining competence than it has been in the history of nursing. A nurse's basic formal preparation to enter the profession is not sufficient for continued competence. The roles of professional and advanced practice nurses are evolving so rapidly that continuing education programs are in a constant state of revision. Now more than ever, formal and informal professional development is needed for nurses to not only survive but thrive in the current health care delivery marketplace. One can safely predict that the need for relevant, accessible, and affordable formal programs will increase over time.

This chapter is based on the following assumptions: nurses need continuing professional development throughout their careers; professional development needs exceed those that can be accomplished through self-instruction; employers are responsible for identifying required competencies as they evolve and for providing opportunities for acquiring competencies; and the commitment to professional development must be shared by employer and employee.

In this chapter, professional development is conceptualized broadly as any organized program that facilitates maintenance and enhancement of nursing competence in providing quality patient care, and making decisions about the provisions of care. It includes the cognitive, psychomotor, and affective abilities needed for direct patient care as well as the abilities needed to manage resources and persons providing care, collaborate with other health and allied health disciplines, and generate nursing care data.

This chapter explores the purposes of professional development at differing points in nursing careers, the locus of professional development functions in organizations, adult learning theories, and linkages between service and educational institutions.

■ PURPOSES OF PROFESSIONAL DEVELOPMENT PROGRAMS

One reality faced by nurse administrators is the disparity in clinical competence among nurse clinicians. Whether attributed to formal education, experience, disposition, or innate ability, differences in level of clinical performance exist. Before planning any professional development program, its purpose and target population need to be identified. After educational needs of the target population have been assessed, effective planning, implementation, and evaluation can proceed.

Education and training programs in service agencies usually target either new or continuing nurse employees. Internal programs usually include orientation, cross training, training for newly created positions, certification/recertification in competencies, or management and leadership (Marquis & Huston, 1992). Many programs also provide offerings for nurses in the broader community, and some serve as regional providers. Cost–benefit assessments have shown positive relationships between a well-trained and educated staff, increased productivity, and quality outcomes. Positive relationships have also been found between employer-sponsored professional development opportunities, increased employee satisfaction, and decreased turnover (Hawkins, 1992).

New Nurse Employees

Orientation is a critical factor in professional development. It is often cited as one of the most important variables in agency attrition rates and general socialization into the nursing profession. The quality and effectiveness of orientation programs is as variable as the service agencies in which they are offered. Their goals also vary, from a basic orientation about organizational structure, policies, and procedures, to clarification of mutual expectations, assessment of competence and learning needs, and establishment of plans for career development.

Different organizational structures are used to achieve orientation goals. The traditional approach is a structured centralized program. Research supports the decentralized and centralized/decentralized combination as structures having the greatest potential for efficiency and effectiveness. These structures delegate all or some responsibility and authority for orientation to managers and staff of designated units, which may or may not be the unit where the employee will work. The efficiency and effectiveness of these approaches, as well as the ideal goal(s) of orientation programs, are ongoing nursing issues. High nurse–patient ratios, increased responsibilities for delegation and supervision of paraprofessionals, increased patient acuity levels, and frequent reorganization of care units are current factors impacting these programs.

In a frequently referenced study, McCloskey and McCain (1987) explored satisfaction, commitment, and professionalism of 320 nurses newly employed in a large metropolitan hospital. Findings from this longitudinal study (1983–1986) indicate that all nurses, new graduates and experienced clinicians, entered a new employment agency with expectations of career development, participation in decision making, and other job rewards. They found that organizational satisfaction, commitment, and professionalism decreased for all nurses in the study during the first 6 months of employment. Researchers attributed these decreases to discrepancies between initial expectations and actual experiences.

One purpose of orientation programs is to inform nurses of the realities and expectations of nursing practice within respective institutions and to plan for career development based on assessment of competencies. A successful orientation program improves the fit between new employee expectations and institutional opportunities for fulfillment.

Preceptor Programs

Preceptor programs couple a new nurse employee with an experienced employee (one-to-one) who is responsible for orientation to the agency and nursing unit. The preceptor serves as a role model and liaison between the agency and the new employee. Objectives for education and training of the new employee are based on mutual identification of learning needs. The preceptor has responsibility for education and training of the new employee and patient care, usually with a reduced patient load. She or he paves the way for successful adjustment by introducing and explaining organizational values, informal communication channels, and nuances of the workplace. Bellinger and McCloskey (1992) found that preceptors were particularly beneficial for nurses with limited education and experience and contributed significantly to social integration and group cohesiveness for novice and experienced new employees.

Preceptor programs require monetary and personnel resources and must be well planned and coordinated to be effective. Preceptors must be oriented to the role and given sufficient teaching time and resources. Reward systems should explicitly and equitably reward preceptors. Regardless of the reward system, some nurses may not want to be preceptors. Assuming that all qualified nurses should be interested in becoming preceptors and using administrative pressure to convince them to do so is a mistake that will jeopardize the success of any program.

Continuing Nurse Employees

There are many changes within an agency that necessitate continuous updating of a nurse's education and training. External changes may also affect nurses' educational needs due to changes in nurse practice acts or certification requirements. The most basic reason for professional development is maintenance of clinical competence. Clinical competence is defined relative to standards of care for designated patient populations. Throughout a nurse's career, clinical competence must be reestablished as one assumes new functions and responsibilities or as advances in practice occur. Organizational goals associated with offering educational programs during these transitions are not only to provide for gains in knowledge and skills for employees, but also to support organizational commitment and job satisfaction.

Attempts to identify and meet the ongoing professional developmental needs of the experienced nurse clinician have been less well developed by service agencies. Controversies include: mandatory versus voluntary continuing education; nurse's motivation for participation; sources of education and training; teaching strategies; and payment by employer or employee (Luchat, Zerbe, & Scott, 1992). The underlying theme in these issues is, who is responsible for career development—the nurse clinician, her employer, or both? The answer remains elusive, but there is a definite trend for agencies to provide support for career growth through monetary reimbursement and flexibility in scheduling to pursue educational goals and/or new internal positions or joint appointments through collaborative arrangements.

Mercy Hospital in Portland, Maine, developed an innovative approach to continuing professional development by organizing a "practice field for team learning" (Robichaud, 1992, p. 320). This approach is "designed to recognize and reward expert nurses for their skilled practical knowledge, discretionary judgment, caring practices and moral agency" (p. 320). Based on practices of personal mastery, mental models, and building shared vision, this model is a nontraditional approach to combining individual professional development and overall organizational development.

Professional commitment and motivation to continually improve one's ability to provide quality patient care needs to be sustained and enhanced throughout a nurse's career. Socialization to and rewards for meeting this expectation should be addressed beginning in orientation and reinforced through the performance management system. Studies support that career development is one contributing factor to job satisfaction (Angelini, 1995; Bellinger & McCloskey, 1992; Francke & Erkens, 1994).

Sources of education and training external to a nurse's place of employment are educational institutions, professional organizations, private providers, and a wide variety of media from books to the Internet. Offerings may be in the form of workshops, seminars, conferences, independent studies/learning modules, or formal courses. Advances in delivery methods, such as distance learning and computer-assisted instruction, have increased development opportunities for nurses, particularly those in smaller isolated agencies (Billings & Bachmeier, 1994). Cannon and associates (1994), in a nonrandomized statewide telephone survey of 535 registered nurses, found that the majority (359) desired academic credit for participation in continuing education programs. Although not the current norm, this may be an indication of future demands.

■ LOCUS OF PROFESSIONAL DEVELOPMENT FUNCTIONS

The locus of professional development programs is related to the structure of the parent institution and available resources. Consideration of the target population's learning needs in determining locus of responsibility for professional development is a more recent phenomenon. Impetus for this consideration has eminated from two general areas: management literature and adult learning and development literature.

A centralized department remains the dominant organizational structure for professional development units. Given the bureaucratic nature of health care organizations, this is not surprising. The advantages of a centralized department are (1) use of fewer human resources, thus decreasing planning and coordination time; (2) increased control of curriculum; and (3) decreased up-front costs. These advantages, however, must be considered in terms of their long-term effects in achieving the goals of education and training.

Decentralization—the dispersement of functions, authority, and power—is more consistent with the human relations theory of management that advocates the importance of social and psychological factors in determining organizational structure. This theory facilitates a more open system of organization, one that is continually adapting to change in its environment and achieves a steady state or dynamic balance of changes (Morgan, 1997). There is a current trend toward decentralization of professional development in health care delivery agencies. This reflects a growing awareness that a change in organizational structure is needed to accommodate the many rapid changes that are occurring in health care. Professional development units have been taxed by demands for education and training of clinicians in the many technological and managerial changes taking place.

Orientation of new employees has traditionally been a two-step process: centralized formal classes and decentralized informal introduction to the job. However, many health care organizations have decentralized their professional development departments and involved more nurse clinicians in the planning, implementation, and evaluation of programs. With support from nurse educators, nurse clinicians are presenting in-service classes to their peers and acting as preceptors for those entering their work group. In fact, in her classic research, Benner (1984) found the most effective educators were those who had recently had similar learning experiences. Thus, a staff nurse with 2 years' experience is better suited to be a preceptor of a new graduate than an expert nurse with 20 years of experience.

■ NURSES AS ADULT LEARNERS

When planning curricula for nursing educational and training programs, the educator needs a firm foundation in both learning theory and adult learning characteristics. When writing objectives, the educator also needs to consider characteristics of both the content and the learner. Objectives focus on content that is to be learned or behaviors indicating that learning has been achieved.

Objectives can be broadly classified according to Bloom's (1956) taxonomy of educational objectives: cognitive, affective, and psychomotor. Cognitive objectives address behaviors depicting intellectual skills and abilities at the levels of knowledge, understanding, application, analysis, synthesis, and evaluation (Reilly & Obermann, 1990). An example of a cognitive objective for the evaluation level is:

> By the fourth class, each student will critique three research articles utilizing Cherry's five principles of research critiques.

Affective objectives are based on behaviors that demonstrate changes in sensitivity, attitudes, and values. This domain of objectives includes receiving, responding, valuing, organizing, and characterizing by a value. An example of an affective objective for valuing is:

> At the conclusion of the seminar on values clarification, each student will verbally judge the relevancy of seminar content to his or her current job responsibilities.

Psychomotor objectives address motor skills and manipulative behaviors. Psychomotor behaviors are divided into four levels: observing, imitating, practicing, and adapting. An example of a psychomotor objective for adapting is:

> At the end of the second class, each student will demonstrate, in selected simulated situations, body mechanics appropriate to the effective delivery of a formal speech.

Educational objectives should encompass three components, the learner, the behavioral change sought, and the content related to the behavioral change. Targeted behavioral changes in the learner must be based on knowledge of the learner's baseline behavior (Reilly & Obermann, 1990).

Learning Theories

Learning theory is a subfield of psychology. This broad subject has two competing main streams of theory: neo-behaviorist and Gestalt.

Neo-behaviorists are the current researchers using Skinner's principles of stimulus–response as the basis of learning. Neo-behaviorists believe "learning is a more or less permanent change of behavior that occurs as a result of practice. Key concepts are stimuli and responses. The process of learning can be understood by studying the relationship of processions of stimuli and responses and what occurs between them that results in desirable behaviors" (Bigge, 1976, p. 86).

Educators with a behaviorist orientation base their teaching efforts on the manipulation of external variables or stimuli to elicit a desired response from the learner. Members of this school of thought advocate control of the learning situation by the teacher, view students as passive receptors for stimuli, do not consider purpose or goal activities of students, do not recognize the value of past experiences and their influence on learning, and recognize extrinsic motivation as the compelling force in learning.

This theoretical approach may be useful for nursing instructors designing training programs to introduce knowledge and skills that are novel to the learner. Examples are how to use new equipment or other totally new information. This approach stresses the importance of presenting each step and requiring return demonstrations. Learning experiences using this approach are standardized, and each learner goes through the same experience.

Gestalt theorists offer a contrasting view of how people learn. Learning is viewed as a process of developing new insights or modifying old ones. Gestalt educators believe learning occurs through goal insight, continuity of life space, and experiences that facilitate learning. The prior experiences and knowledge of students are utilized as an integral part of the teaching–learning process. Their view of the student is that he or she is active, motivated by intrinsic and extrinsic factors, learns by discovery and problem solving, and learns best in an environment that enhances his or her self-esteem and provides for his or her comfort (Knowles, 1990). This theoretical approach leads the educator to examine individual differences among learners and to allow for flexibility in designing learning experiences.

Cognitive Style

One important way that people vary, regardless of age, is learning style or cognitive style. This has been called a theory of learning how to learn. "Helping people to gain insight into their cognitive patterns, methodological preferences, strengths and weaknesses, and to overcome blocks to learning effectiveness is the key to helping people learn" (Smith & Haverkamp, 1977, p. 4).

Assessment of cognitive style helps the educator to plan more effective teaching–learning strategies. Dolphin and Holtzclaw (1983) state that "the needs for diversity in teaching strategies becomes more apparent when a combination of several divergent cognitive styles emerge within the same group of learners" (p. 68). Educators also need to be aware of their own cognitive style. Research shows that educators tend to primarily use the style they prefer. Thus, assessing both the educator's and the student's cognitive style and providing a variety of learning strategies connotes a particular philosophy of teaching in which instruction is viewed as an active two-way communication process involving the direct and indirect exchange of knowledge, skill, and affect.

Adult Learning Theory

Another characteristic of nurses is that they are all adults. In her classic article on the differences between adults and youth, Zahn (1967) states that many differences are related to age and these differences play a significant role in how adults learn. She delineates some of these differences as: (1) a physical decline in speed of performance, reaction time, sight, and hearing; (2) psychological changes in values, goals, responsibilities, self-image, and quantity of experiences; and (3) cognitive–intellectual changes in stability of learning abilities when time limits are controlled. Although cognitive abilities do not decline with age, the educator must consider the need for additional reaction time when planning adult learning activities. The difficulty encountered when relearning a procedure or content—cognitive dissonance—may also necessitate additional time for "unlearning" while incorporating new knowledge and skills.

Psychological differences between children and adults are due to developmental stage and differences in life experiences. The earliest developmental theories did not address adults. The three major adult developmental theories are Havighurst's life cycle theory, Erickson's successive developmental crises, and Buhler's biological clock theory. Havighurst alerts the educator of adults to consider chronologically related dominant concerns (tasks) that are based on biological development and personal and social expectations. Erickson separates the developmental needs of adulthood into three stages: young adult (18 to 29 years), adults (30 to 65 years), and senior adults (over 65 years). Thus, adults in different stages may have different motivation in choosing learning experiences. Buhler directs the instructor to consider that adults, unlike children, choose learning experiences for pragmatic applications rather than undifferentiated future use. Adults use a present orientation in evaluating learning experiences.

Malcolm Knowles is the leading adult learning theorist. His primary concept is that learning for adults should be based on "androgogy" rather than "pedagogy," which was originally developed for teaching children. Following are the five assumptions of androgogy.

1. Adult learners are self-directed.
2. Adults are a resource for their own learning (experience).
3. Adults have learning needs based on social development and roles (readiness).
4. Adults need immediacy of application (time perspective).
5. Adults have a problem-centered orientation to learning (Knowles, 1984; 1990, p. 116).

For adults, unlike children, learning experiences are often based on personal choice. Adults seek learning experiences to augment what they already know (Knowles, 1990). They may be motivated by external forces, such as occupational obsolescence, changing societal roles, economic advancement, or advances in knowledge. They may also be motivated by internal desires such as professional growth, self-improvement, or social interaction. Any or all of these motives may apply to nurse clinicians and should be understood in planning flexible and relevant professional development programs.

Concepts from Gestalt learning theory, cognitive style research, and adult learning theory should be used together in designing individualized learning experiences for nurses. This is most applicable when content focuses on cognitive and affective objectives. Affective objectives are best achieved through active involvement in simulations of affective situations, such as role playing or keeping journals.

The Learning Experience

A final factor to consider in planning a learning experience for nurses is the environment. Knowles (1990) indicates that an environment that facilitates physical comfort, privacy, informality, and lack of distractions promotes learning. He also proposes that the quality and amount of interaction between educator and learner is a crucial factor in the success of learning efforts by adults. An atmosphere of respect, trust, mutual helpfulness, freedom of expression, and acceptance of differences promotes learning. The environment is important regardless of content being presented or teaching strategy chosen.

Teaching modalities available to the educator include independent learning modules, one-to-one coaching as in a preceptorship, informal group inservices led by peers, or formal classes of varying group sizes. Advances in communications technology have expanded access to multimedia, distance learning, and interactive learning options. Choice depends on resources, learning theory perspective, domain of learning objectives, learner characteristics, institutional goals, and demand. Important points for the educator to consider in planning adult learning experiences are (1) creating a physical environment conducive to learning, (2) making adjustments based on adult characteristics, and (3) remembering that the interpersonal aspect of learning is one important factor in the success of the educational experience.

■ CREATIVE LINKAGES BETWEEN SERVICE AND EDUCATION

Facilitating achievement of professional objectives is crucial to the development of nurse clinicians within specified agencies as well as to the entire nursing profession. Ultimately, this will only be achieved through collaboration between formal education and service (Pew Commission, 1995). Both formal affiliations and collaborative endeavors are advocated as the key to strength of the nursing profession by the American Association of Colleges of Nursing, National Commission on Nursing, and the National Institutes of Health, Committee on Nursing and Nursing Education. These relationships may range from informal networking between educators and clinicians to formal institutional mergers. The forms of relationships are limited only by the creativity and commitment of educators and clinicians.

Provision of professional development education is only one purpose of these collaborations. They usually have multiple goals which use synergy to enhance research, extend advanced practice of nursing, expand professional development, improve education, and increase political action (Bell, 1996; Hall & McHugh, 1995; Mundinger, 1995). Collaborative partnerships maximize limited resources and create new channels of communication that break down barriers between nursing practice, education, research, and policy.

One example of an innovative collaboration is the Southern Massachusetts Nursing coalition. This collaborative effort is designed to assist acute care nurses to make the transition to home care. As an alliance of five acute care hospitals, three home care agencies, and a university college of nursing, it provides the continuing education and financial and social support critical to education of nursing personnel. College faculty and home care clinical preceptors provide opportunities for participants to assess and "confront transitional problems" within socially supportive settings while increasing their marketability in a rapidly changing health care environment (O'Neill, 1996, p. 64).

Ideally, information emanating from such relationships should influence basic nursing education programs as well as professional development programs for clinicians. If this were the rule instead of the exception, perhaps the conflict in expectations and role confusion of new graduates would be diminished. Instead, Kramer's (1981) insights concerning "reality shock" of new graduates continue to be applicable, and lines of effective communication between education and service remain inadequate.

According to Walker (1985) the desire to improve communication channels and collaborative efforts is the first step in achieving communication and collaboration. This desire must be coupled with what she describes as attitudes for partnership: a commitment to the total profession, realistic expectations, willingness to accept responsibility for helping each other, and flexibility. Although these prerequisite attitudes are believed to create a conducive mental set, they do not explain how bridges of communication and collaboration can actually be established.

Styles (1984) provided one of the first frameworks for analyzing collaboration between education and service. It provides a useful background for developing and examining collaborative models. Her continuum of collaborative modes (Table 13–1) depicts stages of unity that reflect progressive frequency of interaction on topics of mutual interest, reciprocal advising, mutual approval before acting, and unified policies on selected issues (p. 22).

The Rural Elderly Enhancement Project (REEP) in Alabama is an example of a broad-based partnership between citizens and health and human services professionals (Farley, 1995). As a shared decision-making model, its goal was to develop rural health and human service systems that were family

TABLE 13–1. Stages of Unity

Stage 1	No relationship	Stage 4	Consent
Stage 2	Communication between independent functions	Stage 5	Unified policy joint functions
Stage 3	Consultation	Stage 6	Unified Structure

From Styles, M. (1984). Reflections on collaboration and unification. *Image, 16* (1), 22.

centered, coordinated, and accessible (p. 226). The challenges and subsequent achievements of nurses and other team members in establishing and implementing this partnership demanded changes in the usual modes of operating professional development for each discipline. Programs for all participants were needed to address issues of multidisciplinary team development; sharing power among professionals, citizens, and paraprofessionals; and problem solving skills. Sharing limited power and authority and working with other disciplines in less-structured health care environments, particularly with empowered citizens, requires a great deal of ongoing personal and professional growth.

The Leadership for Primary Care Project (LPHC), a collaborative effort between the University of Illinois at Chicago Colleges of Nursing and Medicine, was developed to establish an ongoing partnership between the university and the community. LPHC fellows were primary health care leaders who were "socially responsible, culturally sensitive, effective communicators, politically savvy and visionary change agents" (McElmurry et al., 1995, p. 232). An expected outcome of participation in this collaborative leadership development program was that fellows would be prepared and motivated to "promulgate the philosophy, concepts and strategies of community participation in their practice, educational and research activities" (p. 231). This 2-year project, an example of one of the more sophisticated professional development efforts, included five teaching modules: primary health care, leadership development, community development, health care system organization, and information resources and data organization. It also required its fellows to develop a primary heath care project.

All the professional nursing organizations in the tricouncil, the National League for Nursing, the American Nurses Association, the American Organization of Nurse Executives, and the American Association of Colleges of Nursing, have position statements supporting collaboration. Conflicts and adversarial stances between education and service, however, continue. Kramer (1981) attributed this to differences in institutional goals and products, abdication of responsibility for collaboration with service by nurse educators, and the unclear, unrealistic expectations of nursing service. She pointed out the primary barrier to collaboration was that "the product of nursing service is care . . . and the product of nursing education is an educated individual" (p. 645). Although the argument can be made that these products do not need to be incongruent, differences in philosophies and priorities continue to be powerful constraints.

Efforts to bridge the gap between service and educational organizations, thus promoting professional interaction, have increased. Unification and affiliative models are being examined for feasibility by more institutions. Unified institutions now have National League for Nursing accredited programs. An example of an affiliative model is that between the University of Massachusetts Boston College of Nursing and the Hebrew Rehabilitation Center for the Aged (HRCA). Established in 1995, this model began as a formal arrangement whereby staff and faculty would work collaboratively to meet the teaching, research, and continuing education needs of the HRCA and college. HRCA staff taught selected undergraduate and graduate courses and college faculty and graduate students offered in-service/continuing education programs at HRCA. Staff and faculty worked together to identify research needs, plan, and conduct research that addressed health care needs of the elderly. After 1 year, benefits of this collaborative effort have grown to encompass more avenues to enhance preparation of nurses to care for the elderly and to expand clinical research to learn more about health needs and nursing interventions for the elderly. Graduate and undergraduate students are being supported by scholarships and have wider participation in research, practice, and continuing education programs.

Creation of advisory boards between education and service institutions has increased. Adjunct faculty–staff appointments are more common in both service and educational institutions. Individual consultation, faculty practice, and guest lectures are evidence of increased interaction between nurse clinicians and educators. Problems are not rare, but enough success is documented to be encouraging.

A collaborative project designed to develop professional expertise in the delivery of "boundaryless" community-based primary care is the Center for Community Health Education, Research and Service (CCHERS). Comprised of universities, health centers, the public health department, and hospital and communities in the Boston, Massachusetts area, this W. K. Kellogg Community Partnership Initiative is a shared governance model of education and health care delivery. Nursing and medical students and other health care professionals learn and work together to "provide primary care clinical services, educate health professions' students, engage in community-based research and develop services addressing community needs" (Meservey, 1995, p. 235).

Learning to work together as interdisciplinary health care delivery teams is critical to the effective and efficient provision of care in the new millennium. Unfortunately, the organizational and interdisciplinary team building skills necessary for success—such as negotiation, conflict resolution, critical thinking, participatory planning, and management—have not been included in most traditional health professions' curricula. Consequently, professional development programs and projects must be designed to bridge the gap and provide opportunities for on-the-job training.

Collaborative Teaching

Many college and university nursing programs now use nurses in service agencies as preceptors for the last clinical experience for undergraduate students, RN-to-BSN programs, and graduate clinical experiences. A preceptor is a nurse clinician or manager who serves in a dual role of clinician and educator. In a collaborative role, he or she works on a one-to-one basis with nursing students and assumes part of the responsibility for their education and training (Henry & Ensunak, 1991). By serving as a positive role model and providing support, encouragement, learning opportunities, and progressively less supervision, the preceptor fosters self-confidence, accountability, and independence in a reality-based setting.

By gaining a clearer understanding of the education process, establishing closer relationships and communication lines between educators and those in practice, sharing ideas and insights, and assuming responsibility for future colleagues, the student nurse preceptor contributes to the total profession and develops an increasing sense of self-worth (Bellinger & McClosky, 1992).

This model, however, has limitations. Nurses in patient care administration and educators must clarify the cost and benefits for a just exhange. Education, training, flexibility in scheduling, salary differentials, and other rewards for increased workload are a few of the variables that will affect success of the preceptorship program. Tuition waivers and faculty participation in projects and in-service programs are examples of some of the recent efforts to address costs associated with this collaborative teaching model.

Dougherty and Cook (1994) describe the partnership arrangement developed between Bronx Municipal Hospital Center (BMHC), Columbia University School of Nursing (CUSN), and the State of New York in response to escalating pediatric and adult primary health care needs and diminished health care personnel resources. The increased use of nurse practitioners (NPs) in primary care supplemented decreased numbers of resident physicians and contributed to meeting the demands of cost-effective managed care. Through strategic planning, the strengths and weaknesses of BMHC and CUSN were matched and "needs per clinical site and preceptors for primary care masters programs could be partially met by medical and nursing staff at BMHC. BMHC's need to initiate a program to increase their number of NPs expeditiously could be met by CUSN" (p. 302).

Strumpf's (1994) presentation on innovation in gerontological practices as models for health care delivery cites the use of nurse practitioners and clinical specialists in the development of teaching nursing homes as the "most significant experiment to improve nursing home care in the last decade" (p. 52). This outcome was facilitated by increased collaborations between university schools of nursing and nursing homes, which enhanced student education, professional development, strengthened clinical expertise of staff, and helped move many nursing homes from a custodial to therapeutic care model.

Many schools of nursing, including Johns Hopkins University, also collaboratively negotiate contracts for both faculty practice in service agencies and clinical instruction by advanced practice nurses in service agencies. These contractual arrangements enrich both the practice and teaching of nurses with primary appointments in both types of organizations.

Although not truly collaborative, internships and externships do enhance communication between service and education and promote socialization of new nurses into practicing clinicians (Sorensen, 1990). Internships and externships lengthen traditional orientation programs, adding more formal classes and a preceptorship. The former is focused on nurse clinicians, primarily new graduates learning to be staff nurses and employees preparing for specialized practice. The latter is targeted for nursing students. Students meeting selected criteria are employed during summers, evenings, and weekends, with the expectation that they will work in that agency or institution after graduation and completion of the registered nurse examination. Both internships and externships usually have goals related to reduction of orientation time/cost, stress, and attrition, while increasing motivation, organizational commitment, and productivity. Each may differ in organizational structure, design, curriculum, and length. Both are often highlighted in recruitment and marketing efforts.

Mentoring, a system in which an experienced adult befriends and guides a less-experienced adult, can also be viewed as a collaborative effort to promote professional development (Jowers & Herr, 1990). Mentors may be in education or service and are part of the "patron system . . . conceptualized as a continuum of sponsorship activities that can assist a person to advance within a given organization or profession" (Campbell & Heider, 1986, p. 110). This collaborative effort is less widely used than others previously mentioned, but is receiving increased attention and advocacy. Jowers and Herr (1990) indicate that the career advice, education, and social support provided by mentors assists protégés to develop confidence and take professional risks, which accelerates career growth. Angelini (1995) studied models and strategies of mentoring in the career development of hospital staff nurses. She concludes that mentoring is a "multi-dimensional process . . . [that is] perceived as a large part of career development. . . . [It takes] on primary importance at the clinical bedside (p. 95). Contract courses are an additional collaborative effort. They provide college or university credit that may lead to a degree or certification at the undergraduate or graduate level. Courses are taught by college or university faculty and offered within or near the designated health care institution or agency. The educational institution contracts with the service institution to offer specified courses, within a selected time frame, to a certain number of nurses. Efforts to establish contract courses would appear to indicate some mutual valuing of these programs.

Outreach continuing education programs may be offered by service institutions, schools of nursing, or independent continuing education providers. Some offerings may be by contract, at the work site, and limited to corporate employees, although the majority are offered elsewhere and open to others. Increasingly, both research conferences and continuing education programs are being offered through joint sponsorship. Often this is evidence of a beginning collaborative relationship between service and educational institutions.

Professional development of nurse clinicians is a more complex endeavor than is commonly recognized. Understanding the varied factors that contribute to success or failure of these programs helps place this complexity in perspective. Adult educators and program planners responsible for professional development are faced with constantly changing education and training needs of clinicians who vary in their interest in any form of continuing education. Program planners are responsible for identifying learning needs, designing programs to meet them, and motivating clinicians to attend and learn.

Establishing relevance is generally accepted as a key element in motivating voluntary attendance and participation in continuing education and professional development programs. Relevance must be considered from the viewpoints of the learner, service agency, and educational institution. Nursing careers today must include lifelong learning, which often includes returning for higher degrees or other formal preparation. Organizational collaboration at all levels enhances the capability of service and education institutions to provide nurses with cutting-edge knowledge and skills that enhance patient care delivery.

■ BIOGRAPHICAL SKETCH

Brenda S. Cherry is professor and Dean of the College of Nursing, University of Massachusetts, Boston. Brenda received her BSN degree in 1968 from North Carolina A&T State University; her MSN from the College of Nursing, University of Nebraska Medical Center in 1977; and her PhD from the University of Nebraska–Lincoln in 1981. Her work experiences include staff nurse and charge positions in the U.S. Army Nurse Corp, civil service, and private health agencies. Since 1977, she has held positions as nurse educator and educational administrator in baccalaureate and masters degree nursing programs. Her participation in professional organizations includes American Nurses Association, National League for Nursing, Sigma Theta Tau, American Association of Colleges of Nursing, and the Massachusetts chapters of the National Black Nurses Association and the American Council on Education. Her professional service activities include membership on advisory boards and committees, participation in continuing education programs, and consultation with educational and health-related organizations. Dr. Cherry has recently been selected to the editorial board of the *Journal of Professional Nursing*.

■ SUGGESTED READINGS

Professional Development Programs

American Association of Colleges of Nursing. (1994). Position statement: Interdisciplinary education and practice. *Journal of Professional Nursing, 12* (2), 119–123.

Anvaripour, P., Bezold, C., & Weissman, G. (1990). A nursing department can and should plan for the future. *Nursing and Health Care, 11,* 207–209.

Benner, P., Tanner, C., & Chesla, C. (1992). From beginner to expert: Gaining a differentiated clinical world in critical care nursing. *Advances in Nursing Science, 14* (3), 13–28.

Camp-Sorrell, D., & O'Sullivan, P. (1991). Effects of continuing education—Pain assessment and documentation. *Career Nursing, 14,* 49–54.

De Tornyay, R. (1994). Creating the teachers of tomorrow's professionals. *Inquiry, 4,* (31), 283–288.

Larson, E.L. (1995). The need for interdisciplinary education for health professionals. *Nursing Outlook, 43,* 180–185.

Lehna, C., & Byrne, A. (1995). An example of a successful collaboration effort between a nurse educator and a hospice clinical nurse specialist/director. *Journal of Professional Nursing, 11* (3), 175–182.

Osteile, M., & O'Callaghan, D. (1996). The changing health care environment: Impact on curriculum and faculty. *Nursing & Health Care, 17* (2), 78–81.

Osterweis, M., McLaughlin, C., Manasse, H., Jr., & Hopper, C. (Eds.). (1996). The U.S. health workforce—Power, politics and policy. Washington, DC: Association of Academic Health Centers.

Wyatt, G., & Dimmer, S. (1992). A planning model for continuing education presenters. *Journal of Continuing Education in Nursing, 23* (4), 161–167.

Adult Education

Cayne, J. (1995). Portfolios: A developmental influence? *Journal of Advanced Nursing, 21,* 395–405.

Francke, A., Garssen, L., & Huijer, A.-S.H. (1995). Determinants of changes in nurses' behavior after continuing education: A literature review. *Journal of Advanced Nursing, 21,* 371–377.

Heinrich, K., & Galdstone, C. (1992). Orientation programs for nurse-adult learners: Fostering a sense of community. *Nurse Educator, 17* (1), 8–11.

Miller, B., Adams, D., & Beck, L. (1993). A behavioral inventory for professionalism in nursing. *Journal of Professional Nursing, 9* (5), 290–295.

Rogers, E., & Webb, C. (1991). Effective teacher characteristics identified by adult learners in nursing. *Journal of Continuing Education in Nursing, 22* (1), 21–23.

Schmidt, K., & Fisher, I. (1992). Effective development and utilization of self-learning models. *Journal of Continuing Education in Nursing, 23* (2), 54–59.

Suitor-Scheller, M. (1993). A qualitative analysis of factors in the work environment that influence nurses' use of knowledge gained from programs. *Journal of Continuing Education in Nursing, 24* (3), 114–122.

Vogel, G., Ruppel, D., & Kaufmann, C. (1991). Learning needs assessment as a vehicle for integrating staff development into a professional practice model. *Journal of Continuing Education in Nursing, 22* (5), 192–197.

Waddel, D. (1992). The effect of continuing education on nursing practice: A meta analysis. *Journal of Continuing Education in Nursing, 23* (4), 164–168.

Wilkinson, J. (1996). The C word: A curriculum for the future. *Nursing and Health Care, 17* (2), 72–77.

Creative Linkages of Service and Education to Increase Professional Development

Coburn, J., & Sturdevant, N. (1992). The acquisition of delegation skills: Collaboration between education and service. *Nurse Educator, 17* (6), 32–34.

Dahl, S., Gustafson, C., & McCullagh, M. (1993). Collaborating to develop a community-based health service for rural homeless persons. *Journal of Nursing Administration, 23* (4), 41–45.

Dufault, M., Bartlett, B., Dagrosa, C., & Joseph, D. (1992). A state-wide consortium initiative to establish an undergraduate clinical internship program. *Journal of Professional Nursing, 8,* 239–244.

Fagin, C.M. (1992). Collaboration between nurses and physicians: No longer a choice. *Academic Medicine, 67,* 295–303.

Hegyvary, S. (1991). Collaborative relationships for education and practice. *Journal of Professional Nursing, 7* (3), 148.

Henery, V., Schmitz, K., Reif, L., & Rudie, P. (1992). Collaboration: Integrating practice and research. *Public Health Nursing, 9* (4), 218–222.

Porter-O'Grady, T. (1994). Building partnership in health care: Creating whole systems change. *Nursing and Health Care, 15* (1), 34–38.

Sharp, N. (1992). Community partnerships in health professions education. *Nursing Management, 23,* 14–15.

■ REFERENCES

Angelini, D. (1995). Mentoring in the career development of hospital staff nurses: Models and strategies. *Journal of Professional Nursing, 11* (2), 89–97.

Bell, R. (1996). Promoting collaboration in community health nursing. *Perspectives on Community, 17* (4), 186–188.

Bellinger, S., and McCloskey, J. (1992). Are preceptors for orientation of new nurses effective? *Journal of Professional Nursing, 8* (6), 321–327.

Benner, P.G. (1984). *From novice to expert: Excellence and power in clinical nursing practice.* Menlo Park, CA: Addison-Wesley.

Bigge, M.L. (1976). *Learning theories for teachers* (3rd ed.). New York: Harper & Row.

Billings, D., and Bachmeier, B. (1994). Teaching and learning at a distance: A review of the nursing literature. In L. Ryan (Ed.), *Review of research in nursing education* (pp. 1–32). New York: National League for Nursing.

Bloom, B.S. (1956). *Taxonomy of educational objectives.* New York: David McKay.

Campbell, H., & Heider, N. (1986). Do nurses need mentors? *Image, 18* (3), 110–113.

Cannon, C., Paulanka, B., & Beam, S. (1994). A statewide assessment of preferences of registered nurses desiring academic credit-bearing continuing education. *Journal of Professional Nursing, 10* (4), 229–235.

Dolphin, P.G., & Holtzclaw, B. (1983). *Continuing education in nursing: Strategies for lifelong learning.* Reston, VA: Reston Publishing.

Dougherty, M., & Cook, S. (1994). Innovative strategic planning to meet expanding primary health care needs. *Nursing and Health Care, 15* (6), 298–302.

Farley, S. (1995). Leadership for citizen–professional partnerships. *Nursing and Health Care, 16* (4), 226–228.

Francke, A., & Erkens, T. (1994). Confluent education: An integrative approach for nursing continuing education. *Journal of Advanced Nursing, 19* (2), 354–361.

Hall, E., & McHugh, M. (1995). Family practice health care. *Nursing and Health Care, 16* (5), 270–275.

Hawkins, J. (1992). Empowering the new graduate: A renewed professionalism for nursing. *Journal of Professional Nursing, 8* (5), 308–312.

Henry, S., & Ensunak, K. (1991). Preceptorship in nursing service and education. In P. Baj & G. Clayton (Eds.), *Review of research in nursing education* (Vol. 3, pp. 51–72). New York: National League for Nursing.

Jowers, L., & Herr, K. (1990). A review of literature on mentor–protégé relationships. In P. Baj & G. Clayton (Eds.), *Review of Research in Nursing Education* (Vol. 3, pp. 49–77). New York: National League for Nursing.

Knowles, M. (1984). *Androgogy in action: Applying modern principles of adult learning* (pp. 417–422). San Francisco: Jossey-Bass.

Knowles, M. (1990). *The adult learner. A neglected species* (4th ed.). Houston, TX: Gulf Publishing.

Kramer, M. (1981). Why does reality shock continue? In J. McCloskey & H. Grace (Eds.), *Current issues in nursing* (pp. 644–653). Boston: Blackwell Scientific Publications.

Luchat, M., Zerbe, M., & Scott, C. (1992). A new clinical educator role: Bridging the education–practice gap. *Journal of Nursing Staff Development, 8,* pp. 55–57.

Marquis, B., & Huston, C. (1992). *Leadership roles and management functions in nursing.* Philadelphia: Lippincott.

McCloskey, J., & McCain, B. (1987). Satisfaction, commitment and professionalism of newly employed nurses. *Image, 19* (1), 20–27.

McElmurry, B., Tyska, C., Gugenheim, A., et al. (1995). Leadership for primary health care. *Nursing and Health Care, 16* (4), 229–233.

Meservey, P. (1995). Fostering collaboration in a boundaryless organization. *Nursing and Health Care, 16* (4), 234–236.

Morgan, G. (1997). *Images of organization* (2nd ed.). Thousand Oaks, CA: Sage.

Mundinger, M. (1995). Advanced practice nursing is the answer—What is the question? *Nursing and Health Care, 16* (5), 254–259.

O'Neill, E., & Pennington, E. (1996). Preparing acute care nurses. *Nursing and Health Care,* 17 (2), 62–65.

Pew Health Professions Commission. (1995). *Critical challenges: Revitalizing the health professions for the twenty-first century.* San Francisco: U.C.S.F. Center for the Health Professions.

Reilly, D., & Obermann, M. (1990). *Behavioral objectives: Evaluation in nursing* (3rd. ed.). New York: National League for Nursing.

Robichaud, A.M. (1992). Professional practice: A microcosm for learning. *Journal of Professional Nursing,* 8 (6), 320.

Rosenlieb, C. (1993). A profile of preceptorships in baccalaureate degree nursing programs for registered nurses. In N. Diekelmann & M. Rather (Eds.), *Transforming R.N. education* (pp. 256–272). New York: National League for Nursing.

Smith, R., & Haverkamp, K. (1977). Toward a theory of learning how to learn. *Adult Education, 28* (1), 3–21.

Sorensen, G. (1990). A residency program. In M. Wandelt & B. Thomas (Eds.), *Innovations in nursing education administration.* New York: National League for Nursing.

Strumpf, N.E. (1994). Innovative gerontological practices as models for health care delivery. *Nursing and Health Care,* 15 (10), 522–527.

Styles, M. (1984). Reflections on collaboration and unification. *Image, 16* (1), 21–23.

Walker, D. (1985). Nursing education and service: The payoffs of partnership. *Nursing and Health Care, 6* (4), 189–191.

Zahn, J. (1967, Winter). Differences between adults and youth affecting learning. *Adult Education,* 67–77.

CASE 13–1 Sustaining a Family Research Team in an
Academic Health Center

Charmaine Kleiber

The three missions of academic health care settings are service, education, and research. The role of the nursing department in the service arena is clear; nurses provide the bulk of services rendered in the hospital setting. Nursing education has also had a clear role in university health care centers; hospital departments of nursing maintain collaborative relationships with various schools and colleges of nursing to provide clinical sites and clinical mentors for all levels of nursing students. The role of the nursing department in the area of research is more ambiguous. Fostering research-based practice and research utilization are well-accepted activities of nursing departments. The conduct of research is often, however, the first activity to be abandoned when budgets are tight and staffing is short.

At University of Iowa Hospitals and Clinics (UIHC), an active nursing research team has been in existence for 7 years. The Family Intervention Research (FIR) team has weathered downsizing and redesigning of the hospital, and relocation of members, sabbaticals, illnesses, births, and deaths. Over the years, the team has received more than $8,000 in funding for research studies, has published nine articles in peer-reviewed journals, and has presented research findings at 22 conferences. The purpose of this case is to describe this remarkable team of nurse researchers

and how it has managed to continue to be productive during these turbulent times.

■ **HISTORY OF THE FAMILY
INTERVENTION RESEARCH TEAM**

The seeds of the FIR team were planted in 1989 when two faculty from the University of Iowa College of Nursing and one advanced practice nurse from the adult critical care units of UIHC collaborated to conduct a qualitative study of family responses to a critical care hospitalization of another family member. Their study revealed new information about the extreme and troubling emotional responses of family members, including children, to hospitalization in an intensive care unit (ICU). Two of the investigators were motivated to form a research team to continue investigation and develop nursing interventions for families related to the critical care environment. In 1990, two pediatric advanced practice nurses, two additional adult advanced practice nurses, and another nursing professor from the College of Nursing were formally invited to join the team. The team evolved over the years, with members dropping out for various reasons such as sabbatical, illness, or increased family responsibilities; new members were invited to join as additional team support was needed. Five

CASE 13–1 *Continued*

of the original team members remain active members. Additional information about how the group was formed and how individual members function is reported elsewhere (Johnson et al., 1993).

The work of the FIR team has centered around the needs of all family members during the critical care hospitalization of a loved one. The first study undertaken by the team was designed to investigate how the feelings and behaviors of adult family members changed over the course of the ICU hospitalization. In that study, family members from five separate ICUs were asked to keep daily diaries of feelings and activities such as eating, sleeping, and coping behaviors. The amount of data generated through these diaries was impossible to describe in one article, so the material was broken out into three categories: family roles, behaviors, and emotions during the ICU hospitalization of a loved one. This division of data resulted in manageable chunks of material that could be covered in journal articles. It also allowed three different members of the team to take responsibility as first author of the manuscripts. When a large team is working on a project and all members are contributing fairly equally to the progress of the work, it is important to share the honor of first and second author positions. The FIR team has been very successful in assuring that all members have the opportunity for individual recognition for the shared work, through either publication or presentations at regional and national meetings.

The second team initiative was to investigate the effects of child visitation in adult critical care units. The idea for the study came from the adult unit advanced practice nurses on the FIR team who were concerned with restricted child visitation practices in the hospital. An experimental design was utilized in which children in the control group were not allowed to visit, and children in the experimental group were allowed to visit in the ICU after receiving specific information about what to expect. A graduate student in nursing who joined the team to gain research experience collected most of the data. She went on to take responsibility for data analysis and subsequently used the project for her thesis. A key factor in allowing this student to have so much control over the study was that her advisor was a member of FIR and had been involved in the study from its conception. The other team members felt comfortable that this student would have excellent mentoring regarding this research project. Still, the study remained the "property" of the FIR team because it had been originated and initiated within the team. All team members were listed as authors in the published results.

The results of the first child visitation study prompted the initiation of a larger multisite study. Because this larger study required traveling for data collection, funding for a research assistant was sought and obtained from the American Association of Critical-Care Nurses. The design of this research project remained essentially the same as the previous study, but it was extended to two community hospitals in order to increase the diversity and size of the sample. The

CASE 13–1 *Continued*

data collection process was plagued with difficulties. There was turnover in some of the nursing leadership positions in the community hospitals, so continuous reeducation was required regarding the purpose of the study. Also, nurses at UIHC had seen the positive results of child visitation in the previous study, and they were reluctant to impose restrictions on child visitation for research purposes. In the end, the team was not able to enroll as many subjects as desired. Enough data were collected, however, to extend the argument that child visitation in adult critical care units is harmless to the patient and may be helpful to the child.

While the child visitation studies were going on, the pediatric specialists within the FIR team became interested in another topic: the information needs of siblings of critically ill children. This interest was spurred by some of the qualitative data collected during the visitation studies. Several parents had spoken very candidly about their discomfort in not knowing what to tell their children about critically ill relatives. This new research topic was discussed at a FIR team meeting. The adult specialist members were not interested in participating in a study on children's information needs, but they encouraged the pediatric specialists to proceed. Thus, three of the FIR team members went on to design a qualitative study and find funding for data collection. The entire FIR team was again offered opportunities to join in on the study at the points of data analysis and manuscript development. The offers for involvement were declined because

the adult-focused members felt that the focus was too narrowly pediatric to fit their interests. Therefore, the author listing on the manuscript reflects only the three pediatric FIR team members who initiated the study and analyzed the data. This episode in the life of the FIR team deserves comment. The members of the team trusted one another to be open, honest, and creative. No restrictions were placed on team members' activities. Members could participate or not, depending on their interests and time restrictions.

The most recent chapter in the FIR team's history involves delving into decision making in the ICU setting. Several of the team members were interested in ethical dilemmas in ICUs, and they saw "professional and family involvement in decision making" as one interesting aspect of ethics. The team has spent 2 years grappling with "decision making." A study has been completed and a manuscript is under development. However, the entire team has a feeling that it has stepped out of its element. No one on the team has a strong background in this area of study; therefore, the group is lacking the spokesperson team member who will pick up the ball and run with it. None of the members has a passion for the subject. On the other hand, all members have a passion for child visitation and the emotional responses of family members to ICU hospitalization. The lesson here is to develop a program of research and stick with it. The FIR team has established a series of studies that have increased knowledge about families of critically ill patients. There are

CASE 13–1 *Continued*

many aspects of child visitation, emotional response to hospitalization, and information needs of siblings that have yet to be explored. The FIR team is in the process of reorienting, and will most likely return to more familiar research ground in the future.

■ WHY SUSTAIN RESEARCH DURING TIMES OF SCARCE RESOURCES?

The challenges to sustaining research activity have been serious. Over 7 years, downsizing at UIHC resulted in increased emphasis on clinical care and managerial responsibilities for the advanced practice nurses, leaving little time for the conduct of research. Demands on the faculty also increased, with all of the College of Nursing team members experiencing increased teaching and research responsibilities. In addition, several of the advanced practice nurses returned to school to begin doctoral work, stretching available time to the limit. Sometimes I marvel that the FIR team continued to function. I think that the success and perseverance of the research team is attributable to the perceived advantages to each of the team members.

One advantage for hospital-based members is the opportunity to work closely with extremely bright and successful nurse researchers from the College of Nursing faculty. Each faculty member brings a unique talent to the group. The ability of these scholars to listen to a discussion of clinical issues and then formulate specific and testable research questions is remarkable. The need for a least one expert in research design on the team cannot be overestimated. The design of the study determines the usefulness and believability of the findings. No matter how well intentioned and worthy the research idea, the study will flounder if the design is muddy or invalid. Nursing faculty also provide access to consultants outside their own areas of expertise, including statistical analysis and grant preparation. College faculty are also knowledgeable regarding funding sources, where to publish studies, and how to present findings at key meetings.

Benefits to faculty include ready access to patient populations for team research, publications as team members, and numerous opportunities for their students to participate in the research process. Having students available to help with literature reviews, data collection, data entry, and data analysis helps to alleviate some of the team's work burden. The students benefit by using pieces of studies to fulfill course or degree requirements. The experienced faculty and advanced practice nurse researchers must be willing to fulfill their roles as mentors by stepping back from the limelight and allowing the beginners to take starring roles in presenting findings. Through continued success with presentations and publications, novice researchers are motivated to advance their formal education and continue with the difficult and tedious work of research. One caution to interagency or interdepartmental teams that include students is to have early discussions on

CASE 13-1 *Continued*

who "owns" the data. If a student must collect, analyze, or present research data as a single author in order to fulfill a requirement, that must be understood by the entire team. Several students have used the FIR team research projects to complete masters degree requirements. Two masters students formally joined the team upon completion of their graduate studies.

A clear advantage to faculty in this arrangement is access to subjects. Also, because the clinically based members know what research is currently being conducted in the critical care units, they are able to guide FIR research initiatives into areas that are likely to be accepted by hospital staff.

Administrative support for research is the most important ingredient to the recipe for success. Why should nurse administrators encourage their advanced practice nurses to be actively involved in research teams? There are several reasons. First, the national trend in health care is toward establishing evidence-based practice. As a profession, nursing is responsible for using the best and most cost-efficient nursing practice to achieve the best possible outcomes. The only way to determine the best practices is through careful examination of evidence using research methods. For example, nurse administrators are instrumental in establishing the policies, such as visiting hours, for their critical care units. What should guide the decision? One might think that the stimulation of having a family member at the bedside would lead to increases in heart rate, blood pressure, and oxygen consump-

tion in the patient. Thinking along those lines would lead to restricting visitation to very ill patients. However, research conducted by the FIR team shows that that line of thinking is not correct. Having family members at the bedside does not result in detrimental physiological changes in the adult patient. Using this evidence to guide policy formation should result in a more flexible, open visiting policy. These are the types of issues that are of interest to nurses in acute care settings.

Second, research can lead to practices that heighten patient and family satisfaction. For example, more liberal visiting hours for children visiting critically ill relatives were implemented at UIHC directly because of the research conducted by the FIR team. Now that our clientele is accustomed to our policies, we hear complaints about some other hospitals with more restrictive visiting hours. People would rather have a loved one hospitalized in an institution that is responsive to the needs of the family as well as the patient. Consumer demand will be instrumental in swinging major health insurance contracts. Those institutions that have a mechanism for investigating the best practices for families and patients will have an edge in the marketplace.

A third reason for administrative support of research activity among hospital advanced practice nurses is to enhance the hospital's reputation. The national recognition that can be attained through publication and presentation of research findings can enhance the attractiveness of an institution and help draw top-notch candidates for open positions.

CASE 13–1 *Continued*

■ TIPS FOR OVERCOMING DIFFICULTIES

When the conduct of research is a goal of an academic health center department of nursing, the nurse administrators must assure that advanced practice nurses are able to set aside adequate time for research activities. Administrators must make it very clear that, for these nurses, research is part of their job description and "nursing work." Therefore, advanced practice nurses cannot be assigned 100 percent to direct patient care duties; a certain percentage of time must be allocated for meetings, library searches, grant writing, data collection, data analysis, and writing. Research takes time, and, if it is an organizational priority and goal, it is not right to expect that it be done during "off" hours.

Advanced practice nurses need to actively seek to preserve their research role. As bedside caregiver positions are eliminated in an effort to decrease cost, the advanced practice nurse may be expected to spend more and more time in direct patient care activities, serving in case management and clinical consultant roles. It is easy for the clinical aspects of the advanced practice role to fill in all available time, choking out the possibilities for research time.

The FIR team had several staff nurses join in various aspects of studies, but always in a student role. The inclusion of staff in research teams should be encouraged, as long as scheduling difficulties are understood by all members. For staff nurses, unless there is grant money to underwrite their time, research involvement is a volunteer activity that provides professional development. Some staff nurses found involvement in the team to be exciting and went on to become members, but others found it so difficult to arrange time away from patient care duties that they did not feel that they could commit to full membership.

Team members should anticipate the need to divide work into achievable chunks. For example, in the best of all possible worlds, manuscripts are written by just one or two people in order to assure flow in writing style and continuity of thought. Sometimes that just is not practical. It may be necessary to divide writing responsibilities into five or six sections and assign each section to a different person in order to get it done. The first author then has the responsibility to edit the manuscript for cohesion. A manuscript that is a little choppy is better than no manuscript at all!

A recent article by Byrne and associates (1996) offers advice to beginning nurse researchers. This author strongly seconds one of their suggestions: stick to topics you love. In the present day health care environment, the conduct of research will require sacrifices on the part of each team member. The reality is that at least some of the work will be done outside of regular work hours. If the team is not thoroughly committed to the research topic, it will be difficult to generate volunteerism. Remember, there are a lot of great research questions out there and no team can answer them all, so pick the question you care about the most and stick to it.

CASE 13–1 *Continued*

When the ball has been dropped and no one will pick it up, it is time to switch research topics or just take a breather. Research teams have a rhythm and life of their own. They are not always peppy and productive. Long periods of stagnation do not necessarily mean that the team is dead. However, each person on the team should take responsibility to assume the "mover" role every now and then. Sometimes all the team needs is a little shove to get going again.

Grab opportunities when they arise. If a research proposal deadline is approaching and you think you have a fundable idea, write the proposal and submit it. The worst that can happen is that you will obtain free advice from the reviewers on how to improve the study proposal. You will never know if your idea is fundable unless you submit a grant proposal.

The intention of this case study is to encourage the formation of other research teams in academic health centers. Hopefully, the experiences of the FIR team can assist others to create successful programs of research and to avoid obstacles that can stymie even the best of teams.

■ BIOGRAPHICAL SKETCH

Charmaine Kleiber is an Advanced Practice Nurse for Research in Children's and Women's Services at The University of Iowa Hospitals and Clinics. She is also a doctoral candidate in Administrative Nursing at the University of Iowa College of Nursing. Charmaine obtained her BSN from the University of Kansas, her MS in nursing from the University of Colorado, and her Pediatric Nurse Practitioner certificate from the University of Iowa. Most of her work experience has been in advanced practice nursing care of children. Ms. Kleiber is a member of Sigma Theta Tau, the Society of Pediatric Nurses, the Association for the Care of Children's Health, the National Association of Pediatric Nurses Associates and Practitioners, and the Midwestern Nursing Research Society. She has authored and co-authored research and research utilization articles that have been published in peer reviewed journals.

■ ACKNOWLEDGMENT

Past and present FIR team members: Kitty Buckwalter, Marty Craft-Rosenberg, Ellen Cram, Kathleen Fawcett, Margo Halm, Susan Johnson, Charmaine Kleiber, Karen Megivern, Lou Ann Montgomery, Anita Nicholson, Marita Titler, Janet Williams.

■ REFERENCES

Byrne, M.M., Kangas, S.K., & Warren, N. (1996). Advice for beginning nurse researchers. *Image, 28,* 165–167.

Johnson, S.K., Halm, M.A., Titler, M.G., Craft, M., Kleiber, C., Montgomery, L.A., Nicholson, A., Buckwalter, K., & Cram, E. (1993). Group functioning of a collaborative family research team. *Clinical Nurse Specialist, 7,* 184–191.

CASE 13–2 From Staff Nurse to Charge Nurse—Introducing a Management Viewpoint

Michelle Sly Smith and Sally A. Zuel

In today's health care environment, the role of unit manager has increasingly become multifaceted. The task of running the unit with a new skill mix, with less staff, and with higher patient acuity requires expertise in areas such as time management, organization, communication, and interpersonal skills, to mention just a few. The challenges of patient care do not end at the end of the manager's day; thus, a charge person is required to ensure that the other shifts function smoothly. The charge nurse position is a pivotal link to nursing leadership. The presence of a charge person is imperative to the operation of the unit as "assigning nurses to care for specific patients is a unit-based management function that is performed more frequently than almost any other . . . " (Bostrom & Suter, 1992, p. 32).

The charge person is in a unique position as he or she typically represents hospital management on off-shifts and on weekends (Harris & Martin-Hylwa, 1992). The charge person is the channel for: (1) role modeling practice, including policy and procedural expectations; (2) articulating administrative and management goals and objectives; (3) operationalizing, with the assistance of staff, administrative and management goals and objectives; (4) unit problem solving; (5) clinical support; and (6) fostering open communication (Harris & Martin-Hylwa, 1992). The charge person, then,

becomes an extension and a reflection of the unit manager and should be selected with great care.

A charge person who functions at an optimal level will have an impact on unit morale, staff cohesiveness, and the job performance of others. In addition, relationships with other professionals and the efficiency and effectiveness of resource utilization can be enhanced.

How does a unit manager choose the perfect candidate to fill this important position? Hamel (1995) states that "steps must be taken to identify those nurses with the greatest management potential and then continually educate them on management tactics" (p. 25). However, be warned that "a great nurse is not always a great manager" (Hamel, 1995, p. 25). The unit manager should be cognizant of the potential charge person's education, experience, competence, and interpersonal relationships with the unit's existing personnel (Harris & Martin-Hylwa, 1992).

Once an individual who has management potential has been identified, the unit manager should begin to assess other strengths of the candidate. The candidate should possess a sound knowledge of hospital policy and procedures, clinical competence to care for the unit's population, skill to function during emergency situations, an ability to foster motivation among others, a desire to teach others, an ability to delegate properly, and strong

CASE 13–2 *Continued*

communication and interpersonal skills. Typically, the potential charge person is the leader on off-shifts and is the person that other staff members look to when problem solving.

One aim of a study conducted by Bostrom and Suter (1992) was to identify factors that nurses used in assigning patient care. Items that were found to be of the most importance when making assignments included: (1) information from the patient acuity system, (2) clinical judgment, (3) experience of the nurse in relation to type of patient and with a particular patient, (4) employment and licensure status of the nurse, (5) presence of nonnursing support staff, (6) the location of the patient on the unit, and (7) other duties of the nurse. In addition, the match of the nurse and patient, as well as potential admissions, discharges, and unit staffing were found to be important. Bostrom and Suter (1992) found that experienced charge nurses utilized more factors in making assignments than did less-experienced charge nurses. However, patient acuity information was less of a consideration for experienced charge nurses during the delegation of patient care.

The study found that charge nurses demonstrated diverse means of making patient care assignments. It is important to recognize this diversity, as there is not always a single way to make assignments; rather, individualization may be necessary within the charge position. The unit manager can examine strengths of potential charge nurses based on the list of decision-making factors outlined in this study.

Our organization has incorporated charge nurse expectations into registered nurse (RN) job descriptions. The novice nurse is introduced to this new role during clinical orientation by observing charge nurses who function effectively in the role. At a later time, the nurse is expected to assume this leadership position. Although this provides an opportunity for managers to review all staff members' ability to perform as charge nurses, it fails to recognize that some individuals cannot function effectively in the charge position.

A charge nurse education program was instituted to assist our staff in meeting the expectations of the charge nurse role. The Joint Commission on Accreditation of Healthcare Organizations' (JCAHO) standards (1994) provided an additional impetus for program development. The program was designed to: (1) provide novice charge nurses with basic information related to the role, (2) act as a refresher for those staff members who routinely function as charge nurses, and (3) further develop management potential of charge nurses. We felt that the development of personnel within this role was a quality approach to ensuring effective nurse leaders within the organization.

We began to explore the charge nurse education process by forming a planning committee to address the needs of charge nurses. This committee was composed of nurses from various areas within the hospital, as well as staff development personnel. During the initial meeting, we considered the desired outcomes of the program, discussed

CASE 13–2 *Continued*

teaching strategies, and identified organizational resources. Conflict resolution, delegation, chain-of-command, time management, goal setting, stress management, communication skills, problem solving, budgetary concerns, ethics, team building, and guest relations were among the topics considered pertinent to the role. It was decided that the best way to prioritize this list was through a needs assessment tool.

The needs assessment was devised and sent to the nursing staff. From the list of priorities identified by nursing staff, the planning committee chose to focus on the following topics: (1) conflict/power struggles, (2) dealing with difficult people and situations, (3) stress management, (4) team building, (5) delegation skills, and (6) time management.

From a management perspective, it was preferable to offer the charge nurse education program in two, 4-hour blocks to accommodate a larger audience. Our first 4-hour session covered the following content: conflict/power struggles, dealing with difficult people and situations, and stress management. The second 4-hour session focused on patient acuity and staffing, delegation, and decision making. Participants were given handouts, additional readings, and bibliography lists for each content area.

In order to entice participants, this program was submitted and approved for continuing education hours. Several planning committee meetings focused on the development of course objectives as well as the identification of speakers. The choice of speakers was very important to the success of this program. The

speakers needed to be seen as role models and leaders by their co-workers. The speakers included management- and staff-level personnel who possessed knowledge related to a particular topic.

Our first session began with a discussion of behavior and leadership styles and their impact on interpersonal relationships and conflict resolution. Participants were asked to complete a leadership style questionnaire prior to the course. The instructor facilitated discussion of the various styles of behavior and participants were asked to identify their own style. Each leadership style identified by the participants was then reviewed. Through small group activities, participants were able to recognize how these topics interrelated and could be utilized in resolving conflict.

The second session emphasized aspects of dealing with difficult people and situations. Case studies were utilized for discussion and appropriate/inappropriate interventions identified. At this point, participants were encouraged to share past experiences. Effective strategies for dealing with difficult people and situations were analyzed. Humor, when used appropriately, was cited as being a particularly useful tool.

The final session of the first day focused on stress and stress management. The outcome of this session was to assist individuals to identify strategies and solutions to reduce stress. A medical psychologist presented information on the physiological and psychological effects of stress. Exercises were conducted to assist in decreasing stress levels. Participants could then take these strategies back for use on their units.

CASE 13–2 *Continued*

The second day started with information on delegation. The content included delegation principles based on the nursing process and effective time-management strategies. Emphasis was placed on the appropriate use of delegation, including responsibility and accountability for delegated tasks. Effective communication was identified as a critical need for optimum delegation. Participants were then asked to complete a post-test, which reviewed highlights of the presentation.

Staffing plans and the institution's patient acuity system were reviewed. This particular topic represented the most troublesome area for the charge nurses. Staff members and charge nurses were unfamiliar with: (1) their own unit's staffing plan, (2) the relationship of the patient acuity system to their staffing plan, and (3) the mechanism for facilitating changes within the patient acuity system. Our goal was to share how staffing assignments were made, utilizing patient acuity data. It was our hope that with this information, participants would be able to examine their own acuity numbers and validate staffing needs on off-shifts and weekends.

The presentation on decision making incorporated aspects of the nursing process into the traditional problem-solving process. Various factors that influence decision making were reviewed. These included each person's value system, life experiences, individual preferences, and organizational climate. Small group discussion revolved around activities conducted during a shift, with emphasis on managing time and setting priorities. Several policies related to the charge nurse role were presented.

Initial program evaluations indicated that group participants valued information on staffing patterns based on acuity, conflict resolution, staff support, effective communication, and humor. Participants were able to identify activities that they planned to do as a result of their learning. Management and staff identified a preference for conducting the course, with similar content, in a day (8 hours) versus two, 4-hour sessions on separate days.

The next program was offered as an 8-hour session. Based on the evaluations, content remained unchanged except for the addition of a presentation on humor and inclusion of case studies within the decision-making section. The humor presentation introduced various techniques that participants could apply in many settings. Group members were asked to share ways that they had employed humor within their role. Various props were an integral part of small group activities. The appropriate application of humor was discussed and examples identified.

With the 8-hour program, participants identified their favorite topics as dealing with difficult people and situations, humor, and stress management. This program has been so well received by management and staff that it has been presented in its entirety multiple times.

An evaluation of course effectiveness was mailed to participants and members of management 6 to 12 months after the

CASE 13–2 *Continued*

course. Staff members who attended the course stated that delegation, conflict resolution, and communication were areas of improved job performance. An increase in self-esteem and assertiveness, with an overall feeling of accomplishment and self-satisfaction, have been identified by participants as benefits of this program. An additional outcome of the course was that participants were more cognizant of the breadth of the charge nurse role and scope of duties.

Overall, managers felt that the charge nurse education program was worthwhile. They noted that the program presented the necessary information for staff members to function effectively in the charge role. However, some managers felt that the program was more beneficial to staff with less than 1 year of experience as compared to seasoned veterans. This difference was not detected from a participant evaluation standpoint.

Implementation of a charge nurse education program and the professional development of personnel within the charge role is crucial to the viability of an organization during these turbulent times. The managed care environment is a fiercely competitive one. Health care providers vying for contracts must be able to demonstrate efficiency and effectiveness. Management must realize that the charge nurse's effectiveness not only has an impact on the operation of their unit, but has far-reaching implications. The organization's customers, internal and external, benefit from the efficiency and productivity of key people within the structure.

Charge nurses are in the perfect position to influence the acquisition of managed care contracts. Businesses interested in contracting with a health care provider are concerned not only with the cost of care, but also with the quality of care. What do patients say about the health care provider? Are patients satisfied with the care they received? Patient satisfaction survey data have become powerful benchmarking tools for making decisions within the managed care environment. The staff member most likely to impact the patient's perception of the care rendered is not the physician; it is the nurse. The charge nurse, operating within this philosophy, is a vital link in assuring that quality care is provided.

Our organization has developed a quality statement that lays the foundation for our performance improvement plan and associated activities. The premise of the statement, "quality is doing the right things right the first time, every time" is rather basic. When an organization begins to examine the number of processes involved in the provision of health care to a single patient, the results are staggering. Inefficiency, misuse of resources, duplication of services, and ineffectiveness plague many of these processes. The charge nurse can act as a gatekeeper in relation to these problems. Charge nurses, with management and administrative support, can assist in identifying excess steps within a process. We must examine the work we do and the way in which it is done. We must begin to question processes that no longer function effectively. Streamlining processes is a crucial step in assuring the

CASE 13–2 *Continued*

delivery of quality patient care as well as ensuring the health of an organization. Without both the freedom to question processes and the authority to institute changes, charge nurses cannot function to their full potential.

As an organization, we strive to promote performance improvement to our external customers through prevention of delays, reduction of stress, avoidance of complications, and reduction of costs. The expert charge nurse, through the coordination and delegation of the staff, can facilitate all of these goals. External customers experience less stress when problems or complications are alleviated or addressed rapidly. Through proper assignment and appropriate delegation, the potential for problems is lessened. Ultimately, this lowers cost for the customers and the facility as the best-qualified person is providing care. Patients' perception of their care will be positive when they are comfortable and satisfied with the care received. Satisfied customers will be more likely to return to the organization for future health needs. In addition, these customers are vehicles for good public relations for the organization, as word of mouth is an important mechanism for deciding which health care provider to utilize.

An effective charge nurse also provides benefits to internal customers. Individuals who are nurtured within this position are better prepared and more knowledgeable of expectations of the role. Charge nurses develop rapport with others in the same role, enhancing communication across departmental and unit boundaries. Effective communica-

tion, and an overall view of and respect for the responsibilities of the other departments, enhances working relationships. The provision of health care as a team facilitates the smooth operation of the organization.

Charge nurses receive compensation from a variety of sources. First, the charge nurse is identified as the leader of a well-functioning team (unit). Second, management and administrative support promote individual development through empowerment. Third, the charge nurse receives positive feedback from internal and external customers. These benefits encourage staff to take greater pride in their work, as well as motivating them to improve performance.

The complexities of modern health care require that organizations have a sense of strategic mission and a vision for the future. Furthermore, individuals in administrative and management positions must assure that the mission and vision are communicated and that practice is centered on movement toward these ends.

An organization that strives to create an atmosphere of trust in which barriers are eliminated and teamwork is promoted will reap rewards from this type of program. For this program's content to be utilized effectively, charge nurses must feel free to be able to act on solutions to problem solving without fear of repercussions from management. In essence, the organization must create an environment in which empowerment is embraced. In today's health care world, with decentralization and collapsing

CASE 13–2 *Continued*

management structures, employee empowerment must be maximized for effective utilization of all resources.

■ BIOGRAPHICAL SKETCHES

Michelle Sly Smith is Hospice Services Director, Hospice of the Wabash Valley, Terre Haute, Indiana. She was formerly Orientation Coordinator, Educational Services, Union Hospital, in Terre Haute. In 1988, she received a BSN from the University of Evansville in Indiana. In 1995, she earned an MSN from Indiana State University in Terre Haute. She is certified in Nursing Continuing Education and Staff Development through the American Nurses Credentialing Center. She is a member of Sigma Theta Tau, Lambda Sigma Chapter. In addition, she is a member of the National Nursing Staff Development Organization, the Indiana Nursing Staff Development Organization, and the Hospice Organization. Ms. Smith's previous experiences include clinical and management positions in medical–surgical nursing.

Sally A. Zuel is Orientation Coordinator, Educational Services, Union Hospital, in Terre Haute, Indiana. Her previous experience includes the following positions: CPR Coordinator, staff and management positions in medical–surgical nursing, Affiliate Faculty for the Indiana Affiliate of the American Heart Association for Basic Cardiac Life Support, Pediatric Life Support, and Advanced Cardiac Life Support. She received a BSN degree in Nursing from Indiana State University,

in Terre Haute. She obtained an MSN in 1996 from Indiana State University. Ms. Zuel is certified in Nursing Continuing Education and Staff Development through the American Nurses Credentialing Center. She is a member of Sigma Theta Tau, Lambda Sigma Chapter. In addition, she is a member of the National Nursing Staff Development Organization and the Indiana Nursing Staff Development Organization.

■ SUGGESTED READINGS

Belasco, J.A. (1990). *Teaching the elephant to dance*. New York: Plume.

Blanchard, K., Burrows, H., & Onken, W. (1989). *The one minute manager meets the monkey*. New York: Morrow.

Braun, K., Christle, D., Walker, D., & Tiwanak, G. (1991). Verbal abuse of nurses and non-nurses. *Nursing Management, 22* (3), 72–76.

Byham, W.C. (1988). *Zapp! The lightning of empowerment*. New York: Harmony.

Byham, W.C. (1993). *Zapp! The lightning of empowerment in health care: How to improve patient care, increase job satisfaction, and lower health care costs*. New York: Development Dimensions International, Inc.

Cox, H. (1991). Verbal abuse nationwide, part I: Oppressed group behavior. *Nursing Management, 22* (2), 32–35.

Cox, H. (1991). Verbal abuse nationwide, part II: Impact and modifications. *Nursing Management, 22* (3), 66–69.

Cronrath, P.R. (1991). Building teams through solving problems. *Nursing Management, 22* (9), 120Q-OR–120X-OR.

DePree, M. (1989). *Leadership is an art*. New York: Doubleday.

CASE 13–2 *Continued*

Hansten, R.I. (1991). Delegation: Learning when and how to let go. *Nursing, 21* (4), 126–129.

Hodes, J.R., & Van Crombrugghe, P. (1990). Nurse–physician relationships. *Nursing Management, 21* (7), 73–75.

Koerner, J.G., & Karpiuk, K.L. (1994). *Implementing differentiated nursing practice transformation by design*. Gaithersburg, MD: Aspen.

Lewis-Ford, B.K. (1993). Management techniques: Coping with difficult people. *Nursing Management, 24* (3), 36–38.

Marquis, B.L., & Huston, C.L. (1994, Spring/Summer). Decisions, decisions, decisions. *Advanced Practice Nurse,* 46–49.

O'Brien, D.D. (1993). Delegate? Who? Me? *Journal of Post Anesthesia Nursing, 8* (4), 233–234.

■ REFERENCES

Bostrom, J., & Suter, W.N. (1992). Charge nurse decision making about patient assignment. *Nursing Administration Quarterly, 16* (4), 32–38.

Hamel, G. (1995, March). The perils of staff promotion take, for example, choosing a charge nurse . . . *Nursing Homes,* 25–27.

Harris, A.M., & Martin-Hylwa, E. (1992). Assistant head nurse: Today's catalytic manager. *Nursing Management, 23* (1), 40–43.

Joint Commission on Accreditation of Healthcare Organizations. (1994). *Comprehensive accreditation manual for hospitals*. Oakbrook Terrace, IL: JCAHO.

14

Performance Management

Betsy Frank

In a fast-changing health care delivery system, human resource management takes on a new importance. When monetary resources are scarce, administrators must maximize utilization of the human talents within their organizations. A well-designed performance management system will do just that. Performance management encompasses more than the traditional performance appraisal system. It involves all that mediates the interactive process between work motivation of the individual and the performance rewards and developmental opportunities provided by the organization. Figure 14–1 provides a graphic illustration of the performance management system.

This chapter opens with an overview of what motivates people to work. It then explores the purposes and options in developing a performance management system. The goal for performance management is to improve work performance in a way that positively impacts health care delivery.

■ OVERVIEW OF WORK MOTIVATION

The quest to understand what motivates people in the work environment is long-standing. Motivation theories seek to explain what energizes behavior, not the behavior itself. Theories and research on motivation can be divided into three categories: reinforcement, needs based, and cognitive.

Reinforcement as a Motivator

The earliest theorists viewed pay as the principal motivator for work and efficiency as the primary goal of work processes. In his 1911 work, *The Principles of Scientific Management,* Taylor posited that workers were motivated primarily by the extrinsic reward, pay. He then developed methods to identify the most efficient and effective methods for doing specific tasks and

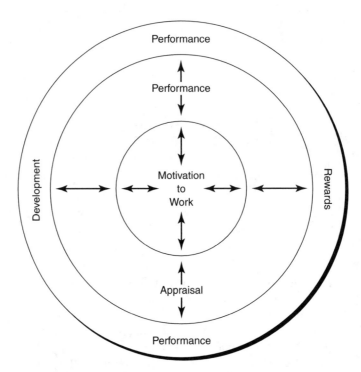

FIGURE 14–1. Performance management is an interactive process between work motivation, performance appraisal, and performance rewards and development.

recommended paying more to workers if a specified productivity standard was exceeded.

Reinforcement theories go one step beyond Taylor to include the external reward (stimulus), the rate of work (response), and the consequences of the rate (positive or negative outcome). The landmark research on how to manipulate these three variables to increase productivity was done by Thorndike (1911) and Skinner (1969). This theoretical framework continues to be used today to design bonus reward systems such as those seen in health maintenance organizations. Physicians, nurse practitioners, and physicians assistants may receive bonuses if they deliver a certain volume of patient services while holding costs down. According to D'Aunno and Fottler (1994), such a system of rewards often has no input from providers. They also point out that this simplistic view of human motivation ignores emotional and cognitive responses to the work environment.

Human Needs as Motivators

Maslow's (1954) hierarchy of needs is well known to nurses and other health care workers. His work grew out of a recognition that human beings have intrinsic needs that influence their work behavior. His contention is that once lower-level physiological and security needs are met, workers are motivated by the need for belonging, self-esteem, and self-actualization. Maslow asserts that higher-order needs are associated with higher quality work. His hierarchy assists managers to identify priorities for change; for instance, nurses and others cannot attend to higher quality of care if their need for sleep is not met due to excessive work hours or frequent change of shifts.

Alderfer (1972) adapted Maslow's framework in response to the criticism that needs may not be as hierarchical and unchanging over time as Maslow proposed. He grouped needs into three categories—existence, relatedness, and growth. Alderfer recognized that individuals may be motivated by more than one need at a time and that the primary need for a person may change over time due to changes in external circumstances. For instance, nurses may value pay or self-actualization at different times in their lives.

Herzberg (1966), another prominent needs theorist, emphasizes that intrinsic and extrinsic needs are both important for different reasons. According to Herzberg's two-factor theory, job satisfaction comes from intrinsic factors and job dissatisfaction, from extrinsic (or hygiene) factors. Job satisfaction and dissatisfaction may occur simultaneously. Motivators or intrinsic factors are the need for achievement, recognition, the nature of the work itself, responsibility, and advancement. Extrinsic or hygiene factors are interpersonal relationships with peers, subordinates, and supervisors; technical supervision; organizational policies; working conditions; pay; and personal life circumstances. Satisfaction with motivators will help retain employees; dissatisfaction with hygiene factors will influence an employee's decision to leave an organization.

Herzberg's work has been much criticized. One frequent comment made by those who have tried to test his theory is that it is verified mainly by using his critical incident methodology. Nevertheless, much research, particularly in the nursing literature, supports the fact that it is primarily intrinsic factors that serve as satisfiers or motivators and hygiene factors that serve as dissatisfiers (Blegen, 1993; Pierce, Hazel, & Mion, 1996). For managers, the implication is that dissatisfaction with supervision, working conditions, and the like must be kept at a minimum and opportunities for growth made available if good employees are to be retained in the organization.

The next step in understanding work motivation came from McClelland (1971), another needs based theorist. He emphasized the differences among workers, the importance of one's personal life in defining needs in one's work life, and that there is no one "magic answer" to job satisfaction or productivity. McClelland grouped needs into categories of achievement, power, and affiliation and posited that their primacy varies by employee. Some persons have more need for task accomplishment, whereas others have more need for responsibility and control over their environment. Others have stronger affiliation needs. All three needs are obtained through experience in one's personal and work lives. By matching individuals with an environment that supports their needs, individual capabilities can be maximized.

Cognitive Views of Motivation

Cognitive theories add issues of worker and organizational expectations to the study of motivation. Vroom (1964) labeled his theory the expectancy model. In this view, behavior in the workplace is a function of expectancies or beliefs about the probability that certain actions, such as coordinating a quality improvement project team, will lead to a certain outcome, such as promotion within a clinical nursing ladder. Valence is the value or desirability placed on the expected outcome. For a person to be highly motivated, the expectancies and valences must both be high. In other words, an employee must not only believe that certain efforts will be rewarded, but the employee must also highly value the expected reward. Thus, managers are challenged to match expected and valued rewards with employee expectations. Within one work group, nurses may be motivated by career advancement, pay, personal development, or flexibility in their schedule. Each will judge outcomes by different values. All these nurses may deliver the same quality of nursing care, are valuable to the organization, and should be rewarded accordingly.

Goal-setting theory (Locke & Latham, 1990) also is relevant to employee work motivation. It is often discussed as a means to increase worker productivity. If nurses and other health care employees set goals to which they are committed, then such goals can motivate behavior in the workplace. For goals to serve as motivators, they must be mutually set, provide challenge, be seen as attainable, and include appropriate feedback and rewards for goal attainment.

Job Satisfaction

Many researchers have sought to identify the essential elements of work satisfaction, assuming this will provide understanding of worker productivity and job retention. One or another theory of work motivation is normally the framework guiding the study of job satisfaction. No matter what the theoretical basis for the study, certain themes have emerged to describe the factors relevant to job satisfaction (Drews & Fisher, 1996). Blegen (1993) conducted a meta-analysis of 48 studies of nurse job satisfaction which had a total of more than 15,000 subjects. Autonomy, task variety or the work itself, and positive interpersonal relationships were positively linked with job satisfaction; stress and routinization were negatively related to job satisfaction. Pay was not tested in this meta-analysis because it did not appear frequently enough in the studies.

Because job dissatisfaction has been linked with turnover and absenteeism, both of which are costly to the organization, managers continue to be interested in work environments which promote worker job satisfaction. Certain organizational processes, such as shared governance, seem to promote professional autonomy and subsequent job satisfaction (Relf, 1995). These organizational processes are extremely important since an effective organization needs to promote a climate where employees work beyond minimum expectations. Managers who have a participative management style may also foster a supportive work environment and have staff who express more job satisfaction than staff who work with more authoritarian managers (Nakata & Saylor, 1994).

Whether or not job satisfaction causes employee productivity and positive patient care outcomes is uncertain. Research has not supported a causal relationship between job satisfaction and productivity. In fact, Steers and Black (1994) suggest that the direction may be just the opposite—productivity leads to job satisfaction when the rewards are viewed as commensurate with the job done, which leads to higher productivity and so on. Herzberg would interpret this cycle as maximizing the satisfiers and minimizing the dissatisfiers. If the relationship between productivity and job satisfaction is indeed iterative, then organizational effectiveness should be enhanced by this strategy.

■ PERFORMANCE MANAGEMENT

Performance management encompasses the majority of the human resource management process (see Fig. 14–2). The performance management system includes the organizational processes used to motivate employees. The purposes of this system for the individual are job performance recognition, compensation, job productivity, and planning for professional development. The purposes for the organization are job analysis, managing compensation, training needs analysis, manpower requirement definition, and systematic identification of individuals for promotion, transfer, discipline, or termination. Unlike the traditional appraisal system, performance management is job, not personality based, involves continual evaluation of job performance rather than at preset times, and is participative. Employees, supervisors, and the organization are all involved in facilitating performance improvement (Benjamin & Penland, 1995).

Individual Job Performance Recognition

One of the first questions managers in an organization must ask in designing their performance management system is, "What behavior do I wish to motivate?" An organization without an answer to this question would be like a hospital that hires an assortment of nurses, technicians, and clerks and then decides what health services to provide. To be effective, conserve effort, and not create ill feelings, rewards must be consistent with management's goals and policies. If the goal is to promote group cohesiveness and safe care, then the performance management system should not emphasize individual effort, but instead should reward group stability and cooperation. For example, promotions should be given by seniority, and rewards offered for assisting others or other collaborative efforts. Group bonuses could be given for achievement of goals such as staffing within a budget goal. On the other hand, if the goal

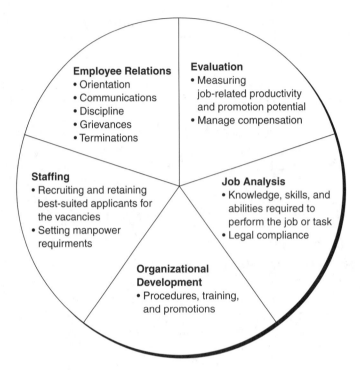

FIGURE 14–2. Functions of human resource management.

is attracting and retaining individual "stars," then performance management should include promotions and other rewards by merit criteria alone, with individual evaluations based on merit performance. The goals of most organizations fall between these two extremes, and so do the reward systems. If, however, the performance management system is not clearly linked to both the reward system and individual motivation the whole process is likely to be viewed as suspect by employees and frequently changed by management because "it doesn't work."

Compensation

Using the performance appraisal for compensation decisions is an important yet often contentious matter within health care and other organizations. The two major options are (1) compensation by qualifications and tenure, and (2) compensation by performance. Many organizations hire by job classification, specifying certain qualifications of experience and education, and then give raises based on tenure and, perhaps, additional education acquired during that tenure. These compensation decisions are pro forma and are largely separate from the evaluation of performance process. The major criticism of these systems is the automatic reward of low performers and lack of incentives for high performance.

When pay-for-performance systems are in place, decisions become more complex. Pay-for-performance schemes are predicated on the fact that better-than-average performance should be rewarded accordingly and that these rewards will, in turn, serve as motivators for future performance. To many, this approach is seen as more just, as it reflects actual differences among employee performances. Lawler's research (1994) supports the fact that if pay decisions, in an employee's view, have a direct connection to performance or are in what he calls the "line of sight," pay will serve as a motivator. Those subscribing to Herzberg's point of view would suggest that pay will only be a dissatisfier when an employee perceives that he or she is undervalued. Kohn (1993) agrees, stating that pay-for-performance rewards only short-term individual performance gains and does not provide long-term improvement in job behavior. According to Kohn, incentives such as opportunities for growth and promotions, which are recognition for achievements, are better motivators for long-term productivity gains. Kohn and others also contend that pay-for-performance systems set up competitive environments that do not promote group cohesiveness and teamwork.

To answer that particular criticism, some organizations have instituted group work team reward systems, often called gain sharing. For example, a hospital might have a system to monetarily reward units when they meet continuous quality improvement targets that result in institutional savings.

Job Productivity

Job-related, productivity-oriented performance appraisal systems designed to assess achievement of observable behavior are becoming the standard for performance appraisal in health care organizations. These appraisals, which are competency based and originate in the job analysis and job descriptions, permit both management and the individual to see how well a specific job has been performed over a given time. They might include items such as, "Does this nurse incorporate knowledge of physiological needs and changes associated with the developmental stages of the patient, with special attention to blood administration?" These systems are usually organized by a conceptual framework such as the nursing process or identified job dimensions in the job description. Increasingly clinician performance appraisal includes both clinical and organizational functions.

Trait-oriented evaluation items are effective, albeit more subjective, in evaluating promotability potential. Trait questions are oriented to the employee rather than the job or productivity. A typical question might be, "Does this nurse express an active interest in performing functions of greater responsibility?" Those who rate highest would be more likely to be considered as candidates for promotion.

Planning for Professional Development

Clinical professionals, project managers, and line managers perform functions that extend over a period of time or are outcome oriented. Annually, the employee and the supervisor should reach a consensus as to the accomplishments expected of the individuals and plans for his or her professional development. These expectations are then summarized in a listing of goals for job functions. For example, a clinical nurse might set a goal that she would serve on a task force to develop and implement a critical pathway within 6 months. At the end of that period, the results are measured and discrepancies noted. The performance appraisal is the formal means through which goal achievement is evaluated. This is sometimes referred to as management by objectives (MBO).

Employee performance appraisal data help to identify those employees who should be targeted for development opportunities. For example, a particular nurse may have been identified as an outstanding patient educator. She could be asked to coordinate a system-wide effort to improve patient education.

Transfer, demotion, discipline, or termination should be related to performance appraisal, thus indicating that the employee is either unable or unwilling to do the work. Management's responsibility is then to determine whether the problem is the result of individual employee difficulties or one that requires system-wide changes. Being *unable* may mean the nurse is willing to do the job, but needs more training; it may also mean a nurse is in a job that is a poor fit with his or her capabilities. Being *unwilling* may mean the nurse lacks motivation, which interferes with meeting performance expectations. Facilitating motivation through personal work adjustments is one solution to this problem. However, an astute manager will also look to the system to see if larger issues are present. Many situational factors may make higher performance extremely difficult. For instance, a high vacancy rate, inadequate clerical support, shortages of supplies, poorly trained subordinates, unclear reporting relationships, excessive paperwork, and a lack of proper equipment all may negatively impact employee performance. Usually these factors impact an entire unit's performance uniformly. Perhaps restructuring the work environment will once again allow intrinsic motivators to energize all nurses so that the majority's performance exceeds expectations.

■ PERFORMANCE MANAGEMENT SYSTEMS

Various systems for evaluating performance have been used for more than 100 years. Performance appraisals began when factories began to specialize the workforce and develop a management hierarchy. One of the earliest and simplest means of recognizing performance was for the foreman to hang a flag over the workbench of the employee having the highest productivity for the previous day. Many employee recognition schemes in use today emulate this activity and recognize the value of nonmonetary rewards.

An additional level of sophistication was added through the development of time and motion studies to prepare work standards for measuring expectations and distributing resources. Workers often received monetary bonuses when productivity was above the work standard. A third major advancement came during World War II, when the military developed trait-oriented appraisals to identify potential leaders for accelerated promotion. This recognized that promotion may require evaluation of more than efficiency in present work. Today, performance management systems are complex and include many types of rewards.

External Requirements for a Performance Management System

Three external environmental forces greatly influence an organization's performance management system: legal regulations, accreditation requirements, and collective bargaining agreements. One organizational goal is to choose employees based on merit and not personal criteria. Regulations for ensuring this goal are issued by the Equal Employment Opportunity Commission (EEOC). In order to prevent discrimination in the workplace, an organization needs to ensure that its performance management system is based on analysis of the job required, necessary behaviors for performance, and systematic feedback at least annually to employees. This is more extensively discussed in Chapter 3, "Legal Aspects of Patient Care Administration."

The Joint Commission on Accreditation of Healthcare Organizations (JCAHO) has further helped in the development of objective appraisal systems that can be used for hiring, orienting, training, and evaluating personnel. Its 1996 standards state, "Competency assessments of . . . individuals clearly address the ages of the patients they serve and the success with which employees produce the expected outcomes from clinical interventions" (Joint Commission, 1996). In other words, the organization has an obligation to determine and evaluate the competencies necessary to deliver quality patient care. The individual also has the obligation to deliver competent care, as defined by the employing institution, which takes into consideration the age of the patients served.

Collective bargaining agreements also influence the direction performance management systems take. Union contracts may specify job qualifications and processes for hiring, promotion, discipline, reward, and appeal activities. It is vital that all patient care administrators be familiar with all provisions of a collective bargaining agreement.

Job Analysis, Work Standards, and Job Descriptions

Specific responsibilities, duties, and competencies are associated with every job. Position or job descriptions originate in the job analyses that outline the type of work and worker characteristics required to fulfill an organization's mission. Job analysis allows decisions about recruiting, selecting, training, appraising, compensating, and human resource planning (Norton & Chrissman, 1992). For professional employees, the work standards that are incorporated into the job descriptions should originate with standards of practice set forth by professional organizations such as the American Nurses Association or governmental bodies such as the practice guidelines by the Agency for Health Care Policy and Research (AHCPR). An example of a work standard for a registered nurse would be, "Interprets assessment data in terms of the patient's age-related needs." A job description for a nurse manager might include, "Prepares yearly budget in accordance with institutional guidelines." In essence, the job description should specify expected performance. Thus, both employee and employer know exactly what is expected on the job. Additionally, a well-written job description can serve as an orientation guide for new employees. Finally, competencies within job descriptions can be used for preemployment assessments.

Staffing, Organizational Development, and Training

Systematic, aggregated data from the performance management system can identify system-wide needs for changes in staffing levels, staff mix, or particular job skills needed in one area. High turnover under one manager may indicate a need for a "closer look" by higher management. Low performance by staff from several units in one area may indicate a training need for staff.

Performance appraisal data are also a part of an organization's continuous quality improvement efforts (Boudreaux, 1994). Individuals who need extra training can be identified and group data can be used to analyze what performance standards must be improved system wide. It is the contention of total quality management experts that most performance problems are system problems, not problems of individual effort. Additionally, Baard and Neville (1996) suggest that deficiencies in competencies should be viewed as opportunities for problem solving and performance improvement. Therefore, system improvements might have to be made along with improvement in individual efforts. For example, if group data show that the majority of nurses fail to meet the standard for patient teaching, the system should be analyzed to see what facilitates and inhibits this care requirement. Appropriate changes can be put in place and data collected and analyzed 6 months later to see if improvements have been made.

■ COMPONENTS OF A PERFORMANCE APPRAISAL SYSTEM

Performance appraisal begins when an employee is first hired, continues cyclically, and ends when the employee leaves the organization. Figure 14–3 provides a graphic description of system requirements.

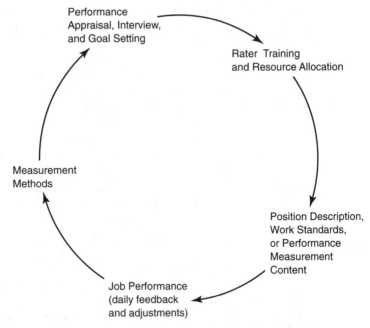

FIGURE 14–3. Components of a performance appraisal system.

Performance Measurement Content

The job analysis should identify competencies required for job performance, and the job description should incorporate work standards outlining the knowledge, skills, and abilities necessary for job performance organized by conceptual framework, job functions, or job dimensions. This is the major source for determining what to measure for performance appraisal and for determining staffing and training needs.

The objectives of the performance appraisal are to identify those behavioral elements of job performance or those employee traits that are deemed critical by management, and then to measure those elements. The important words here are *identify* and *measure*. Therein lies the problem. Few individual jobs are exactly alike and identifying critical elements shared by disparate jobs is difficult. Furthermore, various evaluators have different perceptions of quality performance and ideas about what makes one employee better than another. For example, one nurse manager may perceive that the primary function of a staff nurse is to oversee or provide the treatment of a patient in accordance with the physician's instructions. Another head nurse may believe that the principal function is to ensure the patient's well-being. It is important that the appraisal instrument specify performance expectations and behaviors to reduce the likelihood that individual definitions will be applied. A performance appraisal tool based on competencies helps to alleviate some of this subjectivity.

Whatever process and tools are chosen for measurement, the first goal is to measure the critical elements of job performance. For example, if there is an interest in identifying the most productive nurses, do the questions and rating scales cause these persons to get the highest ratings? Developing a valid appraisal instrument requires that a direct correlation be made between the position description, work standards, and evaluation questions or rating scale. If the answer to a question cannot be justified as indicative of present or future job success, then the question is not valid.

Construct validity is related to how accurately the instrument can measure the variable that the evaluator perceives to be important. As individuals, we may have different perceptions as to reality or truth (the "construct") of a variable. For example, the patient load may be a work standard in evaluating a family nurse practitioner in an ambulatory care clinic. Evaluators might disagree as to what constitutes a "normal patient load." At one extreme is the proponent who advocates measuring only the raw number of case contacts without regard to any patient or work situation characteristics. At the other extreme is the proponent who advocates extensive description of the unique aspects of each case without regard for the number of cases handled. To be a valid instrument, the performance appraisal tool must indicate a specific "normal workload" that incorporates both raw numbers and situational and patient factors that influence workload. If you agree that determination of relevant factors and weights is problematic, then you can appreciate how difficult it is to achieve construct validity.

Measurement deficiency occurs when critical elements that influence the appraisal question or item are not considered. For example, when evaluating the productivity of a primary nurse on a medical unit, a hospital should have an interest in both the quality and quantity of work. A nurse should process a new physician's orders expeditiously, but not so fast as to overlook critical indices. Not to consider both factors fully, probably in separate questions, would be a measurement deficiency in the appraisal instrument.

Measurement contamination occurs when irrelevant information is allowed to influence the construct. Each employee modifies the position to some extent due to style, interests, or special competencies or shortcomings. This overall modification is also reflected in the performance of specific tasks. For example, a nurse might have exceptionally neat handwriting; however, if data are put directly into the computer, handwriting has only marginal importance. If the evaluator includes handwriting in the construct of patient care documentation, this is measurement contamination.

The Measurement Process

Most organizations specify that performance appraisals of new employees be conducted 3 to 6 months after the initial hire and then yearly thereafter. Between performance appraisal interviews, nurse managers need to provide verbal and written positive and negative feedback as well as anecdotal records for each employee documenting their adherence to work standards and progress in achieving their goals. Most employees try to perform their assigned jobs in a manner they perceive as competent and productive. Sometimes their perceptions of job requirements do not coincide with those of their supervisor. In these instances, the supervisor must discuss these discrepancies with the employee, and follow through with the appropriate process to improve performance. This process may include counseling the employee, disciplining the employee, providing opportunities for training in the correct procedures, or providing closer supervision as the employee masters a competency.

Both positive and negative (corrective) feedback should be a normal part of the daily supervisor–employee relationship. Employees must identify job problems to their supervisor; likewise, supervisors must inform employees when employee performance requires improvement. For example, if a registered nurse's car has broken down, forcing her temporarily to switch to sometimes unreliable public transportation, the nurse should inform her supervisor. Likewise, if a patient complains of rude behavior on the part of nursing personnel, the nurse manager should seek to determine the source of the complaint and take corrective action.

Measurement Methods

The most common methods of performance appraisal measurement are ranking, checklists, rating scales, and narratives.

Ranking

The performance appraisal instrument that is the simplest, cheapest, and easiest to administer is based on the supervisor *ranking all personnel in a given group*. To be equitable, all employees should be performing the same general function or be in the same job classification. The strength of this method is that management achieves a rank order that can be readily converted to compute salary increases. That is, those employees with the highest ranking receive the largest salary increases. Fair administration requires the appraiser be very familiar with all behavior of those being ranked. Weaknesses of this method are (1) the need for objective ordinal measures, and (2) its presumption that there is a measurable difference between each of the employees being evaluated. This may lead to supervisory frustration and employee hostility. Another weakness is that a work unit may become competitive and work group members may sabotage others to raise their own rank. Two ranking techniques that are often used are straight ranking and forced distribution.

The *straight ranking* technique uses selected factors and requires the supervisor to rank from high to low all employees in the work unit. A typical ranking question might be, "In productivity, this nurse ranks (number) out of (number) nurses with similar duties and responsibilities."

The *forced distribution* technique allocates a certain percentage of the workforce to each group to achieve a bell-shaped distribution; that is, 5 percent outstanding, 20 percent above average, 50 percent satisfactory, 20 percent acceptable, and 5 percent unsatisfactory. Although this format tends to soften the harsh numerical ranking of each employee used in straight ranking, it has the same strengths and shortcomings as the straight-ranking method. In addition, studies have found that most conscientious workers perceive themselves to be above average. Thus, evaluating the majority of the employees as satisfactory (average) or below may have an adverse effect on an individual's motivation to be productive and commitment to remain with the organization. This has been a major drawback found in implementing most merit-based compensation systems.

Checklists

The checklist-style performance appraisal is used to achieve a profile of the employee based on selected characteristics, traits, or behaviors. Lists prepared by specialists select words and phrases that minimize rater bias and are job related. The nurse manager can then check off the item that most closely describes personnel under his or her supervision. Each item has a "yes" or "no" evaluation scale. The shortcoming of this approach is that it assumes that yes or no responses adequately evaluate the employee and that the supervisor has good observation skills. Inasmuch as the checklist produces an employee profile that may be compared to a desired standard, the checklist is most useful for assessing training needs and promotion.

The *simple checklist* is composed of numerous words or phrases describing various employee behaviors or traits. The rater is asked to check all those that describe the employee on each checklist. Descriptors are often clustered to represent different aspects of one dimension of behavior. The simple checklist has been used widely for documenting competencies. Table 14–1 illustrates a competency checklist.

The *weighted checklist* tends to arrange choices in order of perceived desirability or assign a "hidden" prioritized value to each item used in totaling the score. After the rater completes the checklist, those items checked are multiplied by their respective weights and totaled for a cumulative score that describes a particular profile. Table 14–2 illustrates a weighted checklist for initiative. Validity of items and weights requires rigorous psychometric development. The cost of this has limited applications of this method.

The *forced checklist* requires the rater to read a number of pairs of words or phrases and select the most appropriate item from each pair that describes the employee. Sometimes there are all possible pairs of a set of characteristics. Another variation is a checklist that requires the evaluator to rate the degree to which an employee demonstrates a characteristic using two extreme descriptions. The purpose of changing combinations and forced selections is to describe the employee's true performance or strength in

TABLE 14–1. Union Hospital Competency Assessment Review for Nursing Service

Name: _____ Unit: _____ 4C - RN _____ Date of Review: _____ Evaluator _____

1. AGE-SPECIFIC PROCEDURAL/EQUIPMENT ASSESSMENT

PROCEDURE/SKILL	NEONATE/ INFANT			PEDIATRIC			ADOLESCENT			ADULT			OLDER ADULT			ALL AGES			NOT AGE-RELATED		
	Y	N	NA	Y	N	NA	Y	N	NA	Y	N	NA	Y	N	NA	Y	N	NA	Y	N	NA
1. Demonstrates ability to assess and interpret findings relative to the developmental age of the patient/client.																					
2. Utilizes appropriate verbal skills for comprehension of patient/family/caretaker when providing information, instruction, and when answering questions.																					
3. Demonstrates respect for patient's need to be involved in plan of care.																					
a. Presents information in age-appropriate terms.																					
b. Respects patient's need for independence and control over decisions made.																					
c. Provides for maximization of self-care.																					
4. Involves patient/family in decision making related to plan of care.																					
a. Demonstrates awareness of cultural differences when presenting information to family members.																					
b. Documents appropriately.																					
5. Incorporates knowledge of physiological needs/changes associated with the developmental stages of the patient with special attention to:																					
a. Generic Skills:																					
(1) Abbott Life Care pump																					
(2) Accuchek skills																					
(3) IV and saline lock																					
(4) Oral airways																					
(5) O_2 therapy per venti-mask, initiation																					
(6) O_2 therapy per cannula, initiation																					
(7) Crash cart																					
(8) Suction set-up (receptal system)																					
(9) Patient restraint																					
(10) Administration of medications																					
(11) IVPB infusion through central venous catheter																					

Y, yes; N, no; NA, not applicable.
Courtesy of Union Hospital, Terre Haute, Indiana.

TABLE 14–2. Weighted Checklist

Please check three items that best describe the employee.

		HIDDEN WEIGHT
_____	Person I would expect to take charge in an emergency.	(10)
_____	Does what is expected of the job.	(5)
_____	Limits work to his/her position description.	(3)
_____	Anxious to assume greater responsibility.	(9)
_____	Seeks shortcuts.	(4)
_____	Seeks new and better ways to do the job.	(8)
_____	Occasionally does more than is expected.	(6)

certain characteristics and to be able to compare employees on the same selections. Table 14–3 illustrates a forced checklist to evaluate work attitude.

Rating Scale

The most common performance appraisal instrument is the *rating scale*. In general, rating scales consist of a series of phrases or sentences that describe various situations. The employee is evaluated on the scale as to how he or she fits the model for appropriate action or behavior. Figure 14–4 presents a simple Likert-type scale for rating performance. The evaluator marks the evaluation along a continuum. Notice how the organization featured in Figure 14–4 has combined its performance appraisal tool and its job description.

TABLE 14–3. Forced Checklist

In each of the sets below, choose the items that are the most and least descriptive of the employee.

MOST DESCRIPTIVE	LEAST DESCRIPTIVE	ITEM
_____	_____	Talks easily to patients.
_____	_____	Does not talk to patients when checking charts.
_____	_____	Knows patients' first names.
_____	_____	Prefers to work the night shift.
_____	_____	Always on time for duty.
_____	_____	Stays after shift to finish paperwork and other details.
_____	_____	Satisfactory attendance.
_____	_____	Sometimes hard to find at the work station.

JOB DESCRIPTION/PERFORMANCE EVALUATION
UNION HOSPITAL, INC.
Terre Haute, Indiana 47804

PURPOSE: The Job Description gives direction regarding job duties, personal traits, physical demands, and educational requirements. The job description serves as the tool for performance evaluation. Evaluations are to be completed after six (6) months, and then annually.

JOB TITLE: REGISTERED NURSE/GRADUATE NURSE

DEPARTMENT: Nursing Services

RESPONSIBLE TO: Nursing Care Manager

SCORING CODES:
4 = Exceeds Criteria Consistently
3 = Meets Criteria
2 = Needs Improvement
1 = Unsatisfactory
0 = No Effort Demonstrated

CN-2	CN-3	CN-4
NURSING PROCESS Assessment	NURSING PROCESS Assessment	NURSING PROCESS Assessment

1. Performs comprehensive assessments to include identification of actual or potential physical, psychosocial, teaching, safety, infection control and environmental needs.
  a. Interprets assessment data in terms of the patient's age-related needs.
	1. Performs comprehensive assessments to include identification of actual or potential physical, psychosocial, teaching, safety, infection control and environmental needs.
	  a. Interprets assessment data in terms of the patient's age-related needs.
		1. Performs comprehensive assessments to include identification of actual or potential physical, psychosocial, teaching, safety, infection control and environmental needs.
		  a. Interprets assessment data in terms of the patient's age-related needs.
		  b. Applies unit-specific advanced assessment skills and knowledge to patients with complex medical and nursing care needs.

Originated: June, 1989
Revised: July, 1993 & Feb., 1994

FIGURE 14–4. Job description/performance evaluation. *(Courtesy of Union Hospital, Terre Haute, Indiana.)*

The rating scale method is highly dependent on the observational skills of the evaluator. Another problem may be length. If the scale tries to measure all relevant behaviors, it is likely to become time-consuming and cumbersome.

A more sophisticated instrument is the behavioral anchored rating scale (BARS), which is developed by collecting observations of workers as they do their work. Each behavior is listed as a question and discrete responses to the question are provided. Development using this approach is costly, but some organizations adopt it for its accuracy. Another version of the rating scale is the summated behavioral observation scale (BOS), which is shorter than the BARS because a summary behaviors is used.

Narratives

The *narrative description* instrument describes an employee's performance or characteristics and is particularly useful in assessing training needs, promotability, labor relations conditions, employee development, and manpower requirements. Appraisal instruments frequently require supervisors to write narrative statements describing their perceptions of how the job was performed or descriptions of events that occurred during the reporting period. Although such instruments provide an excellent means of achieving an in-depth and general assessment of the employee, they are time-consuming and heavily dependent on the writing and analytical skills of the supervisor. They also may not result in comparable data for determining compensation changes.

The *essay-style performance appraisal* asks certain general questions and then requires the supervisor to comment on how well the employee appears to relate to each question. For example, "How effectively could this nurse supervise a 24-patient unit?" A short paragraph is written describing why the supervisor believes the nurse can or cannot handle this responsibility. If several qualified observers make a similar valid assessment of the employee, the essay performance appraisal becomes an excellent way for management to identify which persons have supervisory potential or which persons require additional training. This type of appraisal may only be appropriate if the observation of current duties is predictive of future performance in a different job.

The *critical incident performance appraisal* requires summary statements, both positive and negative, about the employee's performance in accomplishing specific tasks or responsibilities. Table 14–4 shows two examples.

The critical incident method requires the supervisor to maintain a logbook and record of events as they occur. This process overcomes evaluator subjectivity through the straightforward reporting of events. However, the critical incident method has two human shortcomings: (1) employees become anxious when they know their supervisor is keeping a log of their behavior, and (2) supervisors are hesitant to report activity that might reflect negatively on their own supervisory skills. The critical incident method also requires systematic allocation of time to record entries on every individual at regular intervals.

TABLE 14–4. Critical Incident Notations

01/25/96. Nurse demonstrated initiative and knowledge of patient teaching needs when he realized patient could not read printed instructions for discharge medications. He arranged for instructions to be audiotaped.

02/15/96. Nurse required considerable supervisory assistance to calm down patient who believed that his mail was being withheld. Nurse's admonition of patient only made matters worse.

The *field review* evaluation is conducted by a third party, often a staff specialist whose sole function is to prepare evaluations. The supervisor, employee, and co-workers are interviewed and comments regarding the employee's performance or character traits are melded into a summary. Because the field review writer is independent of the work unit, he or she is apt to be more candid, less biased in the evaluation, and more reflective of overall organizational norms. On the negative side, the field review method is the most costly and time-consuming of all performance appraisal techniques. These characteristics make application rare.

Appraisal Interview

Employees want to know how well they are performing their jobs. To know this, they need feedback about how others perceive their endeavors. They also need to validate their own perceptions as to their contribution to the organization. The performance appraisal interview provides an excellent opportunity for management and employees to formally provide this feedback. A performance appraisal interview should have no surprises. It should be a summing up of the employee's performance over the entire period being evaluated. The competent supervisor should have provided frequent feedback to the employee, both complimentary and constructive. In a similar manner, the employee should have kept the supervisor informed of his or her performance concerns and aspirations. The employee can also point out job stresses and suggest ways in which the supervisor and staff could improve work conditions. If organizational priorities or policies have changed, the appraisal interview is not the place for the employee to find out about them. With this framework in place, trust develops allowing both participants to hear what the other has to say and making the time more fruitful. As a part of goal setting, the employee exercises autonomy by choosing appropriate courses of action based on the appraisal data. The interview can also be a place where relatedness needs are fulfilled if managers convey the attitude that performance appraisal is a team effort, not an adversarial exercise (Baard & Neville, 1996).

The supervisor who prepares the appraisal is usually the management representative designated to conduct the interview. Sometimes the interview is done by peers if a system of shared governance exists. In whatever manner it is conducted, the performance appraisal interview should be a formal, private meeting, set up in advance to permit ample time for discussion, in which both parties know the purpose and the agenda.

Some supervisors or employees find the appraisal interview to be a confrontational and threatening experience. It becomes a "show and sell" activity. When the employee comes into the office, he or she finds the completed performance appraisal form in the center of the table. The employee is asked to read the form, invited to ask questions or comment, and then requested to sign the form. The supervisor has to "sell" the evaluation to the employee. If the appraisal form is not absolutely final, the employee is placed in the position of having to challenge the performance appraisal and the supervisor of having to defend it. Adopting the principles of performance management guards against this less than positive scenario.

When a performance appraisal rates the employee as either outstanding or unsatisfactory, both parties have probably discussed the work performance during the year and the evaluation is readily accepted. With the majority of personnel in the work unit, however, those who have worked hard to perform their duties efficiently and effectively and believe they have done everything satisfactorily, have probably had less feedback. Wording of the performance appraisal and discussion of the value of the person's performance is especially important. Presenting employees with an "average" appraisal should be avoided. Even if the employees accept such a rating, it will provide little to make them feel that they have made a contribution to the organization and that they are recognized and appreciated.

The best performance appraisal interviews are conducted before the completion of the rating form. This does not suggest any less formality or preparation for the interview. Rather, both parties discuss the duties and responsibilities in the position description, the work standards, the relative weight given to each duty, and how well the employee fulfilled his or her assignments. Included in the discussion is an evaluation of how closely last year's goals were met and the development of next year's goals. If the performance appraisal contains trait-oriented questions, these can be discussed in relation to job requirements and promotion potential. Other opportunities for growth may also be discussed. Issues, about which the supervisor may not be aware, may be introduced and considered. After the interview, the supervisor completes the performance appraisal rating form and may further discuss the rating with the employee. Even if another formal interview is not scheduled, the employee needs to see what was written and have an opportunity to formally comment. This approach to performance appraisal makes the interview a discussion between two colleagues rather than a confrontation between two adversaries.

All performance appraisal systems need to provide opportunities for differences between the supervisor's and the employee's rating to be aired and considered. Some agencies have a formal appeal process.

Rater Training and Resource Allocation

In order for the performance appraisal system to be implemented to provide fair, objective assessments and results that can be utilized effectively, training is needed for both raters and ratees (Steers & Black, 1994). Ratees need to understand how measurement content was determined, what processes are used to ensure reliable and objective assessment, and their role in providing information and feedback on the summary appraisal and in goal setting and goal achievement. Raters also need training in the process, legal regulations and requirements, collective bargaining agreements, standards for measurement and processes, and access to aggregated data. Everyone needs to be committed to equity in distributing rewards and recognition for each person's contribution to the organization.

One goal is consistency across raters and over time. Will the appraisal instrument produce the same results every time if completed by several evaluators observing the same behavior or traits? Or, will the same evaluator give the same ratings for the same behavior or traits every time if the appraisal instrument is completed on several occasions? For instance, when assessing competency in discharge planning, different raters should come to the same conclusion regarding whether or not a nurse consistently meets the criteria for what is defined as adequate discharge planning. When selecting, using, or reviewing results one must always be aware of the reliability factor, irrespective of which performance appraisal instrument is used.

Human interaction and its related bias is probably the greatest barrier encountered when trying to assess a performance appraisal program. The *halo effect* occurs when the rater allows one highly evaluated item to influence inappropriately a high evaluation in other areas. For example, a nurse who always has an exceptionally neat and energetic appearance might also be rated high in job competency even though her nursing skills are only average. Conversely, the *horn effect* occurs when one low evaluation causes all the other appraisal items to have a lower mark. Sometimes, a very recent event may unduly influence either a higher or lower mark, causing the *recency effect.* A common shortcoming is the *generalization effect,* which occurs when a nurse is evaluated based on the whole unit's performance instead of his or her own. This is a more likely occurrence on a "problem unit" or a "star unit," and may result in overly harsh ratings for everyone as a form of discipline or overly generous ratings for everyone as a reward. Another human bias problem is *self-reflection;* a nurse manager may rate all the staff high to show how good his or her own performance is. Sometimes, the supervisor, not wanting to create ill will within a work unit, will exhibit a bias for *central tendency* and rate everyone at about the central midpoint. One way to avoid these errors is to constantly check and remind yourself that appraisals evaluating individuals must be based on job-related criteria over the time period being examined. A moment's reflection looking at all the appraisals on a unit and reviewing these potential errors should assist in minimizing bias.

Another method for increasing objectivity in performance appraisal is to increase the number of people participating in the review (Ewen, 1994). Some agencies use peer review to provide another perspective. The most extensive process is called 360-degree performance appraisal (Tornow, 1993). In this approach, all who are concerned with the employee's performance have a voice in the appraisal process. For example, nurse managers could be evaluated by staff, other managers, physicians, and their immediate supervisors. A more thorough evaluation is the outcome, in contrast to an evaluation conducted only by the immediate supervisor. However, this process is very time consuming. It has been used to evaluate people at a key juncture in their career or those in sensitive positions, when cooperation between several different stakeholder groups is vital.

■ SUMMARY

In summary, performance management systems have applicability to a wide array of human resource functions. Their goals are equitable rewards and recognition for each person's contribution to the work of the organization, objectively administered using valid tools. Administratively, management seeks tools that meet legal and other requirements and are valid, easy to use, supported by training and adequate resources, and perceived as valid and reliable by those being rated.

Performance appraisal is a critical component of the performance management system. How well it is accomplished may have a broad impact on employee productivity and job satisfaction. Hiring and retaining employees who are not performing at their best compromises the organization's survival in a turbulent health care environment. Ultimately a well-run performance management system is not only efficient, but cost-effective as well.

■ BIOGRAPHICAL SKETCH

Betsy Frank is an Associate Professor and Chair of the Department of Health Restoration at Indiana State University School of Nursing in Terre Haute, Indiana. She received her BSN from the Ohio State University in 1968, an MN from the University of Washington in 1970, and a PhD from the University of Utah in 1982. Her work experiences include staff nurse, clinical specialist, acting assistant director of nursing, and nurse educator. She is active in the Council for Research in Nursing Education (a council within the National League for Nursing), Sigma Theta Tau, the Indiana State Nurses Association, and The Council on Graduate Education for Administration in Nursing.

■ SUGGESTED READINGS

Anderson, G.C. (1993). Managing performance appraisal systems. Oxford, United Kingdom: Blackwell.

Antonioni, D. (1994). Improve the performance management process before discontinuing performance appraisals. *Compensation & Benefits Review, 26* (3), 29–37.

Herzberg, F. (1976). *The managerial choice: To be efficient and to be human.* Homewood, IL: Dow-Jones Irwin.

Knox, S., & Gregg, A.C. (1994). Balancing nonmonetary and monetary rewards: A contemporary paradigm for nursing. *Seminars for Nurse Managers, 2,* 140–147.

McCoy, T.J. (1992). *Compensation and motivation.* New York: AMACOM.

Murphy, K.R., & Cleveland, J.N. (1995). *Understanding performance appraisal: Social, organizational, and goal-based perspectives.* Thousand Oaks, CA: Sage.

Steers, R.M., & Porter, L.W. (1991). *Motivation and work behavior.* New York: McGraw-Hill.

■ REFERENCES

Alderfer, C.P. (1972). *Existence, relatedness, and growth.* New York: Free Press.

Baard, P.P., & Neville, S.M. (1996). The intrinsically motivated nurse: Help and hindrance from evaluation feedback sessions. *Journal of Nursing Administration, 26* (7/8), 19–26.

Benjamin, S., & Penland, T. (1995). How developmental supervision and performance management improve effectiveness. *Health Care Supervisor, 14* (2), 19–28.

Blegen, M.A. (1993). Nurse's job satisfaction: A meta-analysis of related variables. *Nursing Research, 42,* 36–40.

Boudreaux, G. (1994). Response: What TQM says about performance appraisal. *Compensation & Benefits Review, 26* (3), 20–24.

D'Aunno, T.A., & Fottler, M.D. (1994). Motivating people. In S.M. Shortell & A.D. Kaluzney (Eds.), *Health care management: Organization design and behavior* (pp. 57–84). Albany, NY: Delmar.

Drews, T.T., & Fisher, M.L. (1996). Job satisfaction and intent to stay: RNs' perception. *Nursing Management, 27* (3), 58.

Ewen, A.J. (1994). Multisource assessment increases healthcare employee satisfaction. *Journal of American Health Information Management Association, 56* (5), 56–60.

Herzberg, F. (1966). *Work and the nature of man.* New York: Mentor.

Joint Commission on Accreditation of Healthcare Organizations. (1996). *Comprehensive accreditation manual for hospitals.* Oakbrook Terrace, IL: JCAHO.

Kohn, A. (1993). *Punished by rewards.* Boston: Houghton Mifflin.

Lawler, E.E. III. (1994). *Motivation in work organizations.* San Francisco: Jossey-Bass.

Locke, E.A., & Latham, G.P. (1990). *A theory of goal setting and task performance.* Englewood Cliffs, NJ: Prentice-Hall.

Maslow, A.H. (1970). *Motivation and personality* (2nd ed.). New York: Harper & Row.

McClelland, D.C. (1971). *Assessing human motivation.* New York: General Learning Press.

Nakata, J.A., & Saylor, C. (1994). Management style and staff nurse satisfaction in a changing environment. *Nursing Administration Quarterly, 18* (3), 51–57.

Norton, S.D., & Chrissman, S. (1992). Staffing, recruiting, and selecting. In P.J. Decker & E.J. Sullivan (Eds.), *Nursing administration: A micro/macro approach for effective nurse executives*. Norwalk, CT: Appleton & Lange.

Pierce, L.L., Hazel, C.M., & Mion, L.C. (1996). Effect of a professional practice model on autonomy, job satisfaction and turnover. *Nursing Management, 27* (2), 48M, 48P, 48S–T.

Relf, M. (1995). Increasing job satisfaction and motivation while reducing nursing turnover through implementation of shared governance. *Critical Care Nurse Quarterly, 18* (3), 7–13.

Skinner, B.F. (1969). *Contingencies of reinforcement: A theoretical analysis*. New York: Appleton-Century-Crofts.

Steers, R.M., & Black, J.S. (1994). *Organizational behavior* (5th ed.). New York: HarperCollins.

Taylor, F.W. (1911). *The principles of scientific management*. New York: Harper & Row.

Thorndike, E.L. (1911). *Animal intelligence*. New York: Macmillan.

Tornow, W.W. (Ed.). (1993). 360-degree feedback [Special issue]. *Human Resource Management, 32,* (2&3), 221–9.

Vroom, V. (1964). *Work and motivation*. New York: Wiley.

CASE 14–1 Changing Rewards to Match Expectations

Carolyn A. Taylor

The auditorium was crowded with hospital staff, and a festive atmosphere enveloped the room. Tables overflowed with finger foods, fruit and vegetable trays, dip, punch, and a gigantic cake. The group waited for the start of a reception to celebrate the completion of our first year under the new Performance Share program and the distribution of checks to hospital staff. Our President/CEO stepped up to the podium, flanked by other key administrators, all poised to display the Performance Share distribution, which had been blown up into a large replica of a check for the total amount. The employees waited anxiously for their individual checks, which would validate the reality of the moment.

Our health system includes a 442-bed teaching hospital, home health agency, adult day care program, ambulatory services, and an extensive community outreach health promotion program located in suburban Maryland within the greater Washington, D.C., metropolitan area. Holy Cross Hospital has an excellent reputation in the community for the provision of quality care to a diverse population.

In the late 1980s, Holy Cross experienced a complete change in the executive administration, signaling a change in management style for the entire institution. The previous administration exhibited a traditional style with a top-down approach to management. One-way communication was the norm, and there

was no empowerment of staff to participate in operational activities or to share in the hospital's financial success. The new administration's move to a participatory style of management at its outset would prepare the way for the Performance Share program and other innovative empowerment-oriented opportunities for the staff.

The health care environment around us was dismal at best. Hospitals were downsizing, right sizing, reengineering, laying off staff, merging, experiencing competitive buyouts, and closing their doors. Managed care penetration was increasing, and the name of the game was cost containment, quality, and competition. Employees were all aware of the new Performance Share program. Quarterly reports had indicated there might be a bonus, but most employees were still unsure whether it would be more than a token program. It seemed unbelievable that in the midst of jobs being touted as a precious privilege, Holy Cross would be distributing more than token amounts of money to the majority of the staff.

The President/CEO started the program by taking the time to thank staff for all the hard work that had gone into making the Performance Share program a successful venture. Then he announced the amount of money that would be distributed. The amount was based on specific criteria that had been predetermined at the outset of the program. The check was for over $1 million!

CASE 14–1 *Continued*

This total brought thunderous applause from the employees. The managers of each department were asked to pick up the bundle of checks for their staff, and to distribute them in person to each employee.

Everyone was walking on air and the hospital was buzzing with the news of Performance Share. Some staff were already asking what they could do to assure next year's success. Others were totally surprised at the amount of their individual share. The dispensing of the checks served the purpose of validating the reality of our efforts to change rewards to match expectations. The energy generated from this one event lasted over 6 months. That was over 2 years ago. But how did we get to that point?

■ PERFORMANCE SHARE

During the 1970s, all staff received the same annual compensation increases, ranging as high as 13 to 15 percent. Rates were set by top management agreement and there was never a notion of variation by merit. When the new administration entered in the late 1980s, the cost-containment environment did not provide hospitals with large annual surpluses to provide continued, significant across-the-board increases. Services were expanding, and Holy Cross was becoming more than a hospital. In addition, the lack of connection between pay and performance seemed a disincentive for outstanding performance. Yet, the new administration wanted to preserve the team spirit and caring atmosphere that were hallmarks of the institution.

The Senior Executive Team held a retreat to plan a strategy for restructuring rewards in a way that would be aligned with employee expectations and performance and would reinforce the hospital's mission. The new system needed to be simple, fair, and easy to understand for all levels of employees; possess discreet goals; and encourage clinicians, support staff, and business staff to work closely together.

The specific objectives were to establish a program to reward employees for superior performance and to support the hospital's "One Team One Spirit" initiative. This phrase is in our mission statement and sums up our vision for Holy Cross employees to establish and work toward mutual goals as a team and in the same "Spirit." The Senior Executive Team's annual Leadership Agenda had, as a high priority, compensation reform to align rewards and expectations.

As an outcome of the retreat, two parallel programs were proposed. One aimed to provide individual rewards through merit compensation increases linked to annual performance evaluations. The other, entitled Performance Share, provided annual organization-wide bonuses for all employees when Holy Cross was able to meet certain standards of performance. This was how we planned to operationalize our "One Team One Spirit" initiative.

The next step was to plan how to spread the word. How could all employees understand the purposes of both proposals? What mechanisms and train-

CASE 14–1 *Continued*

ing were needed to see that both programs were implemented in a fair and efficient way? To carry out this work, we formed an employee implementation committee. This committee consisted of a diverse group of employees from all areas of the hospital who provided advisement on the program's policies, procedures, training, and publicity. We needed an organization-wide perspective on this initiative. This committee was key in making the proposals work.

The Performance Share program pays everyone a bonus of 1 percent or more of their annual salary when the hospital meets or exceeds certain system-wide goals set at the beginning of each fiscal year. The bonus is in addition to the employee's salary and in addition to any increase associated with the employee's performance evaluation. The system-wide goals, each linked to a mission priority, are set at the beginning of each fiscal year by the Senior Executive Team and approved by the Board of Trustees. These goals are identified by benchmarks from the competitive environment, feedback on customer expectations, and quality improvement initiatives. The three mission priorities are: organizational effectiveness, service excellence, and operational excellence. We tried to word mission priorities in ways all employees could understand. For each mission priority goal, a realistic threshold is set, based on past performance, to define the minimum level that needs to be achieved for all employees to earn the Performance Share bonus for that year. Our purpose is to set challenging but achievable goals that are relevant

to all employees across the organization. Employees are informed of the three mission priority goals for the year and the thresholds in simple, understandable language.

The first mission priority, organizational effectiveness, is a measure of our health system's financial success. Performance on this goal sets the amount in the potential pool for distribution if all goals are met. A budget target for Net Income is set by the Senior Management Team at the beginning of each fiscal year. This is the amount of revenue remaining after all of our expenses are paid. Reaching this goal sets aside the equivalent of 1 percent of all salaries in an account for potential distribution through Performance Share. Anything gained over the budget target is called Excess Net Income. Twenty-five percent of all Excess Net Income will also go into the Performance Share account.

Our second mission priority is service excellence. This priority is best represented by how our customers feel about our service. Customer satisfaction is very important to us. Our patients are surveyed about the services we provide by a national organization and the results are categorized into three main areas.

- How satisfied they were overall.
- How likely they are to return to Holy Cross.
- How likely they are to recommend Holy Cross to others.

Patient responses are recorded on a 4-point scale, with 4 being the highest rating. This may be operationalized for the

CASE 14–1 *Continued*

year as a global hospital average score or as average score improvement in a specific area that our quality improvement process has identified as problematic and relating to behavior of all staff; For example, courtesy to patients and families.

The third priority is operational excellence. The goals are chosen based on performance improvement monitoring, benchmarks and national professional standards, and comparison to our nearby competitors. One year we used three measures: procedure and/or treatment errors, falls, and occupational injury rates. The first measure is procedure and/or treatment errors. We only monitored errors that required us to redo a procedure or that could have potentially harmed a patient. The second measure was injuries to patients and visitors due to falls. For this measure only the falls that resulted in actual injury were counted. The third measure was occupational injury rate. This measure includes all reported injuries due to any cause that is job related. All of these performance areas were already being monitored by our quality improvement program. For instance, the occupational injury rate was calculated by dividing the number of occupational injuries we had by the total number of productive hours worked per month. A threshold level of average achievement for the year was set for each of the three measures in relationship to previous performance. For each goal, we also had Quality Improvement Teams that analyzed past performance and created several initiatives to improve performance. The overall score

for the mission priority was a weighted average of the three rates. The Senior Management Team set the weights based on the relative importance of improvement in the three areas of performance for that year.

Each year, priorities will again be set by the Senior Executive Team. As our market and competitive pressures warrant change and our system services evolve, mission priorities and the program will be adapted to support these changes. Once the goals are set at the beginning of the fiscal year, they are not changed for that year.

Employee Eligibility

Both regular and part-time employees in all departments including contracted employees in Environmental Services are eligible for the Performance Share program if they meet the following criteria:

- Have 3 months of service.
- Work the equivalent of 20 hours per week.
- Are employed when checks are distributed.
- Received at least a "meets expectations" at their last individual performance evaluation.
- Have no unresolved, written corrective actions pending at the end of the fiscal year.

Evaluation

The process for evaluating results is called the hospital "performance evaluation." We purposely use the same words we use for individual evaluations. The

CASE 14–1 *Continued*

Performance Share score sheet was developed to provide easy-to-understand feedback much like the forms we use for individual evaluations of employee performance. Each mission priority goal receives a score, and the combined total of all the scores indicates overall performance. Once per quarter, the Senior Executive Team issues a Performance Share report, which includes this score sheet detailing how the hospital is doing and projecting what bonus, if any will be paid if the same performance level continues. In essence, the better we perform the bigger the reward we earn. It is emphasized to all that the bonus is not guaranteed. We have to meet or exceed our goals in order to earn the reward.

The program has been extremely successful and employees eagerly await the results of each quarter's Performance Share report. The report is mailed to their homes. It consists of a letter from the President/CEO providing an organizational update on changes such as new programs, construction progress report, or care delivery system changes. Also included in this letter is some discussion of the performance targets and the areas that need more emphasis, along with those in which we are doing well. Other items included in the report are the key strategic initiatives and their goals for the fiscal year, and quarterly statistical highlights on progress toward goals shown in graphs. The report on Performance Share is also included with the score sheet, a summary of the financial operating results, and a snapshot of where we are now and what we are doing to try to achieve our goals. This report provides all employees with a comprehensive update. Our assumption is that all employees are interested in Holy Cross, its plans for the future, its financial health, and the reasons for current changes. We believe this helps them to see how their work contributes to the system's success. At the end of the year, each employee will have a very good notion of where we stand and whether our performance will result in a personal bonus.

We are in our third year of the Performance Share Program. Expectations have been met in two successive years and employees have been rewarded with bonus checks. Performance Share is not the only change in benefits that has been instituted under the new administration.

■ PAID TIME OFF

Another program that has been successful is the Paid Time Off (PTO) program. The goal of this program was to recognize the diversity of individual employee needs in order to manage time off more effectively and, thereby, reduce unscheduled time off. In order to achieve this goal, categories of time off were discontinued. Instead, everyone would have a "pool" of time to use for all purposes. This would include holidays, vacation, personal time, and sick leave. The end result was that employees would not have to be sick or have a personal crisis to use all their "paid time off" benefits. On average, employees would have more time off with the new program. Paid time off would accumulate by days worked, just as before.

CASE 14–1 *Continued*

Transition

The new PTO pool created for each employee consisted of: (1) current accumulated vacation days, (2) 2 new days, and (3) 7 days of sick leave. Employees would accumulate PTO days on a sliding scale that increased with tenure at Holy Cross. This was consistent with previous policy that those with more tenure had more vacation days. The nine paid holidays a year currently given would be added to the employee's PTO pool as they occurred, resulting in no loss of paid holidays. Any sick days presently accumulated over seven would be kept in an account that could be used only for future illnesses.

Procedures

The bottom line is that the PTO can be used for any purpose the employee desires. Lame excuses are no longer needed to "justify" a sick day. All employees are encouraged to schedule time off in advance to help the team remain productive overall. The same procedures established before the PTO program are followed for longer vacations and high-priority holidays to distribute work and time off fairly among the team members. Scheduled time off does not have to be taken as full days; allowing hours off allows employees to go to a medical or other appointment and not "use up" a full day. Employees must use at least 100 hours of PTO each year. This is to prevent burnout and ensure that all employees take some personal time away from the stresses of work. An employee can also "save" up to 880 hours and sell it back for cash when he or she leaves the organization. As an incentive to "save hours," employees earn interest over time on unused PTO time. The program applies to both full-time and part-time employees, but not to on-call only or temporary employees. PTO time can only be used after 3 months of employment. No PTO time can be used "in advance"; PTO time must be earned in order to use it.

For disabilities over 30 days and less than 150 days, the hospital has a short-term disability program. After 30 days of illness and when all PTO days have been exhausted, the short-term disability plan reimburses 60 percent of pay; this continues until the long-term disability plan kicks in at 5 months.

The Senior Executive Team has seen closer embodiment of the "One Team One Spirit" vision at Holy Cross since the changes in performance appraisal and benefits. The direct communication with each employee about organizational goals, initiatives, and expectations by both middle management and top management has clarified employee expectations and the issues and challenges facing the system. The involvement of representatives from all departments in designing how to implement and communicate the new changes has increased the sense of contribution by each employee in facilitating implementation. We expect each employee to contribute to our financial, customer satisfaction, and operational effectiveness. By changing how compensation and benefits are distributed we have at-

CASE 14–1 *Continued*

tempted to align rewards and expectations. Employees have expressed satisfaction with the recognition of different personal needs of employees and the new flexibility that the Paid Time Off (PTO) program has provided. Those with young children can take a few hours off for a special school event, those with elderly family members can take time off to take them for medical appointments, others can more flexibly plan for recreational activities. The new individual performance appraisal system has clarified the value of outstanding performance to the organization. The Performance Share program has emphasized the need to all work together in turbulent times for the system to not only survive, but thrive. The yearly celebrations visibly mark our successes.

■ BIOGRAPHICAL SKETCH

Carolyn A. Taylor is assistant vice president INOVA Health Systems, associate administrator/chief nurse executive for INOVA Alexandria and INOVA Mount Vernon Hospitals. She previously served in the position of Director, Maternal Child Health Services at Holy Cross Hospital in Silver Spring, Maryland. Ms. Taylor had the responsibility of providing leadership for the largest birthing service in the state of Maryland (the second-largest in the region). She is active in many professional associations and serves on state-wide task forces and committees committed to enhancing the health care of women and children. Ms. Taylor acts as a preceptor for nursing administration graduate students from several universities and is a faculty associate at George Mason University and The John Hopkins University. She also frequently presents at local and regional conferences on women's health issues, managed care, management and leadership, and financial planning for nurses.

15

Evaluation, Quality, and Outcomes

Barbara Barth Frink

The practices and policies of health care are the subject of daily news in the United States. Rapid changes in health care systems, the reorganization of provider groups, the effectiveness or noneffectiveness of certain operations or interventions are as likely to be featured in the *Wall Street Journal,* the *New York Times,* or your local paper as in the *Journal of the American Medical Association* or the *New England Journal of Medicine.* Television news and the burgeoning effect of the Internet contribute to a new public and consumer awareness of health care issues, both financial and clinical.

Regardless of your location of practice, it is highly likely that there have been recent changes in relationships among health care organizations in your locale. Former competitors are aligned, or in business together, and agencies—newly created or never before noticed—have become competitors. These business and relationship changes in communities influence how we think about quality, clinical processes of care, and outcomes. The newly formed "integrated delivery systems" create a different framework for thinking about measurement and quality and outcomes. How do you define the "episode of care"? When is it appropriate to measure outcomes? New market relationships including mergers, consortia, consolidations, or integrations rapidly convert today's outcome data into tomorrow's baseline data.

The purpose of this chapter is to describe essential components of clinical program evaluation for patient care administrators or senior clinicians in the context of clinical performance improvement and outcomes management. Components include: conceptual components of quality and outcomes, issues in risk adjustment, requirements for information systems to support quality, and principles of program evaluation.

I use the term "patient care administrator" in an inclusive sense. Persons in nursing administration roles have varying levels of responsibilities in clinical care. Nursing administration often encompasses the management of patient care services beyond that of nursing care delivery, as coordination of services is an integral part of any nursing role. If you have a strong clinical background, it will enrich your understanding and skills in conducting clinical program evaluation. If you have been more focused on health care management, linking with strong senior clinicians in your administrative practice will contribute greatly to the conduct of clinical program evaluation.

■ CONTEMPORARY CONTEXT FOR ADMINISTRATIVE PRACTICE

Changing relationships among providers, payors, and patients are creating new challenges for clinicians and patient care administrators. At both national and local levels, health care programs, delivery methods, and providers are the focus of inquiry concerning quality, cost, outcomes, efficiency, effectiveness, and equity. Demands for data to support claims of quality and outcome are escalating. This is a direct effect arising from the national emphasis on health care cost escalation and subsequent attempts to control costs through national policies (Gaus, 1995; Steinwachs, 1992).

The financial underwriting of health care services by employers, third-party payors, and the federal government provided a major incentive during the "cost containment era" in health care (1970–1983) to identify methods that would assist all parties, including patients, to make rational decisions regarding health care and health care resources. The strategy of collecting, analyzing, and publishing clinical care process data and resulting clinical and financial outcomes has been used to influence medical/clinical practices and direct or rationalize distribution of human and financial health care resources (Relman, 1988; Roper et al., 1988).

Linking your practice and program evaluations to the strategic imperatives of your organization can be critical to establishing the credibility and value of the evaluation results. At a minimum, understanding the strategic imperatives facing your organization is a vital part of conducting relevant and compelling clinical program evaluations. Identifying key areas that form the context for the evaluation can be done by asking questions such as: What are the market forces (local, state, and national) affecting the delivery system in which you practice? What is the managed care penetration of the local market? What are the key characteristics of provider groups in your region? What percentage of the case mix in your practice and organization is covered by indemnity plans, capitation, or global fee contracts? In which clinical care areas is your delivery system excelling? Who are the key stakeholder groups affecting your organization's strategies? Answers to these and similar questions help to define the strategic direction of the organization or practice, and provide the context for the clinical program evaluation.

■ STRATEGIES

Key strategies for competing in a managed care environment are to: (1) reduce variation in clinical care processes, (2) maintain a clinical and financial risk management program, (3) improve clinical and service quality, and (4) measure and manage outcomes. Well-conducted and disseminated clinical program evaluations are one mechanism whereby these strategies can be implemented. The patient care administrator must understand the theoretical concepts underlying quality: clinical care structures, processes, outcomes, effectiveness, equity, and efficiency.

The following competencies are not intended to be all-inclusive, but will provide the administrator or senior clinician with a reference point for competence and continued development. These core competencies should enable nurse administrators and senior clinicians to assume leadership in demonstrating clinical and service quality, provide valid information for sound fiscal planning, and contribute to positive outcomes for patients and organizations. Patient care administrators must be able to:

- Define, procure, or evaluate information systems required to support evidence-based care, and/or clinical performance improvement.
- Lead clinical or system interdisciplinary performance improvement teams that can demonstrate positive patient outcomes and system efficiencies.
- Evaluate the effectiveness of practice or system changes on patient and system clinical and financial outcomes.
- Participate in descriptive, analytical, or evaluation research on effectiveness and outcomes.
- Recognize the influence of public and health policy on the health care system.

■ CONCEPTUAL COMPONENTS OF QUALITY AND OUTCOMES

The theoretical framework supporting the work on quality, effectiveness, and clinical outcomes is health services research. The basic concepts are not new. Nightingale (1863) is reported to be one of the first administrators of clinical services to use statistics demonstrating the relationship of practice to outcomes. Her use of graphical display in presenting statistical data is still instructive today. Health services research as a discipline has developed considerably since the 1970s. The study of interventions and their effect on clinical outcomes, effectiveness, and quality, and the evaluation of practice guidelines and clinical/critical pathways are major areas of current health services research (Aydin, Bolton, & Weingarten, 1995). The Institute of Medicine defines health services research as "inquiry to produce knowledge about the structure, processes, or effects of personal health services" (1979, p. 14). Personal health services are composed of provider–consumer relationships and are, therefore, within the scope of the health care (medical) system. Theories from economic, behavioral, sociological, and biological science contribute to the conduct of health services research.

As the field has developed over the last 20 years, some of the language and terminology has changed or become more refined. Because health services research is primarily the domain of academic researchers and has its own language that is not widely used in practice, this chapter will use the terminology of quality, effectiveness, and outcomes, which are used by both researchers and those with a clinical, administrative, and/or policy orientation.

Although the term *patient outcomes* is generally spoken of as an entity unto itself, it is important to understand that clinical patient outcomes come from combining two very different philosophical and academic traditions in health care. The first is the biomedical/basic science model and the second is the social science/health economic model. "This fundamental difference in the scientific roots of patient outcomes adds to the complexity of using outcome data to improve clinical performance and to conduct outcomes research" (Frink & Strassner, 1996, p. 201). Differing interpretations of outcomes data may be influenced by these different scientific traditions, which may also, in turn, influence performance improvement activities (Brooten & Naylor, 1995). Wilson and Cleary (1995) provide an excellent discussion of the influences of these different scientific roots on shaping issues related to linking clinical outcomes to quality of life outcomes.

The biomedical model of health care has intellectual roots in biology, biochemistry, and physiology (see Fig. 15–1). Randomized clinical trials of new practices are the preferred research methodology of this model. Desired bio-

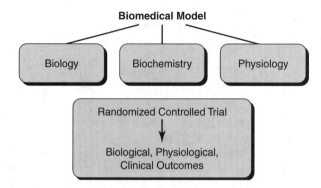

FIGURE 15–1. The biomedical model of outcomes. *(Source: Courtesy of Barbara Frink, The Johns Hopkins Hospital, Baltimore, MD; adapted from Wilson & Cleary [1995].)*

logical, physiological, and clinical outcomes are those supported by research using this biomedical model (Heithoff & Lohr, 1990; Wilson & Cleary, 1995).

The social science model, which is sometimes referred to as the quality of life model of health care, has its intellectual roots in sociology, psychology, and economics (see Fig. 15–2). The measurement of complex behavior, feelings, attitudes, dimensions of functioning, and well-being are the primary research methodologies of this tradition. Therefore, patient outcomes such as health status, functional status, or mental status result from the quality of life model of patient outcomes (Wilson & Cleary, 1995).

The most recent health services and health policy emphasis on effectiveness and outcomes research is based on the conceptual work of Donabedian (1966, 1973, 1980, 1982, 1988), Wennberg (Wennberg & Gittelsohn, 1973; Wennberg, 1984; Wennberg et al., 1988; Fisher & Wennberg, 1990), and Brook (Brook et al., 1983; Brook & Lohr, 1985). The work of these researchers has significantly influenced recent national health policy. An analysis of their work is beyond the scope of this chapter; however, the reader will find a rich history of recent policy trends by investigation of these citations. Concepts representing the various researcher's perspectives are found in the following terms: an epidemiology of health (Milio, 1983), an epidemiology of medical care (Brook & Lohr, 1985), clinical evaluation sciences (Wennberg, 1990), outcomes management (Ellwood, 1988), and era of accountability (Relman, 1988).

Health services research is rich in the integration and collaboration of distinct disciplines arising from different scientific traditions. This wealth, however, has given rise to the use of common or similar terms that may have different interpretations, depending on the orientation of the discipline. For that reason, basic definitions are included here as a reference point.

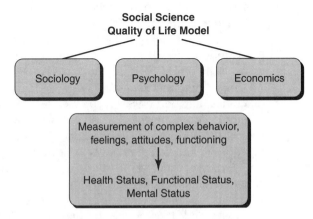

FIGURE 15–2. The social science model of outcomes. *(Source: Courtesy of Barbara Frink, The Johns Hopkins Hospital, Baltimore, MD; adapted from Wilson & Cleary [1995].)*

Definitions

- *Case management*—a multidisciplinary clinical system that uses registered nurses to coordinate the care for specific groups of patients across a continuum of the episode of care. Examples of technology tools of case management are health screening and risk assessment instruments, critical paths, practice guidelines, clinical algorithms, and clinical paths (Frink & Strassner, 1996).
- *Clinical algorithm*—"a flow diagram that consists of branching-logic pathways which permit the application of carefully defined criteria to the task of identifying or classifying different types of [clinical] entities" (Hadorn, 1994, p. 93).
- *Clinical care process management*—a process equivalent to case management. Inherent in "managing" the care process is systematic data collection, outcomes, analysis, feedback, and monitoring with resultant reduction of irrelevant variables and process variation. Thus, operations (management) becomes closely related to research; the link is established between the delivery of care and the outcome (James & Eddy, 1994).
- *Critical paths*—also called care maps, are "extensions of practice guidelines concepts; they are a set of interdisciplinary recommendations for care of a specific condition in a temporal model" for operational environments (Frink & Strassner, 1996, p. 194).
- *Effectiveness*—the actual achieved benefits of health care interventions and services for individuals and populations. The basic principle of effectiveness research is that studying the relationships between structure, process, and outcomes of clinical care will determine the indicators of quality (Aday et al., 1993; Brook & Lohr, 1985).
- *Efficacy*—the benefits that are achievable from care under ideal or controlled conditions, such as a randomized controlled trial (Aday et al., 1993; Heithoff & Lohr, 1990).
- *Outcomes assessment*—the examination of the linkages between structures and processes of care/interventions and both of these to outcomes (Ellwood, 1988).
- *Outcomes management*—the study and improvement of health care outcomes. Ellwood (1988) recommended a plan for outcomes management: (1) Development of standards and guidelines, (2) Routine, widespread measurement of disease-specific clinical outcomes and patient functioning and well-being, (3) Collection of clinical and outcome data on a massive scale, (4) Analysis and dissemination of findings from a continually expanding database" (p. 55).
- *Practice guidelines*—descriptions of "best" or recommended care processes and, thus, a specific mechanism for managing clinical care processes (James & Eddy, 1994). Practice guidelines have varying specificity. Guidelines are developed through application of one or

several formal methodologies; however, the primary focus is on the analytic work: examination of scientific evidence, expert opinion, clinical experience, and decision rules (Woolfe, 1994, p. 105).

- Quality—an attribute of the clinical care process; that is, the right process or care delivered and the extent to which it is correctly delivered. Quality is also the measure of the gap between efficacy and effectiveness: what is achieved versus what is achievable (Aday et al., 1993; Brook & Lohr, 1985).

As you design and/or implement a clinical program evaluation in the context of quality, effectiveness, and outcomes, be explicit in defining your terms. Quality, outcomes, outcomes management, evaluative research, and effectiveness research may be related but are not the same. Similarly, risk, severity, intensity, and case mix are also related concepts, but differ in meaning. Lack of precision in discussions of program evaluation findings with payors, contractors, financial analysts, administrators, and clinicians can have serious consequences.

■ RISK ADJUSTMENT

Although significant attention has been focused, nationally and in health policy circles, on the measurement of patient clinical outcomes and health care outcomes, less attention has been paid to an equally critical factor, that of the adjustment for patient risks for various outcomes (Iezzoni, 1994). Quality, outcomes, and effectiveness studies all require the drawing of inferences about effectiveness of the particular intervention or clinical care process on the clinical outcomes for a patient or a group of patients. There are many complexities in the measurement of such outcomes (Eddy & Hasselblad, 1994), but there are equally as many complexities in being able to account for the patient risk or risk adjustment for those outcomes. Thus, to discuss patient outcomes without also discussing a methodology for risk adjustment is a serious methodological flaw and will likely result in nongeneralizable or noncomparable data.

The primary goal of risk adjustment in quality studies is to account for patient characteristics that may have direct bearing on outcomes, before drawing inferences about the effectiveness or outcomes of care. Risk adjustment in randomized clinical trials (efficacy studies) is controlled by inclusion and exclusion criteria for the studies, as well as by random assignment to control and experimental groups. Randomized trials are most often conducted prospectively while effectiveness studies may be conducted retrospectively. Effectiveness studies that use national data sets, such as Medicare data or Blue Cross data, are conducted retrospectively. Such studies, by definition, do not allow the use of either a standardized protocol or random assignment, and are often population based versus sample based. When using efficacy or effectiveness study results as a "best practice" comparison in a clinical program evaluation, it is important to know what methods were used to stratify the sample or population for risk.

Blumberg (1986) describes the risk adjustment objective as follows, "Risk adjustment is a way to remove or reduce the effects of confounding factors in studies where cases are not randomly assigned to different treatments. The key confounding factors are those aspects of health status that are causally related to the outcome under study" (p. 355).

Severity of Illness

As outcomes data are more in demand for health care decisions, there is an increasing demand for outcomes data that have been risk adjusted. A subset of risk adjustment that is familiar to most clinicians is severity of illness. Most of the current work in severity of illness has been conducted on severity systems that quantify risk of short-term outcomes for acutely ill hospitalized patients (Iezzoni, 1994). However, as health care delivery and clinical care processes have become integrated across different delivery sites, and as providers have begun to assume some financial risk in care, other methods of risk stratification for populations in ambulatory care or geographic communities have been developed (Lawthers et al., 1993; Weiner, Starfield, Steinwachs, & Mumford, 1991).

Severity of illness, although often used as a unidimensional term, is a multidimensional concept. The term *severity* often refers to acute episodes of illness. However, severity measurement systems differ in focus. Stein and associates (1987) classified severity of illness measures in three categories: (1) severity that is focused on the intensity of the resources consumed during a defined episode of illness, such as technology, cost, and length of hospital stay; (2) severity that is based on physiological or clinical definitions, including physiological stability, probability of mortality, and functional status; and (3) severity of illness defined as burden of illness.

Patient care administrators must understand that risk adjustment is a complex field of study and that each severity or risk adjustment system has its own criteria, definitions, and measurement algorithm. Whenever possible, it is prudent to use well-tested, research-based, risk measurement systems in patient outcomes and effectiveness studies. It is also important for the administrator to understand that many risk adjustment systems or severity of illness systems are case-mix specific. That is, they have been designed for the use of a particular patient population, such as oncology, cardiac care, or intensive care specialties, and thus need to be retested if used in broader populations. Clinical outcome information is currently being used by many provider groups, health plans, and regulatory groups to publish report cards that compare cost and clinical performance of providers or health care systems with each other (Joint Commission, 1995; O'Kane, 1996). This new level of competition within health care has increased the focus on understanding risk adjustment systems and applying them appropriately in the practice area.

Examples of key patient characteristics to consider in risk adjustment are primary diagnosis, co-morbidities, measures of severity, functional status, demographics of the population, health status, psychosocial well-being, gender, and age (Iezzoni, 1994). The focus of the effectiveness study or clinical program evaluation will inform the selection of appropriate risk stratification measures. Pauly (1992) reports that the state of the science in the appropriateness and effectiveness of care reveals three major weaknesses: (1) initial severity (of illness) is not accurately measured, (2) the full array of outcomes are not captured, and (3) valid statistical methods are not always applied.

Clinical program evaluation based on principles of evaluation and conducted in the context of quality, effectiveness, and outcomes can be a powerful tool to meet strategic needs in a dynamic health care organization or clinical practice. It is essential that the patient care administrator and senior clinician have an understanding of basic principles of evaluation, as well as specific knowledge of clinical program goals and outcomes.

■ BASIC PRINCIPLES OF PROGRAM EVALUATION

Aspects of traditional program evaluation are reflective of a performance improvement process. According to Salasin and associates (1980), the defining characteristics of program evaluation are:

- Evaluative information is structured and set within a given context.
- The evaluation describes or answers questions about a real-life activity or set of activities according to a theory or criteria.
- Effects are described against standards.
- Evaluation provides a feedback route in a continuing process of program development, implementation, and refinement.
- The evaluation tests activities against values assigned by others.

It is important to determine the organizational level and context of the program evaluation in which you are participating or that you are conducting. When establishing the evaluation team, it is important to select participants who have credibility at the level of the organization in which the evaluation is occurring. There are always stakeholders involved in any evaluation. When defining the evaluation plan, consider key stakeholder issues. Why is the evaluation being conducted? How is the evaluation being conducted? How are the results to be used? Who is interested in the results and why? What resources are available to conduct and disseminate the evaluation findings?

Ideally the evaluation is planned during the program development phase. Expected outcomes of any program evaluation are that there will be decisions made as a result. Examples of possible decision outcomes are:

continue the program in its present format; alter the program; increase or decrease the program budget; change the program or its management to improve the probability of success; alter the program policies; build support with policy makers or other constituent groups (Salasin et al., 1980; Schalock, 1995).

Two other general concepts of program evaluation that may be familiar terms to the reader are formative evaluation and summative evaluation. Formative evaluation occurs throughout the conduct of a program, and summative occurs at the program's end or at a specified completion point (such as one year after implementation). However, summative evaluation can occur at key points within the program evaluation as well (Schalock, 1995).

Formative evaluation is the assessment of potential problems and identification of areas for improvement while the program is being conducted. Description and monitoring of program activities, including measurement of progress toward goal achievement and recommendations for midcourse corrections, are common characteristics of formative evaluation. The key focus of a formative evaluation is program improvement, efficiency, and effectiveness. The reader will quickly identify that these concepts and activities are similar to performance improvement concepts.

In contrast, key characteristics of summative evaluation include a summary of program effectiveness, description of the program, achievement of the program goals, unanticipated outcomes, and comparisons with other programs. Describing the possible consequences if the program you are evaluating had not been implemented can provide a helpful perspective and is often overlooked. Outcomes of a summative evaluation include value judgments regarding the worth of the program and conclusions regarding the effectiveness and the detail of the program accomplishments against some goal (Schalock, 1995).

Another conceptualization of traditional program evaluation is that of Stecher and Davis (1987). This publication is part of an excellent reference module published by Sage. The module includes handbooks, sample instruments, and reference materials for designing, implementing, and evaluating programs (Stecher & Davis, 1987). Stecher and Davis describe five major categories of evaluation models: experimental, goal-oriented, decision-focused, user-oriented, and responsive models. Of these models, the goal oriented is the most similar to performance improvement. For that reason, it may be one of the most valuable to include as a part of a clinical program evaluation.

In the goal-oriented evaluation, program-specific goals and objectives are the criteria for measuring success. Usually the goals are tied to specific outcomes and measurable terms are used to express objectives. The instruments used to measure the concepts are very specific and statistics are used for evaluating the program outcomes. Specific strengths of the goal-oriented evaluation are: (1) logical relationships are established between the objectives and the activities, and (2) emphasis is on the most important aspects of the program. Weaknesses include: (1) the risk of missing unintended outcomes or consequences of the program that fall outside the goals and objectives, and (2) an evaluation that is too narrowly focused (Stecher & Davis, 1987).

■ GUIDING PRINCIPLES FOR CLINICAL PROGRAM EVALUATION

In today's competitive environment, it is of critical importance that senior clinicians and patient care administrators be able to conduct well-defined and valid clinical program evaluations. They must be able to articulate evaluation findings and implications to policy makers at the organizational, regulatory, local, regional, or national level.

Process

Some guiding principles for conducting clinical program evaluations are:

1. Pick areas to evaluate that are of strategic importance in your practice field or organization. Identify the clinical processes or interventions that are high cost, high volume, or high risk. Risk may be defined at the patient, population, or organizational level.
2. Link the evaluation to the purpose, specifications, design, and perhaps even contractual issues of the clinical program itself.
3. Design the evaluation at the same time as the clinical program is designed.
4. Identify the criteria that define success of the program. How will you know if the clinical program was successful and to what degree the goals were achieved? Is the program equally successful in the perspective of each stakeholder group?
5. Consider interdisciplinary and interdepartmental participation in comprising a steering committee or an evaluation team. In addition, it may be appropriate to include financial, clinical, and operations experts as well. Academic health services researchers can be helpful consultants or team members.
6. Consider including recipients of the clinical program services in the evaluation process, whether they be patients representing constituent populations or members of the health care plan. Other parties such as vendors, clients, and third-party payors may provide valuable input to the evaluation.

Methods

The methods of the evaluation should be carefully considered during the design phase. What are the resources that will be required to conduct the evaluation? Consider human resources, material, and technology resources. Technology resources should include specification of the information management for the evaluation. Identify the cost of the resources during the design phase.

Use conceptually, theoretically based measures that are known to be reliable and valid. Generic measures are tested to be broadly applicable across cultures, diseases, conditions, and populations. In contrast, patient or case-mix specific measures are tested to detect "clinically important changes" in the specific case-mix population. Both types of measures have value in clinical practice, research, and policy formulation and analysis (Patrick, 1990).

Outcomes

What is the payoff of the evaluation? Be careful to consider the cost of the evaluation information versus the scope and the power of findings. It is possible to spend as much time evaluating a clinical program as it costs to implement the program! Be sure to include the costs of ongoing formative or summative evaluation in a total cost analysis of the program.

Consider the audiences or stakeholders to whom the outcomes will be reported and what will be done with the findings. Are the findings to be used to improve the clinical program itself? Are they to be implemented to inform policy makers, a governing board, or regulatory agencies? Will the findings be used in a continuous performance improvement process? Is it a summative evaluation that has no further application?

■ INFORMATION SYSTEM INFRASTRUCTURE TO SUPPORT QUALITY AND OUTCOMES

The demand for greater clinical and fiscal accountability is intrinsically linked to information management and system infrastructure. Building an infrastructure to support evidence-based care is a complex interdisciplinary administrative role (Frink & Johnson, 1996). If you are fortunate to practice in a setting where a well-designed infrastructure exists, then knowledge of effective use of data and information systems will enhance your abilities to compete on cost, quality, and outcomes. However, many organizations have an eclectic information systems infrastructure. Often, systems are adequate for departmental transactions, but have little connectivity across departmental lines. System mergers and integrations occur more rapidly than the integration of separate existing information systems. In addition, the databases have been defined around business processes, not clinical processes.

In the past, the business process was the correct focus for defining and monitoring the revenue stream for services. However, as health care financing changes from a revenue base to a cost base, the information needs and required data elements change. Revenue systems are evaluated by the departmental unit of analysis, and information systems are designed accordingly. Success is realized through enhancing and managing the revenue. In a cost environment, where the provider shares or assumes the risk, the departmental unit of analysis is no longer appropriate. The focus moves immediately to the "process" of care, regardless of location of delivery (James & Eddy, 1994). Care processes may cross departmental, institutional, or geographical lines. Information systems must be designed quite differently. They must include clinical, financial, and human resource data systems that are not bound by traditional transaction relationships or location of service. The contribution of such information systems to managing costs and clinical care processes should be evaluated; little evaluative information is currently available (Steinwachs, 1992).

Cost justification of information technologies may fall within your domain as a patient care administrator. Basic principles to consider are: (1) information technologies require both capital and human resources; (2) both system development *and* maintenance require investment; and (3) system justification should include an estimate of risk exposure if the system is not implemented (Frink & Johnson, 1996, p. 4). Risk exposure should not be underestimated. Be as clear as possible in defining the risks if reliable, valid clinical process and outcome data are not available for managing aspects of the case mix or covered lives for which your organization is assuming health care risk.

Clinical program evaluation should include information system infrastructure or support. Objectives for the evaluation may include: the structure of data and data categories; the cost–benefit of data collection, capture, and analysis; and justification of new technologies. Conformity to industry or institutional standards for information system architecture, platform, and design should be clearly documented and departures from standards cost justified (Frink & Johnson, 1996, p. 2).

Networks are another component of the transforming health care environments. Electronic networks and telemedicine spanning rural to urban, primary care to tertiary/quaternary care, and providers to payors, create technological and policy challenges. These systems will not only include transaction processes (such as physician orders; result reports; and admission, discharge, transfers [ADT]), but also clinical algorithms, individualized patient education, and patient-specific clinical databases and repositories. Issues of security, access, equity, and confidentiality require public policy debate and guidelines. Wireless technologies will likely be an integral part of clinical information system infrastructures, providing gateways into the network.

■ SUMMARY

Outcomes research will not necessarily decrease the cost of health care, but it will provide rationality to decisions about what comprises appropriate care, thereby improving efficiency in the use of health care resources and in quality of care (Aaron, 1990; Stobo, 1990). The importance of clinical program evaluation in the context of a very competitive health care environment and quality, effectiveness, and outcomes programs is the major focus of this chapter. Key strategies, core patient care administrator competencies, trends, and scientific roots of effectiveness and outcomes work were presented. Basic principles of program evaluation and clinical program evaluation were reviewed. An adequate information systems infrastructure was presented as a key requirement for conducting both clinical program evaluations and clinical quality outcomes monitoring and research. Health care delivery structures, health care financing mechanisms, clinical care processes, and information system technologies are in a state of change. Patient care administrators and senior clinicians are encouraged to master the basic principles and competencies of clinical quality improvement, requirements for information infrastructure, and clinical program evaluation. In doing so, they will make valuable contributions to the strategic aims of their organization and to the quality of care for patients and families.

■ BIOGRAPHICAL SKETCH

Barbara Barth Frink is the Director of Nursing Systems and Research at The Johns Hopkins Hospital and holds a faculty appointment at The Johns Hopkins University School of Nursing. She has administrative oversight for nursing performance improvement, education, clinical research, systems research, and nursing informatics at the Johns Hopkins Hospital. Dr. Frink was a Special Expert in Nursing Systems at the National Institute of Nursing Research at the National Institutes of Health in 1993–1994, and for several years she was the Director of Nursing Research and Development at the Children's Hospital National Medical Center in Washington, D.C. She received her PhD from the University of Pennsylvania in Nursing Administration with a related field in Decision Sciences. Her masters degree, from Boston College, is in Community Health/Community Mental Health Nursing. Dr. Frink has published in the areas of nursing administration, development of infrastructure to support quality measurement, nursing informatics, and health care technology assessment. Her research interests focus on the clinical and economic outcomes for patients and systems in rapidly changing environments.

■ SUGGESTED READINGS

Aydin, C.E., Bolton, L.B., & Weingarten, S. (Eds.) (1995). *Patient focused care in the hospital: Restructuring and redesign methods to achieve better outcomes.* Washington, DC: Faulkner & Gray.

Brooten, D., & Naylor, M.D. (1995). Nurses' effect on changing patient outcomes. *Journal of Nursing Scholarship, 27,* 95–99.

Program evaluation kit. (1987). Thousand Oaks, CA: Sage.

Schalock, R.L. (1995). *Outcome-based evaluation.* New York: Plenum Press.

■ REFERENCES

Aaron, H.J. (1990). The need for reasonable expectations. In K.A. Heithoff & K.N. Lohr (Eds.), *Effectiveness and outcomes in health care* (pp. 215–217). Washington, DC: National Academy Press.

Aday, L.A., Begley, C.E., Lairson, D.R., & Slater, C.H. (1993). *Evaluating the medical care system: Effectiveness, efficiency, and equity.* Ann Arbor, MI: Health Administration Press.

Aydin, C.E., Bolton, L.B., & Weingarten, S. (1995). Patient focused care, clinical practice guidelines, and outcomes research: Essential links in a changing health care environment. In C.E. Aydin, L.B. Bolton, & S. Weingarten (Eds.), *Patient focused care in the hospital: Restructuring and redesign methods to achieve better outcomes* (pp. 1–13). Washington, DC: Faulkner & Gray.

Blumberg, M.S. (1986). Risk adjusting health care outcomes: A methodologic review. *Medical Care Review, 43* (2), 351–393.

Brook, R., & Lohr, K. (1985). Efficacy, effectiveness, variations, and quality: Boundary-crossing research. *Medical Care, 23 (supp.),* 710–722.

Brook, R., Ware, J., Rogers, W., Keeler, E., Davies, A., Donald, C., Goldberg, G., Lohr, K., Masthay, P., & Newhouse, J. (1983). Does free care improve adults' health? Results from a randomized controlled trial. *New England Journal of Medicine, 309,* 1426–1434, 1453.

Brooten, D., & Naylor, M.D. (1995). Nurses' effect on changing patient outcomes. *Journal of Nursing Scholarship, 27,* 95–99.

Donabedian, A. (1966). Evaluating the quality of medical care. *Milbank Memorial Fund Quarterly, 44* (part 2), 166–206.

Donabedian, A. (1973). *Aspects of medical care administration: Specifying requirements for health care.* Cambridge, MA: Harvard University Press.

Donabedian, A. (1980). *Explorations in quality assessment and monitoring. Volume I, the definition of quality and approaches to its assessment.* Ann Arbor, MI: Health Administration Press.

Donabedian, A. (1982). *Explorations in quality assessment and monitoring. Volume II, the criteria and standards of quality.* Ann Arbor, MI: Health Administration Press.

Donabedian, A. (1988). Quality assessment and assurance: Unity of purpose, diversity of means. *Inquiry, 25,* 173–192.

Eddy, D.M., & Hasselblad, V. (1994). Analyzing indirect evidence. In K.A. McCormick, S.R. Moore, & R. Siegel (Eds.), *Clinical practice guideline development: Methodology perspectives* (pp. 5–13). Rockville, MD: U.S. Department of Health and Human Services.

Ellwood, P. (1988). Shattuck lecture—outcomes management: A technology of patient experience. *New England Journal of Medicine, 318* (23), 1549–1556.

Fisher, E.S., & Wennberg, J.E. (1990). Administrative data in effectiveness studies: The prostatectomy assessment. In K.A. Heithoff & K.N. Lohr (Eds.), *Effectiveness and outcomes in health care.* Washington, DC: National Academy Press.

Frink, B.B., & Johnson, K. (1996). Infrastructure to support guidelines based pediatric care. *Quality improvement workshop proceedings.* Alexandria, VA: National Association of Children's Hospitals and Related Institutions.

Frink, B.B., & Strassner, L. (1996). Variance analysis. In D. Flarey & S.S. Blancett (Eds.), *Handbook of nursing case management: Health care delivery in a world of managed care* (pp. 194–223). Gaithersburg, MD: Aspen.

Gaus, C.R. (1995). Forward. In C.E. Aydin, L.B. Bolton, & S. Weingarten (Eds.), *Patient focused care in the hospital: Restructuring and redesign methods to achieve better outcomes* (pp. ix–x). Washington, DC: Faulkner & Gray.

Hadorn, D.C. (1994). Use of algorithms in clinical guideline development. In K.A. McCormick, S.R. Moore, & R. Siegel (Eds.), *Clinical practice guideline development: Methodology perspectives*. Rockville, MD: U.S. Department of Health and Human Services.

Heithoff, K.A., & Lohr, K.N. (1990). *Effectiveness and outcomes in health care*. Washington, DC: National Academy Press.

Iezzoni, L.I. (1994). *Risk adjustment for measuring health care outcomes*. Ann Arbor, MI: Health Administration Press.

Institute of Medicine. (1979). *Report on health services research*. Washington, DC: National Academy of Sciences.

James, B.C., & Eddy, D.M. (1994). CPI and practice guidelines. In S.D. Horn & D.S.P. Hopkins (Eds.), *Clinical practice improvement: A new technology for developing cost effective quality health care* (pp. 127–140). Washington, DC: Faulkner & Gray.

Joint Commission on Accreditation of Healthcare Organizations. (1995). *An introduction to the management of information standards for health care organizations*. Oakbrook Terrace, IL: JCAHO.

Lawthers, A.G., Palmer, R.H., Edwards, J.E., Fowles, J., Garnick, D.W., & Weiner, J.P. (1993). Developing and evaluating performance measures for ambulatory care quality: A preliminary report of the DEMPAQ project. *The Joint Commission Journal on Quality Improvement, 19* (12), 552–565.

Milio, N. (1983). *Primary care and the public's health*. Lexington, MA: Lexington Books.

Nightingale, F. (1863). *Notes on hospitals* (3rd ed.). London: Longman, Green, Longman, Roberts, & Green.

O'Kane, M.E. (1996). *President's letter. 1996 annual report*. Washington, DC: National Committee for Quality Assurance.

Patrick, D.L. (1990). Assessing health related quality of life outcomes. In K.A. Heithoff & K.N. Lohr (Eds.), *Effectiveness and outcomes in health care* (pp. 137–151). Washington, DC: National Academy Press.

Pauly, M. (1992). Effectiveness research and the impact of financial incentives on outcomes. In S.M. Shortell & U.E. Reinhardt (Eds.), *Improving health policy and management: Nine critical research issues for the 1990s* (pp. 151–193). Ann Arbor, MI: Health Administration Press.

Relman, A. (1988). Assessment and accountability: The third revolution in medical care. *New England Journal of Medicine, 319,* 1220–1222.

Roper, W.L., Winkenwerder, W., Hackbarth, G.M., & Krakauer, H. (1988). Effectiveness in health care: An initiative to evaluate and improve medical practice. *New England Journal of Medicine, 319* (18), 1197–1202.

Salasin et al. (1980). *The evaluation of federal research programs*. McLean, VA: MITRE Corporation.

Schalock, R.L. (1995). *Outcome-based evaluation*. New York: Plenum Press.

Stecher, B.M., & Davis, W.A. (1987). *How to focus a program evaluation*. Newberry Park, CA: Sage.

Stein, R.E., Gortmaker, S.L., Perrin, E.C., Perrin, J., Pless, I.B., Walker, D.K., & Weitzman, M. (1987). Severity of illness: Concepts and measurements. *The Lancet, II* (2), 1506–1509.

Steinwachs, D. (1992). Redesign of delivery systems to enhance productivity. In S.M. Shortell & U.E. Reinhardt (Eds.), *Improving health policy and management: Nine critical research issues for the 1990s* (pp. 275–310). Ann Arbor, MI: Health Administration Press.

Stobo, J.D. (1990). Gaining acceptance for effectiveness and outcomes research. In K.A. Heithoff & K.N. Lohr (Eds.), *Effectiveness and outcomes in health care* (pp. 224–226). Washington, DC: National Academy Press.

Weiner, J.P., Starfield, B.H., Steinwachs, D.M., & Mumford, L.M. (1991). Development and application of a population-oriented measure of ambulatory care case-mix. *Medical Care, 29* (5), 452–472.

Wennberg, J. (1984). Dealing with medical practice variations: A proposal for action. *Health Affairs, 3* (2), 6–32.

Wennberg, J., & Gittelsohn, A. (1973). Small area variations in health care delivery. *Science, 182,* 1102–1108.

Wennberg, L., Mulley, A., Hanley, D., Timothy, R., Fowler, F., Roos, N., Barry, M., McPherson, K., Greener, E.R., Soule, D., Bubolz, T., Fisher, E., & Malenka, D. (1988). An assessment of prostatectomy for benign urinary tract obstruction: Geographic variations and the evaluation of medical care outcomes. *Journal of the American Medical Association, 259,* 3027–3030.

Wennberg, J. (1990). Small area analysis and the medical care outcome problem. In L. Sechrest, B. Starfield, & J. Bunker (Eds.), *Research methodology: Strengthening causal interpretations of nonexperimental data.* Rockville, MD: Agency for health care policy and research.

Wilson, I.B., & Cleary, P.D. (1995). Linking clinical variables with health-related quality of life. *Journal of the American Medical Association, 273,* 59–65.

Woolfe, S.H. (1994). An organized analytic framework for practice guideline development: Using the analytic logic as a guide for reviewing evidence, developing recommendations, and explaining the rationale. In K.A. McCormick, S.R. Moore, & R. Siegel (Eds.), *Clinical practice guideline development: Methodology perspectives* (pp. 105–113). Rockville, MD: U.S. Department of Health and Human Services.

APPLICATION 15–1 Preparing for a JCAHO Accreditation Visit

Donna Richards Sheridan and Carol Ruth Yocum

"The Joint Commission is coming!" These words often elicit a sinking feeling and result in frantic activity by an organization's leaders, including the nurse executives, despite the fact that this event is predictable every 3 years. All too often, the Joint Commission for the Accreditation of Healthcare Organizations (JCAHO) survey preparation activities are accompanied by a sense of doom and feelings of inadequacy, reflected in comments heard from health care leaders, physicians, and clinical staff such as:

- "Like building obsolescence into automobiles, the Joint Commission changes standards every year. How can we ever expect to know them?"
- "What does this standard mean? I cannot understand the jargon."
- "One surveyor said we could comply if we did this, but another surveyor said that wouldn't work."
- "How can we expect to comply with 3,000 standards and still have time to provide quality care to our patients?"

Such fears and frustrations are understandable, considering that after days of intensive scrutiny, the JCAHO visit culminates in a summation conference open to any interested member of the staff, Boards, or public. Additionally, as of 1995, a small fee purchases a copy of any organization's score—the JCAHO Hospital Accreditation Decision Grid. This "report card" states how well the organization met basic accreditation standards. No one likes to look incompetent to peers, the public, competing hospital organizations, and especially managed care brokers. Thus, the challenge becomes—how can the organization's leadership, including the nurse in patient care administration, utilize an administrative process to thrive in a difficult marketplace while meeting accreditation standards? How can routine operating systems incorporate regulatory requirements so that a forthcoming visit by the JCAHO surveyors is met with calm confidence and the outcome is accepted with a sense of pride and accomplishment?

The purpose of this case application is to preclude the need for frantic, last-minute preparation. By defining organizational direction and strategies, then integrating JCAHO standards into daily operations, the ineffective last minute "crunch" is avoided. Illustrations and tools that follow have been tested by nurse executives, health care organization leaders, and quality management professionals. The four steps outlined in Table 15–1 will effectively enhance operational effectiveness while facilitating ongoing successful survey preparation management.

■ GOALS AND ASSOCIATED ORGANIZATIONAL STRUCTURES/PROCESSES

The first step for any leadership group preparing for a successful JCAHO visit is

APPLICATION 15–1 *Continued*

TABLE 15–1. Four Steps for Improving Operational Effectiveness and Preparing for a Successful Survey

---

1. Identify the goal for the survey visit and set up organizational structures/processes essential to success.
2. Integrate common themes of the JCAHO standards into daily operations. Share knowledge throughout the organization.
3. Use survey preparation tools and resources effectively.
4. Approach the survey in an organized and systematic manner.

---

to define your ideal survey goal. Before 1995, the ideal survey goal for most leaders was simply to ensure at the time of the survey that *their* department received no Type 1 Recommendations (Berwick, 1990). The leaders in nursing administration were concerned only with standards that applied to nursing services, the pharmacy director was concerned only about compliance to pharmacy department standards, and so on. Accreditation compliance was easily achieved through this compartmentalized approach. Survey preparation was generally viewed as a clear but onerous task that added to the "real work" of providing care to the patient and "running" the department. Accreditation standards were more tolerable as accountability was confined within departments and the "problem" surfaced only every 3 years.

The Joint Commission, hearing complaints from member organizations, recognized that this triannual flurry of preparation for the accreditation process did not make a difference in how medical and health care services were provided. Care providers and hospital leaders had little motivation to correct long-standing organizational problems. Furthermore, when organized, and accredited under "departmental standards," no incentive existed to provide an efficient patient flow through a variety of services while minimizing cost. Departmental standards actually fueled common management problems such as "turf" issues, fragmentation of care, and resource competition. In response to recognizing that the accreditation standards were having little impact on the goal of positively effecting outcomes of patient care in hospitals, JCAHO looked to the expanding process improvement knowledge from business management practices. Continuous quality improvement processes such as total quality management (Joint Commission, 1996) focused on customer needs and expectations while integrating, rather than departmentalizing, services to meet those customer needs and achieve measurable outcomes. The Joint Commission leadership forged an "Agenda for Change," and "the Joint Commission has worked to bring accreditation in line with a rapidly evolving health care environment that focuses more on outcomes and processes than structures" (Joint Commission, 1995d, p. 24). The "Agenda for Change" has created accreditation standards that are *patient centered* and *performance focused*. The standards are designed to help organizations "focus on the patient, doing the right things well in a multidisciplinary, organization wide manner" (Joint Commission, 1995b, p. 6).

The Joint Commission believes that its standards should:

APPLICATION 15–1 *Continued*

- Focus on those functions and aspects of patient care that are essential to quality patient care and a safe care environment.
- Apply to all organizations and across all services.
- Represent a consensus on the state of the art in the organization performance expected.
- State (to the extent possible) objectives or principles, rather than specific processes, for meeting requirements.
- Be reasonable and achievable.
- Be survivable.

In 1995, the Joint Commission rolled out its completely revised hospital standards. These standards are patient centered, performance focused and organized around functions common to all health care organizations (JCAHO, 1995a).

What, then, is the major impact of the "Agenda for Change" on your organization's choice of an overall goal for the JCAHO survey visit? The "Agenda for Change" shifted how leadership should approach not the just management of the survey, but the very management of the organization.

Accreditation standards *all* now apply to everyone across the entire organizational structure, thus breaking down departmental barriers. Patient-focused standards, presented in a multidisciplinary, organization-wide manner, negate the tunnel vision departmental focus of previous standards. Now, the organization as a whole is responsible for compliance to all the standards in the most current year's *Comprehensive Accreditation*

Manual for Hospitals (CAMH), which includes standards for five patient-focused functions, six organization functions, and three structures with functions. Current standards make a clearer connection "between what a hospital does on a day-to-day basis and the performance expectations expressed in the standards and the intent statements" (Joint Commission, 1995a, p. 31).

Given this new "agenda," the only goal for a successful JCAHO survey is to integrate standards into an organizational management process within daily operations. This process must support leadership, staff, and physicians to demonstrate that the organization as a whole has *a clearly defined strategic plan* that is based on the organization's mission, vision, and values. The plan's strategic priorities (goals) must be efficiently integrated and used throughout the organization at all levels to continuously improve the organization's performance.

Reaching this goal requires leadership commitment to continuously improve the processes of care and systems to support care. The accreditation standards provide guidelines and basic requirements to be addressed. In addition, the standards provide information on a variety of ways an organization will be assessed for compliance, through performance measures, interviews, and review of the medical record. When the strategic planning process guides the organization's performance improvement plan, the strategic priorities (goals) become the basis upon which leaders decide what quality/performance improvement

APPLICATION 15–1 *Continued*

activities need to be undertaken and in what priority, given available resources.

A mission-based strategic planning process begins with the mission and values; considers customer needs, expectations, outcomes, and satisfaction; and evaluates the staff competencies and organizational effectiveness (see Fig. 15–3).

■ INTEGRATION OF THEMES FROM JCAHO STANDARDS INTO DAILY OPERATIONS

Organizational leadership has an ever-increasing role and responsibility for continuous quality improvement and performance improvement within the organization under the new JCAHO standards. Complying with the Leadership Standards requires proof of careful thought through written documentation. Figure 15–3 provides a method of mission-based strategic planning thinking for leadership that identifies all the elements of a planned and systematic approach and links strategic planning to performance improvement. The Leadership Function Flow Chart in the JCAHO *CAMH* (Joint Commission, 1995a, p. 276) can assist leaders to capture their work. The leadership team identifies key events and activities systematically by time. For example, many organizations participate in community needs assessments. That information needs to be used when leaders plan what services the organization will provide. Many organizations do not link the needs with the services, especially in written docu-

mentation. Documentation of the assessment, the services, and their linkage, meets a requirement in the accreditation standards of leadership function. Without this documentation of linkage, an organization may lose "credit" for meeting this standard. The Leadership Process Flow Chart guides leaders in clearly identifying their planning process and communicating the process throughout the organization in an open, collaborative manner that fosters continual improvements.

Additional standards require planning documents that organizational leadership must develop and disseminate within the organization, including

- A mission-based strategic plan
- A hospital-wide plan for the provision of patient care
- The performance improvement plan
- The environment of care management plans

A variety of templates are available from quality management experts to assist leaders in developing and operationalizing these documents. Some organizations prepare "cheat sheets," such as mission statements and fire plans printed on the back of name tags or "catchy" posters strategically placed throughout the facility for quick reference.

Leadership also carries the responsibility for teaching others throughout the organization what the accreditation standards are and how to apply them in daily work. The use of the "common themes" in the standards is one way to make standards more practical and less

APPLICATION 15–1 *Continued*

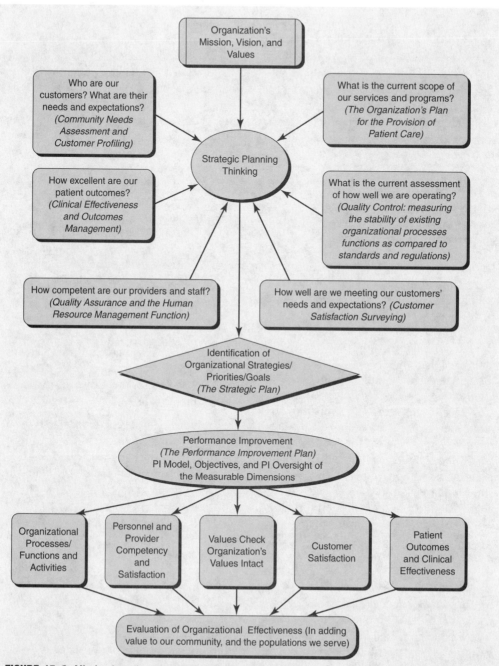

FIGURE 15–3. Mission-based strategic planning process for improving organization performance. *(Source: Yocum, [1996].)*

APPLICATION 15–1 *Continued*

theoretical. Figure 15–4 summarizes the six themes discussed below.

1. Organizational leadership's ongoing commitment to the principles of continuous quality improvement in daily activities, including resource allocation.
2. An organizational culture in which the patient is at the center of the work process despite being served by many practitioners and provided a variety of services.
3. Adherence to a strategic planning model that is mission, vision, and values based and the use of strategic priorities (goals) derived from these three to guide the entire organization's programs and services.
4. The application of the use of interdisciplinary/multidisciplinary team collaboration to create and achieve efficient care processes and improved patient outcomes.
5. A way of doing business within the organization that is one in which all efforts, whether they are for the patient or for organizational operations, are developed, implemented, and managed in a "planned and systematic manner."
6. Use of performance measures (data) as the basis for problem solving and evaluation of effectiveness. In other words, all problem-solving efforts are "data driven."

Data-based problem solving requires that organizational leaders promote the collection and use of performance measures (indicators), and analysis of variation and underlying causes. Leaders must stress measurement in quality improvement/performance improvement as well as in the key processes and/or functions of the organization. For example, if an organization strives to improve efficiency in performance for a patient's preprocedure processing for elective outpatient treatment to increase customer satisfaction, there must be pre- and post-measurement of "performance measures" (indicators) to show that improvement actually occurred. System change, both pre- and post-intervention(s), must be measured by several preselected indicators of success. Such measures may include patient satisfaction, number of visits for preparation for the elective treatment, or the time taken to process a patient through the entire preparation process, always comparing pre- and post-intervention efforts. Data on effectiveness are one of the weakest areas in health care organizational performance improvement programs. Often, either pre- or post-measurement data are missing; thus, true evaluation of the effectiveness of that intervention cannot be captured. Both ongoing routine patient care and operational activities need performance measures (indicators) to measure the stability of existing processes within the organization.

The activity of the organization to "prove" to others that it adheres to the JCAHO standards is dictated within the standards themselves. Proof of compliance must be demonstrated in three

APPLICATION 15–1 *Continued*

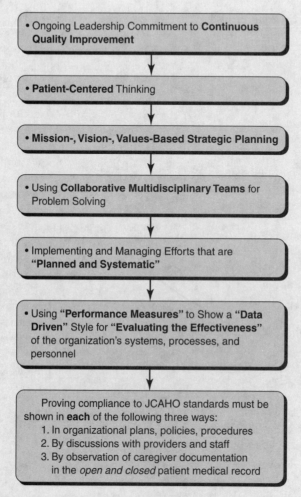

- Ongoing Leadership Commitment to **Continuous Quality Improvement**

- **Patient-Centered** Thinking

- **Mission-, Vision-, Values-Based Strategic Planning**

- Using **Collaborative Multidisciplinary Teams** for Problem Solving

- Implementing and Managing Efforts that are **"Planned and Systematic"**

- Using **"Performance Measures"** to Show a **"Data Driven"** Style for **"Evaluating the Effectiveness"** of the organization's systems, processes, and personnel

Proving compliance to JCAHO standards must be shown in **each** of the following three ways:
1. In organizational plans, policies, procedures
2. By discussions with providers and staff
3. By observation of caregiver documentation in the *open and closed* patient medical record

FIGURE 15–4. The "common themes" found in the JCAHO standards and the survey process. *(Source: Yocum & Sheridan, [1996].)*

ways: First, the organization provides plans, policies, procedures, programs, and descriptions as written, documented proof of compliance. Second, the interviewing of leaders, staff, and physicians throughout the organization corroborates that practice follows organizational document review. Third, the patients' medical records comply with standards of the JCAHO and the plans and policies of the organization. For example, the accreditation standards call for patients to receive informed consent from physicians before any procedure can be performed. The organization must have a policy and procedure to govern the

APPLICATION 15–1 *Continued*

process of informed consent, including the components, the process of obtaining, and the documents used. Leaders, staff, and physicians will then be interviewed to assess whether they practice according to the policy/procedure. The final proof is the patients' medical records showing the consent and how it was obtained. Failure to prove compliance in any of these required three ways usually results in poor scores in the "informed consents" under the Patient Rights Function.

■ EFFECTIVE USE OF SURVEY PREPARATION TOOLS AND RESOURCES

Copious resources are available to enhance JCAHO preparation. This information helps to understand the "intent" of a standard or how to apply it. Below are the *key* resources and tools on standards and preparations that are available to maximize survey scores. The resources in this first listing provide information that will help you learn the relevant standards that you are expected to meet.

- The 1996 *Comprehensive Accreditation Manual for Hospitals* by the Joint Commission is a thick binder that contains the accreditation policies and survey process, the standards, and the intent of the standards for the 11 patient and organizational functions and the 4 structures with functions (Nursing, Medical Staff, Governance, and Management). Also included are the scoring guidelines with minimal compliance ratings, and JCAHO rules for scoring (both aggregation and decision rules). Each standard is followed by "the intent" of the standard (also evaluated during survey), and examples of application of the standard or suggested methods to comply with it. This publication is a "must have."
- *JCAHO Perspectives* (the official Joint Commission newsletter) is published by Mosby-Year Book, Inc. This bimonthly publication highlights standards posing greater compliance challenges. Often, examples of systems or forms used effectively by organizations are shared to further emphasize the "intent" of the standard.
- Professional standards are also found in publications promulgated by such professional organizations as the American Nurses Association, the state's medical association, or other specialty professional organizations.
- State regulations have not been addressed here but are available locally. Some states, such as California, survey using state standards simultaneously with the state medical association and the JCAHO.
- Health Care Finance Association (HCFA) standards should also be reviewed.

Once you have reviewed all the relevant standards, this following listing

APPLICATION 15–1 *Continued*

offers valuable resources to guide preparation for the survey itself. (Remember, the preparation for the next survey informally begins the morning after the surveyers leave.)

- *The Complete Guide to the [current year's] Hospital Survey Process* is a resource tool published by the JCAHO. It is a paperback guidebook detailing the survey process from opening through assessment to closing phases. The tool includes extensive potential questions asked of individuals and teams during the survey, along with guidelines for doing the various performance improvement presentations. These guidelines and sample questions are essential aids for practice sessions before the survey. This publication is also a "must have."
- Many organizations, especially multihospital systems, produce special internal and external survey alerts—alerts on survey changes or "hot spots." These alerts describe the latest problem areas encountered at recently surveyed sister facilities or provide brief tips on various survey topics to aid in preparation for the survey. Figure 15–5 is such an example.
- There are hundreds of other resources (articles, newsletters, and workshops) available from JCAHO and other organizations. Many multihospital systems, such as Daughters of Charity National Health System, have a wealth of resources and

experts available to their constituencies. Other areas of question or concern may be clarified by calling JCAHO information at 1–630–792–5000.

■ AN ORGANIZED AND SYSTEMATIC APPROACH TO THE SURVEY

Compliance with the accreditation standards needs to be integrated into your routine management program and daily operations, and applied to any performance improvement activity, no matter how small. It is a way of thinking and managing. Managers should role model an improvement approach obtaining "standards" for all care or work or service processes. Managers need to always seek measurement of "what is" and strive for improvement. Search the literature benchmarks of best practices for use in determining the relative value of all measurements for accreditation standards, professional standards, or state regulations. A routine approach to every problem must include a database for every problem-solving activity of any individual or any team throughout the organization. In every discussion, address the related "standards" or regulatory requirements. Use research, case reports, historical data accumulated in your agency, and all sources of available data. Recognize standards and regulations as minimum requirements. Set goals to reach beyond the minimums to achieve excellence in patient care outcomes.

An effective survey preparation includes a *formal 2-year cycle* of prepara-

APPLICATION: 15–1 *Continued*

"Hot Spots" in

The JCAHO Patient Focused Function of Assessment of Patients

The assessment process applied to the individual patient must demonstrate a multi-disciplinary collaborative approach that includes all the clinical disciplines that screen, access, or care for the patient. Specific requirements as to what must be documented in the patient's medical record include, but are not limited to, these examples:

The physician must assess the patient and document UPON ADMISSION all the elements listed below in the *Physician History and Physical:*

• Physical Examination Findings
• Psychological Status
• Social Status
• Nutritional Status and Needs
• Functional Status and Rehab Needs
• Need for Discharge Planning

The nurse must assess the patient, including among other elements, an educational assessment and document ALL components listed below as part of that assessment:

• Barriers to the Patient Learning
• Patient's Cultural Beliefs
• Religious Beliefs of the Patient
• Patient Learning Needs

Ponder this question: Is **EACH DISCIPLINE** involved in that patient's care reading and using the results in each others assessments? If not, we do not begin to comply with the multi-disciplinary collaborative approach to the assessment of patients and to the care of patients required by the JCAHO standards.

FIGURE 15–5. Survey education alert: "hot spots" in the JCAHO patient-focused function of Assessment of Patients. *(Source: Yocum & Sheridan, [1996].)*

tion and a *timeline* for a successful survey. A 1-year plan is minimum preparation and may not be effective in fully avoiding Type 1 Recommendations. A 2-year plan provides an effective, ongoing, planned, and systematic approach for checking the organization's compliance level to standards identifying the three roles that are absolutely essential for successful survey preparation—*CEO/Senior Leadership, Survey Coordinator,* and *Accountable Individuals* from Department/Service Directors or assigned "function" leaders. Tasks are identified and arranged in a timeline so that the organization's survey and survey preparation activity key dates can be easily applied.

The nurse executive must assume a leadership role in strategic planning, organizational performance improvement, and accreditation survey preparedness.

APPLICATION 15–1   *Continued*

The expertise of nursing professionals is pivotal to a successful survey, as well as to maintaining a team-oriented health care organizational culture. Contributions of nursing professionals include:

- Experience in collaborative team work.
- Use of a scientific approach, including data-driven decision making.
- Possession of a conceptual framework of the continuum of care.
- Expectations for linking strategies to operations.

Finally, the JCAHO visit culminates in a summation conference open to senior leadership at which the organization receives preliminary accreditation scores on functions and an overall rating called the organization's "grid score" or "report card." Poor scores in any function usually are viewed as a failure in leadership's ability to effectively manage the organization. To prevent this outcome, senior leadership and especially nursing leadership must integrate quality and performance improvement into daily operations. Nurses in patient care administration must demonstrate how to work effectively with interdisciplinary team members to enhance the processes and outcomes of patient care. Only an ongoing systematic interdisciplinary approach to continuous improvement directed toward the strategic goals of the organization will result in a JCAHO visit being met with calm confidence and a survey outcome that generates a sense of team pride and accomplishment. Don't forget to share the survey results

and celebrate your successes to energize your team for the continuous challenges ahead.

■ BIOGRAPHICAL SKETCHES

Donna Richards Sheridan is Vice President, Patient Care and Chief Nurse Executive at St. Francis Memorial Hospital, a division of CHW, in San Francisco. Previously, she worked at Stanford University Hospital and Lucile Salter Packard Children's Hospital in both education and administration roles. She has an MS from the University of California, San Francisco, and an MBA from Pepperdine University. Her doctoral work was in Hospital Corporate Culture. Dr. Sheridan has published two books and four workbooks on a variety of health care topics including: *Economics, Accounting and Finance in Healthcare; People, Policies and Politics; Law, Risk Management and Quality Assurance; Development of the Nurse Manager; How to Write and Publish Articles in Nursing;* and *Transcultural Nursing.* She has been editor of Mosby's bimonthly publication, *Staff Development Insider,* for 5 years and is a member of four editorial boards. She has written numerous articles on topics that include downsizing and surviving in a deregulated industry. Dr. Sheridan has been a consultant on Total Quality Management to several organizations, including Stanford University Hospital, the U.S. Air Force, and the Phoenix V.A. Medical Center. In addition, she has worked as a research consultant to a Kellogg cost-containment grant based in three California

APPLICATION 15–1   *Continued*

medical centers. She is a strategic plan-ning consultant for hospital management teams and is a nationally recognized speaker at professional organizations.

Carol Ruth Yocum has 27 years of health care experience, beginning at the staff nurse level and continuing up through organizational leadership posi-tions. She is masters prepared in Health-Care Administration and certified by the American Nurses Association in two areas, Nursing Administration Advanced and Psychiatric/Mental Health Nursing. She is a member of the National Associa-tion for Healthcare Quality, the Organi-zation of Nurse Executives, and other professional organizations. She has been a Nurse Executive at two organizations, one a nonprofit and the other a for profit patient care delivery system; a Quality Management Director/Clinical Support Services Leader for a large health maintenance organization; and, most recently, a Quality Management Consultant for the Daughters of Charity National Health System, a large national

multisystem, multicare-level health care organization—also serving Catholic Healthcare West Hospitals. Ms. Yocum's specialty is mission-based strategic plan-ning for improving organizational per-formance. Her extensive experience and expertise cover topics ranging from medical staff services quality manage-ment to Asian health care systems.

■ REFERENCES

Berwick, D.M. (1990). *Curing health care: New strategies for quality improvement.* San Francisco: Jossey-Bass.

Joint Commission for the Accreditation of Healthcare Organizations. (1995a). *1996 comprehensive accreditation manual for hospitals.* Oakbrook Terrace, IL: JCAHO.

Joint Commission for the Accreditation of Healthcare Organizations. (1995b). *Joint Commission perspectives.* St. Louis, MO: Mosby.

Joint Commission for the Accreditation of Healthcare Organizations. (1996). *The complete guide to the 1996 hospital survey process.* Oakbrook Terrace, IL: JCAHO.

CASE 15–2 Measuring Outcomes of a Spine Evaluation Service in a Managed Care Setting

Margaret Fisk Mastal and Carshal A. Burris

Kaiser Permanente, a health maintenance organization (HMO) with about 7.5 million members nationwide, has been in the managed care business since the early 1940s. Integrating care and measuring improvements are integral values that are basic to the fabric of the entire Kaiser Permanente organization.

The spine evaluation service described in this case study was implemented in the Washington, D.C., and Baltimore, Maryland, markets, which serve over 500,000 members. This market has 22 medical centers to serve the health care needs of members, in addition to an expanding, sophisticated clinical management information system, which captures data on the care provided, translating it into usable financial, clinical, and other management information for the outcomes measurement process.

Acute low back pain is endemic in American life, costing millions of dollars in lost work time, unnecessary diagnostic testing and treatment, and, for many adults, diminished ability to perform or enjoy usual activities. Across the nation, back problems rank high in reasons for physician visits and are the major cause of disability in adults under 45 years of age (Agency for Health Care Policy and Research, 1994). Nationally it is clear that back problems have unhealthy and costly outcomes for both the consumers and payors of health care.

Kaiser Permanente's Washington and Baltimore markets reflected experiences similar to the national picture. In 1995, acute low back pain of benign origin was among the top five most frequent reasons for member visits: 17,000 members were seen in 27,000 encounters, generating $2.4 million in outpatient visit costs and $1.2 million in expenditures for referrals to specialists and hospitalizations. Each patient averaged 1.4 prescriptions, which cost $900,000 overall, and over one-third had radiological studies (spinal x-rays, magnetic resonance imagery [MRI], or coaxial tomography [CT] studies). Further analysis found large variations among the practice patterns of providers; most were exceeding the practice guidelines established by the Agency for Health Care Policy and Research (AHCPR) (1994). Clearly, this was an opportunity to discover creative ways to improve the management of adults with acute low back problems.

This case study illustrates how a multidisciplinary team identified and measured indicators of success—that is, the outcomes of a spine evaluation service—from both an organizational and a consumer perspective. The goal was to enhance care for adults with persistent acute low back pain in Kaiser Permanente's Washington, D.C–Baltimore, Maryland metropolitan area. The effort provided insights into new ways of

CASE 15–2   *Continued*

thinking about the care rendered, more cost-effective strategies for diagnosis and treatment, and how to build better partnerships among care providers across geographical distances.

■ DEFINING THE POPULATION

Most acute low back pain (95 percent) resolves naturally within 2 to 4 weeks. However, we found that most members in our area wanted and expected instant relief and an immediate return to their normal activities. They became angry with their primary care provider when expectations went unrealized. In an attempt to meet members' expectations for immediate action, providers frequently ordered unnecessary tests and often overprescribed opiate analgesics. Both the members and the providers were frustrated with few positive outcomes.

In consultation with staff working with our clinical management information system, we realized that of the 17,000 members seen in 1995 for acute low back pain, 4,000 (24 percent) incurred multiple visits. This population was the most likely to provoke unnecessary testing, inappropriate specialty referrals, and the overuse of opiate pain-relief medications. Moreover, audits of randomly selected medical records from this group revealed that these members could be classified into two major groups: (1) those who had experienced low back pain for years with complex physical and psychosocial dysfunction indicative of a chronic pain syndrome; and (2) those whose acute low back pain endured for several months. As

the treatment of chronic pain of any sort, including low back pain, requires special treatment modalities, this task force decided to focus on the second group of members whose pain was of less than 6 months duration. This group became the primary emphasis for the spine evaluation service.

■ DEFINING THE SERVICES

Determining what services to provide, and ultimately which indicators would measure success, was largely based on the AHCPR clinical practice guidelines for the care of acute low back problems in adults (AHCPR, 1994). We incorporated these guidelines into the spine evaluation service mission statement:

> The purpose of the Spine Evaluation Service is to organize and manage the delivery of quality, cost-effective care for members with low back pain which does not respond to conservative medical treatment by their primary care provider within four to six weeks. Management includes accurate diagnosis, the use of appropriate diagnostic imaging, coordination of a treatment plan, more appropriate referrals to specialty departments, and a cognitive educational program for the active participation of members in managing their back pain. Members will have between one and four visits with the Spine Evaluation Service team and will be returned to the care of their primary physician with a recommended plan for on-going care.

CASE 15–2 *Continued*

The service was staffed by primary care physicians (internists and family practitioners) and nurses in close professional consultation with physical therapists. Acute low back problems became the purview of primary care with neurological, neurosurgical, and orthopedic intervention occurring only when clinical symptoms and diagnostic studies indicated their intervention was warranted.

The service was piloted in three centers during 1995, and entailed the identification and tracking of indicators that would demonstrate its value: improved health outcomes for members, increased member satisfaction and reduced costs, as well as insights about implementing organizational change.

■ DEFINING AND MEASURING OUTCOMES

In general, indicators for evaluating successful outcomes were grouped into the consumer's perspective and benefits to the organization.

Consumer Perspectives

The members' perspective was found to have two dimensions: (1) their satisfaction with the care provided, and (2) their perception of the physical and psychosocial outcomes of the care they received. Measuring the consumers' perspective was done at two points on the care continuum: at the point of service, and 3 months after their last visit to the spine service.

To evaluate member satisfaction with the care at the point of service, we asked members to complete a short survey form (taking about 1 minute to complete) when they were about to leave that indicated their degree of satisfaction with: (1) wait time for the consult appointment, (2) the length of time they waited to see the physician that day, (3) the courtesy of the physicians and staff during the appointment, (4) their perception of the physicians' understanding of their problem, and (5) the clarity of explanations given them by the physicians about their problem and the plan of treatment.

Over the first 18 months of the program, the members gave us increasingly positive feedback about their satisfaction with their visits and the outcomes. We noticed that as we became more adept and experienced with the program, both the number of survey responses and the members' degree of satisfaction increased. In general, about 70 percent of the members completed the point of service survey, and of these, 50 percent were highly satisfied.

How satisfied the members were in terms of their physical and psychosocial outcomes was measured by asking them to rate their satisfaction with how the treatment decreased their pain, helped them manage their pain, improved their ability to function in their daily activities, and their overall satisfaction with the service. Initially, we sent members a survey in the mail 6 months after they had visited the spine evaluation service and had very poor return rates. We then tried sending the survey 3 months after their last visit and had some increase in the number of

CASE 15–2 *Continued*

completed surveys, but still too few to give us substantive information.

In 1996, we decided to call the members and complete the survey by telephone; this approach met with much greater success. In the Springfield, Virginia, Medical Center, a total of 42 members were seen as new consults in the spine evaluation service during the first quarter. We were able to contact 33 of them and gleaned some new information: 48 percent were "very" or "highly" satisfied with the decrease in their pain, an increased ability to manage their pain, and the improvement in their daily functioning. The majority of members who had only moderate to low satisfaction with return to function were persons who had experienced pain for extended periods of time, that is, months to years; they really fell into the chronic pain category and should not have been seen in this service. Clearly, referral guidelines to the service needed to be reinforced with the referring providers.

We will continue to elicit members' responses by telephone as conversations with them proved insightful to us and increased their satisfaction. However, as pleased as the members utilizing the program were, we needed to measure and evaluate if and how the organization realized benefits from the service. These measures were evaluated against our mission statement, which used the AHCPR guidelines for the care of acute low back problems.

Organizational Perspective

Organizational benefits also had two dimensions: (1) insights that were gained about ways to improve organizational change processes for managing low back pain, and (2) measuring the costs and benefits in terms of members' utilization of pharmacological agents; use of MRI and CT scans; referrals to orthopedics, neurology, neurosurgery, anesthesia, and physical therapy; rate of back surgery; and the number of hospital discharges with diagnostic related group (DRG) #243, Medical Back Problems.

Wisdom gained about implementing changes in the management of low back problems included: (1) the importance of identifying and involving all the stakeholders related to the success of the spine evaluation venture, (2) the need to repeatedly communicate and clarify referral guidelines to primary care providers, and (3) the primacy of developing clinical guidelines for the care of acute low back pain across the continuum of symptoms, from one episode of low back pain to chronic pain, to improve the trajectory of clinical care.

The physicians, nurses, and physical therapists involved in the venture were obvious stakeholders, accessible and open to education and to developing skills to manage the target population more effectively. However, there were other stakeholders that were less obvious and less motivated. For example, the Internal Medicine Service Chiefs and Clinical Coordinators throughout the Baltimore–Washington area were initially unsupportive. The spine evaluation service was staffed in one central place by primary care physicians who were currently functioning in geographically dispersed Internal Medicine and Family

CASE 15–2 *Continued*

Practice departments. Working in the clinic created absences in their "home" outpatient settings with diminished appointment access for their primary patients, resulting in complaints about wait time for appointments. In retrospect, we realized that the resistance initially seen by Internal Medicine Service Chiefs and the Clinical Coordinators was realistic and based on their immediate problems and concerns. This was remedied quickly by providing these stakeholders with information on the purpose of the spine evaluation clinic, the minutes of quarterly spine evaluation service meetings, and the progress and benefits realized by members and the organization. They then were motivated to adjust the distribution of work among physicians to alleviate wait time. They were very interested in the success of the clinic in reducing overall utilization. Identifying and informing all the beneficiaries of the service about our goals and progress was critical to the success of the operation.

The purpose of the program, the services it would provide, and the guidelines for referral, were initially sent to all primary care providers in written form through interoffice mail. It quickly became apparent that they misinterpreted our intent. Instead of sending only those with back pain between 4 to 6 weeks, they also referred those with chronic low back pain. These patients were the primary concern of physicians who found the lack of progress in pain control and daily functioning quite frustrating. The clinic physicians did agree to see and evaluate these patients. They found, as expected, that the usual procedures and educational programs were not meeting the needs of these patients and, in the care plan sent back to the provider, indicated the chronic nature of the back pain and the need for chronic pain management.

The dilemma of clarifying the spinal evaluation service's target population was assisted when our entire referral system was brought online in the latter half of 1995; this allowed providers to directly send referrals electronically to each specialty department. The referral screens included specific guidelines for making referrals. Subsequently, we have noted a decrease in the number of chronic low back pain referrals and an increase in referrals of our targeted population. Further, this system could track and report referral activity in a timely manner, a feature vital to providing feedback to physicians on appropriateness of referrals.

From our examination of data about provider practice patterns and our experiences with inappropriate referrals, we realized that developing and implementing guidelines for the care of members by phase of low back pain would assist in standardizing and coordinating provider practices across large geographical distances. To that end, quarterly meetings in our second year of operations included guideline development sessions, with publication of these guidelines occurring in early 1997.

The guidelines are divided into three phases of the treatment of adults presenting with low back pain: (1) the acute phase, which can persist up to 2 to 4 weeks; (2) the subacute phase, which can persist from 2 weeks up to 6

CASE 15–2 *Continued*

months; and (3) the chronic phase, which persists beyond 6 months and is often accompanied by other complex symptomology. The guidelines include recommendations for the timing of diagnostic procedures such as imaging studies and referrals for spine evaluation or medical specialists. The timing of interventions such as physical pain management strategies, pharmacological agents, surgery, and educational modalities are addressed in the guidelines. Although the impact of these guidelines has not yet been evaluated, informal feedback indicates the physicians are pleased with the guidelines and are using them.

Another outcome was the realization that centralizing a similar program for chronic pain management could reap similar benefits. This program was developed and piloted during 1996 to assist chronic pain patients to cope with pain, reduce it where possible, and improve daily functioning through improving the services, while also reducing ineffective, possibly iatrogenic, unnecessary, and costly treatment. Again a model of intensive, appropriate services and return to their primary physician with treatment recommendations was followed.

■ MEASURING ORGANIZATIONAL BENEFITS

Indicators to measure benefits to the organization were changes in the level of utilization of services associated with acute low back pain problems. For patients with this diagnosis, we enumerated the prescriptions for opiate analgesics, muscle relaxants, and nonsteriodal anti-inflammatory drugs (NSAIDs); the requests for lumbar and sacral x-rays, MRIs, and CTs; the number of referrals to neurology, orthopedics, neurosurgery, and anesthesia; and the number of emergency room visits and the hospital discharges. Our ability to measure, analyze, and evaluate outcomes has grown as the sophistication of our clinical management information system has increased. Because this system was unavailable to us in 1995, cost limited the collection of indicators to manual review at only one site.

Results from those first manual efforts showed promise of improved treatment patterns. The use of opiate analgesics and muscle relaxants decreased 75 percent, prescriptions for NSAIDS increased 60 percent, and requests for MRIs and CTs decreased 80 percent. In short, inappropriate testing and treatment declined and more effective strategies were applied, with an increase in member satisfaction as noted above.

We anticipate more timely, specific information from all sites will be supplied as the clinical management information system grows in capacity to track our indicators and translate results in terms of dollars and cents. Further, we will evaluate differences and similarities between the practice patterns of providers in areas with or without the spine evaluation service regarding the diagnosis and treatment of adults with low back pain.

■ BIOGRAPHICAL SKETCHES

Margaret Fisk Mastal graduated with a diploma in nursing from St. Vincent's

CASE 15–2 *Continued*

Hospital School of Nursing, in New York City. She earned a BSN from the University of Nebraska, and both an MSN and a PhD in Public Policy from George Mason University, in Fairfax, Virginia. Dr. Mastal has had diverse experiences in hospitals as a clinical nurse and nurse administrator in outpatient care, nursing education, and nursing research. She has worked for Kaiser Permanente since 1990, managing a variety of primary care and specialty departments in the ambulatory care setting. Dr. Mastal was appointed to the 1988 Department of Health and Human Services Commission on Nursing, has served in leadership positions in Sigma Theta Tau International Honor Society of Nursing, and currently serves on the Board of Directors for the American Academy of Ambulatory Care Nursing as well as the American Nurses Association Steering Committee on Databases to Support Clinical Practice. She has published numerous articles in professional journals and textbooks on clinical issues, organizational theory, quality improvement, and nursing theory and research.

Carshal A. Burris is the Medical Facility Administrator of the Kaiser Permanente Medical Center, in Springfield, VA. He joined Kaiser Permanente in September 1985. Before joining Kaiser Permanente, Mr. Burris was a member of the Arthur Young Mid Atlantic Health Care Consulting Group. He is a former Master Army Aviator, who retired from the U.S. Army Medical Service in 1982, having served over 30 years in a variety of command and staff assignments at Division, Brigade, Corps, Army, and Department of the Army level medical services. He received his Masters in Health Care Administration degree through the Army Baylor Program.

■ REFERENCES

Al-Assaf, A.F., & Schmele, J.A. (1993). *The textbook of total quality in healthcare.* Delray Beach, FL: St. Lucie Press.

Douglas, D. (1996). Measuring the value of outcomes. *Managed Healthcare News, 12* (7), 22R.

Lewis, B.E. (1995). HMO outcomes research: Lessons from the field. *Journal of Ambulatory Care Management, 18* (1), 47–55.

Phoon, J., Corder, K., & Barter, M. (1995). Managed care and total quality management: A necessary integration. *Journal of Nursing Care Quality, 10* (2), 25–32.

Agency for Health Care Policy and Research. (1994). *Acute low back problems in adults.* Rockville, MD: Department of Health and Human Services.

Index

Absenteeism, 464
Academic health centers, family intervention research in, 445–51
Access to care, legal issues, 81
Accountability, legal issues, 62–63
Accountants, role of, 249
Accounting
  accrual, 299
  cash, 299
  charge-based, 330
  cost, 330
  systems for new ventures, 249
Accreditation standards, 511–12, *See also* Joint Commission for the
Accreditation of Healthcare Organizations (JCAHO)
  "common themes" in, 513, 515, 516
  incorporating into daily operations, 512–17
Accreditation surveys, *See also* Joint Commission for the Accreditation of
Healthcare Organizations (JCAHO)
  formal 2-year preparation cycle, 518–19
  goals and, 512
  "grid scores" or "report cards," 520
  mission-based strategic planning and, 513
  preparing for, 510–21
  strategic planning and, 512
  summation conferences, 520
  systematic approach to, 518–20
  timelines for, 519
Accretion, labor organization recognition by, 72
Accrual accounting, 299
Acculturation models, of group identity, 108
Acquisitions
  growth through, 274
  rate of, 285
Action plans, for organizational change, 153
Activity efficiency measures, 311
Actual costs, 300

Actual expenses, 307
Actual revenues, 306
Acute Care Nurse Practitioners, 401
Acute illness, health policy and, 40
Acute low back pain, spine evaluation service, 522, 523
ADA (Americans with Disabilities Act), 78, 102
Adaptation, leadership as, 409–10
Adjusted patient days, as outcome measure, 384
Administrative conservatorship, 408–9
Administrative decision support systems, 334
Adult learning
  objectives of, 431–32
  theory of, 433–35
Advance directives, 68
Advanced practice nurses (APNs)
  advantages of, 400–401
  antidiscrimination against, 55
  barriers to effective use of, 41–42
  defined by nurse practice acts, 60
  educating public about, 49
  health care access and, 41
  legal authority for, 41
  research by, 445, 449, 450
  traditional paradigm, 41–42
Advertising, 199–200
  broad-market, 199
  expenditures, 199
  name recognition through, 199
  for new ventures, 251–52
Advisory boards, for education/service collaboration, 438
Advocacy groups
  coalitions, policy making process and, 36–37
  health care values and, 42–44
"Advocates for Practitioner Equity Coalition" (APEC), 55
Affective objectives, in adult learning, 432

Affiliative models, for education/service
    collaboration, 437–438
African-Americans, 103
    bicultural issues, 109
    cultural norms, 11, 110, 112
    discrimination claims, 118
    ethic of care and, 11
    segregation of, 102
    stereotypes, 113
    women, ethical theory and, 10–11
Age Discrimination Act (1967), 102
Agency for Health Care Policy and Research
    (AHCPR), 522, 523
"Agenda for Change" (JCAHO), 511, 512
Aging, care of, public policy and, 42
Ain't I A Woman: Black Women and Feminism
    (Hooks), 11
Alderfer, C.P., 463
Ambiguity
    tolerance for
        conflict and, 118
        prejudice and discrimination and, 113
Ambulatory care centers
    employment trends, 202
    machine organizational form in, 273–74
Ambulatory patient groups (APGs), 315
American Marketing Association, Academy for
    Health Services Marketing, 192
American Medical Association (AMA),
    Medicare/Medicaid reforms and, 54–55
American Nurses Association (ANA), 334–35
    Medicare/Medicaid reforms and, 55–56
    Scope and Standards for Nurse
        Administrators (ANA), 18
American Nurses Credentialing Center (ANCC),
    401
Americans with Disabilities Act (ADA), 78,
    102
Analogies, in idea development, 226
Androcentrism, 6
Androgogy, 434
Antidiscrimination amendment, for advanced
    practice nurses, 55
AONE (Association of Nurse Executives),
    157–58
APEC ("Advocates for Practitioner Equity
    Coalition"), 55
APGs (ambulatory patient groups), 315
APNs. See Advanced practice nurses (APNs)

Appeal systems, conflict and, 118
Appraisal interviews, 479–80
Arc, The, 54
Aristotle, 13, 14
Asian-Americans, 103
    cultural norms, 111, 112, 128
Assault, 65
Assessment, organizational. See Organizational
    assessment
Asset valuation, 299
Assignment
    patient care, by charge nurses, 453
    of personnel, defined, 60
    of staff to teams, 165–66
Assimilation, 101–2
    ethics of care and, 9
Association of Nurse Executives (AONE), 157–58
Attitudes, toward work, 369
Attractors, chaos theory and, 277
"At will" employees, 69–70
Authoritarian leadership style, 406–7
Authoritarian personality, prejudice and
    discrimination and, 113
Authority
    delegation of, 412
    as tool of leadership, 411–12, 415
Autonomy
    as core job dimension, 363
    as organizational relationship strategy,
        278–80
Autopoesis
    defined, 276
    in organizations, 276–77
Avoidable costs, 301

Back pain
    acute, low, spine evaluation service, 522, 523
    chronic, spine evaluation service, 527
Bartky, Sandra, 12
Battery, 65
Behavioral anchored rating scale (BARS), 478
Behavioral observation scale (BOS), summated,
    478
Behaviorist learning theory, 432–33
Belief systems, of coalitions, policy making
    and, 36
Benchmarks

external, evaluating financial outcomes with, 388

internal, evaluating financial outcomes with, 387–88

Benefits, *See also* Cost-benefit ratios
cost avoidance, 388–91
determining, 383–84

Benefit segmentation analysis, 195

Beth Israel Medical Center, New York, "A Workplace of Difference" program, 125–30

Bias, in performance evaluation, 481–82

Bicultural individuals, 108–9

Binding arbitration, 75–76

Biological clock theory, of learning, 434

Biomedical model, of health care, 496–97

Blame, conflict and, 117, 118

Bonus reward systems
as motivators, 462
organization-wide, 486

Born effect, 481

Boston College of Nursing, University of Massachusetts, 437–38

"Boundaryless" community-based primary care, 438

Break-even analysis, 302, 303

Break-even volume, 302

Breastfeeding, social marketing of, 197–98

Bridges, William, 164

Broad-market advertising, 199

Brochures, for new ventures, 251–52

Bronx Municipal Hospital Center (BMHC), 439

Budgeted costs, 300

Budgeting
control through, 294
cost control and, 298
defined, 234, 293, 294
importance of, 293
iterative process of, 296, 297–98
supplies, 309–10

Budget manual, 296–97

Budget monitoring, 302–6

Budgets
capital, 297
cash, 297
operating, 297
preparation process, 294–98
corporate strategy development, 294

making projections, 295
operational planning, 295–98
zero-based, 296

Budget variances, tracking, 304

Bureaucracy, in organizations, 275

Bureaucratic work, function of, 273

Business cards, for new ventures, 251–52

Business domain, 214

Businesses, new. *See* Ventures

Business planning, 231–35
budgeting, 235
forecasting, 235
integration of, 235
operational, 234–35
strategic, 232–34
three M's of, 232

Business plans, 236–45
assistance with, 236
contents of, 237–40
defined, 236
developing, 231
length of, 237
production of, 240–41
sample, 242–45
uses of, 237
value of, 227, 236, 237, 250
writing, 237–40

Buyouts, growth through, 274

California Nurses Association, 75

CAMH (*Comprehensive Accreditation Manual for Hospitals*), 512, 517

Cannon, Katie, 10–11

Capital budget, contents of, 297

Capitated systems
outcome measures, 384
productivity measures, 384

Capitation, defined, 316

Capitation payments, 186

Care, *See also* Health care
access to, legal issues, 81
ethics of, 7–10
standards of, 17–18

Career development, responsibility for, 430

Care management, 188
associated services, 252
scope of practice, 252–54

Care maps, 498
Caring
    elements of, 12–13
    ethic of care and, 12
    practice of, 13
Carse, Alisa, 9
Case management
    defined, 498
    as job design, 366
    nurse, cost avoidance benefits, 388–91
    trends, 331
Case manager model, as job design, 366
Case rates, 316
Cash accounting, 299
Cash budget, 297
Cash cows, 196
CCHERS (Center for Health Education Research
        and Service), 438
CD-ROMS, health care information via, 187
Center for Health Education Research and
        Service (CCHERS), 438
Centralized health care, 41
Centralized organizational structure,
        professional development and, 431
Central tendency bias, 481
Chafee, John, 54
Change, See also Organizational change
    acceptance of, shared governance and, 420
    as constant, 159
    dialectical, 278
    evaluating, 281
    integrated health systems, 284–90
    measuring, 281, 381
    organizational theory and, 267–68
    resistance to, 147
    transition to teams, 163–74
    unity of, chaos theory and, 277
Change agents
    nurses as, 157–59
    role of, 373
Change implementers, nurses as, 159
Change management, See also Change theory;
        Organizational change
    analyzing need for change, 150
    commitment and support for, 153
    communication and, 154–55
    in health care organizations, 141–59
    implementation plan, 153
    institutionalization of change, 155

leadership and, 152–53
    learning from experience of others, 148–50
    objectives for success, 153
    organizational goals and, 152
    organizational structure and, 154
    organizational vision and, 150–52
    steps in, 148–55
Change strategists, nurses as, 159
Change theory, 144–47, See also Change
        management; Organizational change
    "big three" model, 147
    Lewin's ice cube metaphor, 144–45, 150
    real time strategic change, 145, 147, 148
    Shewhart's PDCA cycle, 145, 146
Chaos theory, 277
Charge-based accounting, 329–30
Charge nurses, 452–58
    compensation of, 457
    dealing with difficult people and situations,
        454
    decision making by, 455
    delegation by, 455
    education of, 453–57
    effectiveness in managed care environment,
        456–57
    leadership styles, 454
    needs assessment, 454
    selecting, 452–53
    staffing plans and, 455
    stress and stress management, 454
    use of humor by, 454, 455
Charges
    costs and, 382
    methodologies for setting, 317–18
Checklists, as performance appraisal
        instrument, 474–76
Chief nursing officers, patient-focused care and,
        410–11
Chief Operating Officer (COO), nurses as,
        157–58
Children
    critically ill, information needs of siblings,
        447–48
    emotional responses to hospitalization of
        family members, 445–51
Children's Hospital, Boston, 394–402
Child visitation, effects in adult critical care
        units, 446–50
Chronic illness, health policy and, 40

Chronic low back pain, spine evaluation
    service, 527
Civil rights, of employees, 78–80
Civil Rights Act (1964), 77, 78, 102
Claims, conflict and, 117, 118
Classification and acuity system, computerized,
    328
Clients, *See also* Consumers; Patients
    of consultants, 256
    expectations of, 260
    satisfaction with consultants, 259–60
Clinical algorithm, 498
Clinical care process management, 498
Clinical competence
    defined, 429
    professional development and, 427, 428, 429
Clinical ladder model, 366–67
Clinical nurse specialists (CNSs),
    reimbursement in Medicare, 55
Clinical patient outcomes, 496, *See also*
    Outcomes
Clinical program evaluation, 493–506, *See also*
    Program evaluation
    contemporary context, 493
    guiding principles, 503–4
    information system infrastructure supporting,
        504–5
    methods, 503–4
    outcomes, 504
    process of, 503
    risk adjustment and, 500–501
    strategies, 494
    value of, 505–6
Closed systems
    autopoesis and, 277
    models, 268
CNSs (clinical nurse specialists), 55
Coalitions, policy making process and, 36–37
Cognitive dissonance, 434
Cognitive objectives, in adult learning, 431–32
Cognitive style, 433
Cognitive theories, of motivation, 464
Collaboration, between education and service,
    435–41
Collaborative teaching, 438–40
Collective bargaining, 70–73
Collectivism, cultural norms, 111
Collins, Patricia Hill, 11
Colonization

ethic of care and, 11–12
    women and, 11
Color blindness, racioethnic identity and, 107
Columbia University School of Nursing (CUSN),
    439
Committed costs, 300
Common law, settlement of legal disputes
    under, 66
Communication
    conflict resolution and, 119
    education/service collaboration and, 436
    organizational change and, 154–55
    shared governance and, 419
    style, cultural norms and, 112
Community
    educating about nursing issues, 49
    public relations and, 200–201
Community health centers, feminist
    management of, 131–37
Community model, for organizations,
    leadership in, 412–13
Compensation
    of charge nurses, 457
    methods of, 466–67
    performance appraisal and, 466–67
Competition
    analysis of, 193, 194
    direct, 193, 194
    indirect, 193, 194
Complaints, consumer, 195
Complete Guide to the Hospital Survey Process,
    518
*Comprehensive Accreditation Manual for
    Hospitals* (CAMH), 512, 517
Computer-aided diagnostic equipment, FDA
    and, 333
Computer-Based Patient Record Institute, 330
Computerized medical records, 330
Computer management systems, 328–29
Computers, health care information via, 187,
    331–32
Computer system (CS) development, 326
Confidentiality, patient's right to, 68
Conflict
    in declining organizations, 275–76
    hidden, 118
    models, 116–17
    organizational theory and, 280–81
    preventing, 118

Conflict resolution
  cultural diversity issues, 116–20
  ethic of care and, 7
  ethic of justice or rights and, 7
Congruence model, 270–71
Consensus management, shared governance
      and, 418, 422
Conservatorship, administrative, 408–9
Construct validity, in performance appraisal
      systems, 472
Consultants
  billing by, 257
  characteristics, 257–58
  client satisfaction with, 259–60
  defined, 256
  effective, 259
  organizational change and, 282
  reliability of, 260
  roles of, 257
  selecting, 260–62
  in system redesign, 391
  types of, 258–59
Consulting, 256–64
  contract management, 263
  process, phases of, 258–59
Consumer demand
  research and, 449
  responsiveness to, 143
Consumers, See also Clients; Patients
  complaints, 195
  health needs, medical professions and, 40
  marketing analysis, 193–95
  prescription drug marketing to, 199
  proactive, 186–87
Consumer satisfaction
  analysis of, 194–95
  defining and measuring outcomes for, 524–25
Contingency theory of leadership, 406–7
Continuing care retirement centers, strategic
      planning for, 176–83
Continuing education, 429–30
  outreach programs, 440
Continuous quality improvement (CQI)
      strategies, 92
Contractors, See also Consultants
  consultants as, 257
Contracts
  consultants, 257
  employment, 69–70

  management of, 263
Contribution margin, 319
Contributory negligence, of patients, 63
Control, See also Cost control
  as organizational relationship strategy, 278–80
  through budgeting, 294
Controllable costs, 299
COO (chief operating officer), 157–58
Cooperation, as organizational relationship
      strategy, 278–80
Core competencies, for patient care
      administrators, 494
Core job dimensions, 362–63
Corporate culture, intrapreneurs and, 231
Corporate liability, for health care agencies, 63
Corporate risk management, 91–99
Corporate strategy development, budgeting
      and, 294
Corporations, establishing, 248–49
Cosmetic surgery, reimbursement for, 316–17
Cost accounting, 330
  computerized systems, 328
Cost avoidance benefits, evaluating, 388–91
Cost-based pricing, 317
Cost-based systems, 504–5
Cost-benefit ratios, 381–85, 391
Cost-charge ratios, 382
"Cost containment era," of health care, 494
Cost control, 298–310
  asset valuation, 299
  budgeting and, 298
  decision-making concepts, 300–301
  expenses, 306–7
  managerial control, 299–300
  monitoring, 302–6
  operating income, 310
  revenue, 306
  supplies, 309–10
  variances, 308–9
  volume concepts, 301–2
Cost effectiveness
  determining, 324–25
  ratios, 381–85, 391
Cost leadership, as marketing strategy, 197
Cost management, vs. revenue management,
      142–43
Costs
  actual, 300
  avoidable, 301

budgeted, 300
charge data and, 382
committed, 300
controllable, 299
determining, 382–83
direct, 300
escapable, 301
fixed, 301
incremental, 301
indirect, 300
noncommitted, 300
noncontrollable, 299
opportunity, 301
replacement, 300
semifixed, 302
semivariable, 302
step, 302
sunk, 300
total, to patient, 319–20
unit, per service, 324
value and, 320
variable, 301
Countersignature requirements, 355
County health department, marketing program,
        207–12
CQI strategies, 92
Creativity, new ventures and, 226
Credentialing
    liability and, 62
    risk management and, 97–98
Criminal actions, 65
Critical care
    child visitation effects, 446–48
    emotional responses of family members,
        445–51
Critical incident performance appraisal, 478
Critical paths, 498
Cultural assessment, 109–12
Cultural conflict, 103–4, 118
Cultural diversity, 101–21, See also Minority
        groups
    cultural assessment and norms,
        109–12
    cultural expectations, 109
    discrimination and, 113–14
    diversity training, 125–30
    education about, 133–34
    empowerment issues, 134–36
    ethical theory and, 10–12

group identity issues, 105–9
health care delivery issues, 103–5
managing, 114–20
norms, 109–12
patient care sensitivity, 115–16
social change and, 101–3
stereotyping and, 113–14
workplace conflict management, 116–20
Cultural identity
    commitment to, 118
    group identity and, 106, 107
Customer-oriented organizations, 279
Customer satisfaction, 487–88
Customers. See Clients; Consumers; Patients
Cybernetics, 277
    general systems theory, 268

Damages
    general, 66
    nominal, 65
    punitive, 66
    special, 65
Data
    availability of, 391
    defined, 323
Data-based problem solving, 515
Databases, privacy issues, 80
Data management skills, training, 391
Decentralized organizational structure,
        professional development and, 431
Decision making
    by charge nurses, 45
    cost control and, 300–301
    family involvement in, 447
    in health care purchases, 191
    involving nurses in, 372
    in personnel management, 23–28
    shared governance and, 418, 421
Decision support systems, 334
Decline life cycle stage, of organizations,
        275–76
Defamation, 64
Delegation
    charge nurses and, 455
    nurse manager skills, 423
    of personnel, defined, 60
Deliverables, provided by consultants, 258

Democratic leadership style, 406–7
Demographics, cultural diversity and, 103, 125
Deontology, 6, 7
Depreciation, 299
DePree, Max, 413, 414
Deveaux, Monique, 9
Development life cycle stage, of organizations, 272–73
Diagnostic Related Groups (DRGs), 315
Dialectical change, 277–78
Difference dilemma, ethic of care and, 13, 14
Differentiation, as marketing strategy, 197
Direct care time, increasing through job design, 364
Direct charges, pricing and, 319
Direct costs, 300
Direct mail advertising, 200
Disabilities
    discrimination issues, 78
    pregnancy-related, 77
Discipline, by managers, 74–75
Discrimination
    against advanced practice nurses, 55
    against minorities, 113–14
    defined, 113
    in employment, 77–78
Discrimination claims, conflict and, 117–18
Disease management, 188
Distinctive competency, 214
Diversity, cultural. See Cultural diversity
Diversity workshops, 114–15
Division of labor, 359
Dole, Robert J., 54
DRGs (diagnostic related groups), 315
Driving forces, in organizational change, 145
Drug testing, legal issues, 80

Ebonics, 109
Education, See also Professional development; training
    about cultural differences, 133–34
    of charge nurses, 453–57
    collaboration with service, 435–41
    collaborative teaching, 438–40
    of community, about nursing issues, 49
    conflicts with service, 437

of Congressional members, about nursing issues, 49–50
    health care industry change and, 144
    of nurses about policy issues, 51–52
EEOC, 77
Effectiveness, See also Cost-effectiveness ratios
    defined, 498
    determining, 383–84
Effectiveness research, 497
    risk adjustment and, 499–500
Efficacy, defined, 498
Efficacy studies, risk adjustment and, 499–500
Electronic networks, as health care information sources, 505
Emergency care, legal issues, 69
Emergency Medical Treatment and Active Labor Act (1984), 69
Employee benefits, 81
Employee-oriented organizations, 279
Employee Retirement Security Act (1974) (ERISA), 81
Employees, nurturing, 136–37
Employment
    civil rights of employees, 78–80
    discrimination laws, 77–78
    equal opportunity in, 102
    health care reform and, 69–70
    labor contracts, 73–76
    labor organizations, 70–76
    legal issues, 76–80
    maximum hours, 79
    minimum wage, 79
    temporal nature of, 202
    trends, 201–2
    types of, 69–70
    unfair labor practices, 73–74
    workers' compensation, 76–77
    wrongful termination claims, 70
Empowerment
    conflict and, 118
    cultural diversity and, 134–36
    leadership and, 413
Entrepreneurs, See also Intrapreneurs; Ventures
    characteristics of, 226, 228–31
    failure of, 230
    nurses as, 230
Environments
    autopoesis, 276–77
    chaos theory, 277

in congruence model, 270
cybernetics, 277–78
dialectical change, 278
insulation from, 276
learning, 435
organizational, 276–78
Equal Employment Opportunity Commission
    (EEOC), 77
Equal opportunity, in employment, 102
Equal Pay Act (1963), 77, 102
ERISA, 81
Errors. *See* Medical errors
Escapable costs, 301
Essay-style performance appraisal, 478
Ethical dilemmas
    in intensive care units, 447
    in personnel decisions, 23–28
Ethical theory
    ideological use of, 15–16
    Judith Kay, 14–16
    multicultural perspectives, 10–12
    Martha Nussbaum, 13–14
    transformation of, 12–16
    Joan Tronto, 12–13
    value of, 12
Ethic of care, 7–10
    African American culture and, 11
    assimilation approach, 9
    basis of, 7, 19
    colonization and, 11–12
    difficulties in adopting, 8–10
    feminine ethics and, 8
    feminist ethics and, 8–10
    morality and, 14
    in personnel decisions, 23
    political dimension, 8–9
    politics of, 12
    valorization approach, 9–10
Ethic of justice or rights
    assimilation approach, 9
    basis of, 7
    in personnel decisions, 23
Ethics, 3–20, *See also* Morality
    feminist critique of, 6
    of health care marketing, 192
    law and, 16–17
    nursing leadership and, 411
    nursing principles, 18
    politics and, 4, 13, 14

Ethnic identity, 106–8
Evaluation, *See also* Performance appraisal
    systems
    of financial outcomes, 387–91
    of job design, 370
    of organizations, 280–82
    for patient care administrators, 493–506
    of pediatric nurse practitioner program,
        396–400
    of performance management programs,
        488–89
    of shared governance program, 423–24
    of system redesign, 375–76, 379–92
Evidence-based practice, 449
Exclusive bargaining agents, 72
Executive managers, MIS system and, 325
Expectancy model, 464
Expectations
    matching rewards to, 485–91
    outcomes and, 464
Expenses
    actual, 306
    budgeted, 306
    total, 306
    types of, 306–7
    variance, 306
    volume, 306
External benchmarks, evaluating financial
    outcomes with, 388
Externships, 439–40
Extrinsic needs, motivation and, 463
Extrinsic rewards, as motivators, 461–62

Faculty, legal responsibilities, 60–61
Fair Haven Community Health Center, New
    Haven, CT, 131–37
Fair Labor Standards Act (1938) (FLSA), 79
False imprisonment, 65
Family
    decision making involvement, 447
    emotional responses of, 445–51
    intervention research, 445–51
Family Medical Leave Act (1993) (FMLA), 79
Family Nurse Practitioners (PNPs), in Medicare,
    55
Fatalism, cultural norms, 111
FDA, 332–33

Federal Drug Abuse and Treatment Act (1972), 69
Federal Employee Health Act (FEHA), 77
Federal Medication and Concillation Service (FMCS), 75
Feedback
    in appraisal interviews, 479
    as core job dimension, 363
    positive and negative, in performance appraisal systems, 473
Feedback Transformation process, 268
Feminine ethic, ethic of care and, 8
Feminism
    Black women and, 11
    critique of medicine by, 43–44
Feminist ethics
    ethics of care and, 8–10
    feminist theory and, 5–6
    goals, 6, 18
    social-political dimension, 6
    value of, 4
Feminist management, of community health centers, 131–37
Feminist theory, 5–6
    diversity of, 5
    lesbian, 12
    marginal status of women and, 10
    oppression of women and, 16
Fetal abuse, gender bias and, 44
Field review evaluation, 479
Filipino-Americans, cultural norms, 112
Financial outcomes, evaluating, 387–91
Financial ratios, 310–11
Financial skills, 293–311
    budgeting, 293
    budget preparation process, 294–98
    cost concepts and controls, 298–310
    importance of, 293
    patient care program operation and, 313–21
    value of, 310–11
Fixed assets, valuation of, 299
Fixed costs, 301
Fixed expenses, pricing and, 319
Flowcharts, 354
Flow meetings, cultural diversity and, 135
FLSA (Fair Labor Standards Act), 79
FMLA (Family Medical Leave Act), 79
Focus, as marketing strategy, 197
Followers, leadership and, 409–10, 415

Food and Drug Administration (FDA), 332–33
Forced checklists, 474, 476
Forced distribution technique, 474
Force-field analysis, 145, 150, 151
Ford, Martha E., 54
Forecasting
    budgeting and, 294
    defined, 234
Forecasting trend analysis, 295
Formation life cycle stage, of organizations, 272
Formative evaluation, 502
Four P's
    of marketing, 190, 215
    of teams, 169–70, 172
Frederickson, H. George, 4
Free-market system
    health care policy and, 44–45
    leadership and, 413
Fry, Art, 231
Full market coverage, 215
Full-time equivalents (FTEs)
    costs and charges, 383
    in operating budget, 297
Futurists, 159, 163

Gays, discrimination against, 102–3
Gender
    cultural norms, 111, 112
    discrimination on basis of, 102
    effects of, 11
    sexual harassment and, 78–79
    traits, ethics of care and, 8
Gender bias, fetal abuse and, 44
General damages, 66
Generalists, trends, 188
Generalization effect, 481
General systems theory, open systems models and, 268–69
Geriatric care management
    associated services, 252
    business establishment, 247–55
Gestalt learning theory, 433
Gilligan, Carol, 7
Gingrich, Newt, 54
Global contracts, 316
Goal-oriented evaluation, 502–3

Goals
  accreditation visits and, 512
  defining, for organizational change, 152
  motivation and, 464, 465–66
Goal-setting theory, 464
Goodwin House West, Alexandria, Virginia,
      176–83
"Grand moral theory," 7, 10
Graphical user interface (GUI), health care
      applications and, 331
"Gray Panthers," 102
Great man theory of leadership, 406
"Grid scores," JCAHO, 520
Grievances, 75
  resolution of, 88–89
Ground rules, shared governance and, 421
Group identity
  acculturation models, 108
  cultural diversity and, 105–9
  multi-, 106
  stage of development models, 107–8
Group work team reward systems, 467
Growth
  insulation and, 276
  of organizations, 274–75
Growth cycle, of MIS development, 326
Gry, Marilyn, 11
GUI, 331

"Habit of mind" to care, ethic of care and, 12
Hadley, Elizabeth Harrison, 3–4
Halo effect, 481
Handwriting recognition technology, 331
Harassment, in the workplace, 78–79
Hardware, for health care management
      information systems, 329
Hasidic Jewish culture, cultural norms, 128–29
HDOs (health data organizations), 35–36
Healing, from oppression, 15
Health
  broadening definition of, 187
  medical care and, 38–41
Health care, See also Care
  cultural issues, 103–5
  free market and, 44–45
  health assumptions and, 38–41
  politics and, 3–4

social science model, 497
Health care costs
  capitation payments, 186
  reduction in, 186
  spending, federal programs and, 39–40
Health care information
  CD-ROMs, 187
  Internet, 187
  software applications, 187, 331–32
  telehealth (telemedicience), 227, 332, 505
Health Care Management Association, 311
Health care management information systems,
      328, See also Management information
      systems (MISs)
  regulatory and accreditation requirements,
      332–33
Health care marketing. See Marketing
Health care organizations
  academic, family intervention research in,
      445–51
  change management in, 141–59
  changes in, 142–44, 156–57
  consultants employed by, 282
  corporate liability, 63
  ethical images of, 4
  market-driven, 190, 192
  product-driven, 190
  production-driven, 190–91
  professional liability insurance, 63
  professional recruitment and retention, 201–2
  reform, employee relations and, 69–70
  sales-driven, 191
  strategies of, personnel management and, 24
  structure and strategy changes, 187–88
Health care system
  access to, advanced practice nursing and, 41
  consumer changes, 186–87
  current issues, 185–89
  financing, health policy and, 31
  future of, 189
  physician role changes, 188
  recent changes in, 185–86
  transactions, marketing and, 189
Health data organizations (HDOs), state policy
      making process and, 35–36
Healtheon, web site, 187
Health insurance
  individual policies, 249
  regulation of, 81

Health maintenance organizations (HMOs), 522
  consumer analysis, 194
  health care delivery and, 186
Health Plan Employer Data Information Set
    (HEDIS), 189
Health policy, *See also* Policy making; Public
    policy
  centralization of, 41
  consequences of, 37–38
  free market and, 44–45
  health services financing and, 31
  incremental nature of change in, 33–34
  medical profession and, 38–41
  medical self-interest and, 32–33
  new paradigm, 42–46
  nursing and, 31, 45, 46
  nursing values and, 32–33
  politics and, 3–4, 54–57
  process, 31–46
  professions and, 32–33
  states and, 35–36
  theory of policy making, 33–38
  traditional paradigm, 38–42
  values and, 42–44, 45, 46
Health services research, 495–99, *See also*
    Research
  defined, 496
  role of, 495
  terminology, 498–99
HEDIS, 189
Heritage consistence, conflict and, 118
Herman Miller, Inc., 413
Herzberg, F., 463
  job motivation theory, 361–62
Hesburgh, Theodore, 150
Hierarchical leaders, 412, 413
Hierarchy of needs, 462–63
Hierarchy of systems, 277
Hispanics
  cultural norms, 110, 111
  population growth, 103
Historical basis, of fixed assets, 299
History, in congruence model, 270
HIV, 81
HMOs. *See* Health maintenance organizations
    (HMOs)
Holding environment, providing, as leadership
    strategy, 412
"Holding self out" doctrine, 60, 61

Holistic thinking, by inventive organizations,
    149
Holy Cross Hospital, Washington, DC, 485
Home diagnosis, 187
Home health care
  education/service collaboration in, 436
  integrated health systems, 284–90
  Medicare, 38
  trends, 187
Homelessness, policy making and, 34–35
Homosexuals, discrimination against, 102–3
Hooks, Bell, 11
Hospital beds, supply regulation, 45
Hospitals
  consumer demands and, 143
  emotional responses of family members,
    445–51
  employment trends, 201
  health assumptions and, 39
  length of stay, 143, 186
  professional organizational form and, 273
  public-private partnerships, 143
  recent changes, 187–88
  service orientation, 143
  small, machine organizational form in, 273–74
Hostile work environment harassment, 78
"Hot spots," for accreditation visits, 518, 519
Human experience
  elements of, 13–14
  moral claims and, 13
Human immunodeficiency virus (HIV), legal
    issues, 81
Humanistic management, 269
Humanity, common, universal ideas, 13–15
Human needs, as motivators, 462–63
Human resources management, 461, *See also*
    Performance management
Humor, for dealing with difficult people and
    situations, 454, 455
Hygiene factors
  defined, 463
  of work, 361, 363

Ice cube change model, 144–45, 150
ICUs (intensive care units), 445–51
Idea development, for new ventures, 225–27
Identity

cultural, 106, 107, 118
    group, 105–9
Ideonomy, 226
Illness, severity of, outcomes and, 500–501
Immanuel-St. Joseph's-Mayo Health System
        (ISJ), 379–92
Immigration, 101
Implementation
    of job design, 370
    of organizational change, 370
    of plans for organizational change, 153
    of POE system, 345–46
    of strategic planning, 176–83
    of system redesign, 374–76
Implementation specialists, for POE system,
        role of, 342
Importance-Performance-Awareness (IPA)
        mapping, 196
Imprisonment, false, 65
Incident reports, in risk management, 92, 95
Income statement, 304–6
Incremental costs, 301
Indemnity providers, consumer analysis, 194
Indicators (performance measures), 515
Indirect costs, 300
Indirect expenses, pricing and, 319
Individualism, cultural norms, 111
Individual job performance recognition, 465–66
Individual work adjustments, motivation and, 468
Influence, as tool of leadership, 411–13, 415
Information systems, 323–36, See also Health
        care information; Management
        information systems (MISs)
    for clinical program evaluation, 504–5
    cost justification, 505
Information technology
    benefits, 333–34
    nursing practice effects, 334–36
    trends, 331–32
Informed consent, legal issues, 67–69
Innovation
    entrepreneurship and, 226
    sources of, 229–30
Innovative organizational form, 273–74
Inputs, into open systems models, 268
In-service education, about cultural differences,
        133–34
Institute of Medicine (IOM), 45, 495–96
    National Academy of Science, 330

Institutional lawyers, role of, nurse and, 17
Insulation, from environments, 276
Insurance
    health policy and, 44–45
    payments, 314
Insurance industry, 249–50
    regulation of, 81
Integrated health systems, 188
    joining, 284–90
    outcomes and, 493
Integrity, leadership and, 414
Intensive care units (ICUs), emotional
        responses of family members, 445–51
Interaction processes, See also Relationships
    in general systems theory, 268
Interdependence
    ethics of care and, 9
    of teams, 163, 174
Interdisciplinary health care delivery, 438
Internal benchmarks, evaluating financial
        outcomes with, 387–88
Internal Revenue Service (IRS), contractor
        employment guidelines, 70
Internet, 227
    health care information via, 187
    trends, 332
Internships, 439–40
Interpersonal relationships, cultural norms, 112
Interviews, appraisal, 479–80
Intrapreneurs, See also Entrepreneurs; Ventures
    characteristics of, 228–31
    corporate culture and, 231
    nurses as, 230
Intraprise, 413
Intrinsic needs, motivation and, 463
Inventive organizations, characteristics of,
        148–50
Iowa, University of, Hospitals and Clinics
        (UIHC), Family Intervention Research
        team, 445–51
IPA mapping, 196
IRS (Internal Revenue Service), 70

JCAHO Perspective, 517
Jewish culture, cultural norms, 128–29
Job analysis, 469–70, 471
Job descriptions, 470, 471

Job design, 359–71
    defined, 359
    history, 359–63
    implementing, 367–71
    job enlargement, 360–61
    job enrichment, 361–63
    job rotation, 361
    job simplification, 359–60
    in nursing, 364–67
    as ongoing process, 368
    trends, 360
Job dissatisfaction, factors affecting, 464
Job motivation, 361
Job performance, individual, recognition of,
        465–66
Job productivity. *See* Productivity
Job satisfaction
    factors affecting, 464–65
    intrinsic and extrinsic needs and, 463
    of nurse managers, 423
    open systems models and, 269
    productivity and, 465
    professional development and, 430
Johns Hopkins Hospital (JHH), 339
Johns Hopkins Medicine Center for Information
        Services (JHMCIS), 339–56
Johns Hopkins University, 439
Johnson, Kirk, 55
Joint Commission for the Accreditation of
        Healthcare Organizations (JCAHO), 32,
        332, 333, *See also* Accreditation
        standards; Accreditation surveys
    accreditation standards, 511–17
    "Agenda for Change," 511, 512
    charge nurse education program standards,
        453
    defining ideal survey goals for, 510–11
    "grid scores" or "report cards," 520
    Hospital Accreditation Decision Grid, 510
    "hot spots," 518, 519
    preparing for visit from, 510–20
    survey preparation tools and resources, 517–18
Justice, ethic of, 7

Kaiser Permanente, 522–27
Kanter, Rosabeth Moss, 158–59
Kay, Judith, 14–16

Knowles, Malcolm, 434
Koonz, Claudia, 12

Labor contracts
    administration, 74–75
    administration of, 86–87
    legal issues, 73–76
    negotiating, 86
    terminating, 74
Labor management, legal issues, 69–76
Labor organizations
    certification and decertification of, 76
    NLRA and, 70–73
    organizing, 85
    recognition of, 71–72
    relations with, 89–90
    strikes and work actions, 75
Language, native, use of in workplace, 112
Large-scale organizational change, 142
Latinos
    cultural norms, 110, 111
    population growth, 103
Law
    civil rights of employees, 78–80
    discrimination, 77–78
    emerging issues, 80–81
    employment types, 69–70
    ethics and, 16–17
    labor contracts, 73–76
    labor organizations, 70–73, 76
    liability and malpractice, 61–66
    medical records, 66–67
    nursing practice, 59–61
    patient care administration, 59–81
    patient's rights, 67–69
    workers' compensation, 76–77
Leadership, 405–15, *See also* Management
    accreditation standards and, 512, 513, 515
    as adaptive work, 409–10
    authority as tool of, 411–12, 415
    availability of, 414
    by example, 414
    creating, 413–15
    declining organizations and, 276
    defined, 405
    followers and, 409–10, 415
    in health care, 410–11

hierarchical, 412, 413
influence as tool of, 411–13, 415
integrity and, 414
for organizational change, 152–53
purpose and, 414
relationships and, 414–15
roving, 413, 414
symbolic behavior (style), 180
teams and, 163–64, 172, 174
theories of, 406–9
    administrative conservatorship, 408–9
    contingency theory, 406–7
    great man theory, 406
    situational theory, 407
    transactional leadership, 407–8
    transformational leadership, 408
traits, 406
trust and, 413–15
visionary, 408
Leadership Function Flow Chart, 513
Leadership for Primary Care Project (LPHC),
    437
Leadership styles
    authoritarian, 406–7
    charge nurses, 454
    cultural norms, 110–11
    democratic, 406–7
Learning
    in adults, 431–35
    Gestalt theory, 433
    neo-behaviorist theory, 432–33
    policy making process and, 36–37
    styles, 433
Learning environment, 435
    shared governance and, 420
Learning organizations, defined, 142
Leave, job-protected, 79
Legislators, educating about nursing issues, 49–50
Lesbian feminism, 12
Lesbians, discrimination against, 102–3
Letters to the editor, value of writing, 51
Leverage ratios, 311
Lewin, Kurt, 144–45, 150
Liability, legal issues, 61–62
Liability insurance, 63, 250
Libel, 64
Licensed practical nurses (LPNs)
    defined by nurse practice acts, 60
    as supervisors, 73

Licensing boards, disciplinary actions, 61
Licensure
    denial, 61
    probation, 61
    reciprocity, 59
    reinstatment of revoked licenses, 61
    revocation, 61
    suspension, 61
Life cycle stages, of organizations, 271–76
Life cycle theory, of learning, 434
Lincoln, John C., Hospital, Phoenix, AZ, 156–57
Liquidity ratios, 311
Lisa M. v. Henry Mayo Newhall Memorial
    Hospital, 62–63
Locus of control orientation, cultural norms,
    111–12
Logos, for new ventures, 252
Long-term care centers, machine organizational
    form in, 273–74
Loops, in cybernetics, 277–78
LOS data, 388
Loss-prevention techniques, for risk
    management, 98
Lowenstein-Glanville conflict model, 117–18
LPHC (Leadership for Primary Care Project),
    437
LPNs. See Licensed practical nurses (LPNs)

McClelland, D.C., 463
Machine organizational form, 272–73
McKinnon, Catherine, 5
McKinsey 7-S framework, 176–77
Malpractice
    contributory negligence of patient and, 63
    defined, 62
    legal issues, 62–63
    standard of care and, 62–63
Managed care
    charge nurse effectiveness in, 456
    competition strategies, 494
    consumer analysis, 194
    defined, 316, 331
    employment trends, 201, 202
    goals, 331
    health care system changes, 186–87
    legal issues, 75
    trends, 187, 331

Managed care organizations (MCOs), 316

Managed risks, 96

Management, *See also* Leadership
  defined, 405
  humanistic, participative, 269
  MIS system and, 324–25

Management-by-objectives (MBO)
  defined, 468
  model, 381

Management engineering, 360

Management information systems (MISs), *See also* Information Systems, 323–36
  benefits of, 325–26
  cost-effectiveness analysis, 324–25
  defined, 323–24
  growth cycle, 326
  health care, 328
  information technology and, 333–34
  for patient care, 334–36
  selecting, 328–29
  trends, 329–33

Managing Transitions (Bridges), 164

Market-driven health care organizations
  characteristics of, 192
  defined, 190

Marketing, 189–202
  applying principles to work setting, 208, 210
  competitor analysis, 193
  consumer analysis, 193–95
  in county health department, 207–12
  defined, 189–90
  ethics of, 192
  four P's of, 190, 215
  framework for, 209
  health care transactions and, 189
  management process, 215
  the need for marketing to staff, 207
  personal selling, 200
  phases and tasks, 212
  prerequisites for, 213–14
  psychiatric clinical specialist's role in, 213–24
  public relations, 200–201
  quarterly reporting, 216, 220–23
  reinforcement and recognition, 210–11
  responsibility for, 213
  role in strategic planning, 192–97
  self-assessment in, 196
  of services, unique factors, 191
  social, 197–98

  strategic plans, 196–97
  targeted, 199–200, 215, 219
  value of, 213

Marketing plans, 198–201
  advertising, 199–200
  contents, 198
  developing, 215–18, 251–52

Marketing strategies, 215
  identified in business plan, 239–40

Market niche, 227–28

Markets, types of, 190

Market segmentation analysis, 194, 195

Market share, 214

MAR (Medical Administration Record), 346

Maslow, A.H., 462–63

Massachusetts, University of, Boston College of Nursing, 437–38

Maturana, Humberto, 276

Maturity life cycle stage, of organizations, 273–75

Maximum hours of employment, legal issues, 79

Mayo Medical Center, Department of Nursing, 417–24

MBO (management-by-objective), 381, 468

MCOs (managed care organizations), 316

Measurement contamination, in performance appraisal systems, 472

Measurement deficiency, in performance appraisal systems, 472

Mediation
  conflict and, 118
  strikes and, 75

Medicaid, 315–16
  health policy and, 39–40
  politics and, 54–57

Medical conditions, employer inquiries about, 78

Medical devices, functionality of, 64

Medical errors
  procedure errors, 488
  public relations and, 200–201
  treatment errors, 488

Medical professions
  consumer health needs and, 40
  domination of health care policy by, 46
  feminist critique of, 43–44
  health assumptions and, 38–41
  health policy and, 32–33, 38–41

role in health policy, 32–33
self-interest of, 32–33
underrepresentation of women in, 6
Medical records
computerized, 330
confidentiality of, 68–69
erroneous chart entries in, 67
legal issues, 66–67
Medicare
health policy and, 39–40
home health care program, 38
nurse practitioners in, 55–56
payment issues, 314–15
politics and, 54–57
subsidization of medical system by, 39
Medicare Act, 315
Medication Administration Record (MAR), 346
Mentoring, 440
Mercy Hospital, Portland, Maine, 430
Mergers
growth through, 274
rate of, 285
Milestones, defined, 258
Minimum wages, legal issues, 79
Minority groups, *See also* Cultural diversity
cultural issues, 102–3
cultural norms, 109–12
discrimination against, 113–14
group identity, 105–9
health care delivery issues, 103–5
negative intergroup relationships, 113–14
prejudice against, 113–14
segregation of, 102
stereotyping, 113
MIS. *See* Management information systems (MISs)
Missionary organizational form, 272
Mission-based strategic planning, accreditation
standards and, 513, 514, 515
Mission priority goals, for performance
management program, 487–88
Monitoring, budget, 302–6
Monocultural majority, 108
Monocultural minorities, 108
Morality, *See also* Ethics
ethic of care and, 7–8, 14
ethic of justice or rights and, 7
human experience and, 13–14
law and, 17
politics and, 13

Motivation, 461–65
cognitive views of, 464
goals for, 465–66
job satisfaction and, 464–65
personal work adjustments and, 468
theories of, 461–65
Motivators
defined, 463
goals as, 464
human needs as, 462–63
reinforcement as, 461–62
of work, 361
Multiculturalism. *See* Cultural diversity
Multigroup identification, 106
Multiskilling, 26
Murder, of patients, 65

Name recognition, 199
Narayan, Uma, 11–12, 15–16
Narratives, as performance appraisal
instrument, 478–79
National Academy of Science, Institute of
Medicine, 330
National Association of Professional Geriatric
Care Managers, 247, 250, 253, 254
National Association of Public Hospitals
(NAPH), Medicare/Medicaid reforms
and, 55
National chains, 274
National Committee for Quality Assurance
(NCQA), 189
National Council of State Boards of Nursing,
licensing, 59
National Institutes of Health, web site, 187
National Labor-Management Relationship Act
(NLRA), 70–73
amendments (1974), 75
National Labor Relations Board (NLRB), 71, 74
certification by, 76
Natural language processing, 331
NCQA (National Committee for Quality
Assurance), 189
NEA (Nursing Education Act), 56
Needs
as motivators, 462–63
types of, 463
Needs assessment, by charge nurses, 454

Negative variances, 308
Negligence
    by nurses, 63
    contributory, of patient, 63
    legal issues, 63–64
    presumption of, "holding self out" doctrine
        and, 61
    requirements for proving in court, 64
Negotiation
    nurses' role in, 158
    shared governance and, 420–21
Nelson, Hilde Lindemann, 9
Neo-behaviorist learning theory, 432–33
Net revenue, 314
Networks
    as health care information sources, 505
    value of, 50
New employees, orientation programs, 428–29, 431
Niche, creating for new ventures, 227–28
Nightingale, Florence, 227, 495
NIS. 326; *See also* Nursing information systems
        (NISs)
NLRA (National Labor-Management
        Relationship Act), 70–73, 75
NLRB (National Labor Relations Board), 71, 74
NLRB v. Health Care and Retirement Corp., 73
NOLF (Nursing Organization Liaison Forum), 55
*No Longer Patient: Feminist Ethics and Health
        Care* (Sherwin), 5
Nominal damages, 65
Noncommitted costs, 300
Noncontrollable costs, 299
Nonverbal behavior, cultural norms, 110
Normally prevented risks, 96–97
NPs. *See* Nurse practitioners (NPs)
Nurse-administered unit, as job design, 367
Nurse case management, cost avoidance
        benefits, 388–91
Nurse executives
    as change agents, 157–58
    professional status of, 364
    role in accreditation surveys, 519–20
Nurse extender model, as job design, 364–65
Nurse managers
    liability issues, 62
    personnel liablity issues, 60
    shared governance role, 422–23
Nurse-patient relationship, malpractice issues
        and, 62–63

Nurse practice acts, 59–61
    licensure reciprocity, 59
    nurse types defined by, 60
Nurse practitioners (NPs)
    in acute care setting, 394–402
    education/service collaboration and, 439
    in Medicare, 55–56
    reimbursement in Medicare, 55
    tertiary nurse practitioners (TNP), 401
Nurses
    as adult learners, 431–35
    as change agents, 157–59
    computer-based physician order entry system
        benefits, 355–56
    cultural diversity strategies, 129
    financial management by, 310–11
    involving in decision making, 372
    marketing role, 213
    negligence by, 63
    new employees, orientation of, 428–29, 431
    as supervisors, NLRA definition, 73
    turnover, 366–67
    types defined by nurse practice acts, 60
Nurse's Directory of Capitol Connections, 50
Nursing
    competition with other health professions, 33
    education/service collaboration, 435–41
    ethical principles, 18
    ethical responsibilities, 3–20
    health care policy and, 45, 46
    health care services and, 41
    job design in, 364–67
    legal issues, 59–67
    research role, 445
    staffing, quality of care and, 45
    values, health policy and, 32–33
Nursing Education Act (NEA), funding under, 56
Nursing homes, teaching, 439
Nursing Informatics, 326
Nursing information systems (NISs), 326,
        334–36, *See also* Management information
        systems (MISs)
Nursing Organization Liaison Forum (NOLF), 55
Nursing organizations, value of joining, 50–51
Nursing's Social Policy Statement, 3
Nursing students, legal responsibilities, 60
Nurturing
    cultural diversity and, 136–37
    defined, 136

Nussbaum, Martha, 13–14

Objectives, identifying, for organizational
    change, 153
Occupational injury rate, 488
Occupational Safety and Health Act (1970), 76–77
Oligarchy, in organizational maturity stage, 273
Online documentation of medications (ODM),
    346
Open systems models, 268–69
    basic concepts, 268–69
    concepts, 268–69
    congruence model, 269–71
    defined, 267
    environments and, 276–78
    organizational environments, 276–78
    organizational participants, 278–80
    uses of, 267–69
Open system thinking, administrative
    conservatorship and, 408–9
Operating budget, 297
Operating expenses, 305–6
Operating income, 306, 310
Operating margin, 310
Operational manager, MIS system and, 325
Operational planning
    making, 295–98
    process of, 234–35
Opportunity costs, 301
Oppression
    healing from, 15
    resistance to, 15
    of women
        ethic of care and, 9–10
        feminist ethics and, 5, 8
        feminist theory and, 16
OrderNet, 339–56
Organizational assessment, 267–82
    congruence model, 269–71
    open systems models, 268–69
    organizational diagnosis and intervention,
        280–81
    organizational environments, 276–78
    organizational life cycle stages, 271–76
    organizational participants, 278–80
Organizational change, See also Change;
    Change management; Change theory

evaluating, 281, 370–71
health care industry and, 142–44
implementing, 370, 374–76
job design, 368–71
large-scale, 141–59
managing, 141–59
measuring, 281
patient care delivery system redesign,
    156–57
perceiving the need for, 368
planning stage, 368–70
service culture change, 155–56
Organizational life cycle stages, 271–76
    decline, 275–76
    development, 272–73
    formation, 272
    maturity, 273–75
Organizational participants
    customers, 278
    employees, 278
    in open systems theory, 278–80
    shareholders, 278
Organizational strategies
    autonomy, 278–80
    control, 278–80
    cooperation, 278–80
Organizational structure
    assessment of, 279–80
    conflict and, 280–81
    defined, 180–81
    hierarchy, delegation of authority in, 412,
        413
    types of, 278–80
Organizational theory
    open systems models, 267–69
    organizational change and, 267–68
Organizations
    bureaucracy in, 275
    business structure, 248–49
    change experience of, 148–50
    climate, conflict and, 118
    closed, 276
    conflict in, 118, 275–76
    culture, conflict and, 118
    development of, performance management
        and, 470
    diagnosis and evaluation, 280–82
    effectiveness, as mission priority goal, 487
    environments, 276–78

goals definition, 152
growth through mergers or acquisitions, 274
innovative form of, 273–74
inventive, 148–50
leadership of, 152–53
learning, 142
machine form of, 272–73
marketing prerequisites, 213–14
missionary form of, 272
need for change by, 150
performance, mission-based strategic planning and, 513, 514, 515
professional form of, 273–74
reconfiguration of, 271
reinvention of, 141–42
shared values, 182
skills, 182–83
staff, 181–82
strategic planning implementation, 176–83
structure of, 154
symbolic behavior (style), 180
systems, 182
turnarounds in, 276
vision of, 150–52
Orientation programs, for new employees, 428–29, 431
Orphan Drug Act, 37
Outcome measures, selecting, 383–84
Outcomes, 493–506
clinical program evaluation and, 504
consumer perspective, 524–25
defining, 524–27
financial, 387–91
measuring, for spine evaluation service, 522–27
organizational perspective, 525–27
relationship of practice to, 495–99
research, 497
risk adjustment for, 499–501
severity of illness and, 500–501
Outcomes assessment, 498
Outcomes management, 498
Outcomes research
information system supporting, 504–5
value of, 505
Outputs, from open systems models, 268
Outreach continuing education programs, 440
Outsourcing, 69, 201–2
Overtime rates, 79

Paid Time Off (PTO) program, 489–91
Paraprofessionals, job simplification and, 365
Parents, pediatric nurse practitioner program and, 399
Participative management, 419, See also Shared governance
open systems models, 269
performance and, 485
shared governance, 465
Partnerships, establishing, 248
Patient autonomy movement, 43
Patient care
assignments, by charge nurses, 453
culturally sensitive, 115–16
management, information systems for, 334–36
Patient care administration
clinical program evaluation, 493–506
contemporary context, 494
core competencies for, 494
defined, 493–94
legal issues, 59–81
emerging issues, 80–81
employment, 76–80
labor management, 69–76
nursing practice, 59–67
patient's rights, 67–69
Patient days
adjusted, 383
as outcome measure, 383–84
Patient focus, shared governance and, 417–18
Patient-focused care (PFC)
leadership and, 410–11
redesign, 165
Patient-focused standards, 511–12
Patient-focused work transformation, 158
Patient-nurse relationship, malpractice issues and, 62–63
Patient outcomes, 496, See also Outcomes
Patient-physician relationship, legal issues, 68–69
Patient records, computerized, 330
Patients, See also Clients; Consumers
assessing for violent behavior, 64
characteristics, risk adjustment and, 501
contributory negligence, 63
empowerment of, 134–36
murder of, 65
protection from, 64

satisfaction of, managed care decision making and, 456
as stakeholders, 319
Patient Self-Determination Health Act (1990), 68
Patient's rights, legal issues, 67–69
Patron system, 440
Pay-for-performance systems, 467
Payroll system, for new ventures, 249
PDCA cycle, 145
Pediatric advanced practice nurses, research by, 445
Pediatric nurse practitioners (PNPs), 394–402
    advantages of, 400–401
    in Medicare, 55
Peer delegation skills, of nurse managers, 423
Peer review, 479–80, 481
Perceived injurious experiences (PIEs), 117–18
Per diem payments, 316
Performance appraisal systems, 471–82, *See also* Evaluation
    appraisal interviews, 479–80
    bias in, 481–82
    checklists, 474–76
    compensation and, 466–67
    construct validity in, 472
    content, 471–72
    measurement contamination in, 472
    measurement deficiency in, 472
    measurement methods, 473–79
    measurement process, 472–73
    narratives, 478–79
    nurse manager role, 423
    objectives of, 471
    positive and negative feedback, 473
    productivity-oriented, 467
    professional development planning and, 468
    ranking, 473–74
    rater training, 482
    rating scales, 476–78
    requirement, 470, 471
    resource allocation, 482
    subjectivity in, 471, 481–82
    tools for, 471–72
    trait-oriented, 467
Performance management systems, 461–82
    compensation, 466–67
    defined, 465
    evaluation of, 488–89
    external requirements for, 469
    history, 468–69
    individual performance recognition, 465–66
    job analyses, 469–70
    job descriptions, 470
    job productivity, 467
    mission priority goals, 487–88
    motivation, 461–65
    organizational development, 470
    professional development planning, 468
    staffing, 470
    training, 470
    work standards, 470
    work/time off scheduling, 489–91
Performance measures (indicators), 515
Performance Share program, 485–91
Personality types, prejudice and discrimination and, 113
Personal selling, 200
Personal space, cultural norms, 110
Personnel, *See also* Employees; Employment
    nurse manager liability issues, 60
Personnel decisions, moral reasoning in, 23–28
PFC. *See* Patient-focused care (PFC)
Pharmacists, as providers, 187
Phenotype, group identity and, 106
Physician hospital organizations (PHOs), 188, 193–94
Physician order entry (POE) system, 339–56
    committee structure for, 340
    implementation, 345–46, 353
    issues, 353–55
    nursing benefits, 355–56
    pilot phase, 340–42
    project initiative, 339
    project team nurses, 342–43
    roll-out planning, 343–45
Physicians
    changing roles of, 188, 193–94
    employment trends, 201
    health assumptions and, 39
    overvaluation of services, 41
    as stakeholders, 319
    supply regulation, 45
Physician's orders
    countersignature requirements, 355
    legal issues, 67
PIEs (perceived injurious experiences), 117–18
PI (profitability index), 318

Place, in marketing, 215–16
Planning
    for job design, 368–70
    for job design implementation, 369–70
    for organizational change, 368–70
    for system redesign, 374–75
"Playfulness," 11
PNPs. See Pediatric nurse practitioners (PNPs)
POE. See Physician order entry (POE) system
Policy making, See also Health policy; Public
        policy
    consequences of, 37–38
    implementation difficulties and, 35
    incremental change, 33–34
    issue definition and, 34
    learning and, 36–37
    problem causality determination, 34–35, 38
    state role in, 35–36
    theory of, 33–38
Political movements, health care values and,
        42–44
Politicized organizations, conflict in, 276
Politics
    ethics and, 13, 14
    ethics of care and, 8–9
    feminist ethics and, 6
    health care policy and, 3–4, 54–57
    morality and, 13
    nurses' role in, 158
Portable computers, for POE system, 346,
        353
Portfolio analysis, 196
Positioning, 197
Positive margin, 319
Positive variances, 308
Postive variances, revenues, 306
Postmodernism, 12, 15
PPS (prospective payment system), 315
Practice guidelines, 498–99
Preceptors
    collaborative teaching and, 438–39
    defined, 437
    programs, 429
Pre-employment inquiries, about medical
        conditions, 78
Pregnancy Discrimination Act (1978), 102
Pregnancy-related disabilities, 77
Pregnant women, discriminatory treatment of,
        77

Prejudice, 113–14
    cultural, 103
    defined, 113
    reaction to, 129
Prescription drugs, direct-to-consumer
        marketing of, 199
Prevented risks, 96
Prevention, 187
Price regulation, 45
Price variance, 308
Pricing
    cost-based, 317
    in marketing, 215
    methodologies for, 317–18
Primary care
    "boundaryless" community-based, 438
    health policy and, 37
Primary care nursing, as job design, 365–66
Privacy
    legal issues, 80
    patient's right to, 68
Private health insurance
    health policy and, 44–45
    politics and, 55
Private payors, 314
Privileged information, legal issues, 68–69
Probation, 61
Problem identification, job design and,
        368–69
Problem solving
    dialectical change and, 278
    in job design, 369
Procedure errors, 488
Product
    identified in business plan, 239
    in marketing, 215
Product-driven health care organizations, 190
Production-driven health care organizations,
        190–91
Productivity
    evaluating, 384
    goal-setting theory and, 464
    job satisfaction and, 465
    open systems models and, 269
    performance appraisal and, 467
    reinforcement and, 462
Productivity-oriented performance appraisal
        systems, 467
Products, provided by consultants, 258

Professional development, 427-41, *See also*
    Education; Training
  adult learners, 431–35
  in centralized organizations, 431
  charge nurses, 456
  continuing education, 429–30
  in decentralized organizations, 431
  defined, 427
  educator effectiveness, 431
  health care industry change and, 144
  links between service and education, 435–41
  locus of, 430–31
  orientation of new employees, 428–29
  planning for, 468
  preceptor programs, 429
  program types, 428–30
  purpose of, 428–30
  relevance of, 441
  responsibility for, 430
  sources of, 430
  value of, 427
Professional liability insurance, 63, 250
Professional organizational form, 273–74
Professional performance, standards of, 17–18
Profitability index (PI), 318
Profitability ratios, 310, 311
Program evaluation, *See also* Clinical program
    evaluation
  basic principle, 501–3
  characteristics of, 501
  formative evaluation, 502
  goal-oriented, 502–3
  organizational level and context of, 501
  planning, 501–2
  summative evaluation, 502
  value of, 505–6
Projections, making, budgeting and, 295
Project leaders, for POE system, role of, 342
Project managers, for POE system, role of, 342
Project work plan, defined, 258
Promotion, in marketing, 216
Proposals, 262
  requests for, 262
Prospective payment system (PPS), 315
Providing a holding environment, as leadership
    strategy, 412
Psychiatric clinical specialist, marketing role,
    213–24
Psychomotor objectives, in adult learning, 432

PTO (Paid Time Off) program, 489–91
Public hearings, value of attending, 51–52
Public opinion, professional claims and,
    32–33
Public payors, 314
Public policy, *See also* Health policy; Policy
    making
  care of the aging and, 42
  workshops, value of attending, 51
Public-private partnerships, health care
    organization change and, 143
Public relations, 200–201
Punitive damages, 66
Purpose, leadership and, 414

Quality
  conceptual components of, 495–99
  defined, 320, 499
  information system infrastructure supporting,
    504–5
  risk adjustment in, 499
Quality of care
  nursing staffing and, 45
  pediatric nurse practitioner program and,
    399–400
Quality of life health care model, 497
Quality management systems, computerized,
    328
Quid pro quo sexual harassment, 78

Racial identity, 106–8
Randomized clinical trials, 499
Ranking, as performance appraisal instrument,
    473–74
Rape, of patients, 65
Ratee training, for performance appraisals, 481
Rater training, for performance appraisals, 481
Rating scales, as performance appraisal
    instrument, 476–78
Ratios, 381–85
  cost-benefit, 381–85, 391
  cost-charge, 382
  cost-effectiveness, 381–85, 391
  defined, 381
  financial, 310–11

Real time strategic change model, 145, 147, 148
Recency effect, 481
Recognition
    of individual job performance, 465–66
    in marketing, 210–11
Recognition systems, *See also* Performance
        appraisal systems; Performance
        management systems
    history, 468–69
Reconfiguration, of organizations, 271
Recruitment, 201–2
Reengineering, 372, 373–74
Refusal of treatment, legal issues, 67–69
Regional integrated systems, 274
Registered nurses (RNs)
    charge nurse expectations, 453
    countersigning of patient records by, 66
    defined by nurse practice acts, 60
    delegation by, 60
    job simplification, 365
    part-time, 386
    as supervisors, 73
Reinforcement
    in marketing, 210–11
    as a motivator, 461–62
Reinvention of business, 141–42
Relationship, ethic of, 7
Relationships, *See also* Interaction processes
    autonomy, 278–80
    control, 278–80
    cooperation, 278–80
    leaders and, 414–15
    negative intergroup, 113–14
    open systems theory and, 269
    system redesign and, 387
Replacement costs, 300
    of fixed assets, 299
"Report cards," JCAHO, 520
Requests for proposals, 262
Research, *See also* Health services research
    administrative support of, 449–50
    by advanced practice nurses, 445, 449, 450
    family intervention, 445–51
    nursing department role in, 445
    outcomes, 504–5
    proposal writing, 450–51
    value of, 448–49
    women's health research movement, 43–44
Res ipsa loquitor rule, 63

Resource allocation process, 296–97, *See also*
        budgeting
Resource-driven model, 381
Resources, in congruence model, 270
Respect, shared governance and, 419, 420
Respondeat superior, 62
Responsibility, of individuals, shared
        governance and, 419
Restraining forces, in organizational change,
        145
Restraint, unlawful, 65
Retention, 201–2
Retirement centers, implementation of strategic
        planning for, 176–83
Retreat days, for team staff, 166
Revenue-based systems, 504
Revenue budget, 314
Revenue and expense statement, 304–6
Revenue management, vs. cost management,
        142–43
Revenues
    actual, 306
    budgeted, 306
    net, 314
    projected, 306
    total, 306
    types of, 305
    variance, 306
    volume projections, 306
Reward systems
    expectation and, 485–91
    goals and, 465–66
    for group performance, 467
    for individual performance, 465–66
    motivation and, 461–62
Rights
    ethic of, 7
    hierarchy of, 7
Right to work, 74
Risk adjustment, 499–501
Risk management
    credentialing/recredentialing process and,
        97–98
    defined, 91
    health care system, 91–99
    incident reports, 92, 95
    monitoring and evaluation, 98
    recommended actions, 98–99
    risk analysis, 95–96

risk control, 98
risk funding, 98
risk identification, 92–95
risk type and, 96–97
RNs. *See* Registered nurses (RNs)
Roll-out, of POE system
    issues, 353
    planning for, 343–45, 354
Roll-out coordinators, for POE system, role of,
    343
Roving leaders, 414
Rule-based morality, 7
Rural Elderly Enhancement Project (REEP), 436–37
Russia, cultural norms, 129

Sacred cows, congruence models and, 270–71
Safe Medical Devices Act, 64, 332
Sales-driven health care organizations, 190–91
SBA web site, 248
Schweitzer, Albert, 414
Scientific management, 360, 461
Scope of practice, care management, 252–54
Scope of Practice for Nursing Informatics, The
    (ANA), 334–35
Segregation, 102
Self-assessment, 196
Self-care, 187
Self-reflection bias, 481
Semifixed costs, 302
Semivariable costs, 302
Sensitivity training, for cultural diversity, 114–15
Service culture, organizational change, 155–56
Service integration, 284–90
Service-line manager, as job design, 366
Service marketing. *See* Marketing
Service orientation, of hospitals, 143
Service portfolio analysis, 196
Services
    identified in business plan, 239
    provided by consultants, 258
Service units, projections for, 295
7-S framework, 176–77, 182–83
Severity of illness, outcomes and, 500–501
Severity measurement systems, 500
Sexual harassment, 78–79
Shared governance, 372, 417–24
    evaluation of, 423–24

factors affecting success of, 417–19
    job satisfaction and, 464–65
    nurse manager role, 422–24
    strategies for success, 420–22
Shared Medical Systems (SMS), 339
Shared values, in organizations, 182
Shareholder-oriented organizations, 279
Sherwin, Susan, 5, 8
Shewhart, Thomas, 145, 146
Siblings, of critically ill children, information
    needs of, 447–48
Simple checklists, 474
Single facility assumption, 72
Situational theory of leadership, 406–7
Skills
    in organizations, 182–83
    variety of, as core job dimension, 363
Skin color, group identity and, 106
Slander, 64
Sliding scale payments, 316
Small Business Administration (SBA), web site,
    248
Small businesses. *See* Ventures
SMS (Shared Medical Systems), 339
Social change, workplace and, 101–3
Socialization, group identity and, 105
Social marketing, applying to health care, 197–99
Social position, conflict and, 118
Social science model, of health care, 497
Social structures, feminist ethics and, 6
Sociotechnical design, 361, 363
Software
    FDA and, 333
    health care applications, 331–32
    health care information via, 187, 331–32
    for health care management information
        systems, 329
Sole proprietorships, establishing, 248
Southern Massachusetts Nursing Coalition, 436
Space orientation, cultural norms, 110
Special damages, 65
Specialists
    educational programs and, 40
    health policy and, 37
Spine evaluation service
    measuring outcomes for, 522–27
    mission statement, 523
Staff
    defined, 181

Staff (cont.)
  meetings, cultural diversity and, 135
  strategy, 182
  turnover, 136, 366–67, 464, 470
Staffing
  performance management and, 470
  plans, charge nurses and, 455
Stage of development models, group identity
    and, 107–8
Stakeholders
  identifying and involving, 525
  types of, 319–20
Standardized procedures, legal issues, 61
Standards of care, 17–18
  malpractice issues and, 62–63
Standards of professional performance, 17–18
Stangl, Fritz, 12
States, nurse practice acts, 59–61
Statute of limitations, 66
Step costs, 302
Stereotyping
  defined, 113
  reaction to, 129
Straight ranking, 474
Strategic business thinking, for new ventures,
    231–35
Strategic managers, MIS system and, 325
Strategic planning
  accreditation visits and, 512
  budgeting and, 294
  defined, 232
  implementation of, 176–83
  marketing and, 192–97
  process, 232–34
  speed and, 232, 234
Strategic plans
  contents, 198
  marketing element, 196–97
Strategy
  in congruence models, 271
  defined, 177
Stress and stress management, charge nurses
    and, 454
Strikes, 75
Structure, in general systems theory, 268
Style, 180
Subacute care, 188
Successive developmental crises, learning
    theory, 434

Summated behavioral observation scale (BOS),
    478
Summation conferences, following
    accreditation surveys, 520
Summative evaluation, 502
Sunk costs, 300
"Super users," 344
Supervisors
  cultural issues and conflict, 104
  employee relationships, feedback in, 473
  ethics and, 24–28
  Family Medical Leave Act and, 79
  NLRA definition, 72–73
  nurses as, 73
Supplies
  budgeting, 309–10
  defined, 309
Support analysts, for POE system, role of, 342–43
Surveys, consumer, 524–25
Suspension, of licenses, 61
SWOT, 193
Symbolic behavior, 180
System awareness, implementation of system
    redesign and, 375
System redesign, 371–76
  basic beliefs about, 379–80
  beliefs about, 385–87
  defined, 359
  evaluation, 375–76, 379–92
  extension of case management to, 372–73
  implementing, 374–76
  need for, 371–72
  nursing frameworks, 372
  planning, 374–75
  reengineering, 372, 373–74
  shared governance, 372
  total quality management (TQM), 372, 373
Systems
  hierarchy of, 277
  organizational, defined, 181
Systems thinking
  by inventive organizations, 149
  organizational change and, 143–44

Tactical manager, MIS system and, 325
Taft-Harley Act, 74
Taoism, 278

Target markets, 215, 219
  identified in business plan, 239
Task identity, as core job dimension, 363
Task significance, as core job dimension, 363
Taxes, business, 249
TCP (tertiary nurse practitioners), 401
Teaching, *See also* Education; Professional
        development
  collaborative, 438–40
Teaching nursing homes, 439
Teams
  assessment, 166, 167–68
  assigning staff to, 165–66
  confusion stage, 166, 169
  cross-functional, 164
  defined, 164
  development tools, 173
  factors affecting performance, 171
  four P's of, 169–70, 172
  interdependent, 174
  resistance to, 169
  retreat days for, 166
  role of, 163–64
  transition to, 163–74
Technical budget meetings, 297
Telecommunications technology, 332
Telehealth (telemedicine), 227, 332, 505
Tertiary nurse practitioners (TCP), 401
Third-party payors, 314–17, *See also* Medicaid;
        Medicare
  capitation, 316
  case rates (global contracts), 316
  managed care organizations (MCOs), 316
  per diem, 316
  private, 314
  public, 314
  sliding scales, 316
  as stakeholders, 320
Thomas, Bill, 55
360-degree performance appraisal, 482
Time orientation, cultural norms, 110
Tong, Rosemarie, 8
Top managers, MIS system and, 325
Total costs, to patient, 319–20
Total quality management (TQM), 339, 372,
        373, 511
Training, *See also* Education; Professional
        development
  for performance appraisal, 481

performance management and, 470
  for POE system, 343–44
"Train the trainer" approach, 420
Trait-oriented performance appraisal systems,
        467
Traits, leadership, 406
Tranformational leadership, 408
Transactional leadership, 407–8
Transactions, defined, 407
Transformation process, in open systems
        models, 268
Transformative ethic, 12–16, 19
  Judith Kay, 14–16
  Martha Nussbaum, 13–14
  Joan Tronto, 12–13
Transitions
  defined, 164
  leadership for, 172, 174
  to teams, 163–74
Treatment errors, 488
Trend analysis, budgeting and, 295
Tronto, Joan, 12–13, 14
Trust, leadership and, 413–15
Turnarounds, in declining organizations,
        276
Turnover
  job dissatisfaction and, 464
  of nurses, 366–67
  nurturing and, 136
  performance management and, 470

UAPs. *See* Unlicensed assistive personnel
        (UAPs)
Unfair labor practices, 73–74
  resolution of charges, 87–88
Unification models, for education/service
        collaboration, 437
Union security clause, 74
Unions. *See* Labor organizations
Unit costs per service, 324
United Hospital, St. Paul, MN, 165–74
United States Congress, educating,
        49–50
Unit managers, roles and responsibilities,
        452–58
Unit productivity, evaluating, 384
Unlawful restraint, 65

Unlicensed assistive personnel (UAPs)
   defined by nurse practice acts, 60
   health policy and, 45–46
Unperceived injurious experiences (UNPIEs),
   117
Unpreventable risks, 96, 97
Unskilled work
   job enlargement for, 360–61
   job simplification, 359–60
Usage variance, 308–9
Utilitarianism, 6, 7
Utilization rates, projections, 318

Valence, 464
Valorization, ethics of care and, 9
Value, defined, 320
Value analysis, 320
Values
   health care policy and, 42–44, 45, 46
   shared, in organizations, 182
Varela, Francisco, 276
Variable costs, 301
Variance analysis, 308–9
Variances
   price, 308
   revenues, 306
   usage, 308–9
   volume, 308
Ventures, See also Entrepreneurs; Intrapreneurs
   advertising, 251
   assistance for, 230–31
   business plan, 236–45
   care and maintenance, 254–55
   entrepreneurial characteristics, 228–31
   equipment for, 250
   failure of, 230
   financial issue analysis, 313–21
   financing, 225
   fixed costs for, 250
   idea development, 225–27
   intrapreneurial characteristics, 228–31
   marketing plan, 251–52
   niche creation, 227–28
   starting, 225–45
   strategic business thinking, 231–35
Verbal orders
   countersignature requirements, 355

legal issues, 67
Vestal, Kathy, 158
Vicarious liability, 62
Vice President for Patient Services (VPPS),
   nurses as, 157–58
Violence
   patient assessment for, 64
   in the workplace, preventing, 77
Virtue ethics, 14
Vision, organizational, 150–52
Visionary leaders, 408
Visitation, research on, 446–50
Visiting Nurse Association (VNA), Northern
   Virginia, 284–90
Visiting Nurse Association (VNA) Community
   Hospice, 284
Visiting Nurses Home Care (VNHC), 284
Voice recognition technology, 331
Volume, 302–3
Volume projections, revenues, 306
Volume variance, 308
Volunteering, value of, 51
Voting, shared governance and, 418
VPPS (Vice President for Patient Services),
   157–58
Vroom, V., 464

Walker, Margaret, 6
Washington Hospital Center (WHC), 155–56
Waterman's 7-S framework, 182–83
Weighted checklists, 474, 476
Wellness, health care organization change and,
   143
Welsh, Jack, 154
Western Electric, human relations studies, 269
Wireless laptop computers, for POE system,
   346, 353
Women
   colonization and, 11
   as community health center managers,
      131–37
   cultural norms, 111
   discrimination against, 106–7
   domination of, 16
   equal pay issues, 77
   marginal status of, 10
   multicultural perspectives, 10–12

as not yet human, 5, 13
oppression of, 9–10, 16
    feminist ethics and, 5, 8
pregnant, discriminatory treatment of, 77
recognition of, 9
respect for, 9
underrepresentation in medicine, 6
Women's health research movement, 43–44
Women's movement, health care policy and, 43
Work, *See also* Employment; Job design
    attitudes toward, 369
Work actions, 75
Work adjustments, motivation and, 468
Workers' compensation, legal issues, 76–77
Work ethic, new ventures and, 230
Workforce, cultural diversity in, 125
Work group maturity, 407
Worklists, 355

Work motivation. *See* Motivation
Work papers, 258
Workplace
    conflict management, 116–20
    safety regulation, 76–77
"Workplace of Difference, A," 125–30
Work redesign, 75, 80, *See also* Job design
Work sampling, 364
Work standards, 470
Work transformation, patient-focused, 158
World Wide Web, 227
    health information sites, 187
    Small Business Administration, 248
    trends, 332

Zero-based budgets, 296